Additional resources to this book
can be found at:

www.grupoasis.com/book/radiographic_interpretation

To log in, type in the following password:

AIWA5PTLK3

AF901489

ATLAS OF RADIOGRAPHIC INTERPRETATION
in small animals

Plaza Antonio Beltrán Martínez nº 1, planta 8 - letra I
(Centro empresarial El Trovador)
50002 Zaragoza - Spain

First printing: 2014

This book was originally published in Spanish under the title:
Atlas de interpretación radiológica en pequeños animales

ISBN Spanish edition: 978-84-941014-3-4

Translation:
Grupo Asís Biomedia, SL

ISBN: 978-84-941975-1-2
DL: Z 1875-2013

Design, layout and printing:
Servet editorial - Grupo Asís Biomedia, SL
www.grupoasis.com
info@grupoasis.com

Servet is the publishing house of Grupo Asís

Warning:

Veterinary science is constantly evolving, as are pharmacology and the other sciences. Inevitably, it is therefore the responsibility of the veterinary surgeon to determine and verify the dosage, the method of administration, the duration of treatment and any possible contraindications to the treatments given to each individual patient, based on his or her professional experience. Neither the publisher nor the author can be held liable for any damage or harm caused to people, animals or properties resulting from the correct or incorrect application of the information contained in this book.

ATLAS OF RADIOGRAPHIC INTERPRETATION IN SMALL ANIMALS

Includes the most common diagnostic errors

M. ISABEL GARCÍA REAL

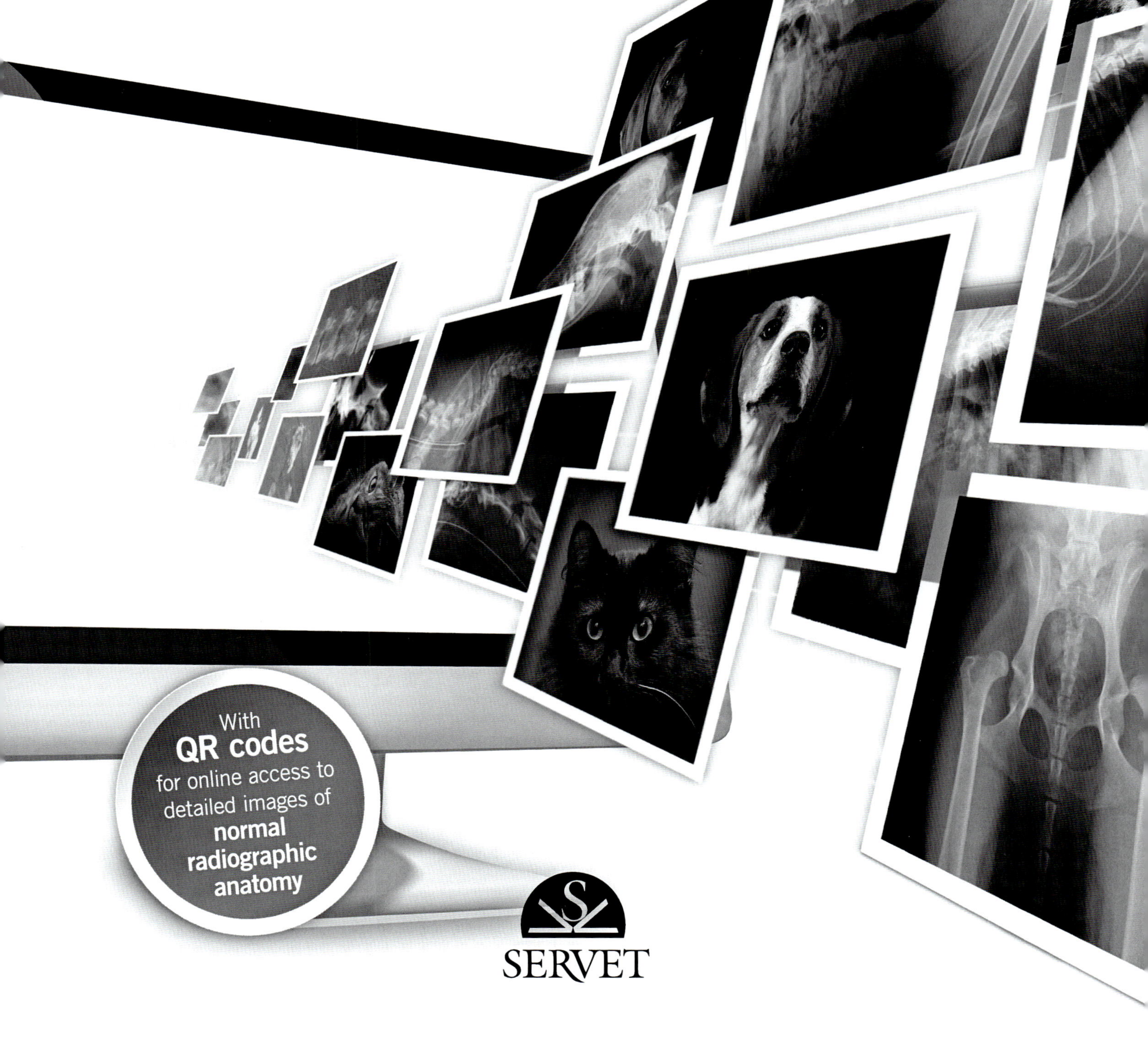

With **QR codes** for online access to detailed images of **normal radiographic anatomy**

SERVET

"Radiographic interpretation: a balance between science and art"

Clifford R. Berry, Donald E. Thrall

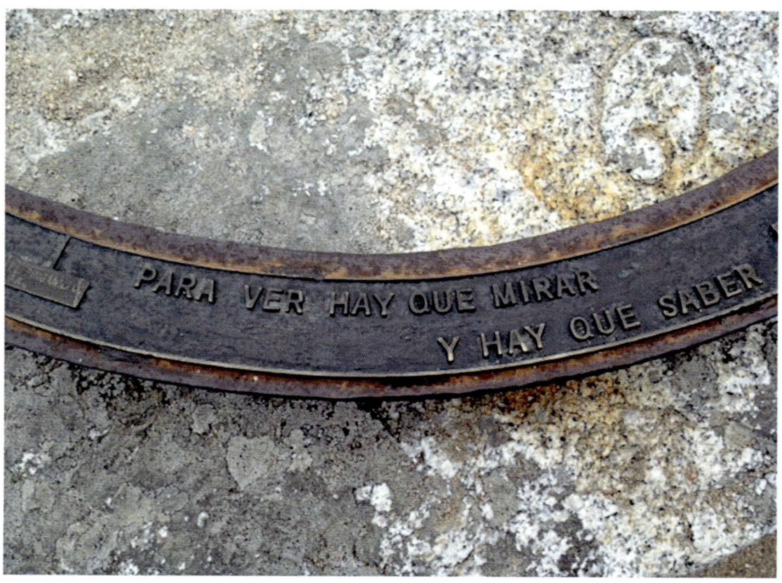

"In order to see, it is necessary to look and it is necessary to know."
Mirador de los Robledos, Sierra de Guadarrama, Madrid

To David, for being the star that most enlightens my life

Acknowledgements

My acknowledgements go to:

My colleagues at the Diagnostic Imaging Service of the Complutense Veterinary Teaching Hospital, because they have all contributed in some way to this book. I would like to make a special mention to Mercedes García Sancho and Enrique García Pérez, as they were the first to interpret some of the radiographs included in this book.

The clinicians at the Complutense Veterinary Teaching Hospital, with whom the Diagnostic Imaging Service makes an "almost" perfect team.

The staff of the Computed Tomography Unit of the *Centro Militar de Veterinaria de la Defensa* (Military Veterinary Medicine Centre), with whom our Service maintains close collaboration and friendship.

The owners and their pets who come to our Hospital, because they are the real source of, and reason for, our work.

Veterinary students, who keep demanding a constant effort of self-improvement from us, so that their training as future vets is increasingly better.

The staff at the San Carlos Teaching Hospital (Dr Casado, Concha, Julio) and Severo Ochoa Hospital (Dr Petrement, Dr Pedro-Viejo, Dr Salcedo, Dr Ramiro, Dr Amigo), for their contribution to making this project possible.

Finally, I would like to especially thank my family and friends, for their great patience with the time I did not spend with them while I was working on this book.

Author

M. ISABEL GARCÍA REAL

She is a Doctor in Veterinary Medicine. She graduated from the Complutense University of Madrid in 1993 and obtained her Ph.D. in 2000. She joined the Department of Animal Medicine and Surgery of the Faculty of Veterinary Medicine of the Complutense University of Madrid in 1993, where she now works as a Professor of Veterinary Diagnostic Imaging.

She has been the Head of the Diagnostic Imaging Service at the Complutense Veterinary Teaching Hospital since 2005 and Director of the Magnetic Resonance Unit of the hospital since its opening in December 2008. Her teaching and research work focuses on radiology, abdominal ultrasounds, CT scans and MRI.

She has been a visiting scholar at the Universities of California (Davis, USA) and Cambridge (United Kingdom) and has completed internships at the Animal Medical Center in New York and the Animal Health Trust (Newmarket, United Kingdom).

She is the author of several national and international publications, and has participated as a speaker in various courses and national and international conferences.

Prologue

Radiography still is the diagnostic imaging technique most frequently used in small animal clinical medicine. That is why those graduate and postgraduate students and professionals who wish to practice clinical medicine need a reference book to use as a guide to radiographic interpretation.

This book fulfils this aim and transmits the author's wide professional experience through the great number of images shown, which cover the most significant diseases and will allow students and veterinary clinicians to recognise the most important and common radiographic signs. In addition, some images are accompanied by diagrams that illustrate the position of the organs, as well as by images obtained with other diagnostic imaging techniques such as ultrasonography, computed tomography and magnetic resonance imaging. It also includes complementary material which can be accessed on the Internet, as well as a section with self-assessment case studies.

I would like to congratulate the author for this atlas, which will be of great value to students and veterinary clinicians.

Amalia Agut Giménez, Diplomate ECVDI
Professor at the Faculty of Animal Medicine and Surgery
(Diagnostic Imaging)
University of Murcia

Preface

In these times when veterinary surgeons have access to advanced diagnostic imaging techniques, such as computed tomography and magnetic resonance imaging, and the use of ultrasonography has become a routine technique, the enormous value that radiography still has as an essential diagnostic tool in small animal clinical medicine is sometimes underestimated.

In my years of experience as a Professor of Diagnostic Imaging (it will be 20 years this year 2013), I have observed a general tendency in veterinary surgeons to try to improve their training in the use of other techniques, mainly ultrasonography, as they often assume that their basic knowledge in radiology is sufficient to carry out their clinical work. My greatest satisfaction as a teacher of continuous professional development courses in radiology has always been to help veterinary professionals discover that a radiograph can give them "much more" than what they initially expect from it. I hope this book will, at least to a certain extent, achieve the same.

I would also like to insist on the fact that it is essential to learn to never settle for a poor radiograph. Being careful with the patient's positioning and the radiographic technique is the first step to a correct interpretation of the images. Although this book does not include specific sections about radiographic technique (there are numerous books that provide a lot of information on this subject available on the market), I have included some recommendations at the beginning of each chapter, in the section titled "Principles of interpretation".

The text also contains numerous references to normal radiographic anatomy and the main non-pathological variations that lead to errors in the interpretation of a radiograph. The chapter "Most common diagnostic errors" includes an extensive review of this and other causes that often lead to incorrect diagnoses.

Through the QR codes that can be found throughout the book, the reader will have access to a complete atlas of normal radiographic anatomy in the dog, in which it is possible to view the normal image of each anatomical region in the standard projections, with and without the clinically relevant anatomical details identified. In addition, the end of each chapter also includes a web link to self-assessment cases.

Atlas of radiographic interpretation in small animals

www.grupoasis.com/book/radiographic_interpretation

For the reader who is not familiarised with the standard orientation of radiographs, it should be reminded that the right and cranial side of the patient always appears at the left of the observer, while the cranial, dorsal or proximal area is shown in the upper part.

My original idea for this book had always been to offer veterinary students and professionals an easy-to-read text that would provide the essential information to interpret radiographs correctly and that, at the same time, would include a large number of radiographic images to illustrate, as much as the book allows it, most of the diseases mentioned in the text. Hence the title *Atlas of radiographic interpretation in small animals*. I hope to have achieved this aim.

M. Isabel García Real
April, 2013

Table of contents

CHAPTER 1 ABDOMEN

CHAPTER 2 NECK AND THORAX

CHAPTER 3 APPENDICULAR SKELETON

CHAPTER 4 SPINE

CHAPTER 5 HEAD

CHAPTER 6 MOST COMMON DIAGNOSTIC ERRORS

ATLAS OF RADIOGRAPHIC INTERPRETATION
in small animals

Abdomen

1

Principles of interpretation

Radiography of the abdomen is one of the most commonly performed diagnostic tests in small animal veterinary practice. The now daily use of ultrasonography has reduced the need for radiographs of the abdomen in many cases, but it is important to highlight that the diagnostic information offered by both techniques is still complementary. For instance, an ultrasound scan is always performed if there is a clinical suspicion of liver disease, but radiography is more accurate when a possible reduction of the size of the liver needs to be confirmed. Another example of the valuable combination of both techniques is found in the assessment of the gastrointestinal tract, where ultrasonography has acquired great relevance over the past few years, without minimising the importance of the diagnostic information offered by radiography in this aspect.

When taking a radiograph of the abdomen, we should include:

- The diaphragm.
- The lumbar spine.
- The abdominal wall.
- The pelvic inlet.

In large breed dogs, the length of the abdomen may exceed the length of the cassette. This therefore requires taking two radiographs to examine the whole abdomen: one centred on its cranial part and the other centred on its caudal part. It is necessary to use an anti-scatter grid (either stationary or Potter-Bucky) when the height of the abdomen exceeds 10 cm once the patient has been placed on the cassette or table. This measure will improve the sharpness of the image by reducing the influence of scattered radiation on the radiograph.

The radiographic projections that are usually used are the lateral and ventrodorsal projections. On occasions, comparing the images of right lateral and left lateral projections may provide additional information, especially in the case of the gastrointestinal tract. Ventrodorsal radiographs are preferred over dorsoventral ones, since the latter are taken in sternal recumbency and the shadows of the organs therefore appear slightly distorted due to compression. If we want to examine the urethra of a male dog, its course will be better viewed by extending the hind limbs in cranial direction.

It is usually possible to identify the liver, spleen, kidneys, bladder, stomach, small intestine, large intestine, abdominal wall and shadow of the diaphragm on a normal radiograph of the abdomen. In male dogs, it is also possible to observe the os penis, the shadow of the prepuce and part of the prostate (fig. 1.1). In normal conditions, it is not possible to identify the pancreas, adrenal glands, gallbladder, ureters, urethra, lymph nodes, blood vessels, ovaries or a non-pregnant uterus.

The main differences between the radiographic image of the abdomen in cats and that in dogs (fig. 1.2) are summarised in table 1.1.

The main limiting factors in the interpretation of radiographs of the abdomen are the superimposition of the numerous anatomical structures contained in the peritoneal cavity and the lack of differentiation between many of them, as most of them have the same radiopacity (soft tissue-fluid). The liver, spleen, kidneys, bladder, etc., all have the same radiographic density, the same tone of grey in the image. The walls of the stomach and intestine also have the same radiopacity as the fluid or mucous content that may be present in the lumen of these organs and it is therefore impossible to identify them on a plain radiograph. The food or gas content of the stomach and gas or faeces in the intestine are more easily identified, precisely because the radiographic density of gas, non-digested or partially digested food and faeces is different from that of the walls and fluid or mucous content of the gastrointestinal tract, as well as from that of most of the surrounding anatomical structures.

TABLE 1.1 Summary of the main differences in the radiographic appearance of the abdomen between the dog and the cat.

	Dog	Cat
Stomach	Pyloric antrum to the right of the median line.	Pyloric antrum on the median line. A layer of fat is sometimes observed on the wall.
Caecum	Generally visible in the right mid-abdomen.	Not identified.
Spleen	Visible on lateral and ventrodorsal radiographs.	Only visible on ventrodorsal radiographs.
Pancreas	Not identified.	The left lobe is sometimes observed on ventrodorsal radiographs.
Adrenal glands	Not identified.	Calcified adrenal glands with a normal size are sometimes observed as an incidental finding.
Os penis	Visible	It is not identified as it is minute in size.
Abdominal fat	More or less homogeneous distribution.	Tendency to a greater accumulation of fat in the area of the falcifom ligament (ventral to the liver), surrounding the intestinal mass (which is centred in the mid-abdomen) and in the retroperitoneal space (facilitates the observation of the kidneys).

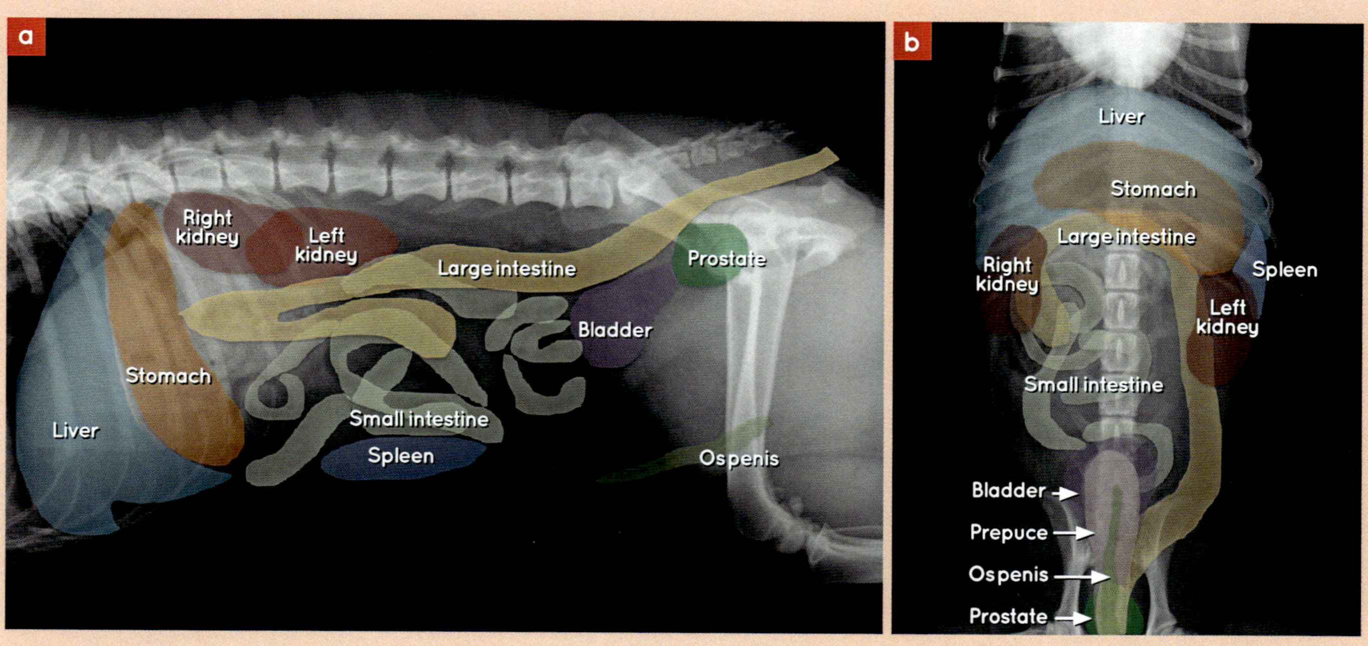

FIGURE 1.1. Lateral (a) and ventrodorsal (b) views of the abdomen of a dog whose main anatomical structures have been identified and highlighted as coloured shadows.

The fat that accumulates in the peritoneum is located between the abdominal organs, which facilitates the differentiation of their contours on the radiograph. The radiographic images of very young or very thin adult animals, which have very little abdominal fat, will show a lack of differentiation of the structures. This may be confused with the image of free fluid or peritoneal reaction. However, an excessive amount of abdominal fat significantly increases X-ray scattering, which may lead to a blurry appearance of the image, even in spite of the use of an anti-scatter grid.

Advanced diagnostic imaging techniques such as computed tomography or magnetic resonance imaging are not often used for the assessment of the abdomen, since the combination of plain or contrast radiography and ultrasonography allows most diagnostic needs to be covered in this anatomical region. Nevertheless, they may be particularly interesting for the evaluation of alterations of the retroperitoneum or blood vessels (e.g. precise diagnosis of portosystemic communications). Both techniques are excellent to examine the pelvic region, as they offer images with great anatomical details of the muscles and bone structures of this area, the rectum, anal sacs, urethra, vagina and vulval vestibule in females, as well as of the prostate, penis and scrotum in males.

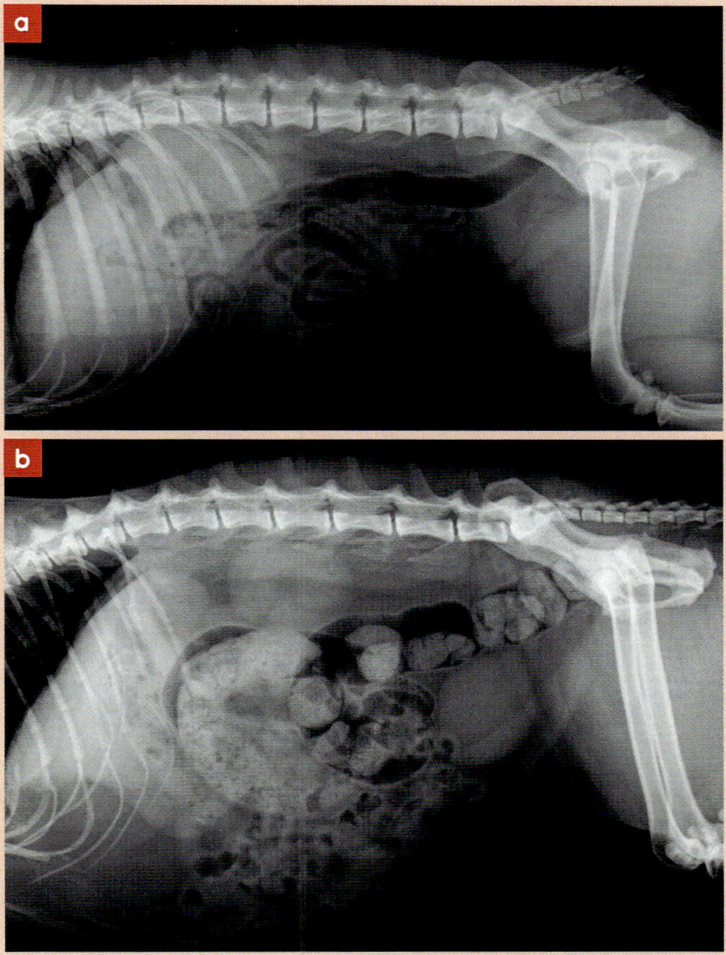

FIGURE 1.2. Lateral radiographs of the normal abdomen of a dog (a) and of a cat (b).

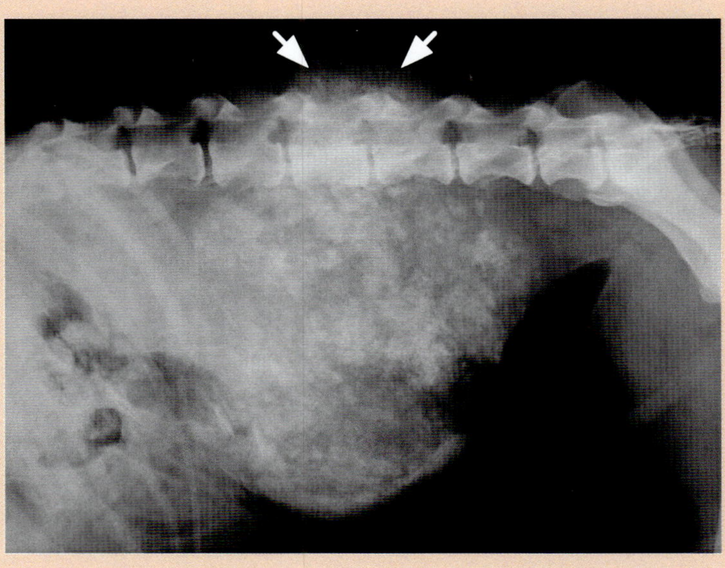

FIGURE 1.3. Lateral radiograph of the abdomen of a dog with a calcified mass located in the abdominal wall. It cannot be confused with an intrabdominal mass, since the dorsal margin of the mass can be seen above the lumbar spine (arrows).

Abdominal wall

The abdominal wall is formed cranially by the diaphragm and costal wall, ventrally and laterally by the abdominal muscles, dorsally by the sublumbar muscles and caudally by the peritoneum.

Radiography allows the detection of alterations in the radiographic density of the wall. The presence of bands of gas lucency is indicative of subcutaneous emphysema, generally associated with penetrating wounds. Lipomas have fat density, while some muscle or skin tumours may appear calcified (fig. 1.3). Areas of calcification that are not associated with masses may also be observed in the wall, for example in patients suffering from Cushing's syndrome with cutaneous calcinosis.

Normal radiographic anatomy of the abdomen
lateral, ventrodorsal and dorsoventral views

http://goo.gl/hnl420

Radiography is also a useful tool in the diagnosis of **hernias**, which may have a congenital origin or occur as a consequence of trauma. Umbilical or inguinal hernias appear as focal distensions of the ventral abdominal wall. Their radiographic density varies in function of the contents of the hernial sac. It is relatively easy to identify the presence of intestinal loops in a hernia, since they appear as structures with a tubular morphology where gas –or faeces in the case of the colon– generally accumulates to a greater or lesser extent. It is also possible to identify the shadow of the bladder if it is distended (fig. 1.4). When the uterus is displaced into the hernial sac, the uterine horns appear as tubular structures with soft-tissue density. These are difficult to differentiate from intestinal loops with fluid or mucous content, unless the uterus is enlarged due to pregnancy or to a pathological dilatation. It is possible to use contrast techniques to confirm the presence of the intestine or bladder in a hernial sac, but it is usually not necessary as ultrasonography is an excellent complementary technique in those cases and allows a fairly precise examination of the defect in the wall and of the structures contained in the hernia.

The **diaphragm** is a musculotendinous sheet that separates the thoracic and abdominal cavities. In normal conditions it is not possible to identify the diaphragm on a plain radiograph, since the liver lies adjacent to it and has the same radiographic density. However, the characteristic morphology of the diaphragm, which is divided into two dorsal crura and a ventral dome, allows us to distinguish its shadow on radiograph. The shadow of the diaphragm will vary according to the chosen radiographic projection (fig. 1.5).

The radiographic image of a diaphragmatic hernia varies in function of the size and location of the defect or rupture in the diaphragm. The most characteristic radiographic sign is the identification of abdominal anatomical structures in the thoracic cavity. A stomach or intestine with gas, food or faeces is easier to identify, while organs with soft-tissue density, such as the liver or spleen, may appear less differentiated (fig. 1.6). In some cases, the abdominal cavity may

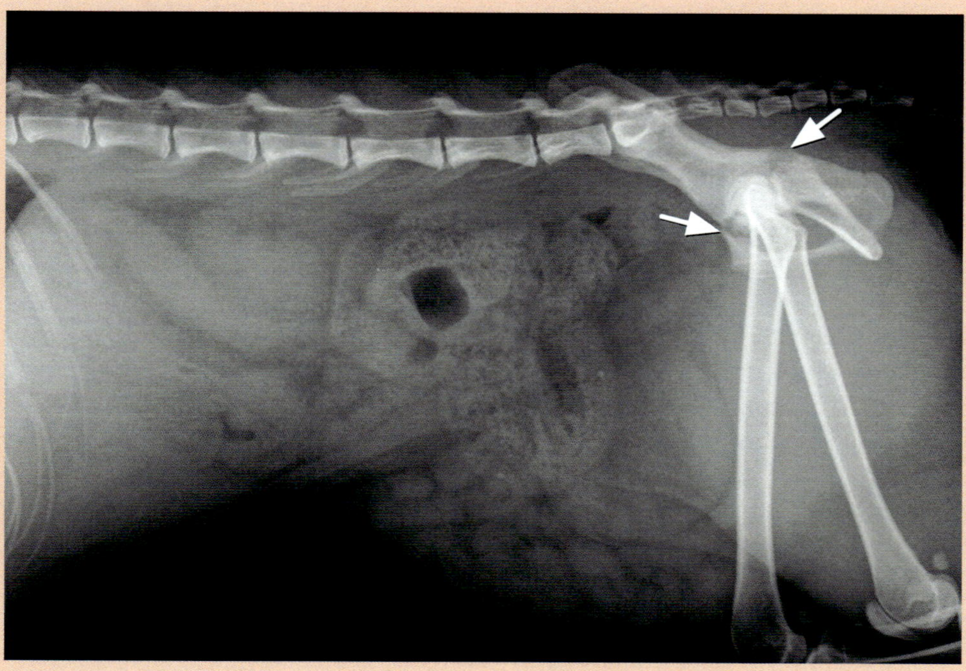

FIGURE 1.4. Lateral radiograph of the abdomen of a cat with an inguinal hernia containing the bladder and segments of the small intestine and colon. Two lines of fracture (arrows) can be observed in the bony pelvis.

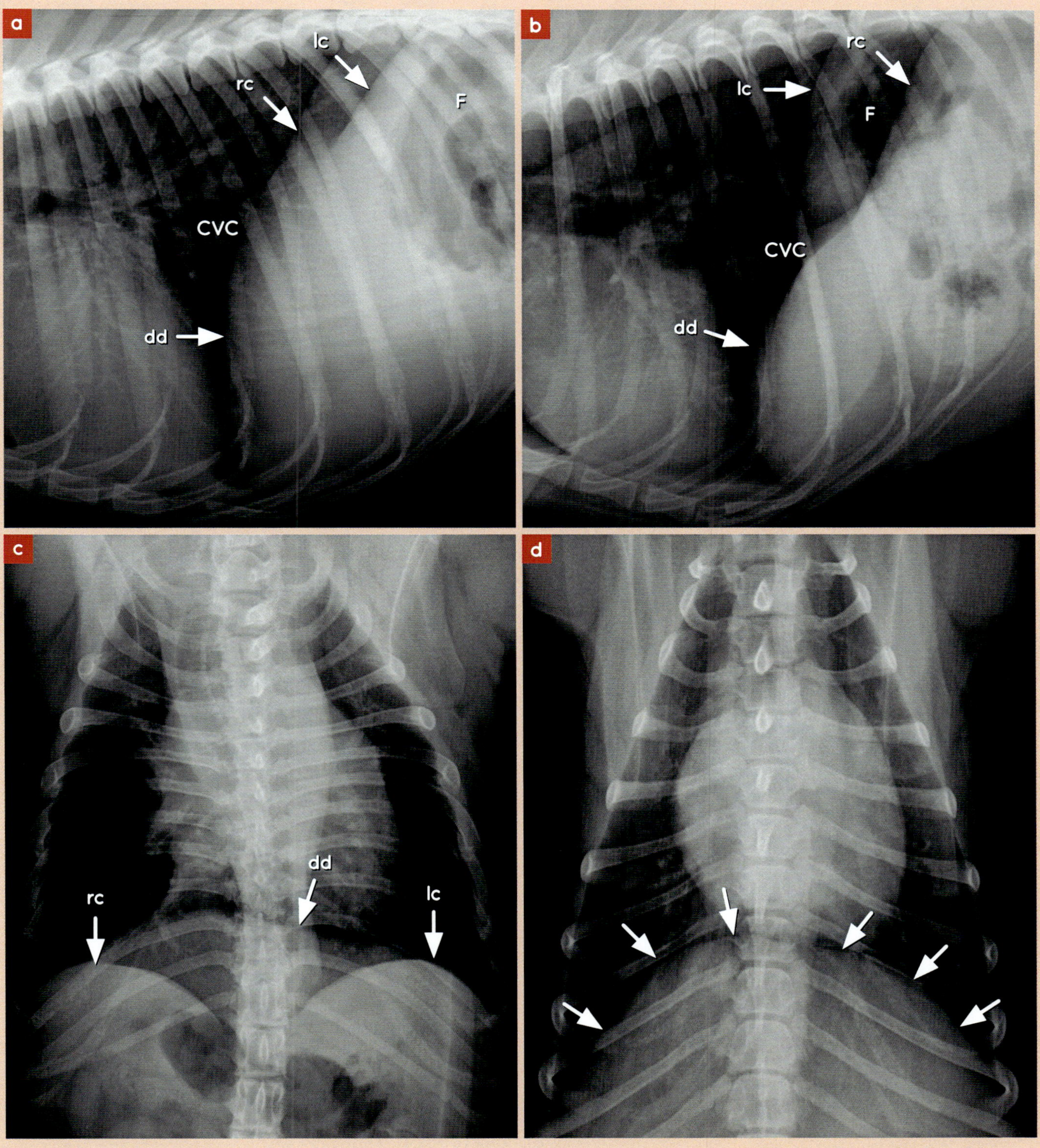

FIGURE 1.5. Right lateral (a), left lateral (b), ventrodorsal (c) and dorsoventral (d) radiographs of the thorax, in which it is possible to see the normal appearance of the diaphragmatic shadow. Right crus of the diaphragm: rc. Left crus of the diaphragm: lc. Diaphragmatic dome: dd. In the right lateral projection, the right crus of the diaphragm is located cranial to the left crus, while in the left lateral projection it is the left crus that has the most cranial position. The two crura of the diaphragm can be differentiated radiographically because the caudal vena cava (CVC) blends with the right crus, while the fundus (F) always appears immediately caudal to the left crus. On the ventrodorsal view, the diaphragmatic shadow may appear as three convex images (the two crura in caudal position and the dome in cranial position), although they are not always easy to identify on radiographs. On the ventrodorsal view, the diaphragmatic shadow always appears as a single convex image (arrows).

appear partially empty of its contents (fig. 1.7). If an associated pleural effusion appears, this may mask the images of the abdominal organs displaced into the thorax. When the defect in the diaphragm is small, it is more difficult to diagnose as there may be no evident radiological signs, for instance, when only a part of the liver protrudes through the defect. Ultrasonography is sometimes useful to provide complementary information, although small diaphragmatic hernias are also difficult to diagnose with this technique.

Perineal hernias (fig. 1.8) occur more frequently in males and may contain the prostate and bladder. Although a positive-contrast cystogram may be performed to confirm the presence of the bladder in the hernial sac, ultrasonography allows the easy identification of all the structures contained in it.

Peritoneal cavity and retroperitoneal space

The peritoneum is a serous membrane essentially composed of connective tissue, which delimits the peritoneal space. The retroperitoneum is the anatomical space located between the dorsal parietal peritoneum and the vertebrae and paraspinal muscles; the kidneys, adrenal glands, ureters, blood vessels and lymph nodes lie in it.

In dogs, abdominal fat essentially accumulates in the mesentery and greater omentum, which are spaces formed by folds of peritoneum. In cats, on the other hand, more fat is accumulated in the falciform ligament (ventral to the liver) and retroperitoneal space than in the mesentery. In obese cats, the small intestinal loops may appear clumped in the centre of the abdomen due to a more peripheral accumulation of intraperitoneal fat (fig. 1.9).

Pneumoperitoneum

It is defined as the presence of free gas in the peritoneal cavity. The most frequent cause is iatrogenic, due to an accumulation of air after a laparotomy, which may remain up to one month in this anatomical space and is progressively absorbed. The pathological causes of pneumoperitoneum are penetrating wounds and the perforation or rupture of abdominal organs containing gas (stomach and intestine).

The radiographic signs of pneumoperitoneum depend on the amount of accumulated gas in the cavity. When gas accumulates in large amounts, a general reduction of abdominal radiopacity and a greater definition of the contour of the organs due to

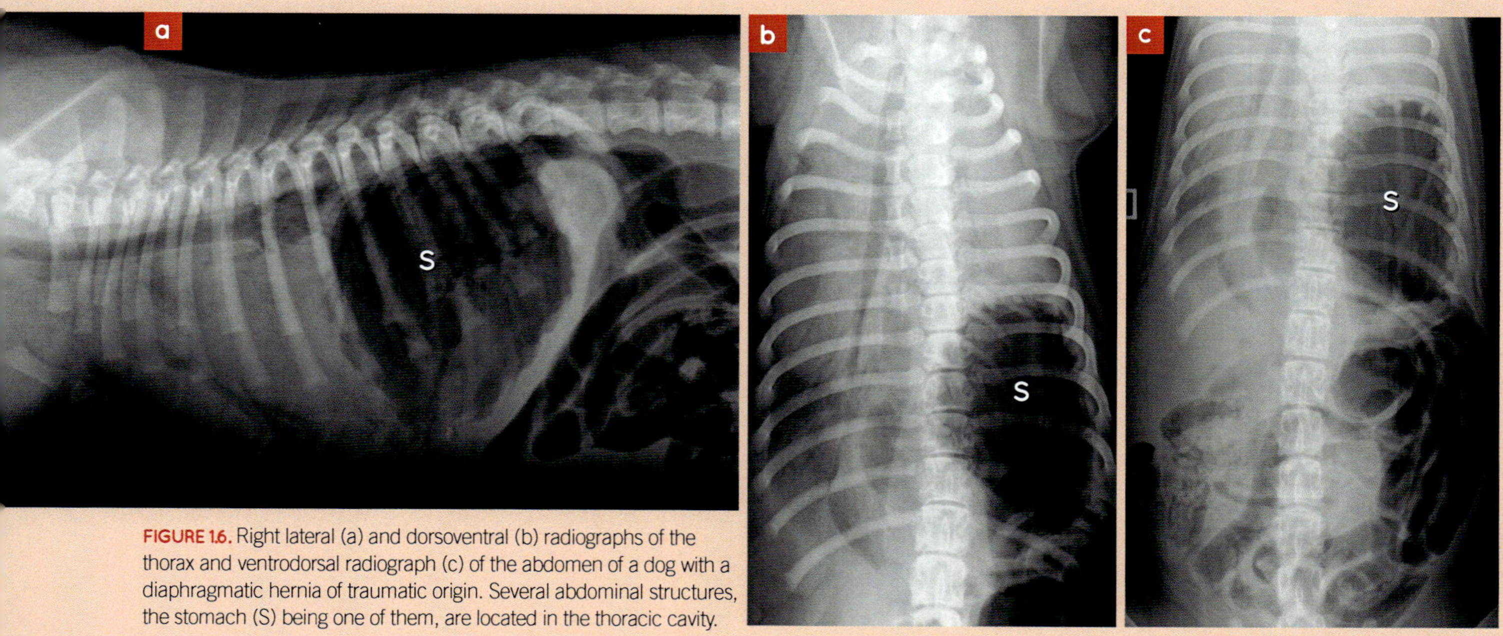

FIGURE 1.6. Right lateral (a) and dorsoventral (b) radiographs of the thorax and ventrodorsal radiograph (c) of the abdomen of a dog with a diaphragmatic hernia of traumatic origin. Several abdominal structures, the stomach (S) being one of them, are located in the thoracic cavity.

the accumulation of gas between them are observed (fig. 1.10). On the other hand, it may be difficult to identify small amounts of free gas, since they are usually mistaken for gas contained in the digestive tract. If gas accumulates between the liver and the diaphragm, the latter can be observed as a thin line of soft-tissue opacity limited cranially by the lung and caudally by free peritoneal gas (fig. 1.11). The observation of this radiological finding confirms the diagnosis of pneumoperitoneum.

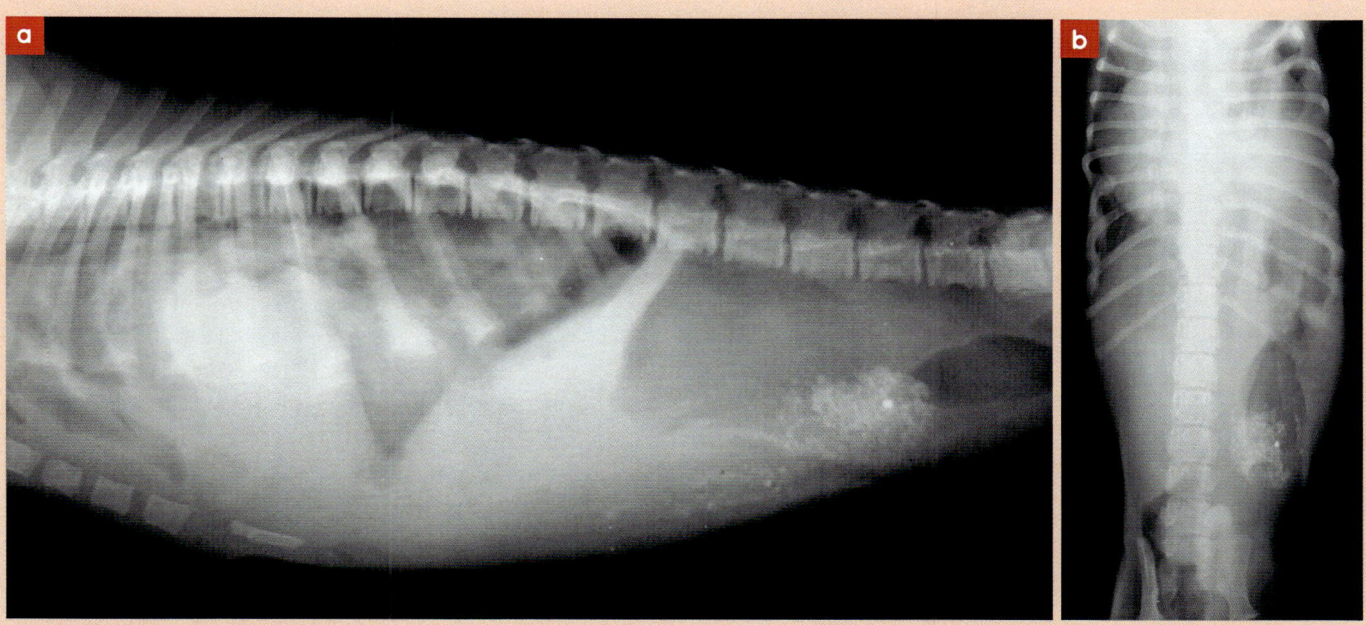

FIGURE 1.7. Right lateral (a) and ventrodorsal (b) radiographs of the abdomen and thorax of a young dog with a diaphragmatic hernia of congenital origin. It is possible to identify intestinal loops with gas content in the thorax, while the abdomen appears partially empty.

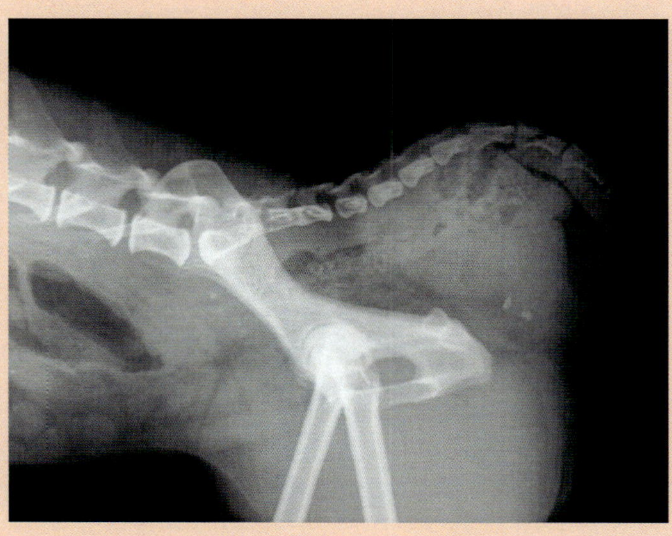

FIGURE 1.8. Lateral radiograph of the caudal abdomen and perineal region of a male dog with a perineal hernia. It is not possible to visualise the shadow of the bladder in the caudal area of the abdomen, as it is located in the hernial sac together with the prostate and part of the rectum.

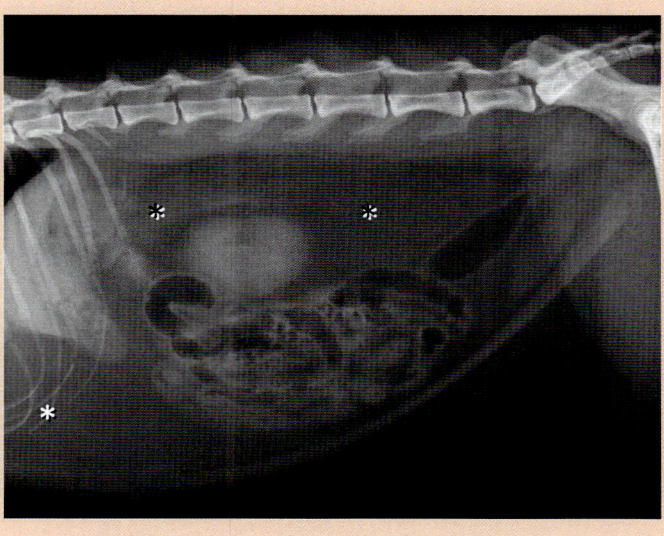

FIGURE 1.9. Lateral radiograph of the abdomen of an obese cat. Cats accumulate more fat in the falciform ligament (ventral to the liver, marked with a white asterisk) and in the retroperitoneal space (marked with black asterisks) than in the mesentery. In obese cats, the intestinal loops appear clumped in the centre of the abdomen due to the greater accumulation of fat in the peripheral areas.

Normal radiographic anatomy of the abdomen
lateral view

http://goo.gl/hnl420

Free fluid

It may be exudate, transudate, blood, urine, bile or lymph. The most common causes of accumulation of free fluid in the peritoneal cavity are:

- Congestive heart failure.
- Hepatic alterations.
- Trauma.
- Renal disease.
- Hypoproteinaemia.
- Peritonitis.
- Abdominal neoplasia.

The most frequent causes of accumulation of free fluid in the retroperitoneal space are:

- Acute kidney injury (the amount of fluid is usually minimal and accumulates next to the affected kidney or kidneys).
- Extravasation of urine of traumatic origin.
- Haemorrhage associated to trauma.
- Coagulopathies.
- Vessel rupture.
- Rupture of highly vascularised retroperitoneal masses.

The radiographic signs of ascites depend on the amount of accumulated fluid in the peritoneal cavity. In general, increased soft-tissue opacity may be observed in the abdomen due to the accumulation of fluid between the abdominal organs. This accumulation of fluid makes the identification of the outline of the organs difficult or impossible, which may be the only evident radiographic sign when the amount of fluid is limited. If the amount is very large, the abdomen will have practically homogeneous soft-tissue opacity, and only the gas, food or faeces contained in the stomach and intestine will be discernible (fig. 1.12). It may be accompanied by more or less marked abdominal distension, depending on the amount of accumulated fluid.

The presence of free fluid in the retroperitoneal space increases radiopacity in this anatomical cavity, together with a loss of detail of the structures contained in it (fig. 1.13). Ultrasonography is more useful than radiography to detect small amounts of free fluid in the retroperitoneum and also allows the collection of samples under ultrasound guidance.

Peritonitis and retroperitonitis

Inflammation of the peritoneum causes a loss of detail of the outline of the abdominal structures that is similar to that caused by free fluid. In fact, ascites and peritonitis cannot be differentiated on a radiograph. When peritonitis is focal, it will only be possible to observe a loss of detail of the structures in the affected area of the abdomen, and the image will thus be very similar to that caused by the presence of small amounts of free fluid in the peritoneal cavity. If peritonitis is generalised, the image will be very similar to that caused by a large amount of free peritoneal fluid, although it is not usually accompanied by abdominal distension (fig. 1.14). However, it is important to bear in mind that peritonitis is often associated with ascites, in which case there will be two causes leading to the same radiographic image (fig. 1.15).

Ultrasonography allows us to clearly distinguish between free fluid, which appears anechoic and improves the identification of the contour of the structures it surrounds, and peritonitis, which is characterised by increased echogenicity of the mesentery (fig. 1.16).

A common cause of focal peritonitis is pancreatitis. A normal pancreas cannot be identified on radiographs, although in obese cats it may be possible to identify its left lobe as an area of soft-tissue density located between the fundus of the stomach, the spleen and the left kidney. When pancreatitis is associated with peritonitis, an irregular increase of soft-tissue opacity in the medial or cranial area of the abdomen may be observed on radiographs (fig. 1.17). The descending duodenum may appear curved and displaced in ventral and lateral direction (fig. 1.18). Pancreatitis is sometimes associated with secondary paralytic ileus, which causes generalised and moderate dilatation of the small intestine.

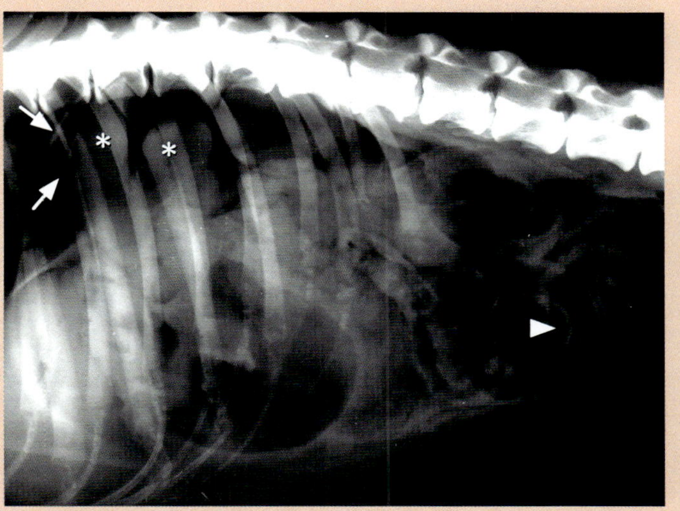

FIGURE 1.10. Lateral radiograph of the abdomen of a dog with a pneumoperitoneum. There is a large amount of intra-abdominal free gas. It is located between the organs, which facilitates the observation of their outline and causes a general reduction of radiopacity of the abdomen. This way, it is possible to identify the liver lobes (asterisks) and the diaphragm (arrows) and to view the external aspect of the gastric and intestinal wall clearly, especially in the segments containing gas, since the soft-tissue opacity of the wall contrasts with the gas lucency on both sides (tip of the arrow).

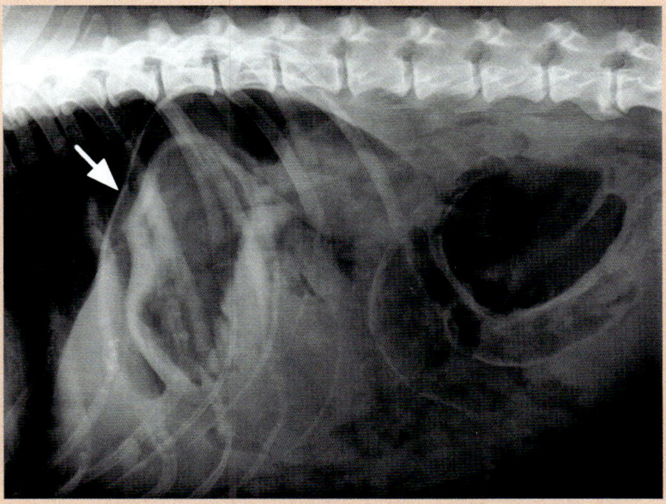

FIGURE 1.11. Lateral radiograph of the abdomen of a dog with a pneumoperitoneum. The amount of intra-abdominal free gas is moderate. When it is located between the diaphragm and the liver, it is possible to identify the diaphragm (arrow), since it contrasts with the gas located cranial and caudal to it, which confirms the pneumoperitoneum.

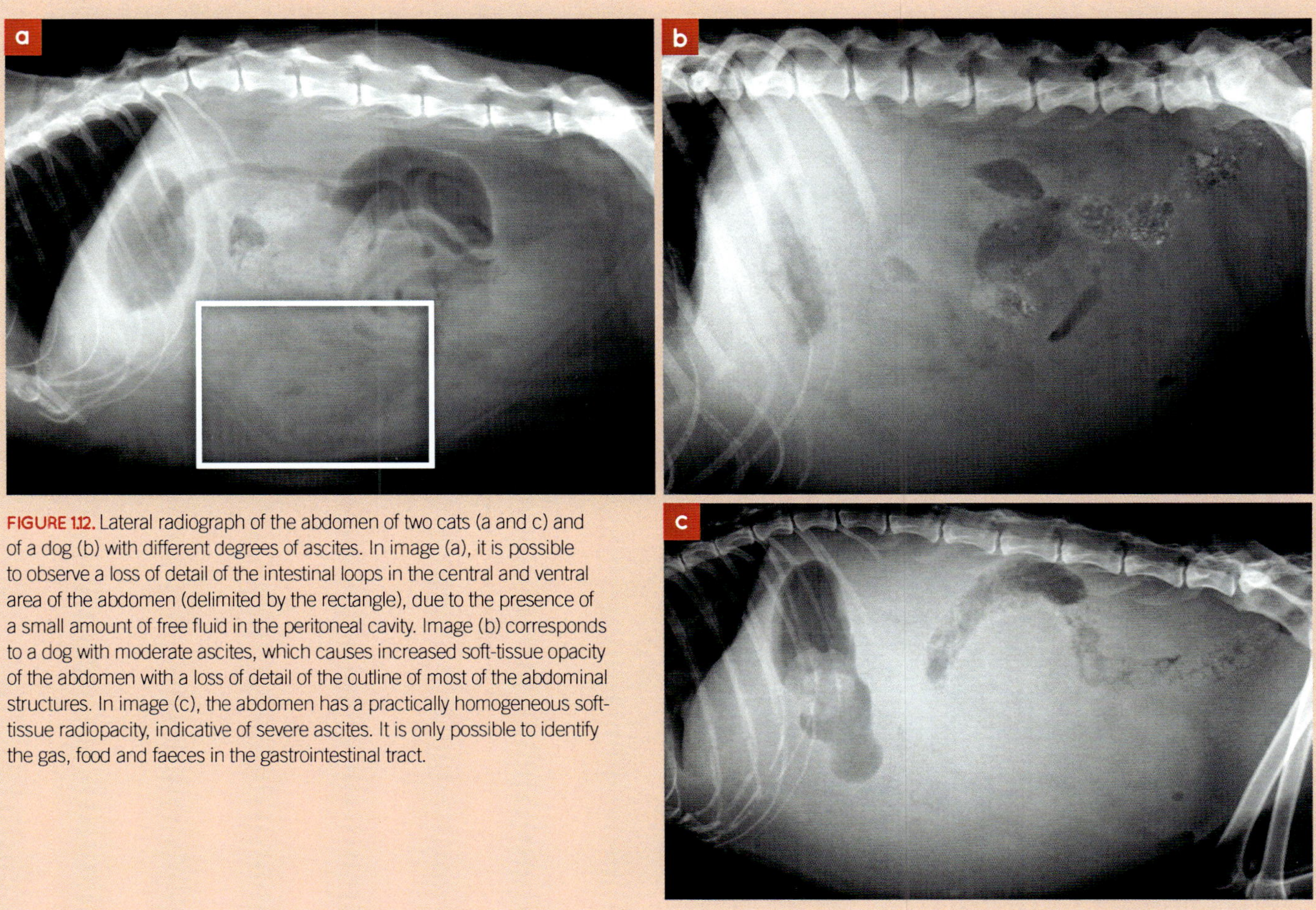

FIGURE 1.12. Lateral radiograph of the abdomen of two cats (a and c) and of a dog (b) with different degrees of ascites. In image (a), it is possible to observe a loss of detail of the intestinal loops in the central and ventral area of the abdomen (delimited by the rectangle), due to the presence of a small amount of free fluid in the peritoneal cavity. Image (b) corresponds to a dog with moderate ascites, which causes increased soft-tissue opacity of the abdomen with a loss of detail of the outline of most of the abdominal structures. In image (c), the abdomen has a practically homogeneous soft-tissue radiopacity, indicative of severe ascites. It is only possible to identify the gas, food and faeces in the gastrointestinal tract.

The most frequent causes of retroperitonitis are the penetration of foreign bodies, penetrating wounds, the extension of local infections (e.g. pyelonephritis) and iatrogenic lesions of the urethra. The most common radiographic finding is increased radiopacity in the retroperitoneal area, with a displacement of the adjacent structures if associated masses appear (e.g. abscess). In chronic cases, signs of spondylitis may appear in lumbar vertebrae, which are characterised by the appearance of bony overgrowths in the ventral margin of the affected vertebral bodies.

Although ultrasonography is useful to detect accumulated fluid, abscesses, alterations of the renal parenchyma, etc., the information it provides is sometimes limited due to the location and size of the lesions. In these cases, the use of computed tomography or magnetic resonance imaging becomes necessary, as they offer detailed anatomical information of the area and both are very sensitive for the detection of most of the pathological alterations that may be found at this level.

Peritoneal carcinomatosis

The neoplastic infiltration of the peritoneum is termed peritoneal carcinomatosis. This may have a very similar image to that of peritonitis and therefore to that of free intra-abdominal fluid. In addition, carcinomatosis often causes ascites. In the ultrasound examination, it is possible to observe thickening and irregular margins of the mesentery and, on occasions, focal hypoechoic lesions in it.

Masses

An abdominal mass appears as a consequence of the increase in size of one or various intra-abdominal structures. This increase in size may be due to pathological causes (neoplasia, hyperplasia, haematoma, abscess, granuloma or cyst, essentially), but also occurs in some physiological processes such as pregnancy, or in iatrogenic diseases such as splenomegaly associated with the administration of barbiturates.

Although it is not usually possible to determine with certainty the origin of an abdominal mass based

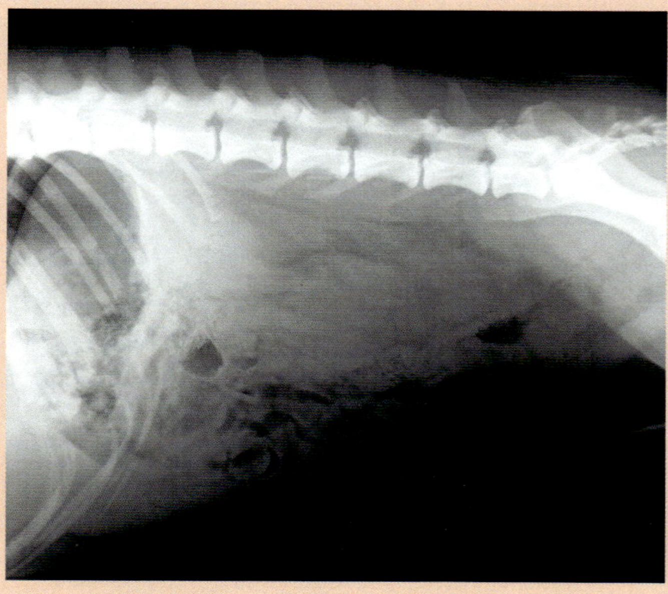

FIGURE 1.13. Lateral radiograph of the abdomen of a dog with free fluid in the retroperitoneal space. An increase in radiopacity in the dorsal area of the abdomen can be observed, with a loss of detail of the renal shadows and ventral displacement of the colon.

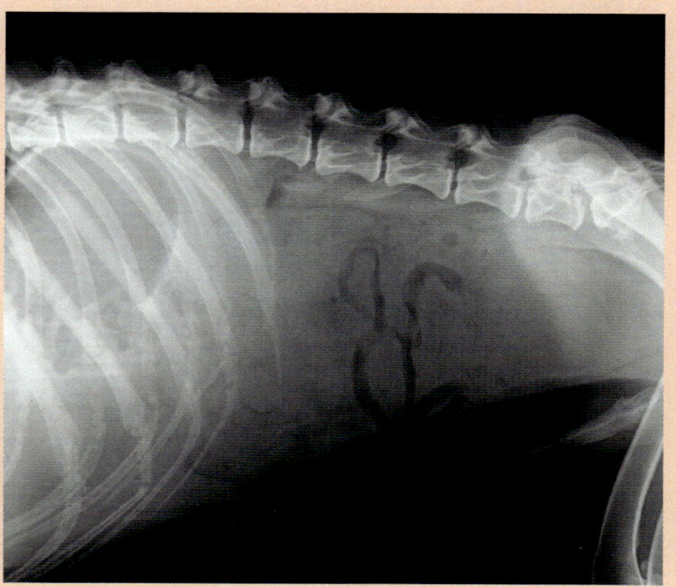

FIGURE 1.14. Lateral radiograph of the abdomen of a dog with peritonitis. Increased soft-tissue opacity may be observed in the abdomen, with a loss of differentiation of the outline of most of the abdominal structures and no abdominal distension. This image cannot be distinguished from that of moderate ascites.

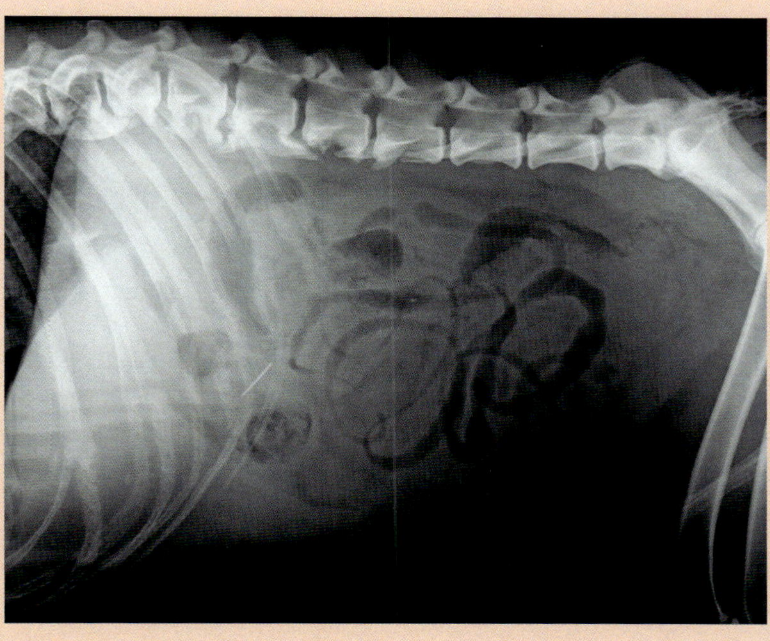

FIGURE 1.15. Lateral radiograph of the abdomen of a dog with peritonitis and ascites due to an intestinal perforation. Increased soft-tissue opacity may be observed in the abdomen, with a loss of differentiation of the outline of most of the abdominal structures and abdominal distension. A sharp metallic foreign body can be seen in the cranial abdomen. Spondylosis deformans of the spine (T11-L4 and L7-S) is worth mentioning as an incidental finding.

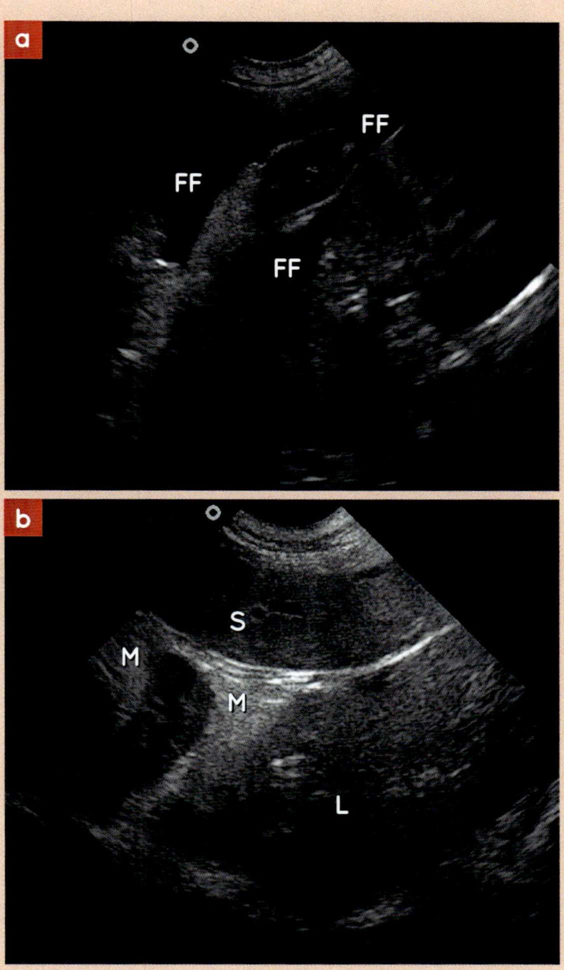

FIGURE 1.16. Ultrasound images of ascites (a) and peritonitis (b). The free fluid (FF) is anechonic and, as opposed to what occurs on a radiograph, it makes the observation of the outline of the organs easier. The inflammation of the peritoneum causes an increase of the echogenicity of the mesentery (M). S: spleen, L: liver.

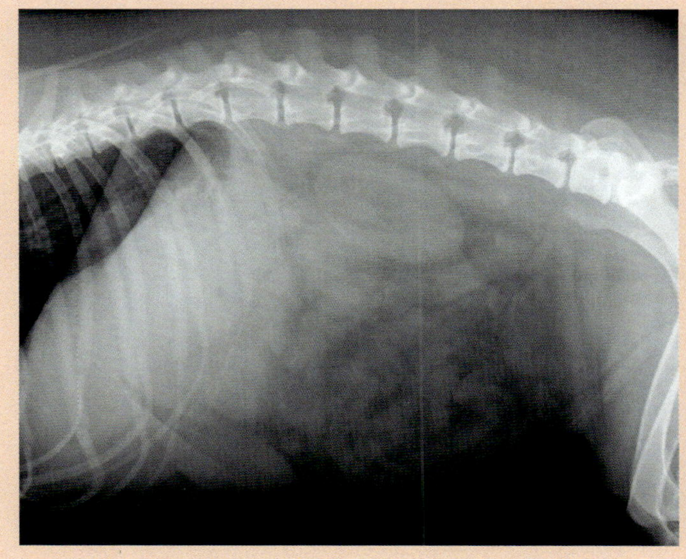

FIGURE 1.17. Lateral radiograph of the abdomen of a dog with peritonitis secondary to pancreatitis. The mottled radiopaque area in the central and ventral region of the abdomen and the loss of differentiation of the outline of the intestinal loops are due to focal peritonitis. Radiographically, it is not possible to distinguish between peritonitis caused by pancreatitis and other potential causes of inflammation or neoplastic infiltrations (carcinomatosis) of the peritoneum.

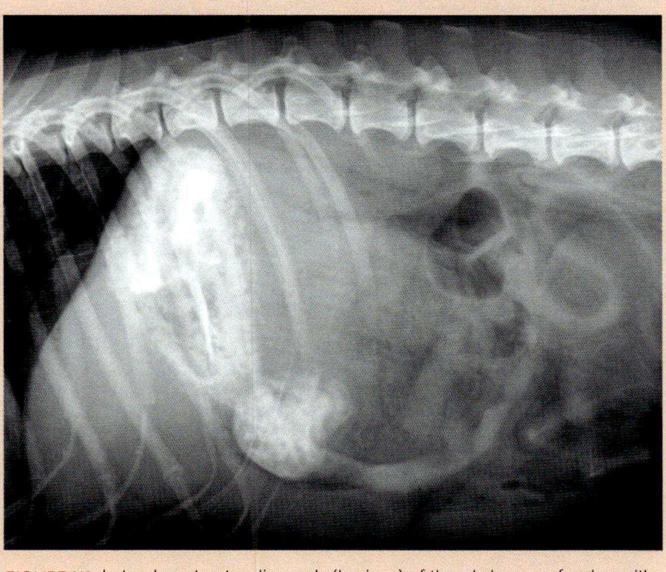

FIGURE 1.18. Lateral contrast radiograph (barium) of the abdomen of a dog with pancreatitis. The presence of the contrast medium in the duodenum shows its displacement and ventral curvature, caused by the inflammatory process of the pancreas. The central area of the abdomen shows a loss of differentiation of the structures due to the peritonitis associated with the process.

Normal radiographic anatomy of the abdomen **lateral view**

http://goo.gl/hnl420

Normal radiographic anatomy of the abdomen **ventrodorsal view**

http://goo.gl/6p7452

only on plain radiographs, its location in the cavity (table 1.2) and the displacement of other abdominal structures it causes may be of great help when establishing a differential diagnosis. For example, a hepatic mass causes a caudal and dorsal displacement of the stomach (fig. 1.19), while a splenic mass usually appears located in the central and ventral area of the abdomen, generally on the left side, and may displace the caecum and the colon in dorsal direction and the small intestine in dorsal and caudal direction (fig. 1.20). Taking radiographs in the two orthogonal projections, lateral and ventrodorsal, provides more complete information in this aspect.

Abdominal masses usually have soft-tissue opacity, although lipomas appear as fat opacity masses. Exceptionally, gas may be identified in an abdominal mass when there are areas of necrosis or when it is related to the digestive tract.

The visibility of a mass on a radiograph depends on its size and on the degree of definition of its margins, which may be significantly reduced when free fluid is present or if the patient also suffers from peritonitis or carcinomatosis, or is very thin. If the margins of a mass cannot be clearly seen in the image, but there is an evident abnormal displacement of the adjacent anatomical structures, we will use the term "mass effect" (fig. 1.21).

Depending on their size, retroperitoneal masses may displace adjacent abdominal structures in ventral direction (fig. 1.22). They may have a renal, adrenal, muscular, lymphatic or vascular origin, essentially. Computed tomography and magnetic resonance imaging allow us to precisely define the borders of the mass and determine whether the adjacent structures are affected (fig. 1.23).

The adrenal glands can only be identified on a radiograph if they are enlarged or calcified. An adrenal origin should be suspected when a mass (with soft-tissue density or partially calcified) is identified craniomedial to a kidney (fig. 1.24). The radiographic finding of a calcified adrenal mass in patients with Cushing's syndrome is very indicative of a neoplasm. However, it should be borne in mind that in cats, the adrenal glands may be calcified with no pathological significance.

TABLE 1.2. Most probable organs of origin according to the location of an abdominal mass.

Location		Organ of origin
Cranial abdomen	Dorsal	■ Liver ■ Stomach ■ Pancreas ■ Kidney ■ Adrenal glands
	Ventral	■ Liver ■ Stomach ■ Pancreas ■ Biliary system
Middle abdomen	Dorsal	■ Kidney ■ Adrenal glands ■ Ovary ■ Retroperitoneal lymph nodes ■ Ureter
	Ventral	■ Spleen ■ Intestine ■ Jejunal lymph nodes* ■ Right lobe of the pancreas* ■ Left kidney* ■ Ovary*
Caudal abdomen	Dorsal	■ Medial iliac lymph nodes ■ Large intestine ■ Ureter
	Ventral	■ Bladder ■ Uterus ■ Prostate ■ Abdominal testicle

* The masses originating in these organs may gravitate towards the ventral part of the abdomen if they are very large.

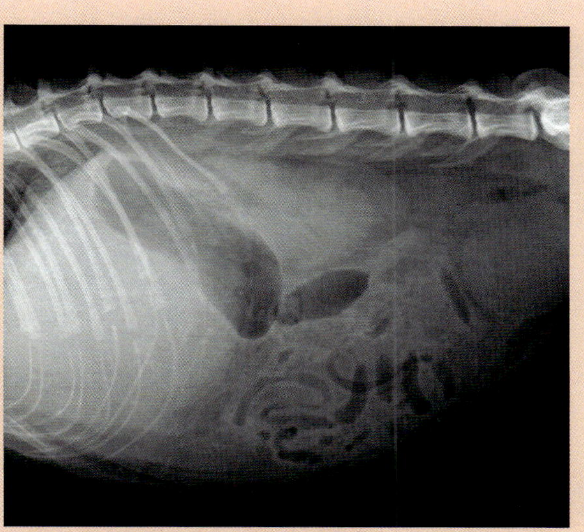

FIGURE 1.19. Lateral radiograph of the abdomen of a cat with a liver mass. The most significant finding is the dorsal and caudal displacement of the stomach. The loss of detail of structures in the central area of the abdomen is due to the presence of free fluid in the peritoneal cavity.

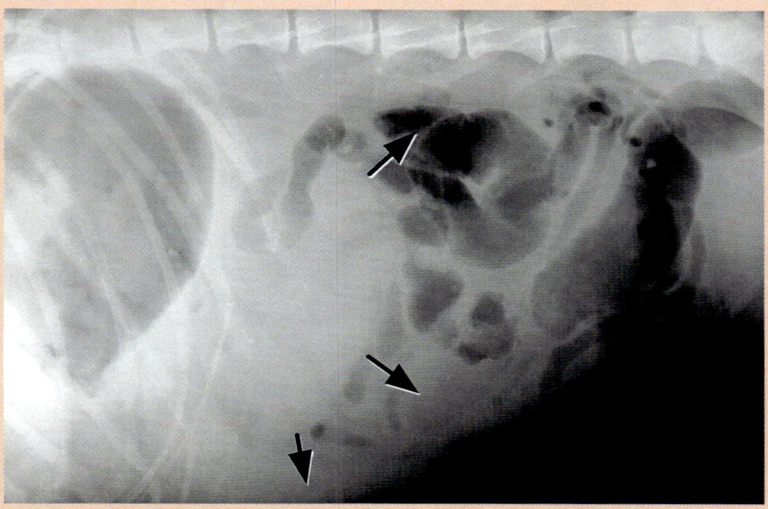

FIGURE 1.21. Lateral radiograph of the abdomen of a dog with a "mass effect" in the cranial area of the abdomen. Immediately caudal to the stomach, it is possible to observe an area of soft-tissue opacity with poorly defined margins, which displaces the adjacent structures dorsally, caudally and ventrally. This finding is due to the presence of a small-sized mass in the central area of the splenic tail.

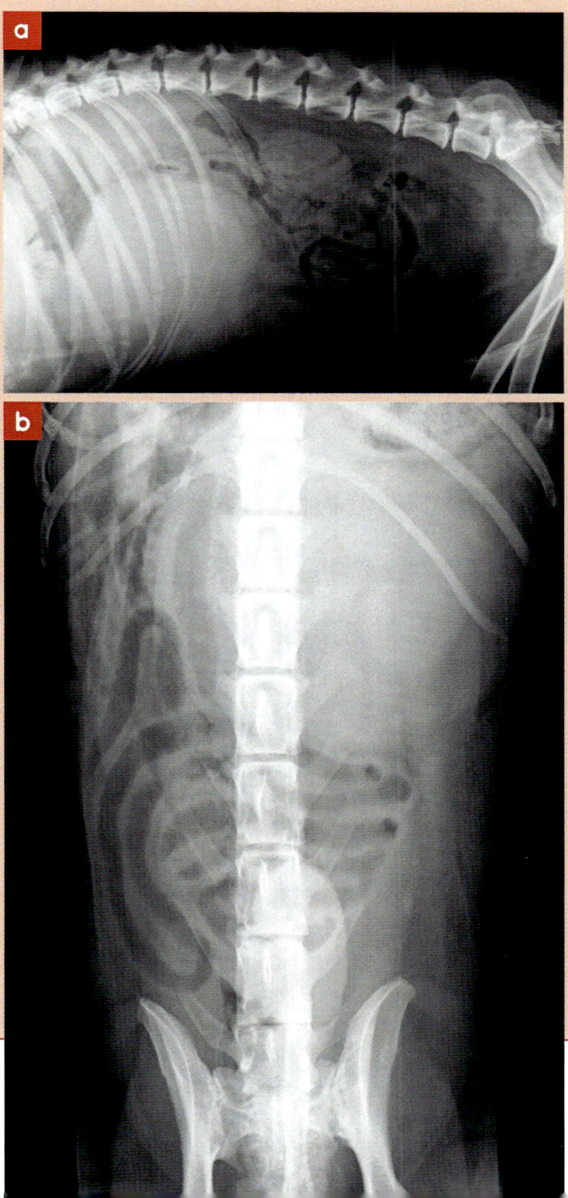

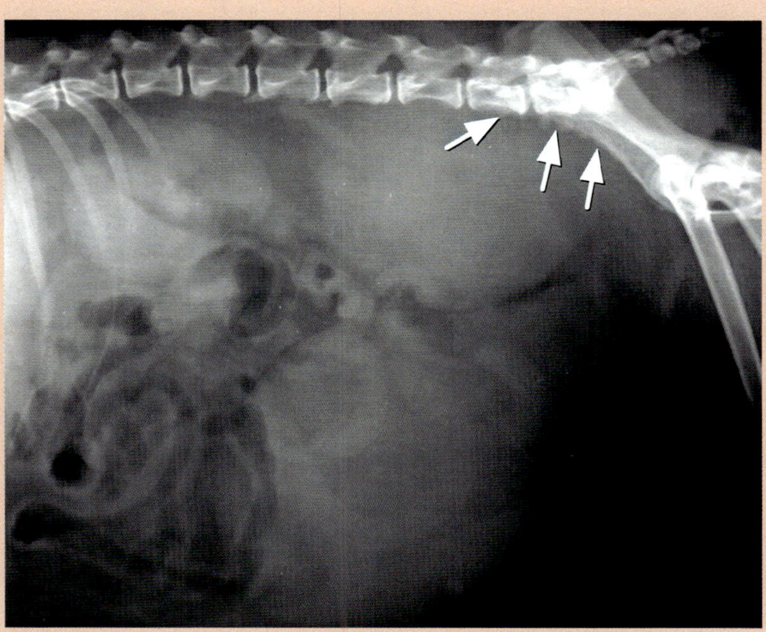

FIGURE 1.22. Lateral radiograph of the abdomen of a dog with a localised tumour in the retroperitoneal space. The mass causes a ventral displacement of the bladder (very distended), descending colon and rectum. In the ventral margin of the last lumbar vertebrae and cranial margin of one of the wings of the ilium, it is possible to identify small bony overgrowths (arrows), compatible with bone metastases. If it were a retroperitoneal abscess instead of a tumour, the bony overgrowths could be due to secondary spondylitis/osteomyelitis.

FIGURE 1.20. Lateral (a) and ventrodorsal (b) radiographs of the abdomen of a dog with a splenic mass, which can be seen in the left cranial area of the abdomen, displacing the colon dorsally and to the right, and the small intestine dorsally, caudally and to the right.

Ultrasonography will allow a more precise assessment of the peritoneal and retroperitoneal masses and in many cases, will enable ultrasound-guided cytology or biopsy.

Liver, spleen and lymph nodes

Liver

On lateral radiographs, the liver occupies a triangular area between the diaphragm and the ventral abdominal wall. Its caudoventral border has an angular shape and does not generally extend beyond the costal arch, or only very slightly. This caudal border is sometimes masked by the splenic shadow. The longitudinal axis of the stomach on this view should be, in normal conditions, perpendicular to the spine or parallel to the ribs. On ventrodorsal radiographs, the liver occupies almost the whole concavity of the diaphragm. Its caudal border appears delimited by the cranial duodenal flexure, the cranial pole of the right kidney and the lesser curvature of the stomach. The left lobes appear superimposed on the fundus on this view (fig. 1.25).

Radiographically, we can detect changes in the size, outline, location and radiographic density of the liver.

When the liver increases in size in a generalised manner, the stomach is displaced caudally.

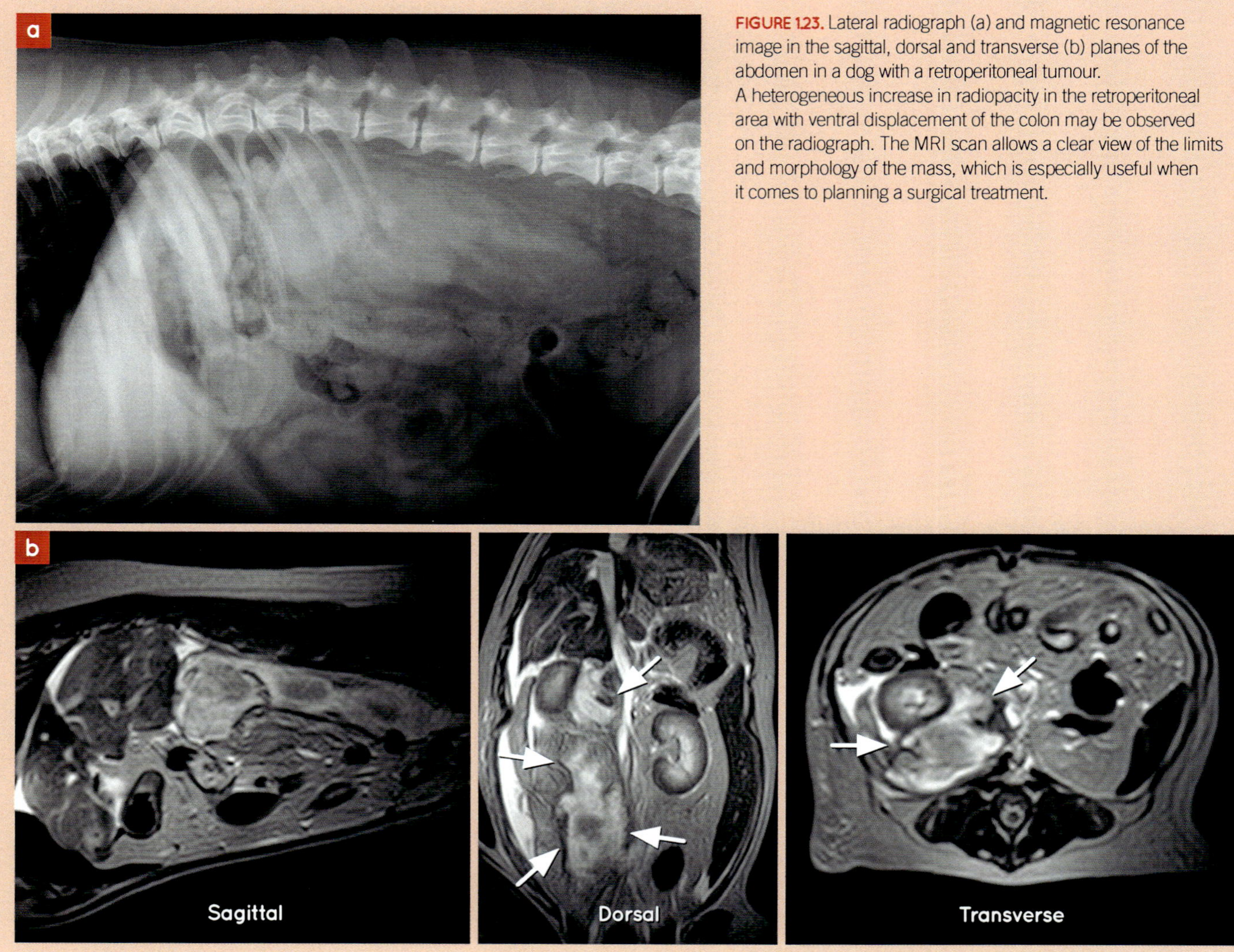

FIGURE 1.23. Lateral radiograph (a) and magnetic resonance image in the sagittal, dorsal and transverse (b) planes of the abdomen in a dog with a retroperitoneal tumour.
A heterogeneous increase in radiopacity in the retroperitoneal area with ventral displacement of the colon may be observed on the radiograph. The MRI scan allows a clear view of the limits and morphology of the mass, which is especially useful when it comes to planning a surgical treatment.

The caudoventral border may appear round and is located farther away from the costal arch (fig. 1.26). If the increase in size is localised, these signs may not be as obvious on the radiograph. The radiographic image of liver masses depend on their size and location in the organ, but if they are large, they occupy the most cranial part of the abdominal cavity and significantly displace the stomach caudally and dorsally (fig. 1.27).

Radiography is a fairly precise tool to detect a reduction of the size of the liver (microhepatia). The axis of the stomach appears displaced cranially and the distance between the margin of the diaphragmatic dome and caudal hepatic border (fig. 1.28).

Doubts about the size of the liver may sometimes arise with ultrasonography, but this technique provides much more information about alterations of the

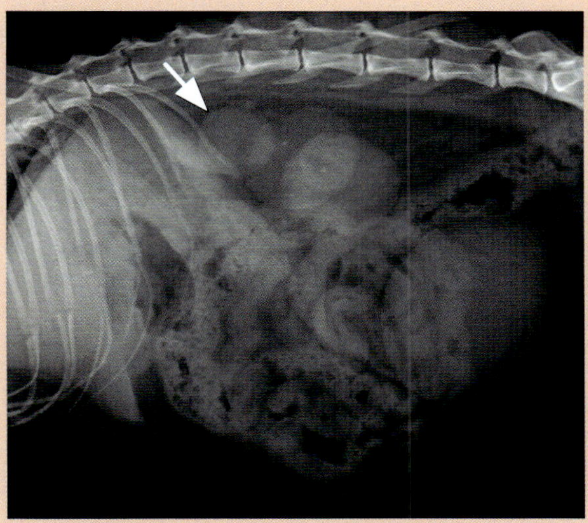

FIGURE 1.24. Lateral radiograph of a cat with an adrenal mass (arrow). Although its size is small, the large amount of retroperitoneal fat allows it to be clearly identified in the image. The fact that it is located cranial to the renal shadows indicates that it is of adrenal origin, although masses of other origins (e.g. glandular) may also appear in this location.

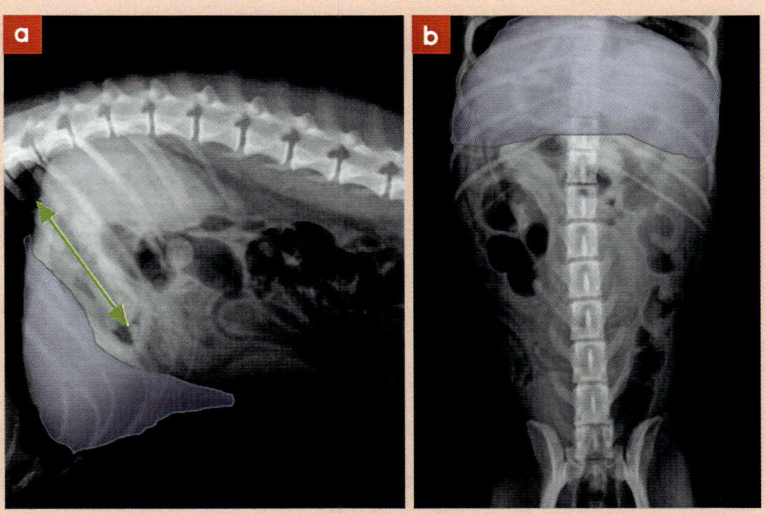

FIGURE 1.25. Lateral (a) and (b) ventrodorsal radiographs of the abdomen of a healthy dog, in which the shadows of the liver are highlighted with blue areas. The green line represents the longitudinal axis of the stomach, drawn from the centre of the fundus to the centre of the pyloric area.

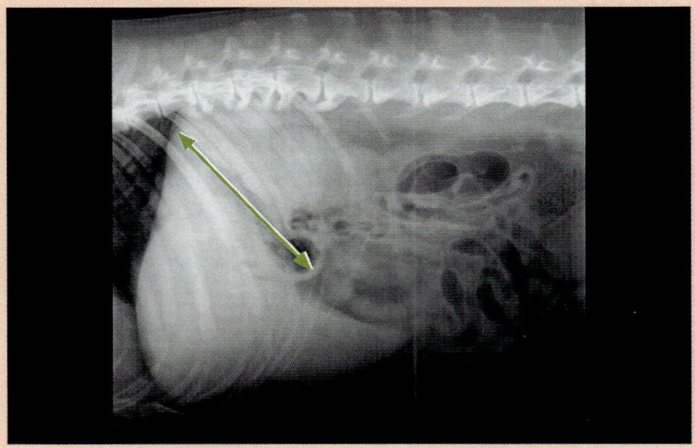

FIGURE 1.26. Lateral radiograph of the cranial abdomen of a dog suffering from hepatomegaly. The axis of the stomach appears displaced caudally and a great part of the caudoventral border extends beyond the costal arch. As an incidental finding, it is possible to observe spondylosis deformans in the T11-L2 segment.

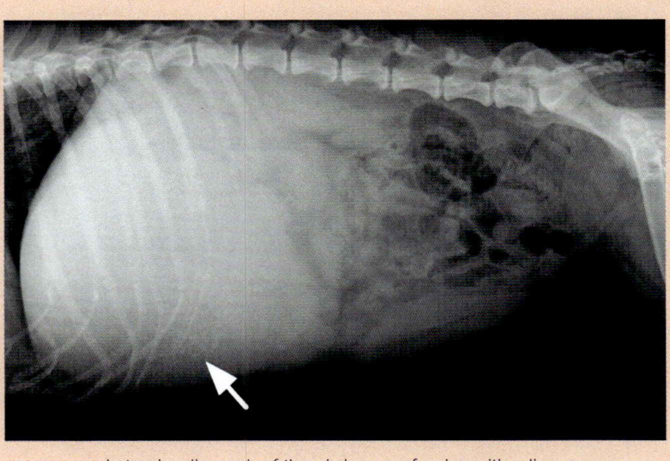

FIGURE 1.27. Lateral radiograph of the abdomen of a dog with a liver mass, which occupies a great part of the cranial abdomen and displaces the stomach, intestine and spleen caudally. The mass shows a region with small areas of calcifications (arrow).

liver parenchyma and margins, which is why both methods are used in a complementary manner to diagnose a reduction of the size of this organ.

It is not uncommon to observe areas of mineral opacity in the liver. Gallbladder sludge or calcified gallbladder stones are often identified on plain radiographs and are in many cases a casual finding (fig. 1.29). If the calcified areas have a linear pattern, the most probable diagnosis is that of calcification of the biliary tract (fig. 1.30), which is sometimes an incidental finding in small breed dogs. Abscesses, haematomas, cysts and tumours may also appear partially calcified in this organ. In addition, the presence of gas may be detected in the liver parenchyma or in the gallbladder and biliary tract. This may be due to an infection caused by anaerobes or, in diabetic patients, by microorganisms that ferment glucose, giving rise to the formation of carbon dioxide. If the morphology of the gas opacity areas is linear, this suggests involvement of the biliary tract (neumobilia), if it is oval, of the gallbladder, and if it is irregular, this is more suggestive of the presence of an abscess or of a tumour with a necrotic centre in the parenchyma. In any case, both calcifications and the presence of gas in this organ can be assessed and confirmed by means of ultrasonography.

Spleen

The spleen is an organ with a relatively variable size and location, especially in dogs. The head of the spleen has a more stable position in the left craniodorsal area of the abdomen, thanks to the gastrosplenic ligament. On radiographs, it appears as a shadow with a triangular morphology superimposed on the last ribs of the left side (fig. 1.31), and it is visible both in dogs and cats. The position of the tail of the spleen, by contrast, may considerably vary. In the case of dogs, it usually appears on lateral radiographs as a triangular or oval shadow located in the medial ventral area of the abdomen, but it is rarely identified in healthy cats. Compared with that of a dog, the spleen of a cat is smaller and shorter.

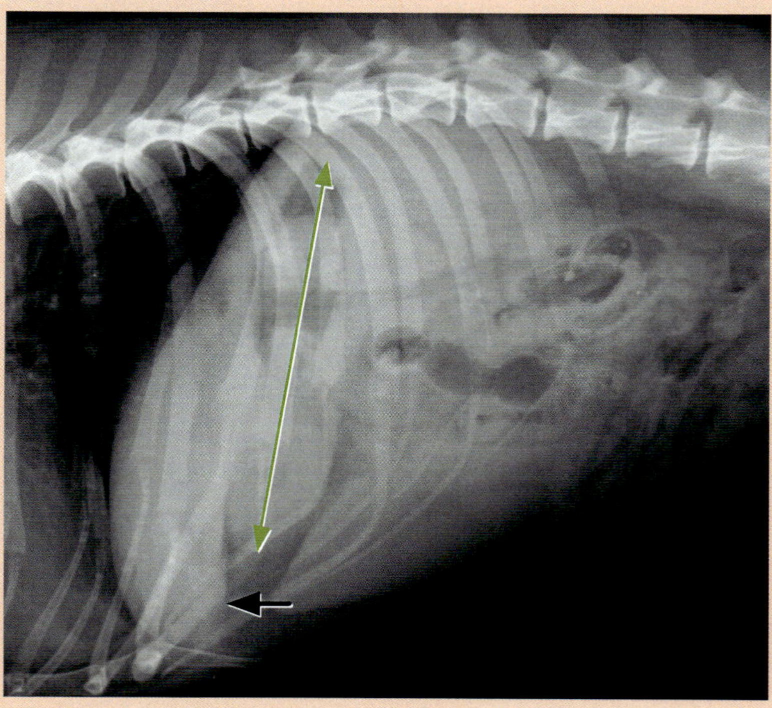

FIGURE 1.28. Lateral radiograph of the abdomen of a dog with an abnormally small liver (microhepatia). The axis of the stomach is displaced in cranial direction and the distance between the dome of the diaphragm and the caudoventral border of the liver appears reduced (indicated by the black arrow).

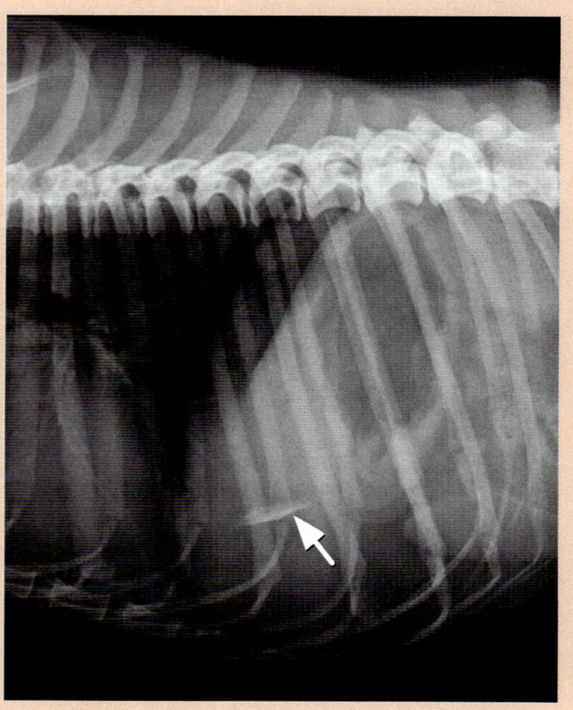

FIGURE 1.29. Enlarged image of the cranial abdomen on a lateral radiograph of a dog with calcified sludge in the gallbladder (arrow).

Normal radiographic anatomy of the abdomen **ventrodorsal view**

http://goo.gl/6p7452

The length of the splenic shadow will vary on lateral radiographs, depending on the position of the tail of the spleen. If the latter is almost completely located in the cranial part of the mid-abdomen, the shadow will be relatively short; if it is in an oblique position in the mid-abdomen, the shadow will be longer; and if it is located along the left side of the animal, the shadow will then be very long on the radiograph (fig. 1.32).

We should not confuse a longer shadow of the spleen with splenomegaly. Splenomegaly is assessed in a subjective manner but is always accompanied by an enlargement (fig. 1.33) and in many cases rounded borders of the organ. It should be borne in mind that healthy German Shepherd dogs have a larger spleen than other breeds of a similar size. In the case of a splenic torsion, the organ usually appears very enlarged, with rounded margins and an abnormal position in the abdomen.

The image of splenic masses varies in function of their size and location (fig. 1.34). If there is a haemorrhage, the tumour margins may appear totally or partially masked, although the displacement of the adjacent viscera will be an evident sign of its presence in the abdominal cavity.

Changes in the radiographic density of the spleen are rare. The organ may show areas of calcification associated with dystrophic calcification of neoplasms, abscesses, granulomas or haematomas. In cases of splenic torsion, gas may also appear in the splenic parenchyma due to the formation of areas of necrosis.

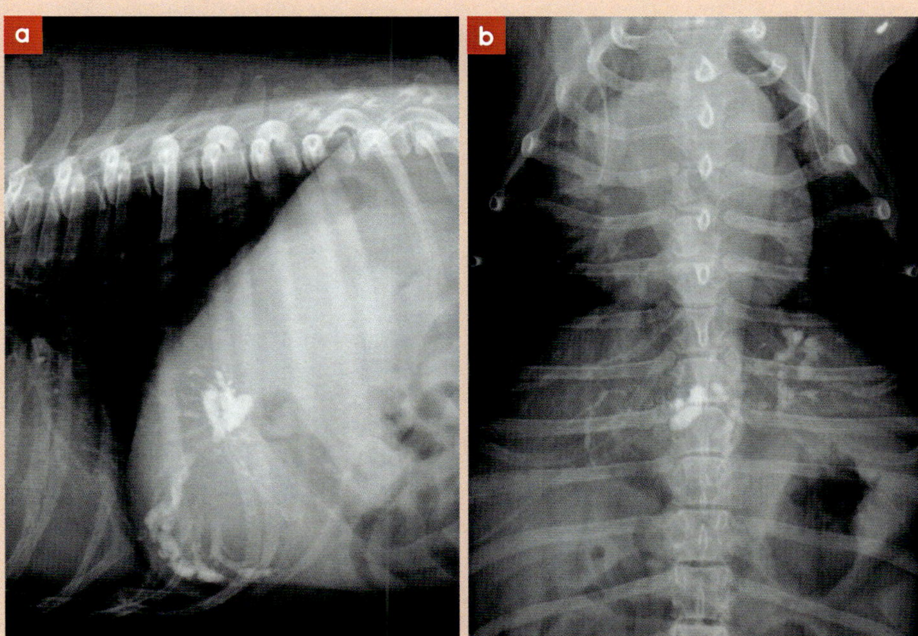

FIGURE 1.30. Enlarged images of two lateral (a) and ventrodorsal (b) radiographs of the cranial abdomen of a dog with calcification of the bile ducts. This finding may be incidental in small breeds.

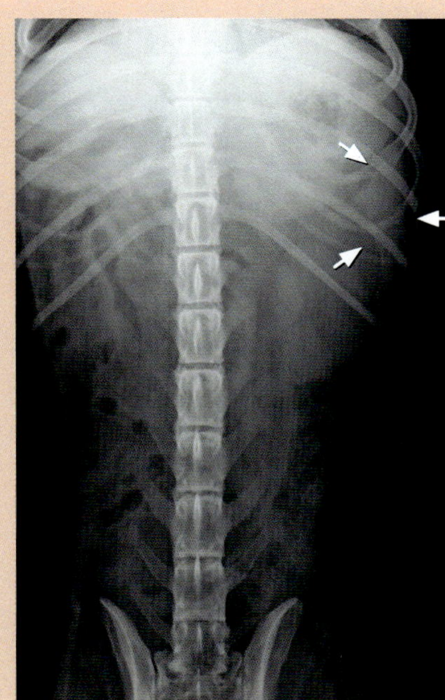

FIGURE 1.31. Ventrodorsal radiograph of the abdomen of a healthy dog. The shadow of the head of the spleen (arrows) has a triangular morphology on this view and is located in the left cranial abdomen, superimposed on the most caudal ribs of the same side.

Lymph nodes

Abdominal lymph nodes are only identified on radiographs when they are enlarged or calcified. The more retroperitoneal fat a patient has, the easier it will be to observe them.

The medial iliac (sublumbar) lymph nodes are the easiest to identify on radiographs of the abdomen when they are enlarged. They are located ventral to the L6 and L7 lumbar vertebrae, although their shadow may extend more cranially if the increase in their size is very marked (fig. 1.35). The enlargement may be due to lymphadenitis, hyperplasia or neoplasia. A tumoral infiltration of these lymph nodes may be primary (e.g. lymphoma) or metastatic (e.g. in the case of localised tumours in the caudal area of the abdomen or in the pelvis).

Urinary system

Conventional radiography is a very important diagnostic technique in the study of diseases of the urinary system, although it has now been replaced to a great extent by ultrasonography, since this latter allows a direct assessment of the internal architecture of the kidneys and bladder. However, contrast radiographic techniques still are the standard method of choice to examine the ureters and urethra.

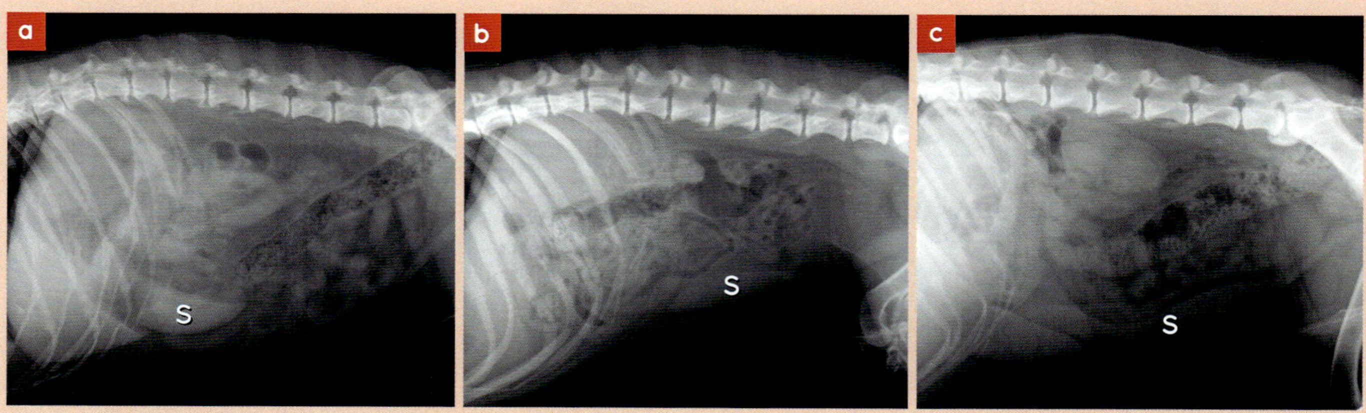

▲ **FIGURE 1.32.** Lateral radiographs of the abdomens of three healthy dogs showing different positions of the tail of the spleen. In image (a), the shadow is short because the tail of the spleen (S) is located in the cranial abdomen. In image (b), the shadow is slightly longer because the tail of the spleen is located obliquely in the mid-abdomen. In image (c), the tail of the spleen is located along the left side of the animal, thus creating a longer shadow on the lateral view. In the three cases, the spleen has a normal size.

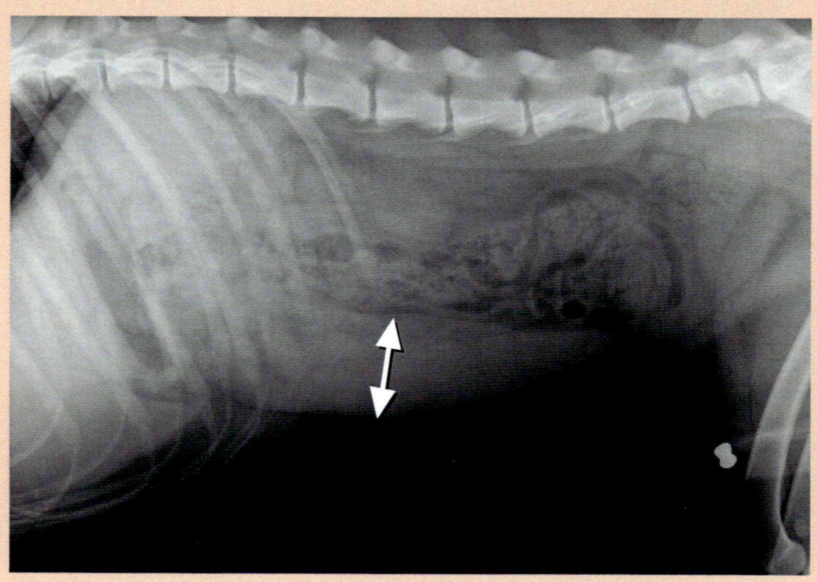

FIGURE 1.33. Lateral radiograph of the abdomen of a dog with splenomegaly. The spleen appears enlarged (arrow), which indicates an increase in the size of the organ. As an incidental finding, it is possible to observe a metallic foreign body (shotgun pellet) in the area of the prepuce, superimposed on the os penis. ▶

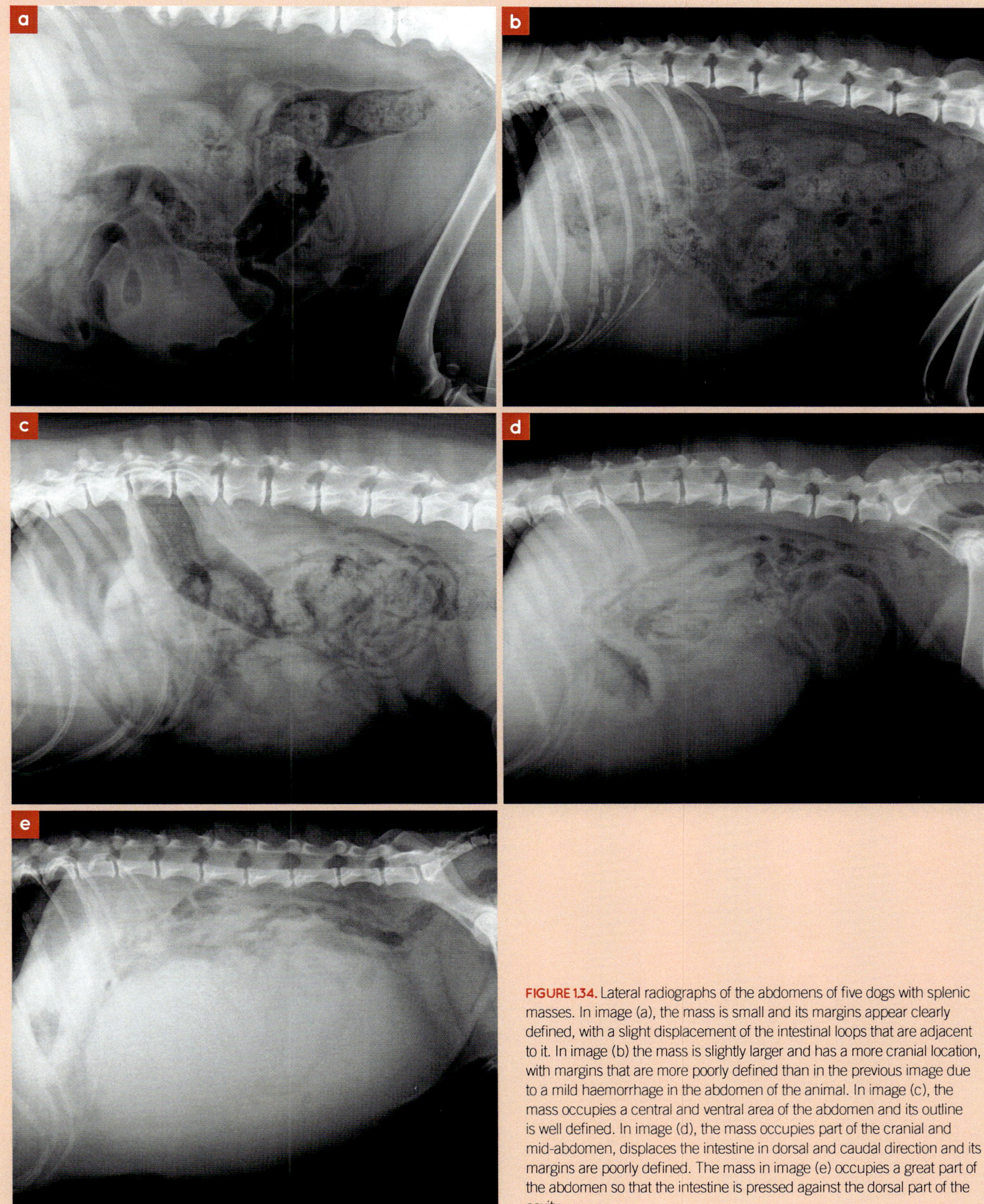

FIGURE 1.34. Lateral radiographs of the abdomens of five dogs with splenic masses. In image (a), the mass is small and its margins appear clearly defined, with a slight displacement of the intestinal loops that are adjacent to it. In image (b) the mass is slightly larger and has a more cranial location, with margins that are more poorly defined than in the previous image due to a mild haemorrhage in the abdomen of the animal. In image (c), the mass occupies a central and ventral area of the abdomen and its outline is well defined. In image (d), the mass occupies part of the cranial and mid-abdomen, displaces the intestine in dorsal and caudal direction and its margins are poorly defined. The mass in image (e) occupies a great part of the abdomen so that the intestine is pressed against the dorsal part of the cavity.

Kidneys

A plain radiograph allows the observation of alterations in the number, size, outline, position and radiographic density of the kidneys, but it does not offer any information about their internal architecture. That is why the diagnostic imaging technique of choice to assess the kidneys is ultrasonography, since this technique does offer detailed information about the normal internal structure and its possible alterations.

The contrast technique used to examine the kidneys and ureters is excretory urography. It involves the intravenous administration of a positive contrast medium that is selectively excreted by the kidneys. With this technique it is possible to obtain a certain amount of information about the internal structure of the kidney (although not as complete as that offered by ultrasonography), and functional information based on the qualitative assessment of the degree of filtration of the contrast agent through the renal parenchyma.

The kidneys are located in the retroperitoneal space. On lateral radiographs, they appear located in the craniodorsal area of the abdomen and partially superimposed, while on ventrodorsal radiographs they are not superimposed on one another but on other structures, which masks the shadow of one or the two kidneys, particularly in dogs. The greater the amount of retroperitoneal fat an animal has, the more defined the renal shadows will be in the image. Cats accumulate more fat in this anatomical location, which significantly improves the visualisation of the kidneys. The anatomical location of the right kidney is more cranial than that of the left one, which allows their differentiation on lateral radiographs.

The evaluation of the size of the renal shadows is based on the comparison of their length with that of the vertebral body of the L2 vertebra. In healthy animals, the maximum length of the renal shadows should be comprised between 2.5 and 3.5 times the length of L2 in dogs (fig. 1.37), and between 2.4 and 3 times its length in cats (fig. 1.38), although lower ranges have been published in older cats with no clinical symptoms of kidney disease (2.1 to 3.2 in non-neutered cats and 1.9 to 2.6 in neutered cats.)

An increase in the size of the renal shadows may be due to very different diseases. A decrease in the size of the kidneys in young animals is usually caused by congenital diseases such as renal dysplasia or hypoplasia, while in adult animals it is usually attributed to chronic renal diseases at an advanced or terminal stage.

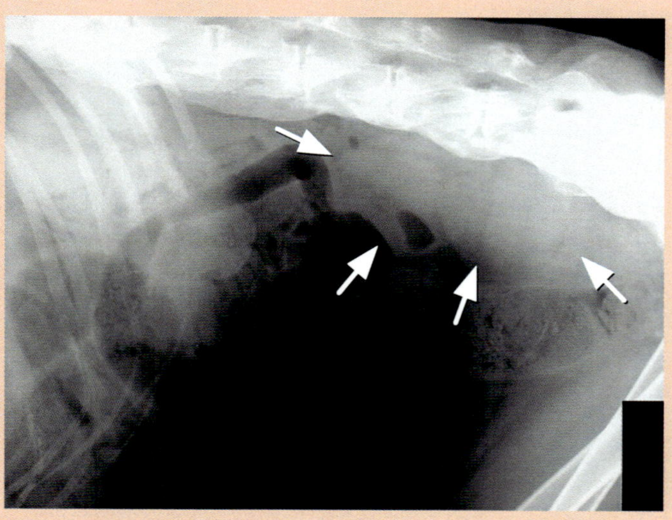

FIGURE 1.35. Enlarged image of the caudal abdomen on a lateral radiograph of a dog with sublumbar lymphadenopathies. Its outline cannot be seen properly due to the presence of surrounding retroperitoneal fat.

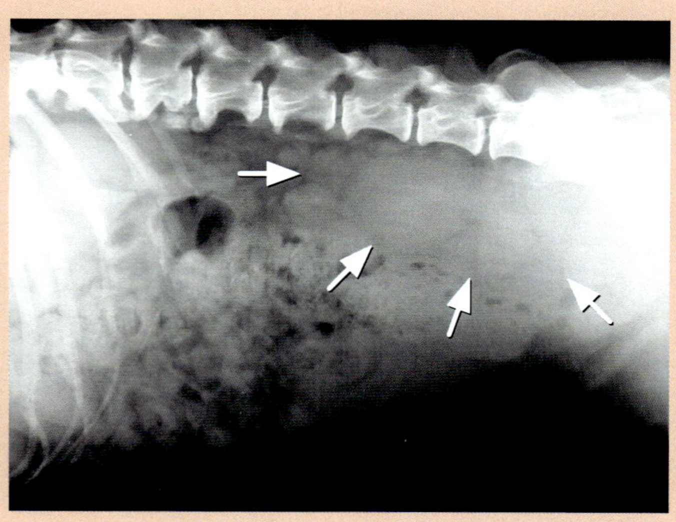

FIGURE 1.36. Lateral radiograph of the abdomen of a dog with very large sublumbar lymphadenopathies due to a lymphoma. The "mass effect" is located ventral to L5-L7 and causes the ventral displacement of the descending colon.

The relative assessment of the kidneys, that is to say, comparing the size, shape and outline of a kidney with those of the other, may be more useful in practice than evaluating the actual size of each kidney. If the two renal shadows appear enlarged, the differential diagnosis will include renal lymphoma (fig. 1.39), bilateral hydronephrosis, polycystic kidney disease, bilateral perinephric cyst (fig. 1.40) and bilateral neoplasia. If the two kidneys appear decreased in size, the most probable cause is chronic interstitial nephritis (fig. 1.41). When one of the shadows maintains a normal size and the other one is enlarged, this suggests neoplasia, renal trauma, unilateral perinephric cyst or unilateral hydornephrosis. Finally, if the

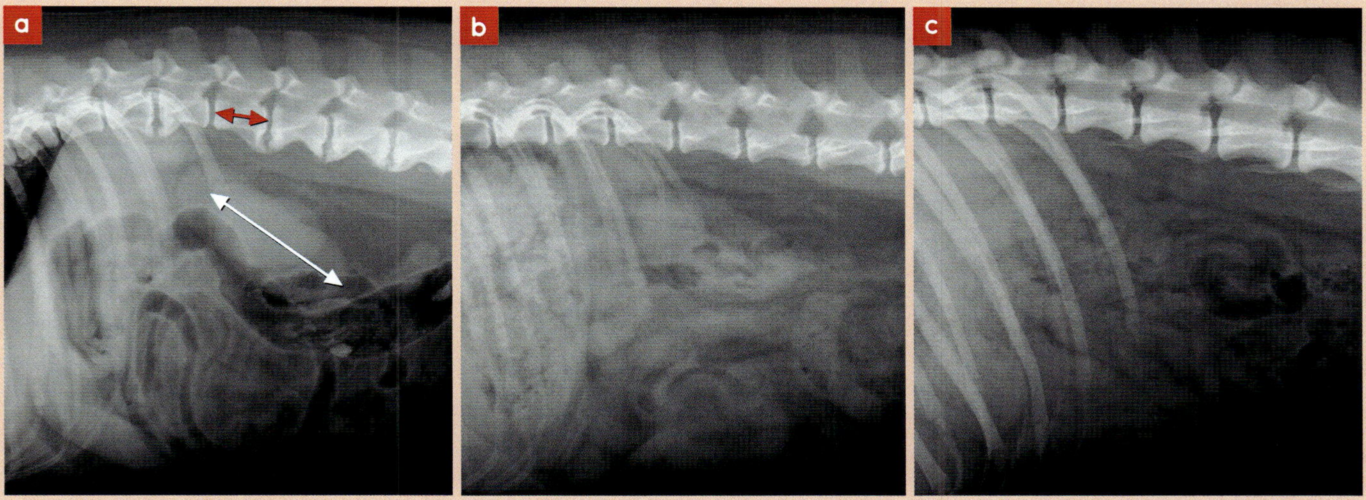

FIGURE 1.37. Enlarged images of the cranial abdomens on lateral radiographs of three dogs with normal kidneys. In image (a), the two renal shadows are perfectly differentiated due to the large amount of retroperitoneal fat of the animal. In normal conditions, the length of the renal shadows (shown in the left kidney with a white arrow), should be comprised between 2.5 and 3.5 times the length of the L2 vertebra (shown with a red arrow). In image (b), only the shadow of the left kidney, which is anatomically located in a more caudal position, is well defined, while the right renal shadow is masked by other structures. In image (c), none of the renal shadows can be clearly distinguished because of the lack of retroperitoneal fat and other superimposed structures.

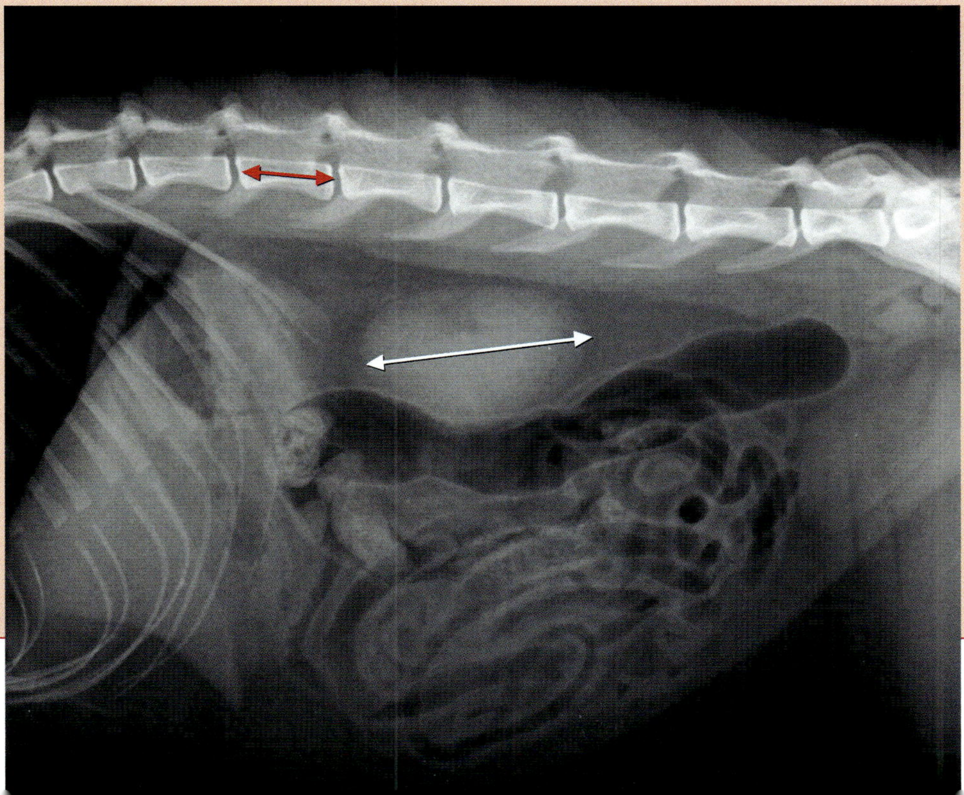

FIGURE 1.38. Lateral radiograph of the abdomen of a cat with normal kidneys. The two renal shadows appear practically superimposed. In general, they are better visualised in cats than in dogs as cats tend to accumulate more fat in the retroperitoneal space. As a general reference for normality, the length of the renal shadows (indicated in the left kidney with a white arrow) should be between 2.4 and 3 times the length of the L2 vertebra (indicated with a red arrow), although lower ranges have been published in older cats (2.1 to 3.2 in non-neutered cats and 1.9 to 2.6 in neutered cats).

Normal radiographic anatomy of the abdomen **ventrodorsal view**

http://goo.gl/6p7452

shadow of a kidney is enlarged and the other one is reduced, the most probable cause is chronic interstitial nephritis in a kidney with compensatory hypertrophy of the other one (fig. 1.42).

Plain radiography also allows the visualisation of alterations in the outline of the kidneys, although ultrasonography is more precise in this aspect. The most common causes of changes in the contour of the kidneys are: polycystic renal disease, neoplasia, abscess, simple cysts, haematoma, cortical infarction or chronic renal disease at an advanced stage (fig. 1.43).

It is uncommon to detect significant anomalies in the position of the kidneys. When they appear displaced from their normal position, this is generally due to an increase in the size or displacement of the structures that are adjacent to the kidneys, although they may also have an abnormal location due to congenital alterations (renal ectopy) or to trauma causing their avulsion.

Calcification of the renal parenchyma due to the presence of calculi (fig. 1.44) or to dystrophic calcification is frequent, especially in older animals. Not all calculi are observed as mineral opacities. Those composed of ammonium urate and cystin have a similar radiopacity to that of soft tissues and fluids, which is why they are usually qualified as radiolucent in plain radiography. Ultrasonography allows the detection of all types of calculi, although if they are small it will be difficult or impossible to distinguish them from calcifications in the renal parenchyma. Excretory urography may offer more precise information in this sense, especially if it is evaluated by means of computed tomography. Dystrophic calcification alone does not usually have any pathological significance, although it sometimes coincides with the appearance of other signs of chronic kidney disease in the patient.

In some healthy cats, it is possible to identify the normal renal pelvis due to the presence of fat in this area, which contrasts with the soft-tissue opacity of the surrounding parenchyma. Negative-contrast or

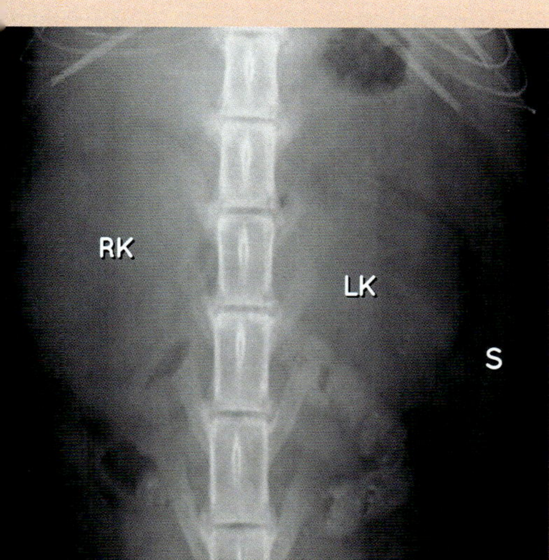

FIGURE 1.39. Enlarged image of the abdomen on a ventral radiograph of a cat with renal lymphoma. The two renal shadows (RK, LK) appear enlarged in size with an irregular contour. The spleen (S) also appears enlarged.

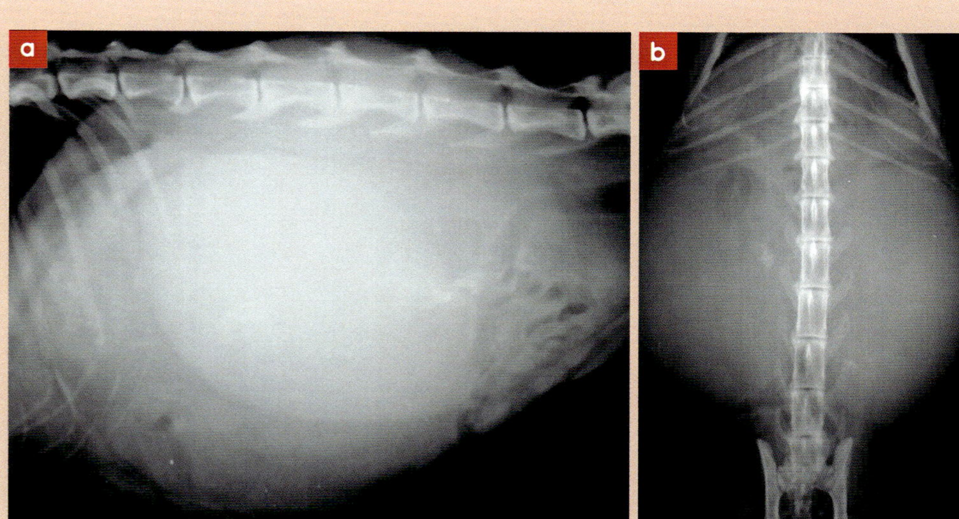

FIGURE 1.40. Lateral (a) and (b) ventrodorsal radiographs of the abdomen of a cat with bilateral perinephric cysts (perinephric pseudocysts). This disease is very uncommon and mainly affects older cats. It is characterised by an accumulation of a large amount of fluid (urine, transudate, lymph, or blood) that totally or partially surrounds one or the two kidneys. In this case, it gives rise to the appearance of large masses in the region of the kidneys.

double-constrat cystography also allows the identification of the presence of gas in the kidneys as a consequence of vesicoureteral reflux. The non-iatrogenic presence of gas in the kidney may suggest the presence of anaerobic bacteria that produce gas.

Patients with chronic renal failure may show secondary signs on plain radiographs, such as dystrophic calcification of the folds of the gastric wall or osteopaenia caused by secondary renal hyperparathryroidism, which essentially affects the maxilla and mandible (see chapter 5).

Excretory urography

Compared with plain radiography, excretory urography provides additional morphological information as well as qualitative information about renal function. Taking into account the information that other imaging techniques can provide, it would currently be recommended to perform excretory urography in cases of urinary incontinence, uroabdomen (suspicion of rupture of the kidney, bladder or ureter), or to investigate haematuria or locate the kidneys in the presence of a retroperitoneal mass. It would be contraindicated in patients suffering from anuria, dehydration

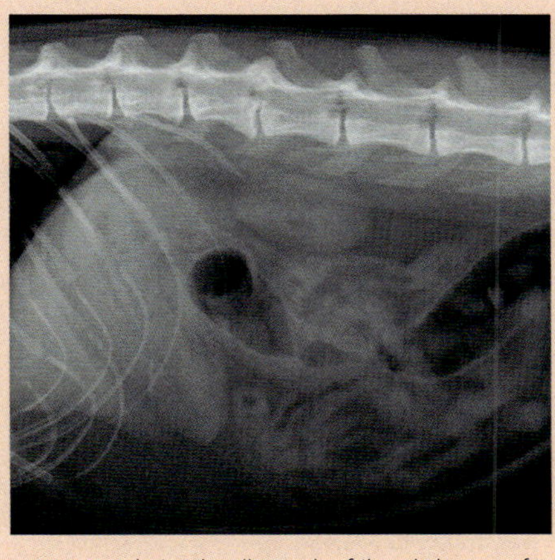

FIGURE 1.41. Lateral radiograph of the abdomen of a cat with abnormally small kidneys.

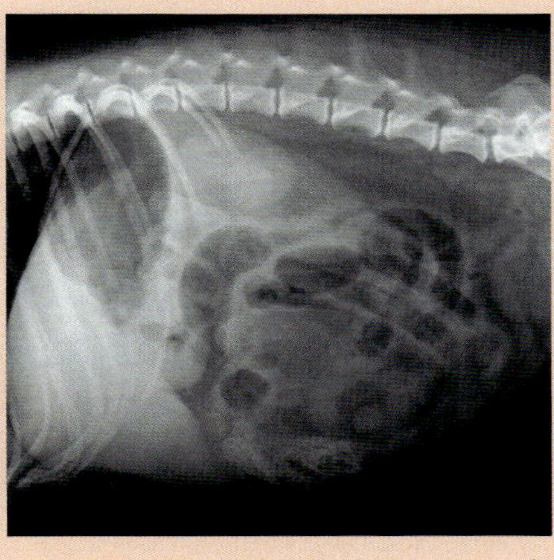

FIGURE 1.42. Lateral radiograph of the abdomen of a dog with an abnormally small right kidney. The left kidney is slightly enlarged, which could be due to compensatory hypertrophy.

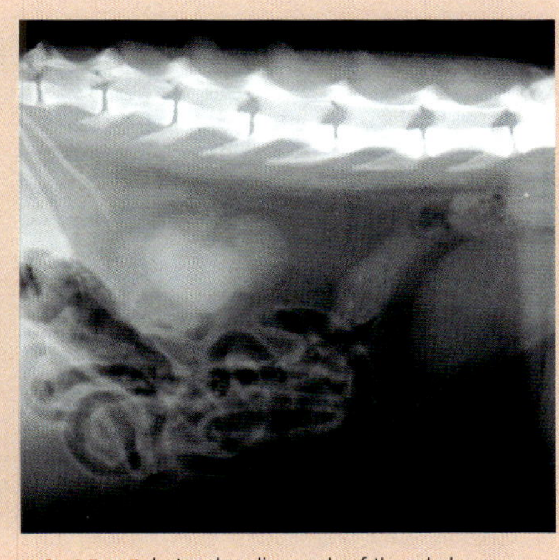

FIGURE 1.43. Lateral radiograph of the abdomen of a cat with an alteration of the contour of the left kidney.

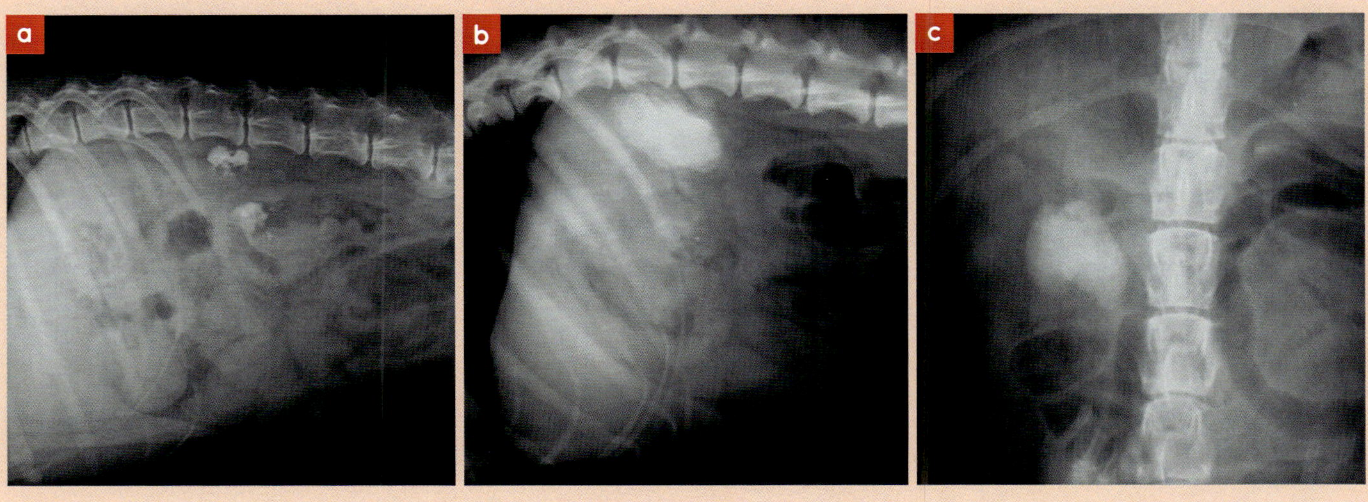

FIGURE 1.44. Enlarged images of the cranial abdomen on lateral (a and b) and ventrodorsal (c) radiographs of three dogs with radiopaque renal calculi.

and allergy to iodine. Excretory urography is not an appropriate technique to specifically examine the bladder, since the contrast medium mixes with urine in this organ and, in addition, an adequate degree of bladder distension is not usually achieved. However, it may be used as an alternative technique to conventional cystography when it is impossible to catheterise the patient.

The intravenous administration of hyperosmotic iodinated contrast media (e.g. diatrizoate or meglumine amidotrizoate) may cause adverse reactions in some patients, although the incidence is low. Nausea and vomiting are the most frequent adverse effects, while systemic hypotension and acute kidney injury induced by the contrast agent are possible, although less probable, complications. There is a risk of anaphylaxis but it is very uncommon. However, the necessary medication to treat it should always be available before starting the procedure and the intravenous catheter should be maintained until the end in case administration of emergency medication is required.

It is recommended to obtain a signed informed consent from the pet's owner every time a contrast technique is performed.

The risk of adverse effects is reduced with the use of low osmolarity, non-ionic iodinated contrast media, such as iohexol or iopamidol, although their much higher cost limits their indication to those patients that have previously been diagnosed with renal disease.

The preparation of the patient prior to an intravenous urogram is very important. The animal should be kept on an empty stomach for 12-24 hours, a mild laxative should be administered and an enema should be performed 2 hours before starting the procedure. This will avoid the loss of information due to superimposition of food or faeces on the renal shadows. If a urinalysis or urine culture is necessary, the sample should be collected before administering the contrast agent, since this may affect the results and inhibit the growth of some bacteria.

It is very convenient to perform urography with the animal under sedation or anaesthesia. This a procedure requires obtaining numerous radiographs in a short time, and the intervals given in the protocol have to be respected, which will be easier if we do not have to restrain the patient manually.

Before administering the contrast medium, lateral and ventrodorsal radiographs should be taken to evaluate the appropriate preparation of the patient (absence of food in the stomach and of faeces in the colon), adjust the exposure values and rule out any evident alterations that would exclude the need to perform a contrast technique. It should be borne in mind that small renal calculi can be detected on a plain radiograph and, in contrast, can be masked by the contrast media.

If the objective is to assess the entry of the ureters into the bladder with precision, it is highly recommended to perform a pneumocystogram before the intravenous administration of the iodinated contrast medium. In order to do so, the bladder should previously be emptied from urine and, next, gas should be introduced (air, carbon dioxide or nitrous oxide) until it is adequately distended. This way, the gas contained in the bladder will clearly contrast with the distal end of the ureters when these are filled the with positive contrast agent during the urography procedure. Oblique lateral radiographs will help to differentiate a ureter from the other.

Although two methods for intravenous administration of the iodinated contrast agent are usually described, slow infusion and bolus administration, it is more common to use the latter, with a dose of 600 to 800 mg of iodine per kg of live weight (mg I/kg). Box 1.1 summarises the protocol to take radiographs. The phases into which a urography procedure is divided (fig. 1.45) are:

1. **Vascular phase**: the renal arteries become radiopaque 5-7 seconds after the start of contrast medium injection, which is why it will only be observed on a radiograph if this is taken at the same time as the contrast medium bolus is injected.
2. **Nephrogram**: the renal parenchyma becomes opaque 10-20 seconds after the start of contrast medium injection, which is when maximum opacification is reached. Opacity will then progressively decline in healthy animals.
3. **Pyelogram**: the renal pelvis and ureters become radiopaque. Their visualisation starts 1-2 minutes after the start of contrast medium injection. In normal conditions, the pelvis has a curvilinear shape and is less than 2 mm long. In some dogs and in most cats it is possible to observe the normal pelvic diverticula, which are less than 1 mm.

TABLE 1.1 Excretory urography protocol

Before the urography procedure

- 12-24 hours before: fasting and mild laxative.
- 2 hours before: enema to empty the colon.
- Plain L and VD radiographs.
- Injection of air into the bladder (if the ureters are to be assessed).

Administration of the contrast medium

- 600-800 mg I/kg in an intravenous bolus.

Sequence of radiographs

- 10-20 seconds: VD.
- 1-2 minutes: VD.
- 5 minutes: VD and L (+ oblique if the ureters are to be assessed)
- 20 minutes*: VD and L (+ oblique is the ureters are to be assessed).
- 40 minutes: VD and L to assess the bladder.
- Additional radiographs may be necessary if no conclusive results have been obtained.

*The ureters are best seen between 5 and 20 minutes after the administration of the contrast medium and additional radiographs may therefore be taken during this interval to evaluate their image more precisely.

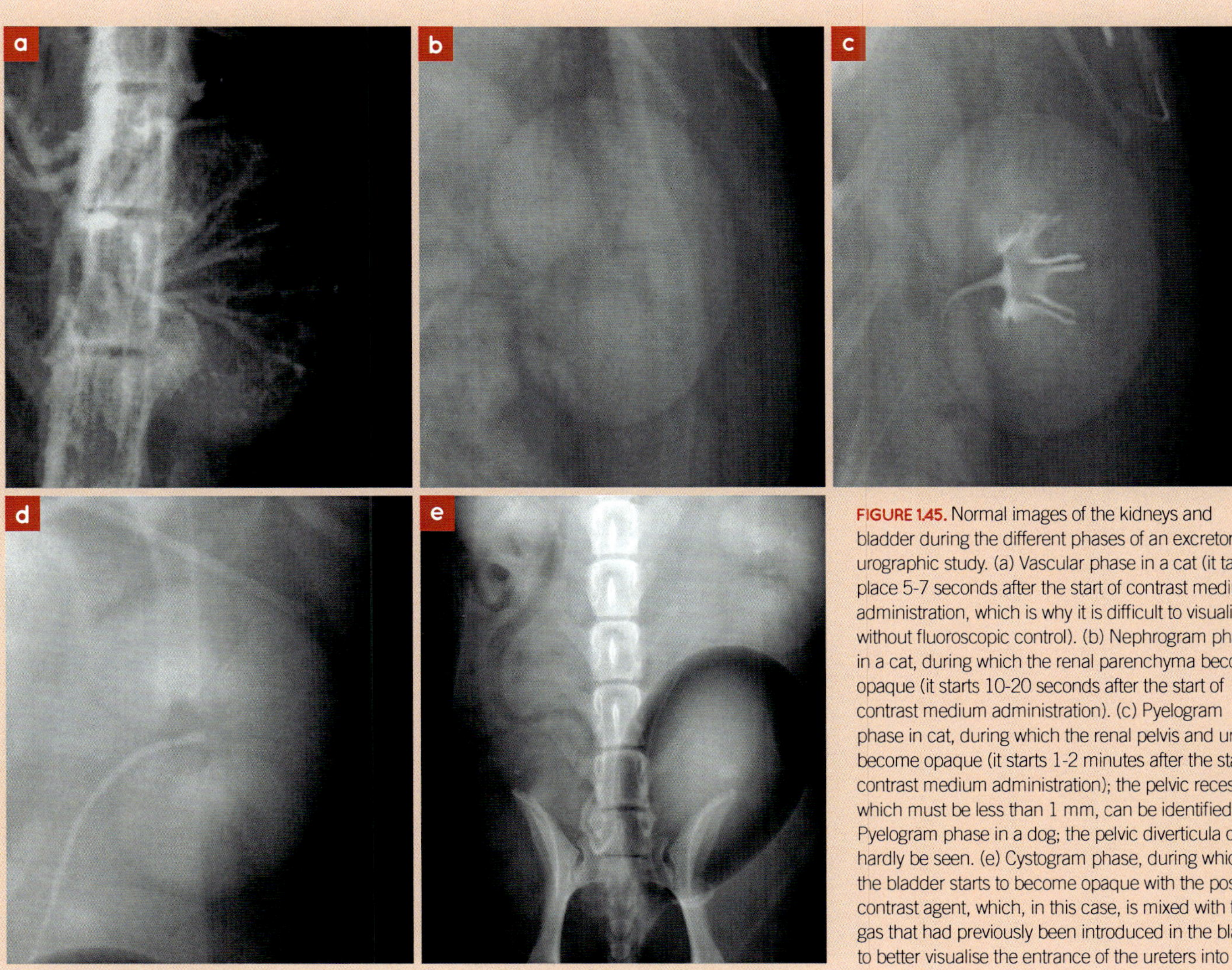

FIGURE 1.45. Normal images of the kidneys and bladder during the different phases of an excretory urographic study. (a) Vascular phase in a cat (it takes place 5-7 seconds after the start of contrast medium administration, which is why it is difficult to visualise without fluoroscopic control). (b) Nephrogram phase in a cat, during which the renal parenchyma becomes opaque (it starts 10-20 seconds after the start of contrast medium administration). (c) Pyelogram phase in cat, during which the renal pelvis and ureters become opaque (it starts 1-2 minutes after the start of contrast medium administration); the pelvic recesses, which must be less than 1 mm, can be identified. (d) Pyelogram phase in a dog; the pelvic diverticula can hardly be seen. (e) Cystogram phase, during which the bladder starts to become opaque with the positive contrast agent, which, in this case, is mixed with the gas that had previously been introduced in the bladder to better visualise the entrance of the ureters into it.

The peristaltic waves that occur in the ureters and contribute to the progress of urine often lead to only one part of the ureter being opaque on each radiograph.

4. **Cystogram**: opacification of the bladder. If air has previously been injected in the bladder to improve the visualisation of the openings of the ureters, the iodinated contrast material will progressively mix with the negative contrast material. If this does not allow an appropriate evaluation of the ureters, it will be useful to empty the bladder and introduce additional negative contrast medium during the course of the study.

The excretion of the contrast medium depends on the degree of glomerular filtration. A delay in the excretion of the contrast medium may be indicative of renal failure, but it is not a precise method for its evaluation. The nephrogram should progressively disappear throughout the procedure, although up to 25 % of normal dogs may still have a detectable nephrogram up to 2 hours after the contrast medium injection.

Some of the abnormal patterns (fig. 1.46) that may be observed on excretory urograms are:

- Lack of renal opacification: insufficient dose of contrast medium, severe renal disease, renal aplasia or atrophy, avulsion or obstruction of the renal artery, extreme hydronephrosis, severe neoplasia.
- Heterogeneous renal opacification: cysts, abscesses, haematomas, neoplasia, infactus, nephritis, pyelonephritis.
- Normal initial opacification, which then persists or increases: severe renal disease, acute renal obstruction, systemic hypotension or acute renal injury caused by the contrast.
- Dilatation of the pelvis and/or ureters.
- Abnormal location of the end of the ureters.
- Filling defects: calculi or blood clots.

Computed tomography optimises the information that can be obtained from excretory urography, since it prevents the loss of information due to superimposition of structures. The dose of contrast medium may be reduced to 400 mg I/kg (important for patients with kidney disease) and allows a more precise calculation of the degree of glomerular filtration.

Percutaneous pyelography

Percutaneous pyelography may be used as an alternative to excretory urography. This technique involves the direct administration of a contrast medium in the

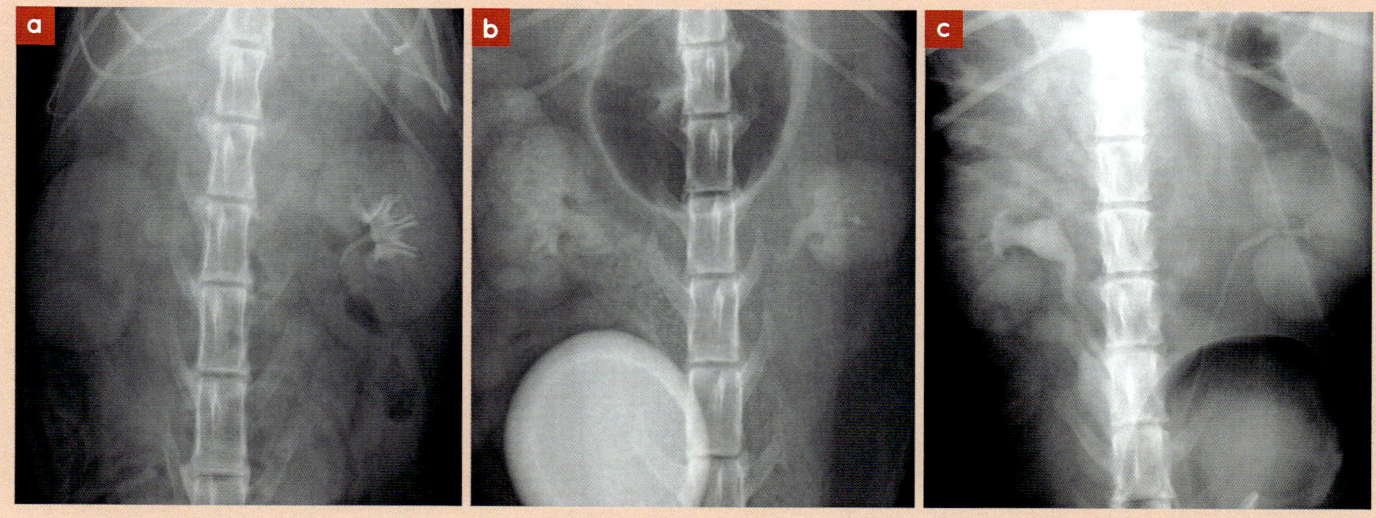

FIGURE 1.46. Abnormal patterns on excretory urograms. (a) Absence of pyelogram in the right kidney 10 minutes after the contrast medium injection, indicative of a marked delay in glomerular filtration. (b) The contrast agent improves the visualisation of the alteration in the outline of both kidneys, the decrease in size of the left kidney and the mild proximal dilatation of the left ureter and moderate dilatation of the right one. (c) Mild dilatation of the renal pelvis and moderate dilatation of the proximal part of the right ureter, which could be due to pyelonephritis or to an obstructive condition of the ureter.

renal pelvis by means of an ultrasound-guided puncture, thus avoiding the adverse effects of intravenous administration. The contrast medium is not diluted and its excretion does not depend on renal function. The main indication of this procedure is the assessment of a ureteral obstruction. The most important potential risk of this test is the possibility of causing haemorrhage in the kidney. It may also cause extravasation of the contrast medium to the peritoneal space, which has no clinical significance, but makes the interpretation of the images difficult. Once the ultrasound-guided puncture has been performed, 1-2 ml of urine first have to be aspirated so as to slowly introduce the same volume of contrast medium, under ultrasound or fluoroscopic control.

Ureters

Normal ureters are not usually identified on a plain radiograph. However, the excellent contrast resolution offered by digital radiography allows, in some cases, the partial visualisation of one or the two ureters in animals with a large amount of retroperitoneal fat (fig. 1.47).

Ultrasonography is of limited use for the examination of the ureters, as it is very complicated to identify their whole course owing to their small diameter and the presence of gas. Visualising the ureteral jet that causes the entry of urine into the bladder, which can be identified with B-mode or Doppler ultrasonography, helps to assess ureteral permeability and locate the vesicoureteral junction.

Conventional excretory urography is the technique of choice to evaluate these structures, due to its low cost and high availability. However, a urographic contrast study using computed tomography is excellent to diagnose any ureteral alteration, since it avoids the loss of information due to the superimposition of structures (it does not require the previous emptying of the colon by means of laxatives and an enema) and images with great spatial resolution of small regions can be obtained. The disadvantages of computed tomography are the low availability of equipment and the high cost of the study.

Excretory urography allows the evaluation of the location, diameter, permeability and integrity of the ureters. With this technique, it is possible to observe tubular structures with a diameter of 2-3 mm, which extend from the renal sinus to the vesical trigone. It is usual not to be able to visualise the whole course of the ureter in one single image due to peristalsis (fig. 1.48). The area of opening of the ureters is better observed if gas is injected into the bladder immediately before the urogram, since the gas that is introduced in the bladder contrasts better with the ureters when

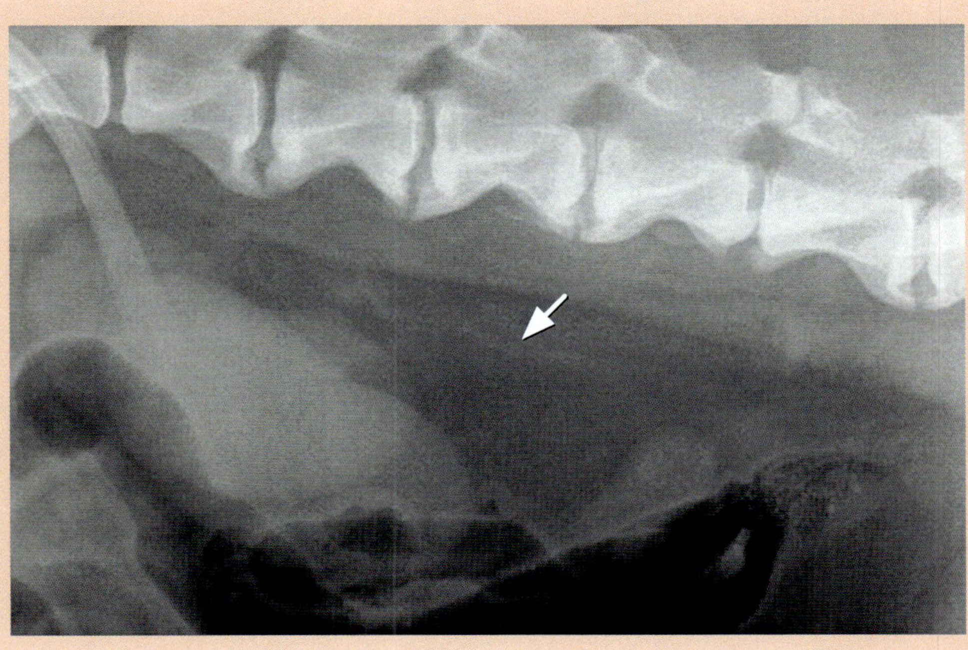

FIGURE 1.47. Enlarged image of a lateral radiograph showing the retroperitoneal region of the abdomen of a healthy dog. The large amount of retroperitoneal fat allows the visualisation in this case of one of the ureters (arrow). This finding is more frequent on digital radiographs, thanks to the greater contrast resolution they have when compared with conventional radiographs.

they are subsequently filled with a positive contrast agent. Oblique lateral views are very useful to differentiate one ureter from the other with certainty in the image (fig. 1.49).

On a plain radiograph it is possible to detect mineral density structures compatible with radiopaque calculi in the area of the ureters (fig. 1.50). However, excretory urography will be necessary to confirm the diagnosis, as we may confuse these structures with calcifications of other tissues or with foreign bodies with mineral density on a plain radiograph.

Exceptionally, it may be possible to identify a ureteral dilatation on plain radiographs, in animals with a large amount of retroperitoneal fat (fig. 1.51), although excretory urography is usually required to establish this diagnosis. The dilatation of the ureters makes their ultrasound examination easier, although it may be complicated to follow their whole course. Ureteral dilatations may have a congenital (megaureter) or acquired (hydroureter) origin. Ureteral obstructions, which may be caused by calculi, clots, stenosis or masses, cause dilatation anterior to the site of obstruction (fig. 1.52). When a ureter is accidentally ligated during an ovariohysterectomy, it rapidly dilates and permanent distension, urinary stasis and a tendency to suffer from recurrent infections may occur. Pyelonephritis may also cause dilatation of the proximal part of the ureter, although it is usually mild in comparison with the dilatation caused by obstructions.

An ectopic ureter is a congenital anomaly, which affects dogs more frequently than cats, especially females. The clinical sign shown by affected animals is urinary incontinence, although it does not always occur in males. The caudal end of one or the two ureters does not open into the normal anatomical location, the vesicular trigone (caudodorsal area of the bladder), but into a different location, which is usually the neck of the bladder or urethra (fig. 1.53), and less frequently, the vagina, uterus or rectum. Ectopic ureters may have a normal diameter or be dilated and have a relatively tortuous course (fig. 1.54). In some cases, an ectopic ureter enters the area of the vesicular trigone but then has an intraparietal course

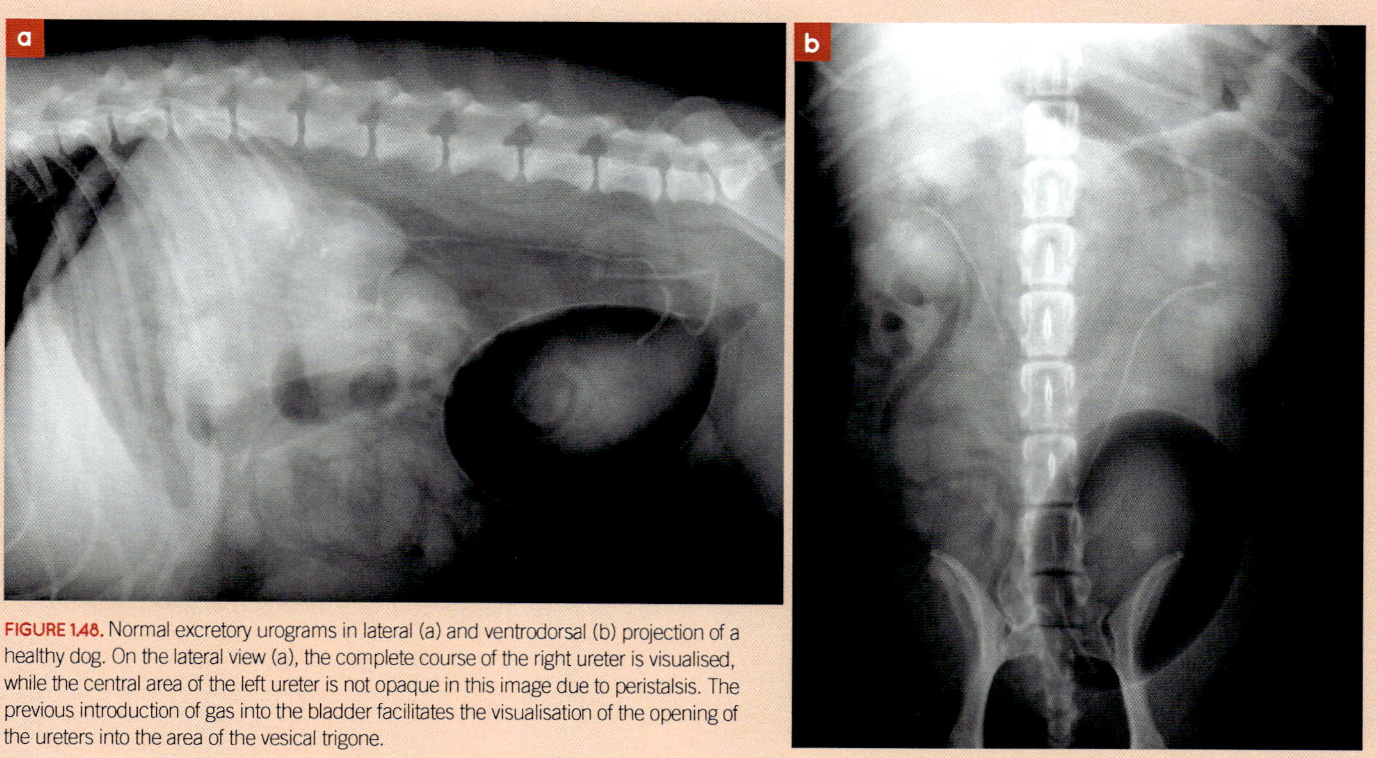

FIGURE 1.48. Normal excretory urograms in lateral (a) and ventrodorsal (b) projection of a healthy dog. On the lateral view (a), the complete course of the right ureter is visualised, while the central area of the left ureter is not opaque in this image due to peristalsis. The previous introduction of gas into the bladder facilitates the visualisation of the opening of the ureters into the area of the vesical trigone.

and opens into an abnormal location, generally the urethra, which can cause confusing images on an excretory urogram, especially if the ureter is not dilated. This intraparietal course, in which the ectopic ureters usually "leave the bladder out", is more frequent in dogs than in cats. Fluoroscopy and ultrasonography may sometimes help to establish a diagnosis. When the excretory urogram is not conclusive, it should be complemented with a retrograde urethrogram in males and retrograde vaginourethrogram in females.

Ureteroceles are focal cystic dilatations of the submucosa of the ureters and usually form at their distal

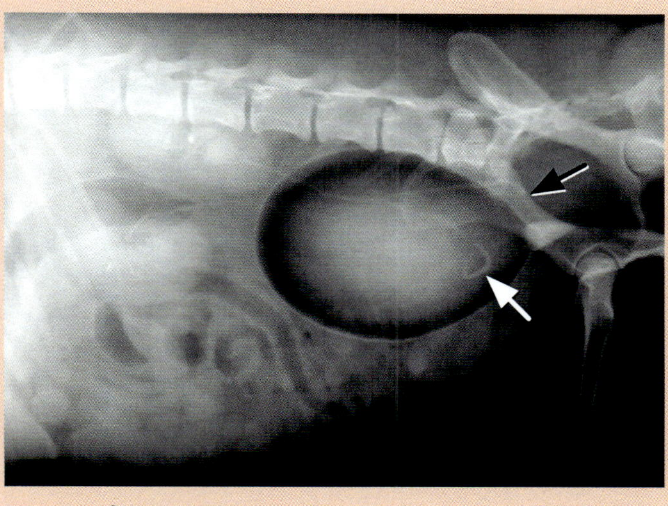

FIGURE 1.49. Oblique lateral excretory urogram of a healthy dog. This projection facilitates the differentiation of the two ureters in the image, in which the ureter located closest to the cassette will have a more ventral position. This image was obtained in right lateral projection, so that the ureter with a more ventral location is the right one (white arrow) and the ureter in a more dorsal position is the left one (black arrow).

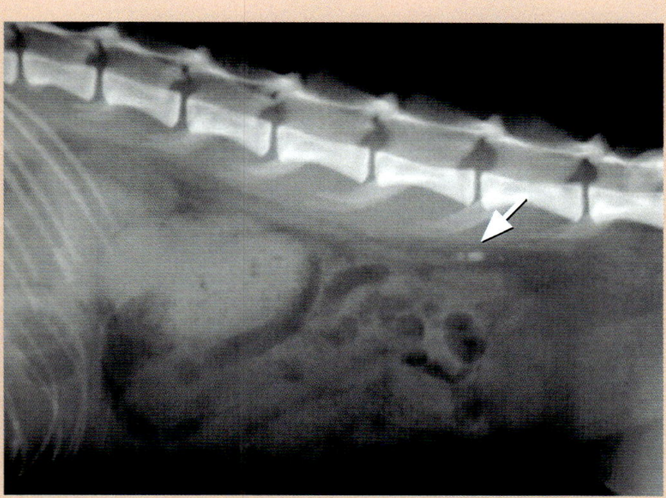

FIGURE 1.50. Lateral abdominal radiograph of a cat with radiopaque calculi in a ureter (arrow). This image may be confused with calcification of other soft tissues or foreign bodies in the intestine and should be confirmed by means excretory urography, where the calculi will create filling defects on the pyelogram.

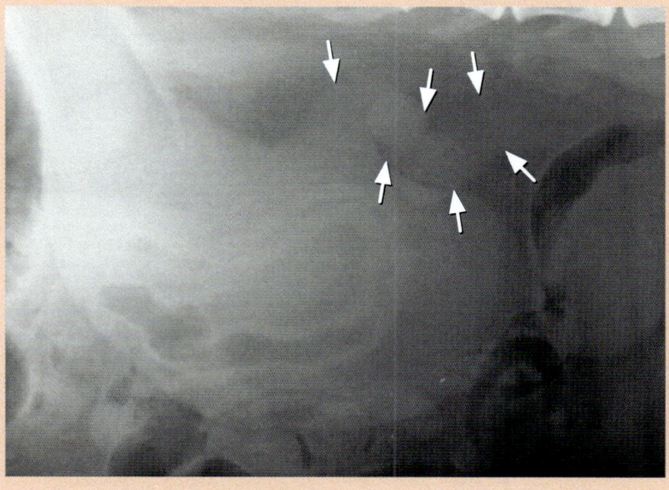

FIGURE 1.51. Enlarged image of the cranial retroperitoneal region on a lateral radiograph of a dog with severe dilatation of the left ureter. Dilated ureters are not usually differentiated on plain radiographs, but in this case the large amount of retroperitoneal fat made their identification easier.

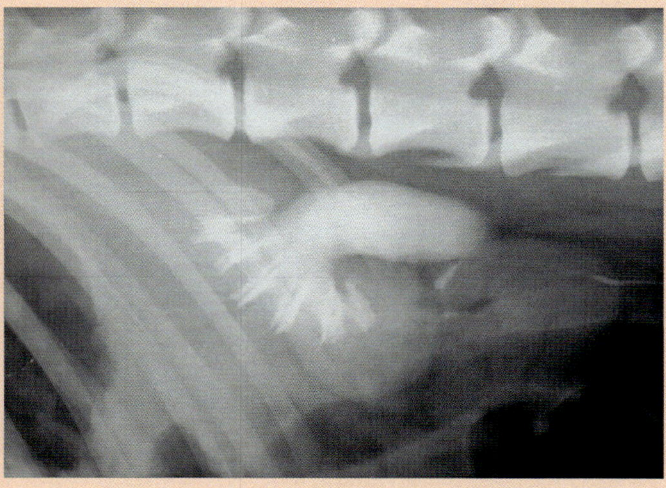

FIGURE 1.52. Enlarged image of a lateral urogram showing the cranial retroperitoneal region of a dog. Severe focal dilatation of the right ureter can be observed. Focal dilatation of the ureters usually occurs as a result of an obstruction caused by calculi, clots, stenosis or masses. Dilatation in these cases is anterior (proximal) to the site of obstruction.

Normal radiographic anatomy of the abdomen **ventrodorsal view**

http://goo.gl/6p7452

end, at the vesicoureteral junction or close to it. They may sometimes project towards the lumen of the bladder or urethra.

They appear more frequently in ectopic ureters. The excretory urogram shows a focal dilatation with accumulation of contrast where they are located.

Ureteral tumours (fig. 1.55) are uncommon and appear as areas of filling defect on the urogram, accompanied by dilatation anterior to the obstructed site when they cause obstruction. Some bladder tumours may extend to the ureter.

When rupture of a ureter occurs, generally due to trauma, signs of the presence of free fluid may be observed in the retroperitoneal space on plain radiographs and extravasation of the contrast to the peritoneum on the excretory urogram, although the exact site of rupture may be difficult to find. A perirenal or paraureteral urinoma, which consists in a retroperitoneal fibrous sac where extravasated urine accumulates (fig. 1.56), may occasionally form as a consequence of the rupture.

Bladder

Plain radiography allows the observation of the size, shape, location and radiographic density of the bladder, but does not provide any information about its internal structure. The bladder wall and urine have the same radiopacity on radiographs and therefore cannot be differentiated in normal conditions. That is why, as for the assessment of the kidneys, the technique of choice for the study of the bladder is ultrasonography, since it offers detailed information of the bladder wall and content.

Cystography is the contrast technique used to complement the diagnostic information provided by plain radiography. The diagnostic superiority of ultrasonography over cystography is indisputable, but not all veterinary clinics have an ultrasound scanner or enough experience to make a correct ultrasound diagnosis. That is why cystography is still used in those cases for the diagnosis of calculi, inflammations, masses and trauma. It the bladder is ruptured, cystography

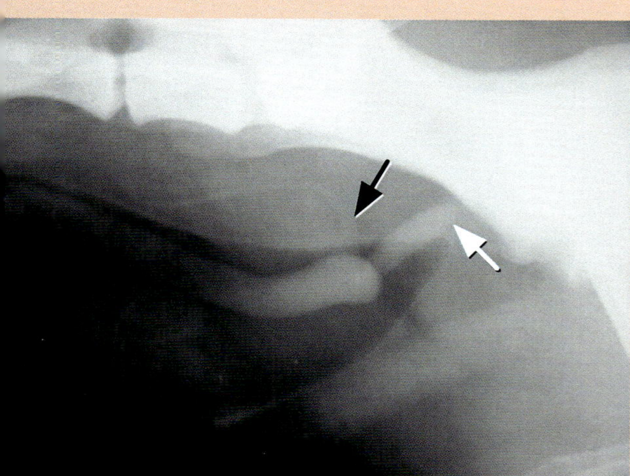

FIGURE 1.53. Enlarged image of a lateral urogram showing the caudal abdomen of a dog, in which a unilateral ectopic ureter may be observed. The ectopic ureter (white arrow) appears dilated and runs beyond the vesical trigone to open into the urethra. The normal ureter (black arrow) has a normal diameter and opens into the vesicular trigone.

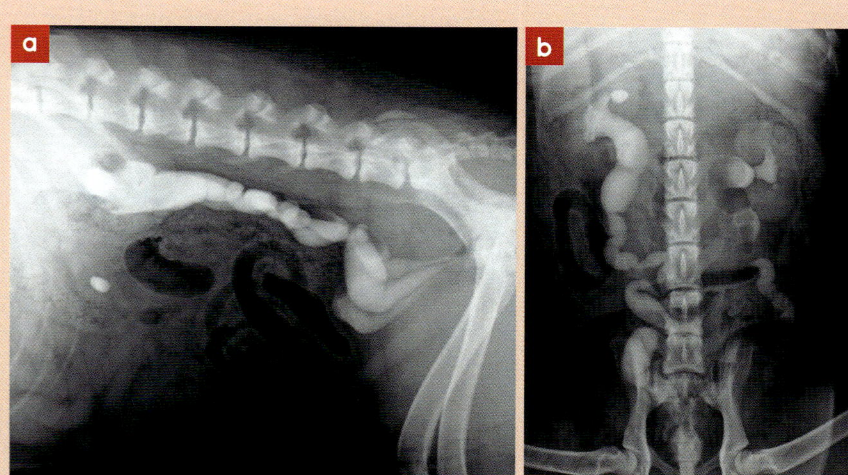

FIGURE 1.54. Lateral (a) and ventrodorsal (b) urograms of a dog, on which a bilateral ectopic ureter is observed. Both ureters appear very dilated, have a tortuous course and open into the area of junction of the neck of the bladder with the urethra, caudal to the vesicular trigone. Both renal pelvises also appear moderately dilated. On the ventrodorsal view (b), it is possible to observe the positive contrast material mixed with gas, as a result of vesicoureteral reflux of the gas introduced into the bladder immediately before the urogram. A small foreign body with mineral density (stone) can be observed in the intestine as an incidental finding.

can provide more precise information than ultrasonography, since ultrasound findings may be uncertain, while the extravasation of the contrast medium to the peritoneal cavity always confirms the diagnosis.

Cystography involves the introduction of a contrast medium (positive, negative or both) in the bladder through a flexible catheter. In order to obtain optimum results, it is important to empty the bladder from urine prior to introducing the contrast material. Sedation or anaesthesia of the patient will facilitate the procedure.

Positive-contrast cystography

Iodinated contrast media, generally diluted at 10 %, are used in doses of 6-12 ml/kg. It is the technique of choice to evaluate anomalous positions of the bladder or a possible rupture of the wall. On the other hand, it may mask small irregularities of the bladder mucosa as well as some abnormal intraluminal contents.

Negative-contrast cystography (pneumocystography)

A negative contrast medium, generally air, is used. When performing this technique, there is a minimal risk of causing gas embolism, which may even lead to the death of the animal. This risk is higher in cats than in dogs and may be reduced by using carbon dioxide or nitrous oxide instead of air, due to the greater solubility of these two substances. Doses of 6-12 ml/kg may be used, or gas may simply be introduced, checking the degree of distension of the bladder by palpation. This is the cheapest and most simple method, but it is the least sensible of the three techniques to detect alterations of the mucosa and small defects in the bladder wall.

Double-contrast cystography

First, a small amount of positive contrast medium is introduced (1-5 ml in dogs and 0.5-1 ml in cats) and then, the bladder is distended with a negative contrast medium. This way, a thin layer of positive contrast material will clearly define the internal margin of the wall. This technique is ideal to examine alterations of the mucosa and the presence of radiolucent calculi in the bladder.

Pathological alterations

On a plain radiograph, the size and the position of the shadow of the bladder vary in function of the amount

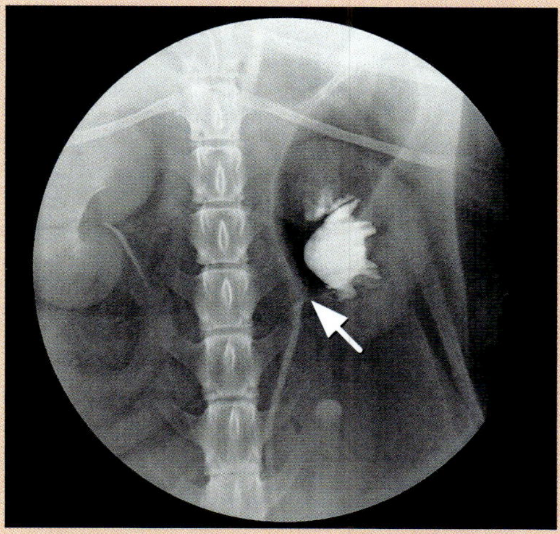

FIGURE 1.55. Enlarged image of a ventrodorsal urogram showing the cranial abdomen of a dog. It is possible to observe a moderate dilatation of the left renal pelvis and a permanent filling defect of the proximal end of the left ureter due to the presence of a ureteral neoplasm in this location.

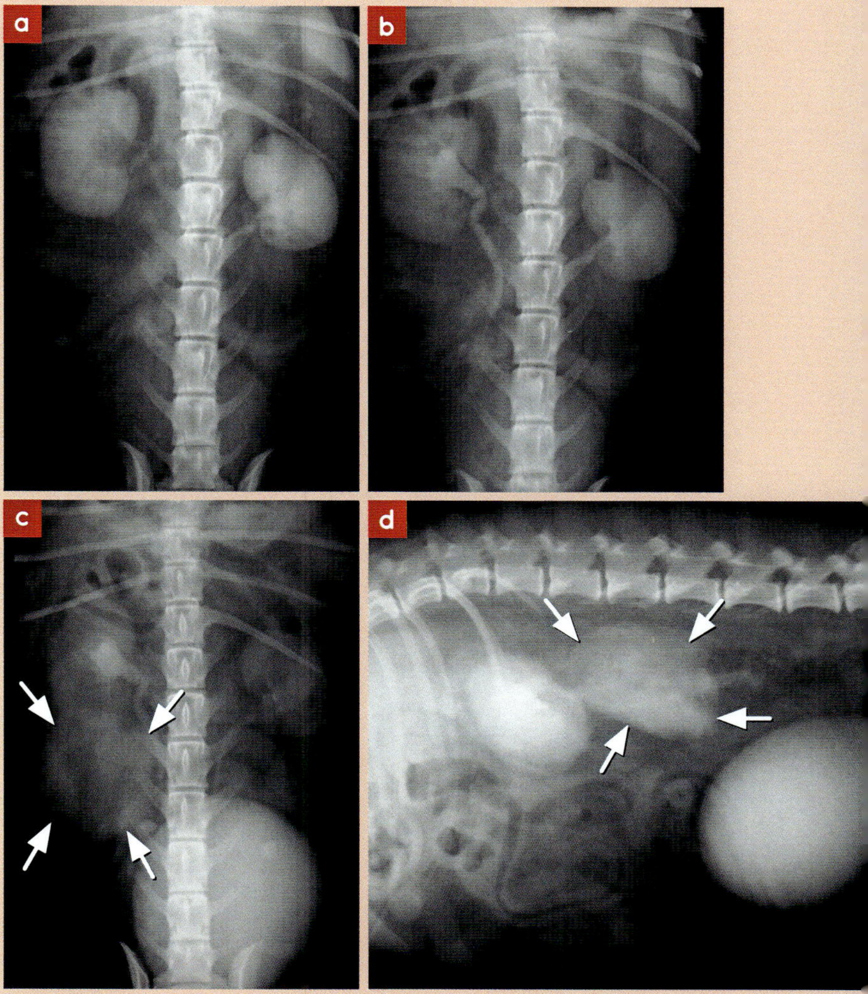

FIGURE 1.56. Ventrodorsal (a, b and c) and lateral (d) urograms showing the cranial abdomen of a dog. A focal accumulation of the contrast medium may be observed in the retroperitoneal space caudal to the right kidney, which also appears enlarged in comparison with the left one, with mild to moderate dilatation of the right renal pelvis and mild to moderate dilatation of the right ureter. The focal accumulation of contrast is due to a paraureteral urinoma (arrows).

of urine it contains. The animals that have not urinated for many hours, whether due to pathological causes or not, may have a very distended bladder, which should not be mistaken for an abdominal mass (fig. 1.57). A scarcely distended bladder will be more difficult to identify, especially when it is superimposed with the intestine or when the animal has very little retroperitoneal fat.

The neck of the bladder may appear located cranial to the pubis or in an intrapelvic position in healthy dogs, especially when the bladder is not very distended. However, the position of the bladder is always intra-abdominal in cats.

The alteration of the bladder that is most often diagnosed by means of radiography is lithiasis. Radiopaque calculi (fig. 1.58) are identified on plain radiographs, although they may be masked by other superimposed structures if they are small (fig. 1.59). Radiolucent calculi (ammonium acid urate and cystine) should be diagnosed by means of ultrasonography or, alternatively, double-contrast cystography (fig. 1.60), as they may be masked with the contrast if medium positive-contrast cystography is used, particularly if they are small in size and number. Radiolucent calculi may have a very similar image to that produced by clots or gas bubbles on a double-contrast cystogram. On the other hand, they are easily identified by means of ultrasonography.

Alterations of the radiographic density of the bladder wall may also be detected on plain radiographs. The appearance of calcified areas in the wall is usually due to its dystrophic calcification (fig. 1.61), which is generally associated with chronic inflammatory processes or neoplasms.

The presence of gas in the bladder lumen is usually iatrogenic, when gas is introduced voluntarily or involuntarily when catheterising the patient (fig. 1.62). In case of emphysematous cystitis, the gas may have an intraparietal (fig. 1.63) or intraluminal location. This type of cystitis is more frequent in diabetic patients, in which the formation of gas is due to microorganisms causing the fermentation of glucose.

The information provided by cystography as regards the thickness of the bladder wall is more limited than that offered by ultrasonography. Double-contrast

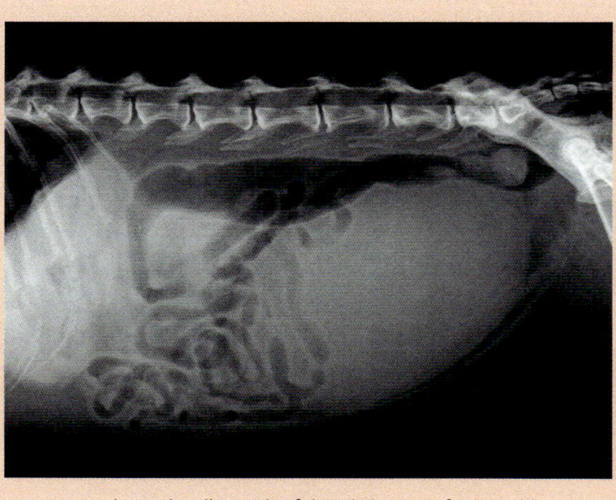

FIGURE 1.57. Lateral radiograph of the abdomen of a cat with severe bladder distension, which causes a dorsal displacement of the colon and a cranial and dorsal displacement of the small intestine.

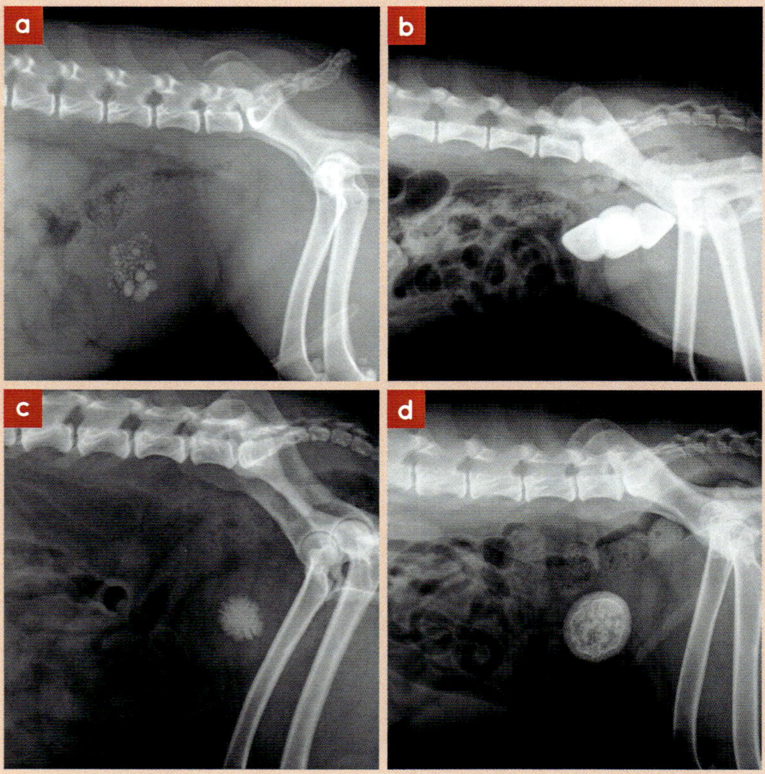

FIGURE 1.58. Enlarged images of the caudal abdomen on lateral radiographs of four dogs with radiopaque calculi in the bladder.

cystography allows the differentiation of small irregularities of the wall that would otherwise go unnoticed if a positive contrast medium or gas alone were used (fig. 1.64). If the irregularities of the wall are more marked, for example in the case of tumours or polypoid cystitis, or if the thickness of the wall is significantly increased, even homogeneously, the three techniques provide useful information. However, double-contrast cystography is always the most recommended method for this type of evaluation.

Generalised cystitis is usually caused by a relatively homogeneous increase in the thickness of the bladder wall (fig. 1.65), although the thickening is sometimes more marked in the cranioventral area of the bladder. Tumours, on the other hand, usually cause a more focal and irregular increase in thickness (fig. 1.66), although it may be similar to that caused by localised or polypoid cystitis, or to the image produced by the presence of clots adhered to the bladder wall. Most bladder tumours form in the bladder trigone and usually

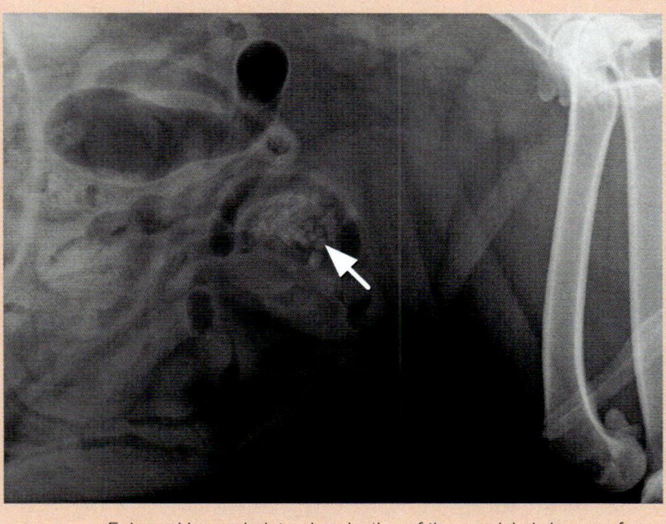

FIGURE 1.59. Enlarged image in lateral projection of the caudal abdomen of a dog with bladder lithiasis. Numerous small-sized calculi are present (arrow), which may go unnoticed due to the superimposition of small intestinal loops.

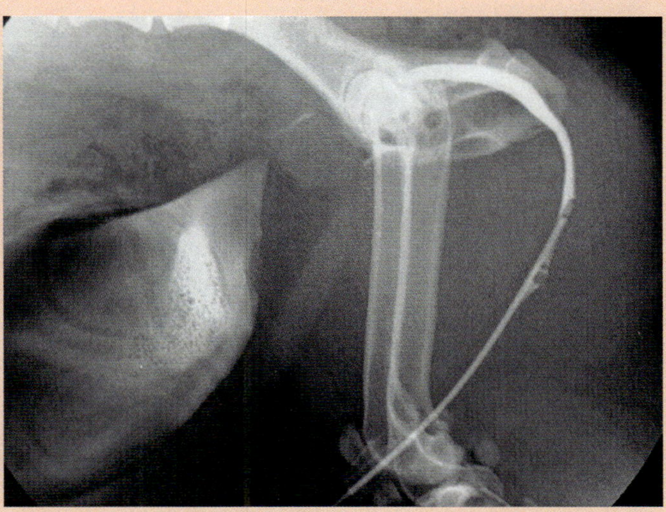

FIGURE 1.60. Enlarged image of a double-contrast cystogram showing the caudal abdomen of a dog. Numerous areas of filling defect compatible with calculi can be observed in the bladder.

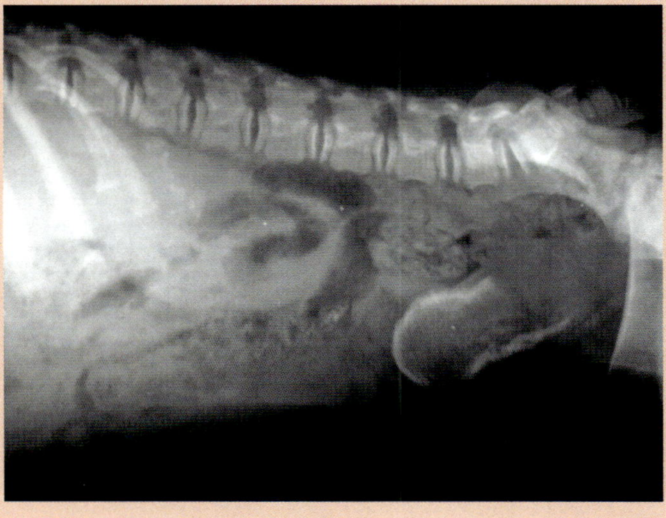

FIGURE 1.61. Lateral radiograph of the abdomen of a young dog with dystrophic calcification of the bladder wall.

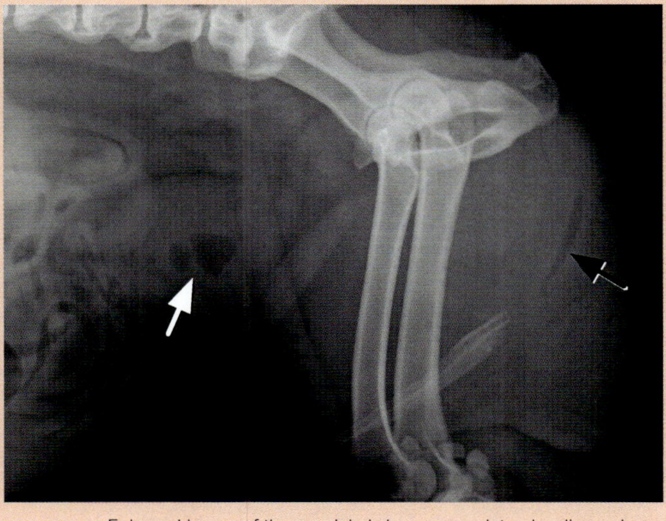

FIGURE 1.62. Enlarged image of the caudal abdomen on a lateral radiograph of a dog with gas in its bladder (white arrow) and urethra (black arrow) due to iatrogenic causes, as a result of a previous catheterisation.

Normal radiographic
anatomy of the abdomen
lateral view

http://goo.gl/hnl420

cause some degree of ureteral or urethral obstruction as they grow.

Ultrasonography allows a better definition of the extension of this type of lesions as well as the collection of samples for cytology or biopsies.

If bladder rupture is suspected, either as a consequence of trauma or due to iatrogenic causes, positive-contrast cystography should be chosen (fig. 1.67), even ahead of ultrasonography. The contrast medium used should be very diluted, as it is irritating for the peritoneum. Although ionic iodinated contrast media may be used for other types of assessments, if a rupture is suspected it is better to choose nonionic iodinated contrast media. Indeed, although all the iodinated contrast agents are absorbed in the peritoneum, ionic contrast agents may worsen a possible bleeding if the lesion is recent. The extravasation of the contrast medium may sometimes not be observed immediately and may appear after 5-10 minutes. The test should therefore not be considered negative until this time has passed. Pneumocystography is not recommended to confirm a bladder rupture, since if this latter is small, the extravasation of the gas to the peritoneum will be slow and may be mistaken for gas contained in the gastrointestinal tract.

Positive-contrast cystography is also more useful than double-contrast cystography to detect anomalous positions of the bladder, for example when it is displaced into a hernial sac or in the case of intrapelvic bladders. In cases of urinary incontinence due to an incompetence of the urethral sphincter mechanism, the animal is able to void its bladder normally, but leaks urine when at rest or during sleep. This anomaly may have a congenital origin in females, which may have a shorter urethra than normal or a bladder with an intrapelvic location (fig. 1.68).

Although they are not very frequent, some anomalies of the urachus may be diagnosed by means of cystography, such as patent urachus (fig. 1.69), patent urachal ligament and urachal diverticula, these latter being more frequent in cats. The animals that suffer from this anomaly of the urachus usually have recurrent bacterial cystitis.

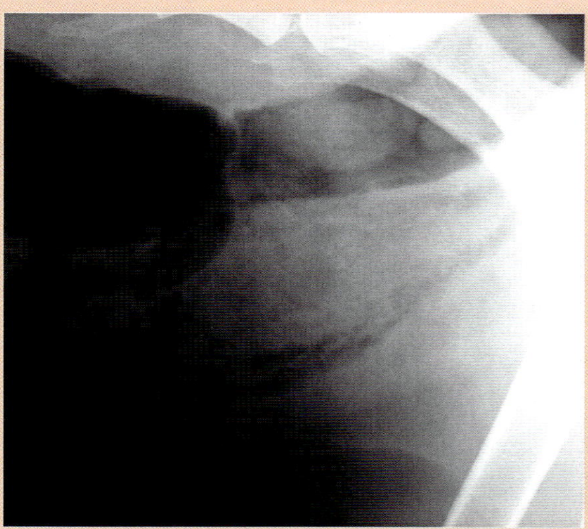

FIGURE 1.63. Enlarged image of the caudal abdomen on a lateral radiograph of a dog with emphysematous cystitis. Areas of gas opacity distributed throughout the bladder wall can be observed. Emphysematous cystitis is more frequent in diabetic patients.

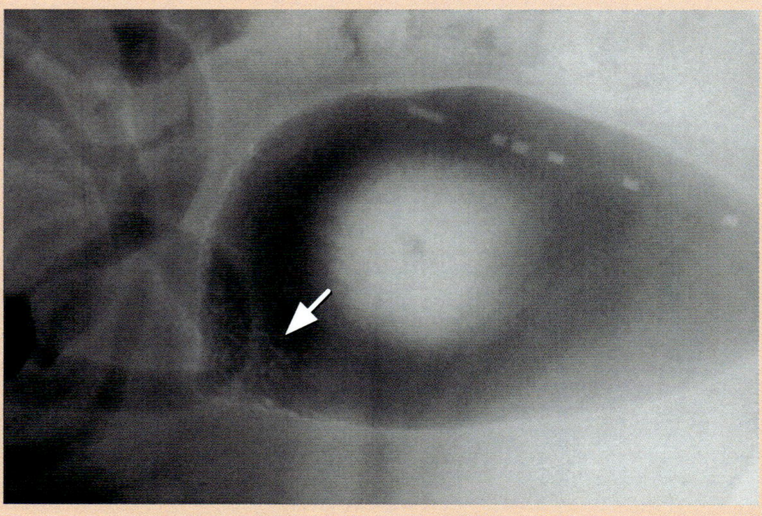

FIGURE 1.64. Enlarged image of a double-contrast cystogram showing the caudal abdomen of a dog. Small areas of accumulation of positive contrast material may be observed in the cranioventral region of the bladder, in addition to a slight deformation of the bladder wall at the same location. These findings are indicative of localised cystitis, although they may also be caused by a tumour (second possible diagnosis).

Urethra

A normal urethra is not identified on plain radiographs and ultrasonography is often not useful either for its evaluation. The technique of choice is therefore **urethrography**. Iodinated contrast media are used and the patient must previously be sedated or anaesthetised.

In order to perform a retrograde urethrogram in a male, a flexible catheter is filled with contrast material (to avoid the introduction of air bubbles) and its end is placed into the penile urethra (fig. 1.70). Tongue forceps can be used to hold the catheter in position and prevent leakage. Next, a small volume of contrast medium (1 ml/kg in dogs and 2-4 ml in total in cats) is

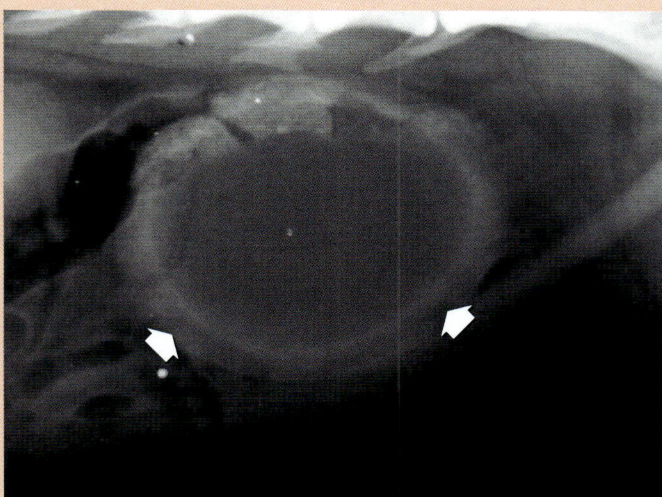

FIGURE 1.65. Enlarged image of a pneumocystogram showing the caudal abdomen of a cat, in which a marked, generalised and regular thickening of the bladder wall can be observed. This image is compatible with generalised cystitis, although it may also be caused by a tumour (second possible diagnosis, although it is unlikely since the tumours that affect the entire bladder wall usually have irregular margins).

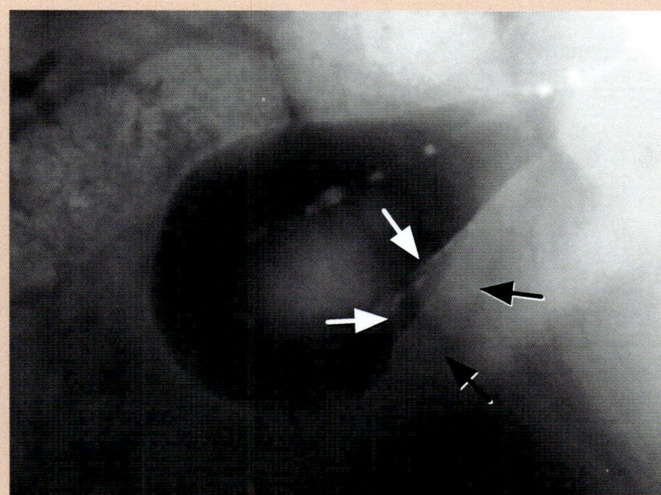

FIGURE 1.66. Enlarged image of a double-contrast cystogram showing the caudal abdomen of a dog, in which a focal thickening of the ventral wall of the bladder can be observed. A thin layer of positive contrast medium clearly delimits the internal margin of the lesion (white arrows). This image is compatible with a bladder neoplasm (other possible diagnoses include localised cystitis and, with much less probability, adhered blood clot).

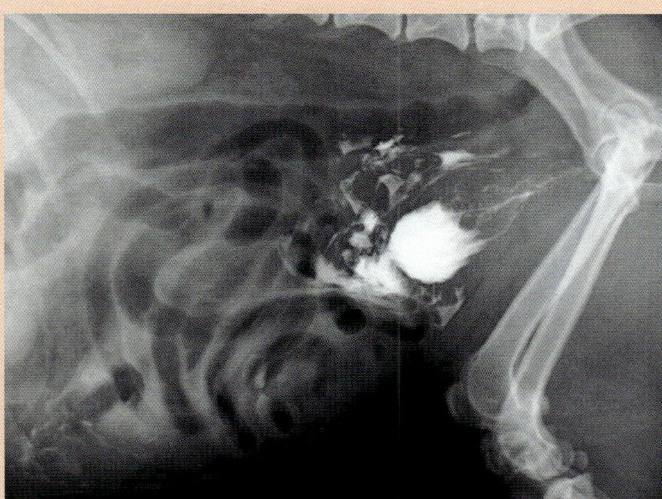

FIGURE 1.67. Lateral positive-contrast urogram showing the abdomen of a dog. Extravasation of the contrast medium to the peritoneal cavity can be observed, which confirms a bladder rupture.

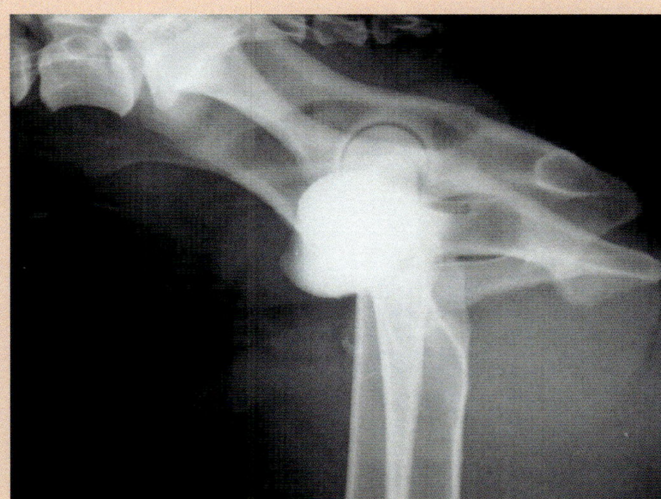

FIGURE 1.68. Enlarged image of the caudal abdomen of a dog after an excretory urogram and positive-contrast cystogram, in which it can be seen that the bladder has an intrapelvic location. This anomaly is a frequent cause of urinary incontinence in young females.

Normal radiographic anatomy of the abdomen **lateral view (cranial extension of hind limbs)**

http://goo.gl/hnl420

introduced without exerting too much pressure, since there is a risk of rupturing the urethra. If fluoroscopy is used, the end of the catheter can be placed in the neck of the bladder to be withdrawn later, at the same time as the contrast medium is injected; this way, the whole course of the urethra is filled and can be visualised in real time on the monitor.

The normal urethra has a larger diameter in the pelvis than in the perineal and penile areas. It is normal to observe an area of narrowing at the level of the ichial arch, which should not be mistaken for pathological stenosis.

In females, the urethra is not usually directly catheterised, since the presence of the catheter in the lumen may mask lesions. A retrograde vaginourethrogram under anaesthesia is therefore performed in these patients. A Foley catheter is placed, with its end cut and filled with contrast material, in the vaginal vestibule. The balloon is inflated and the lips of the vulva are closed with forceps, to avoid leakage of the contrast medium at the moment of its injection. As in males, a dose of 1 ml/kg is used. The contrast medium fills the bladder and the urethra at the same time. This procedure is usually performed as a complementary technique to urography when an ectopic ureter is suspected.

Anterograde urethrography is also used for those cases in which the urethra cannot be catheterised. The animal is previously anaesthetised and an iodinated contrast agent is introduced in the bladder by means of bladder puncture or intravenous urography. Next, the bladder is manually compressed to allow the passage of the contrast medium to the urethra at the same time as the radiograph is taken.

Plain radiography allows the detection of radiopaque calculi in the course of the urethra (fig. 1.71). In male dogs, they are usually located in the perineal and penile urethra. In male cats, calculi or blockages are usually located in the penile urethra, although their radiopacity is often insufficient for them to be detected on a radiograph. Urethral lithiasis is much less frequent in female dogs and cats. In urethrography, calculi will produce images of filling defect in the contrast column, which are easy to mistake for gas bubbles introduced as a result of catheterisation. The os penis sometimes has a separate centre of ossification

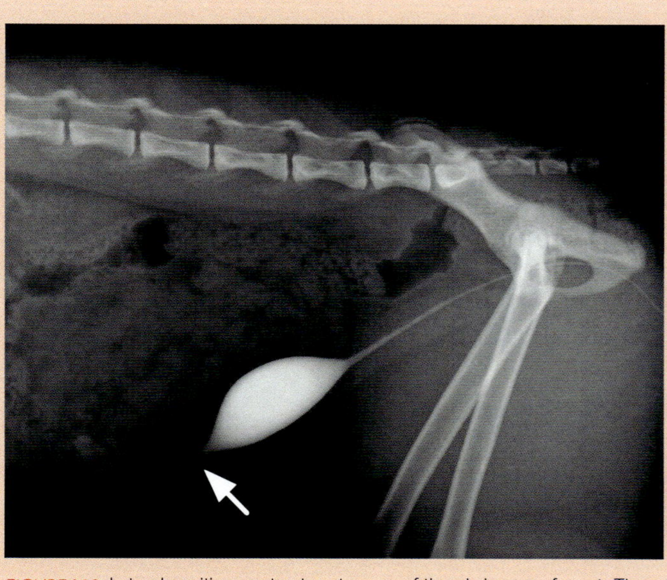

FIGURE 1.69. Lateral positive-contrast cystogram of the abdomen of a cat. The bladder has an ellipsoidal morphology and still has a tube that connects it with the umbilical area (arrow). This image is compatible with patent urachus.

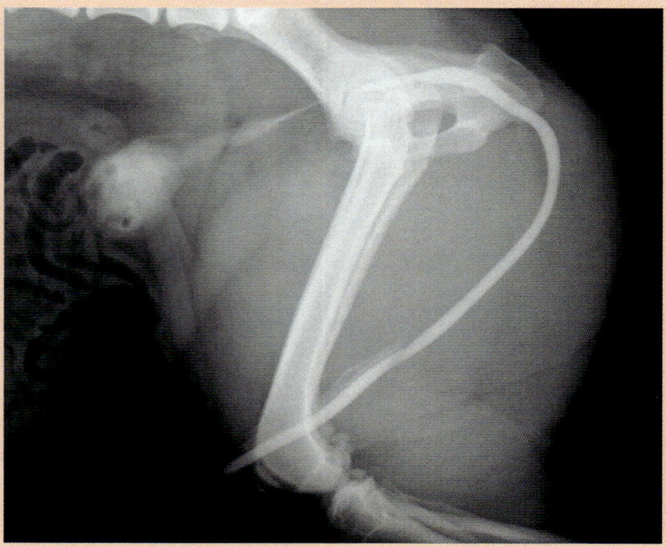

FIGURE 1.70. Enlarged lateral retrograde urethrogram showing the caudal abdomen and perineal region of a healthy dog, with the limbs extended in cranial direction.

at its distal end, which should not be confused with a urethral calculus.

On a urethrogram, the normal urethra has a tubular morphology and smooth margins. Irregular margins suggest neoplasia or severe inflammation of the urethra (fig. 1.72).

Urethral tumours are more frequent in female dogs than in males or cats of both sexes. Computed tomography and magnetic resonance imaging (fig. 1.73) allow a detailed study of the lesion and its possible extension to adjacent tissues or structures.

Stenosis appears as permanent focal narrowings of the urethral diameter. Although they may be associated with tumours or severe inflammation, they are often caused iatrogenically by repeated catheterisation (fig. 1.74).

Urethral ruptures may cause urine leakage into the peritoneal cavity when they affect the proximal part of the urethra, or into the pelvic cavity, perineal area or prepuce when they affect more distal segments. Urethrography allows the identification of extravasation by means of the contrast medium (fig. 1.75). It is a common finding in animals with a hip fracture, dysuria or anuria.

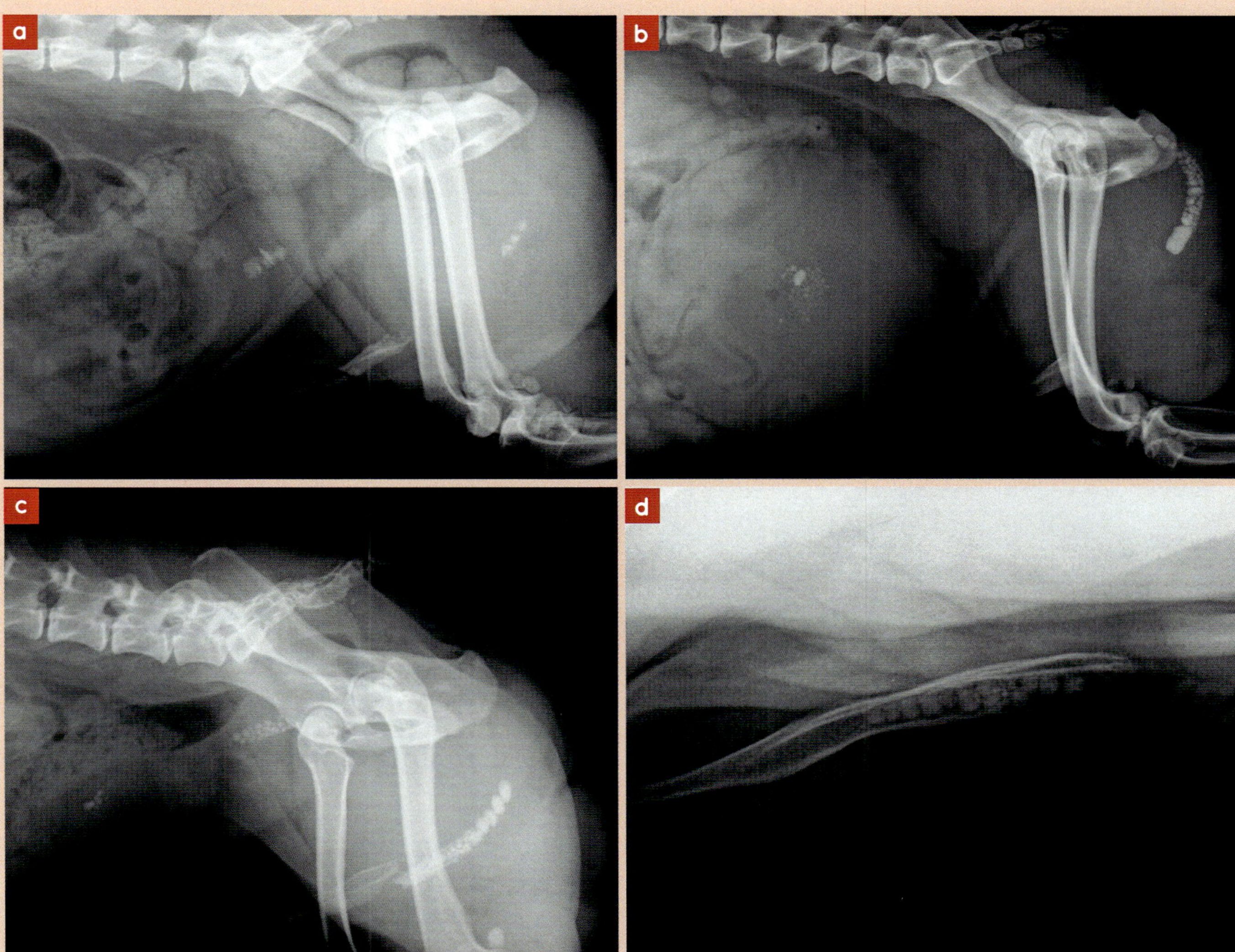

FIGURE 1.71. Enlarged images in lateral projection of the caudal abdomen and perineal region (a, b and c) and penile region (d) of four dogs with radiopaque urethral calculi. (a) Radiopaque calculi with an irregular morphology can be identified in the bladder, perineal segment and penile segment of the urethra. (b) It is possible to observe a marked distension of the bladder, which contains numerous small-sized calculi, as well as numerous calculi in the perineal segment of the urethra, some of which are large. (c) A reduced number of small calculi are present in the bladder and numerous calculi, some of which are large, can be seen in the prostatic and perineal segments of the urethra. (d) Numerous urethral calculi can be identified in the penile segment of the urethra.

Genital system

Genital system of the female

The normal genital system of a female is not identified on a plain radiograph, with the exception of the uterus during the second half of gestation. Ultrasonography is the technique of choice to assess a normal uterus and ovaries, as well as to identify any pathological changes in these structures. However, the number of foetuses and the relationship between the diameter of the foetal head and that of the pelvic canal in term pregnancies are assessed by means of plain radiography, since ultrasonography does not provide precise information in those cases. Retrograde vaginourethrography, which has previously been described (see Urethra section), allows the radiological examination of the morphology of the vagina and vaginal vestibule.

The normal pregnant uterus can be identified on a plain radiograph from day 30 of pregnancy in the dog and between days 25 and 35 in the cat (fig. 1.76), but it will not be possible to differentiate this image from that produced by a pathological distension of the uterus until bone mineralisation can be detected, that is to say at day 45 of pregnancy in the dog and between days 36 and 45 in the cat. It is necessary to bear in mind that these data refer to the days of pregnancy, which do not necessarily coincide with the days that have passed since the time of breeding in the dog, since sperm may remain viable in the uterus up to 7 days before fertilisation. This means

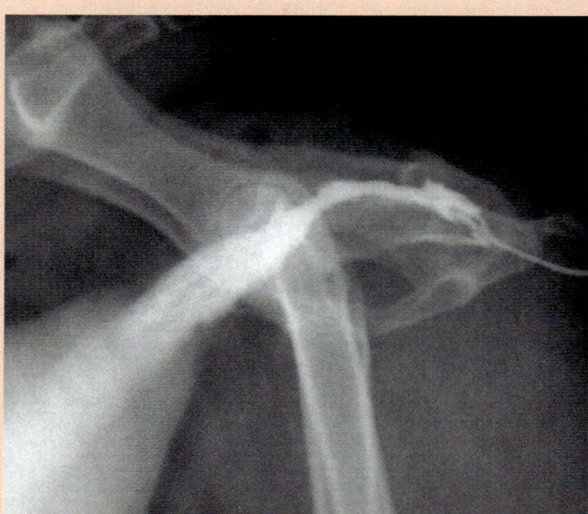

FIGURE 1.72. Enlarged image of a lateral retrograde urethrogram showing the pelvic region of a dog, on which a marked irregularity of the outline of the urethrogram can be observed. This image is compatible with urethral tumour or severe urethritis.

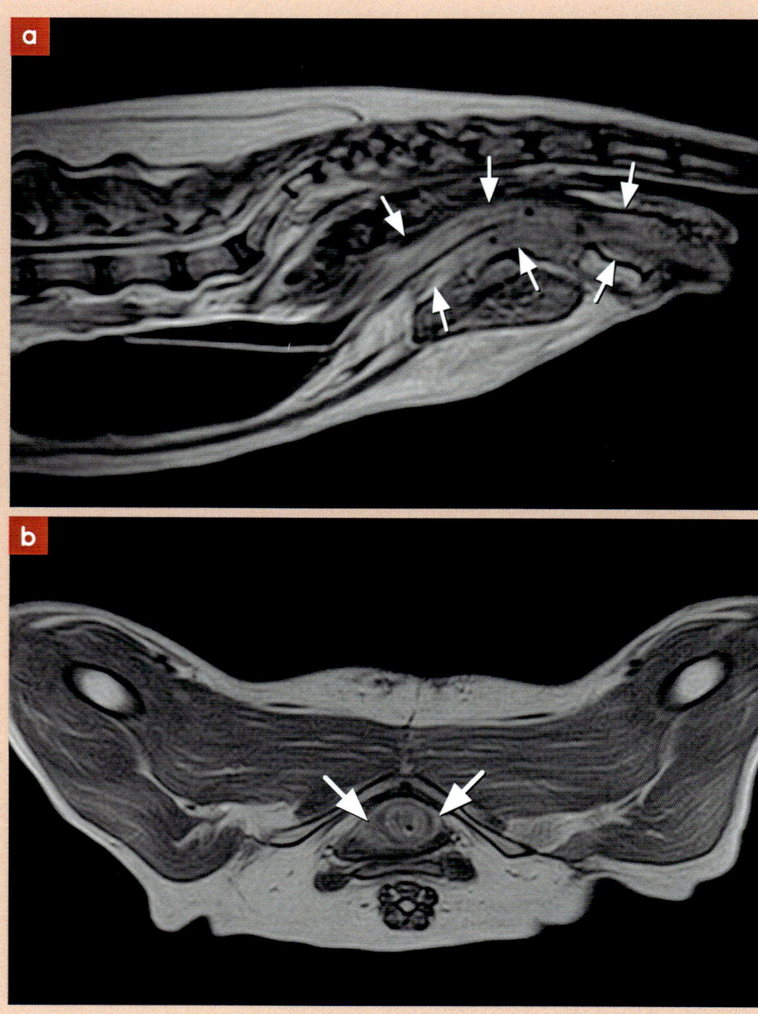

FIGURE 1.73. Post-contrast magnetic resonances images in sagittal (a) and transverse (b) plane of the pelvic region of a dog with a urethral tumour. The urethral wall shows a marked and generalised thickening and is enhanced after the administration of gadolinium. The external limits of the urethral wall are indicated with arrows in both images. Magnetic resonance imaging is an excellent technique for the evaluation of intrapelvic diseases and diseases of the perineal region.

that an absence of foetal bone mineralisation on day 45 post-breeding does not necessarily imply a negative pregnancy diagnosis. However, ultrasonography is much more precise to diagnose a pregnancy, since it is possible to identify the embryonic vesicles from days 18 to 20 of pregnancy in the dog and 15 to 17 in the cat, although it is recommended to confirm the diagnosis a few days later (from day 23), when the heartbeat can be observed.

Ultrasound examinations may however be less precise than radiographs when it comes to counting the number of foetuses. In order to carry out this assessment, it is recommended to take lateral and ventrodorsal radiographs of the abdomen at the end of pregnancy. In order to improve the precision of the diagnosis, the number of heads and that of spines should be counted on both projections, since the superimposition of the foetuses with each other and with other structures may lead to diagnostic errors, especially when there are many of them (fig. 1.77).

Ultrasonography does not enable a precise assessment of the relationship between the size of the foetus and the diameter of the pelvic canal. This measurement should be made using radiography (fig. 1.78). If the cranial diameter of the foetus clearly exceeds the width of the canal on the radiograph, this is considered as an evident sign of dystocia. This usually occurs when the size of the male is much greater than that of the female, especially in pregnancies of one or two foetuses, or in brachycephalic breeds, in

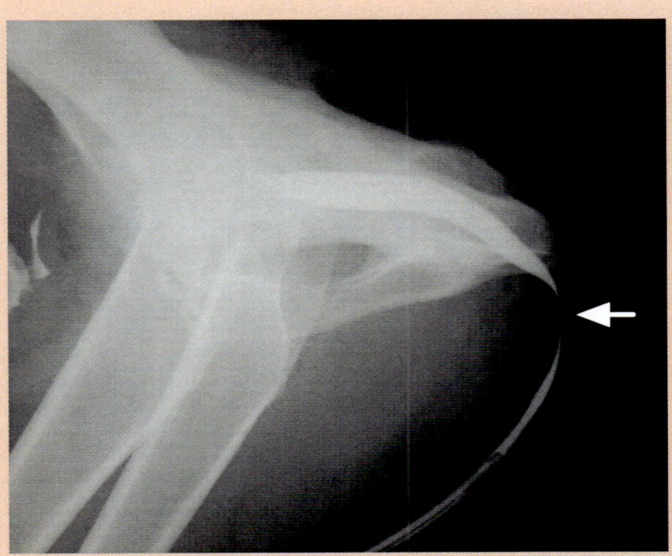

FIGURE 1.74. Enlarged image of a lateral retrograde urogram showing the pelvic region of a male dog, in which it is possible to observe an area of stenosis in the perineal segment of the urethra, secondary to focal urethritis caused by repeated catheterisation.

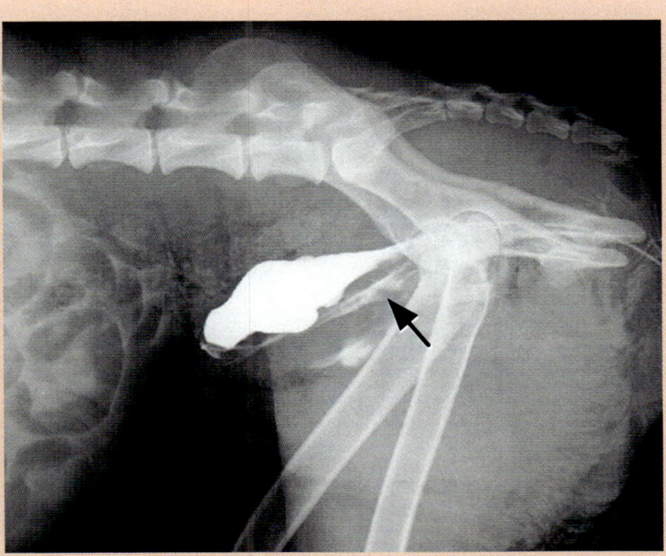

FIGURE 1.75. Lateral retrograde urethrogram showing the caudal abdomen of a female dog with a urethral rupture. The black arrow indicates the extravasation of the contrast medium.

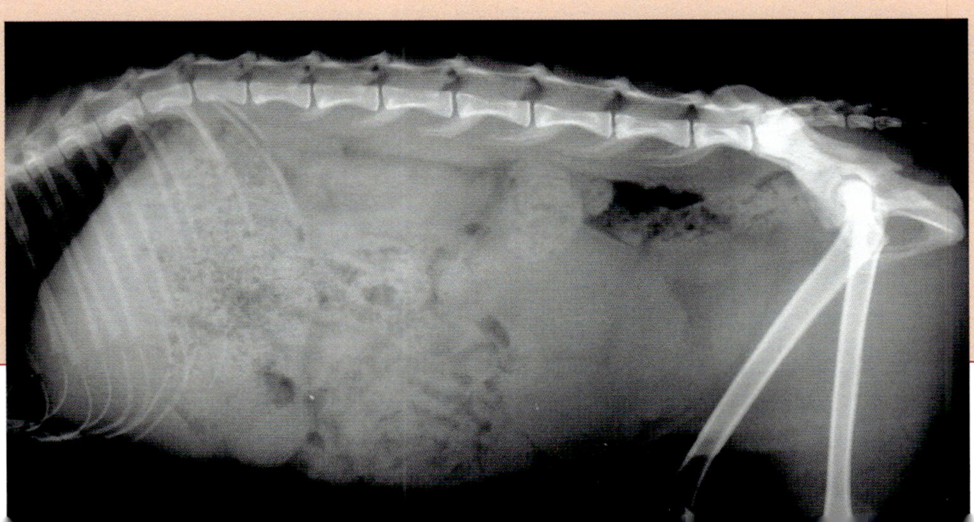

FIGURE 1.76. Lateral radiograph of the abdomen of a cat on day 30 of pregnancy. The dilated uterus appears cranial to the bladder, displacing the colon in dorsal direction and the small intestine in cranial direction. As the bones of the foetuses are not mineralised yet, this image may be confused with dilatation of the uterus due to pathological causes. A fracture of the ischion can also be identified.

which the size of the skull is proportionally greater and the morphology of the maternal pelvis is flatter. Other causes of dystocia observable by means of radiography include morphological alterations of the bony pelvis (fractures of traumatic origin, which can cause a more or less marked narrowing of the pelvic canal, are the most common) or poor foetal position at the time of birth. Radiography allows the observation of the normal uterus after birth, due to its increased size until day 12 postpartum in the dog and day 6 postpartum in the cat. It will also be useful to detect any retained foetuses once the birth is over.

Although ultrasound examinations are much more appropriate to assess a possible foetal death, some signs suggesting this diagnosis may be detected on the radiograph:

- Presence of gas in the foetus or in the lumen of the pregnant uterus (fig. 1.79).
- Anomalous position of the mineralised foetal structures.
- Evident signs of delay in foetal growth (fig. 1.80).

Those cases of endometrial hyperplasia and endometritis that are not accompanied by a great accumulation of fluid in the lumen of the uterus are easily identified on an ultrasound scan, but are not usually detectable on a plain radiograph. However, marked dilatations of the uterus, generally due to pyometra and, on a less frequent basis, to hydrometra, mucometra or haematometra, are easily identified on radiographs. They appear as tubular structures with soft tissue opacity, in many cases with a tortuous course, which occupy the central and caudal part of the abdomen (fig. 1.81). In some cases, the dilatation only affects one or two uterine horns, so the changes may only be observed in one of the sides of the abdomen on ventrodorsal radiographs.

Uterine stump abscesses or granulomas, which may appear as a complication of an ovariohysterectomy, are not usually detected on radiographs, unless they reach a size that is sufficiently large to produce a clear "mass effect" between the bladder and the colon.

Uterine neoplasms are very uncommon and cannot normally be differentiated from masses of another origin on radiographs of the abdomen. Ovarian neoplasms also have a low incidence in small animals. These latter may be uni- or bilateral and are sometimes accompanied by free peritoneal fluid and carcinomatosis, which may mask the image of the mass or masses on the radiograph. They are located caudal to the kidneys and may displace these latter in cranial direction and the intestine in ventral direction if they reach a large size (fig. 1.82). Some ovarian tumours (teratomas and teratocarcinomas) may appear calcified.

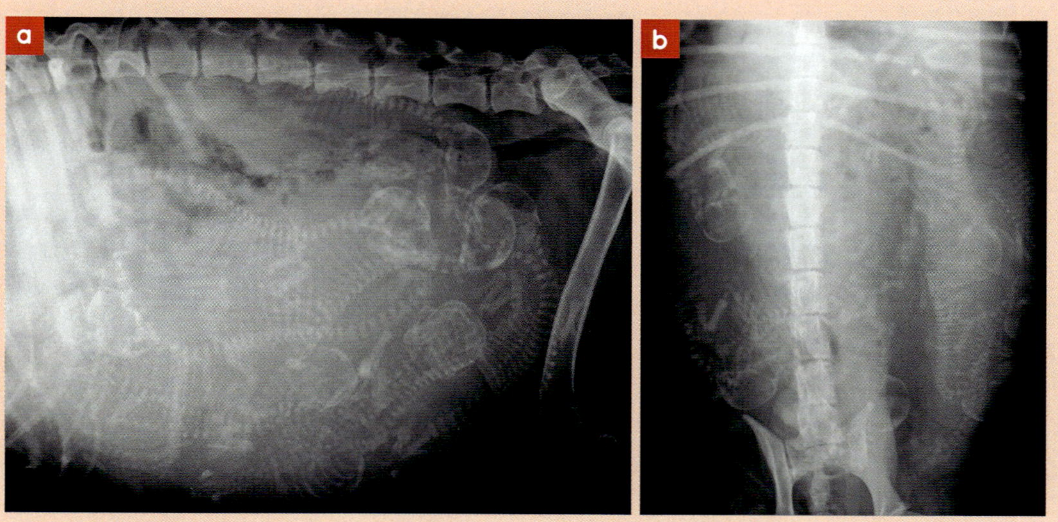

FIGURE 1.77. Lateral (a) and ventrodorsal (b) radiographs of the abdomen of a dog on day 55 of pregnancy with eight foetuses. Radiography is the most precise technique to count the number of foetuses, although the radiographs must be taken on the last days of pregnancy so as to minimise the damage that radiation may cause to the foetuses (the risk is higher during the first third of pregnancy, during the period of organogenesis).

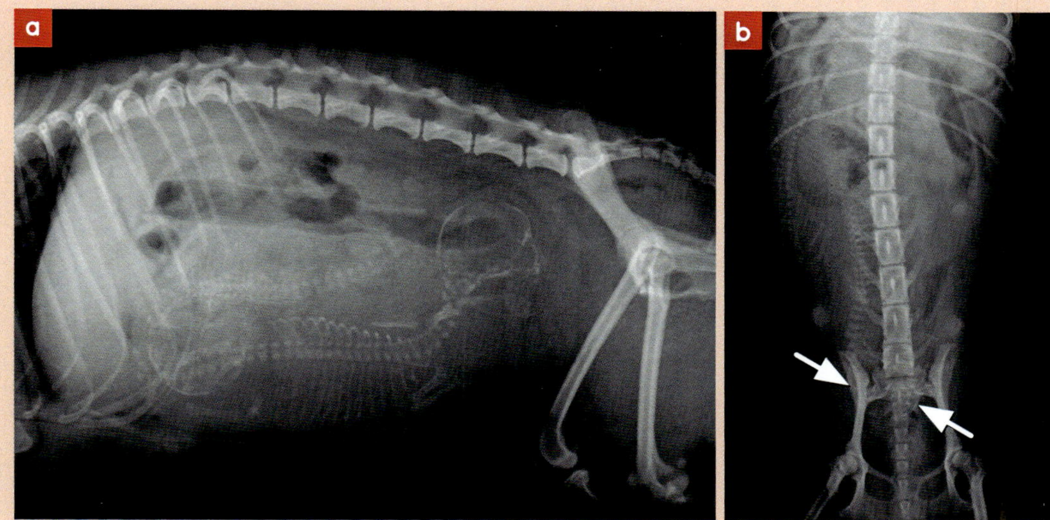

FIGURE 1.78. Lateral (a) and ventrodorsal (b) radiographs of the abdomen of a bitch on day 62 of pregnancy with two foetuses. The ventrodorsal radiograph allows the comparison of the cranial diameter (between the arrows) with the width of the pelvic canal.

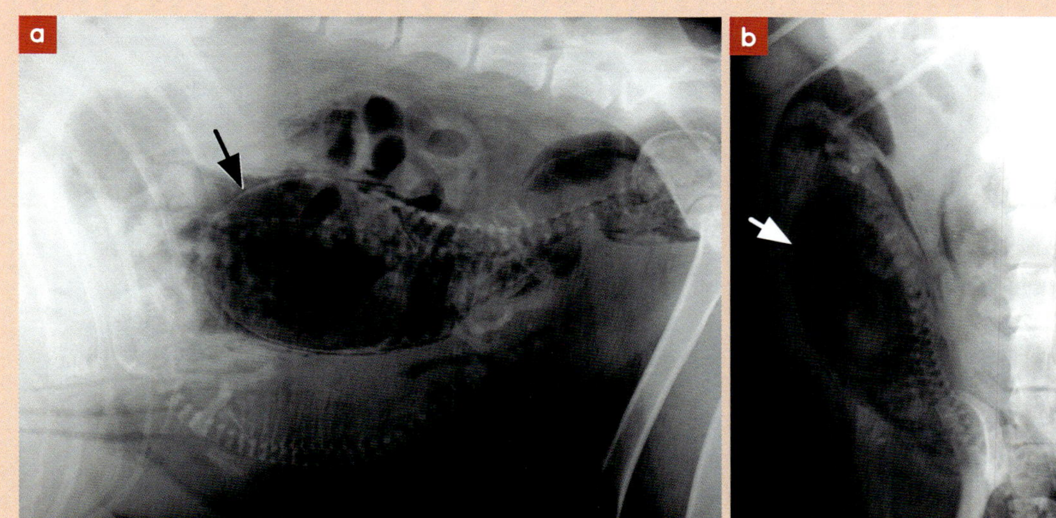

FIGURE 1.79. Enlarged images of the abdomen on lateral (a) and ventrodorsal (b) radiographs of a bitch on day 64 of pregnancy with two foetuses. Intrafoetal and intrauterine gas may be observed and are both indicative of foetal death. The foetal abdominal wall (arrows) may be identified as there is gas on both sides of it.

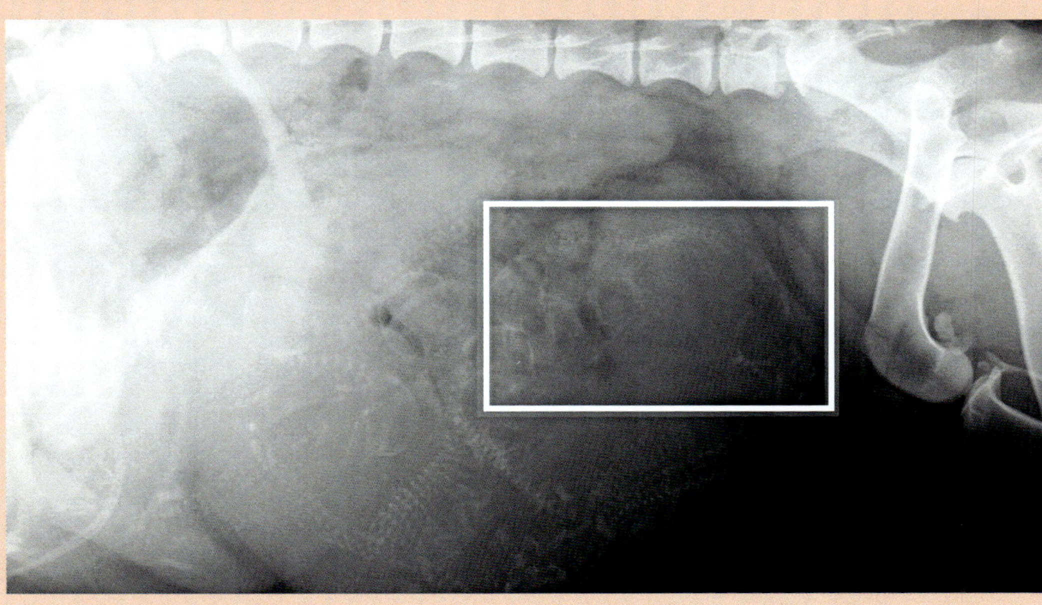

FIGURE 1.80. Lateral radiograph of the abdomen of a bitch on day 50 of pregnancy with seven foetuses. The foetus shown in the rectangle is smaller and the degree of mineralisation is lower compared with other foetuses. This finding may be due to foetal death, although it should be confirmed by means of an ultrasound examination.

Normal radiographic anatomy of the abdomen **lateral view**

http://goo.gl/hnl420

When a vaginourethrogram is performed, it is important to keep the end of the Foley catheter in the vaginal vestibule and not to introduce it in the vagina, as a vaginal rupture may occur when inflating the balloon. The normal vagina has a spindle-shaped morphology and it is common to see a small amount of contrast medium passing to the body of the uterus during oestrus. The vestibulovaginal junction appears as an area of narrowing between the vagina and the vestibule (fig. 1.83).

Vaginal masses (neoplasms, polyps, abscesses, haematomas, infiltration secondary to a urethral tumour) may create filling defects on the vaginogram. Vaginal hypertrophy is more common in brachycephalic breeds and may cause, together with tumours, a marked irregularity in the margins of the vagina.

Ectopic ureters that open into the vagina may be filled with contrast medium during a retrograde vaginourethrography study, although it is recommended to combine this technique with excretory urography for a more precise evaluation of this anomaly.

Vestibulovaginal stenosis is an abnormal narrowing of the vestibulovaginal junction, which may be asymptomatic or predispose to recurrent urinary and genital infections in the affected females. Although it has traditionally been considered that if the height of the vestibulovaginal junction is lower than a third of the height of the vagina on lateral radiographs, this is indicative of stenosis, some research studies suggest that this finding may be incidental in healthy animals.

Genital system of the male

Ultrasonography is the technique of choice to examine the prostate and testicles. The information provided by a radiograph is much more limited.

In dogs, the prostate is located immediately caudal to the neck of the bladder. Its normal position is intrapelvic,

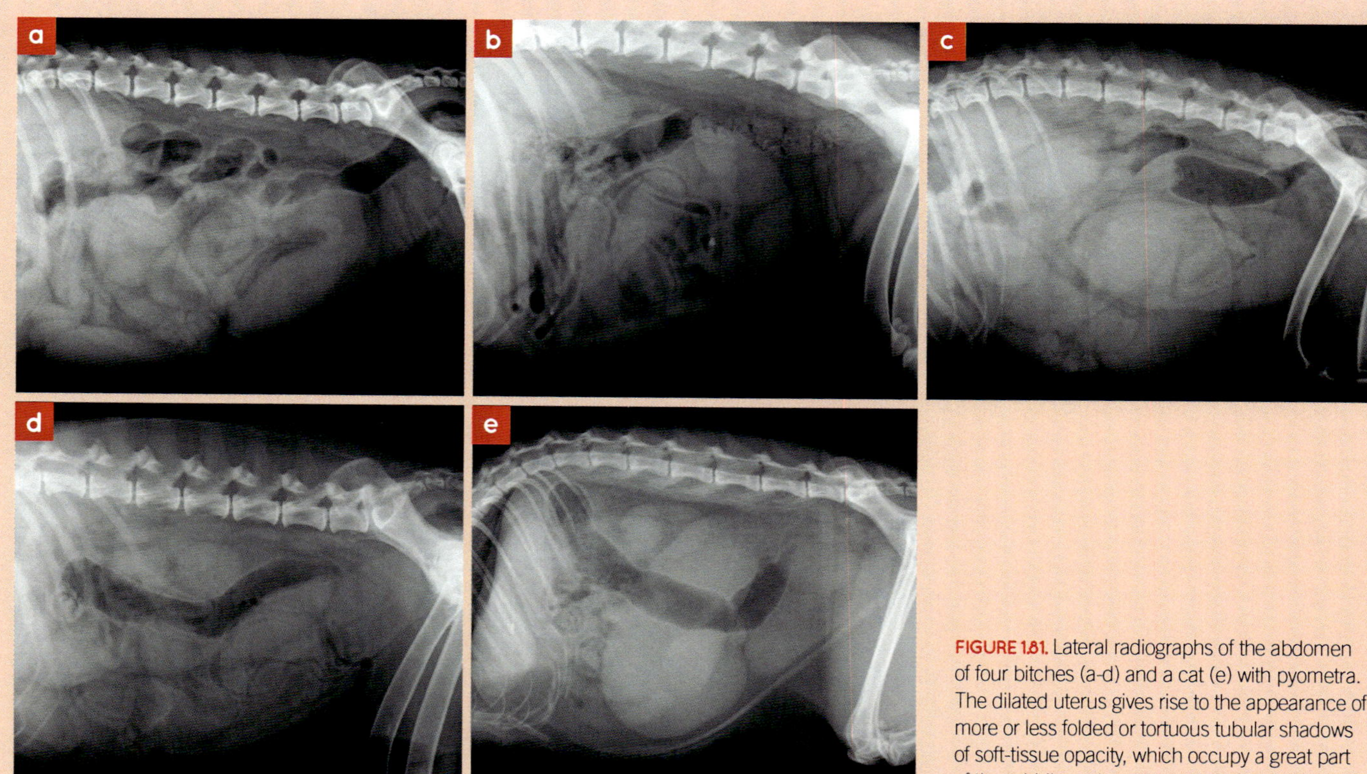

FIGURE 1.81. Lateral radiographs of the abdomen of four bitches (a-d) and a cat (e) with pyometra. The dilated uterus gives rise to the appearance of more or less folded or tortuous tubular shadows of soft-tissue opacity, which occupy a great part of the middle and caudal abdomen.

so its shadow is usually completely or partially masked by the bony pelvis on radiographs of the abdomen.

In cats, the prostate has a more caudal anatomical position than in dogs and its size is very small, which is why it is not identified on radiographs.

In addition, prostatic diseases are extremely rare in cats, so we will only refer to dogs from this point on.

The triangle of fat that accumulates between the caudoventral margin of the bladder and the cranioventral margin of the prostate, which is visible on lateral radiographs, helps to identify the image of this gland on the radiograph (fig. 1.84). The normal prostate is sometimes slightly displaced in cranial direction, especially if the bladder is very distended, which facilitates its evaluation. It is considered that the height of the prostatic shadow in non-neutered healthy males does not exceed 70 % of the distance between the promontory of the sacrum and the pubis on lateral radiographs. In some breeds, such as the Scottish Terrier, the normal prostate may exceed this limit.

Retrograde urethrography enables the evaluation of the image of the prostatic urethra and sometimes provides additional information on the prostatic parenchyma. In a healthy dog, the prostatic urethra has a more or less homogeneous diameter and smooth margins. It is sometimes possible to observe the passage of contrast medium to the normal prostatic parenchyma, when the prostatic ducts are partially filled.

The most frequent cause of an increase in the size of the prostate is benign hyperplasia, which is very common in non-neutered males from 5 years of age. Prostatitis, prostatic abscesses and neoplasms may also cause a more or less marked increase of the size of the gland. In some cases, prostatomegaly is accompanied by a cranial displacement of the gland towards the abdomen (fig. 1.85). If the increase in size is marked, this usually causes compression or dorsal displacement of the rectum, which may be the only evident radiological sign of prostatomegaly if the gland maintains its intrapelvic position (fig. 1.86). When the height of the shadow exceeds 90 % of the distance between the promontory of the sacrum and the pubis, this finding is considered indicative of a mass-type lesion (tumour, abscess, large-sized cyst). If the increase in size is significant, a mass in the caudal abdomen that displaces the adjacent structures in cranial and dorsal direction (fig. 1.87) will appear on the radiograph. When the diameter of the urethra is very

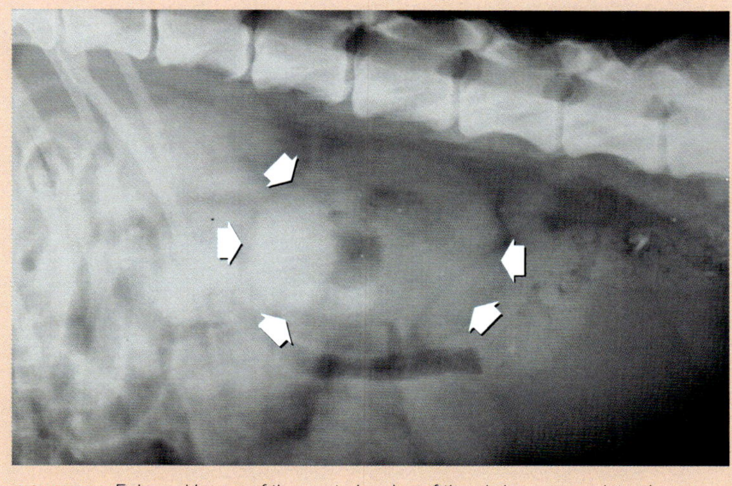

FIGURE 1.82. Enlarged image of the central region of the abdomen on a lateral radiograph of a dog with an ovarian neoplasm. The mass (arrows) is located caudal to the kidneys and displaces the colon in ventral direction.

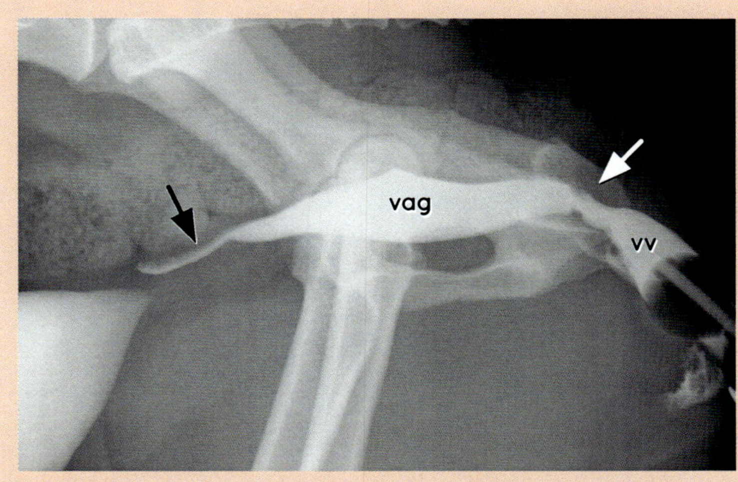

FIGURE 1.83. Normal vaginogram in a dog. The vestibulovaginal junction (white arrow) has a smaller diameter than the vaginal vestibule (vv) and the vagina (vag.). During oestrus, it is normal for a small amount of contrast medium to pass into the uterus (black arrow).

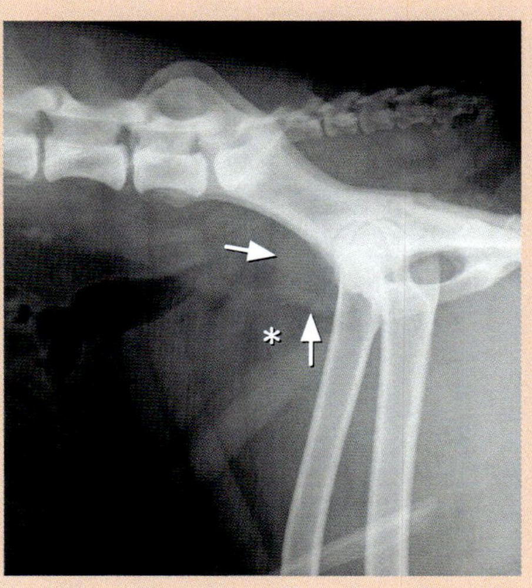

FIGURE 1.84. Enlarged image of the caudal abdomen on a lateral radiograph of a dog, in which the normal prostate is partially visualised. The cranial border of the gland is indicated by arrows. The triangle of fat (asterisk) that is located between the caudoventral border of the bladder and the cranioventral border of the prostate helps to identify the image of this latter on radiographs.

reduced as a consequence of a prostatic disease, the bladder may appear very distended.

In the case of prostatic neoplasms, the outline of the gland may be irregular or appear poorly defined in the image, even if there is sufficient fat surrounding it. As associated findings, it is possible to observe images indicative of an increase in the size of the sublumbar lymph nodes ("mass effect" located ventral to L5-L6-L7) and lesions in the closest bony structures, which suggest metastasis. Bone metastases from prostatic tumours usually appear as proliferative lesions in the ventral margin of the lumbar vertebrae and, in a less frequent manner, in the margin of the sacrum, wings of the ilium and femur. At more advanced stages, they may metastasise to the lungs and other long bones. The appearance of areas of calcification in the prostatic parenchyma is very suggestive of neoplasia (fig. 1.88), although they may also appear in severe chronic prostatitis.

Paraprostatic cysts can reach a large size and are identified on plain radiographs as soft-tissue opacity masses located in the caudal area of the abdomen. Calcification of the wall is sometimes observed. An ultrasound scan or alternatively a cystogram will allow the differentiation of the bladder from masses with an origin located in other abdominal organs (fig. 1.89).

Neutered dogs show prostatic atrophy secondary to orchiectomy, so the identification of the shadow of the prostate on radiographs will be difficult. The same may occur in patients with Sertoli-cell testicular tumour or in those that receive oestrogen therapy.

If the prostatic shadow is large and the urethra appears displaced within it, this finding will be indicative of the presence of a mass-type lesion in the parenchyma of the gland, while if the image of the prostatic urethra shows a marked narrowing or irregularity in its margins (fig. 1.90), this will indicate aggressive disease of the prostate or urethra. The contrast medium may extravasate into cavitary lesions of the prostatic parenchyma that are communicated with the urethra (fig. 1.91). If the morphology of these lesions is very irregular, this is considered compatible with neoplasia.

Radiography provides very limited information about the testicles, scrotum or penis. The only detectable testicular disease would be a mass caused by a very enlarged testicle with an abdominal or inguinal location. In the case of the scrotum, it may be possible to identify the presence of intestinal loops with gas in a scrotal hernia. Deformations, fractures and osteomyelitis of the os penis (fig. 1.92) have also been described.

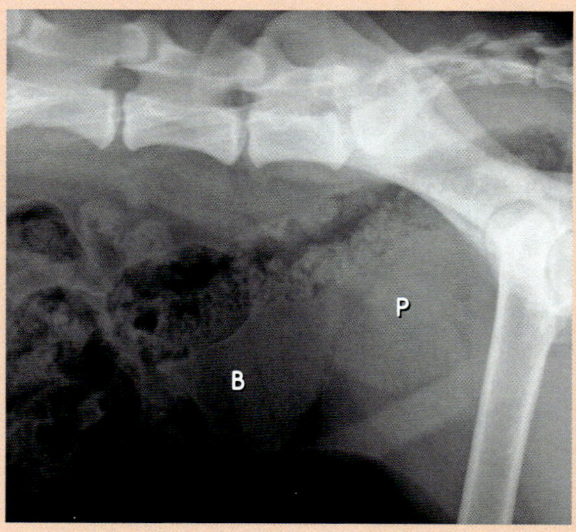

FIGURE 1.85. Enlarged image of the caudal abdomen on a lateral radiograph of a dog with prostatomegaly. The prostate (P), appears enlarged and displaced in cranial direction towards the abdominal cavity. The shadow of the bladder (B) appears cranial to it.

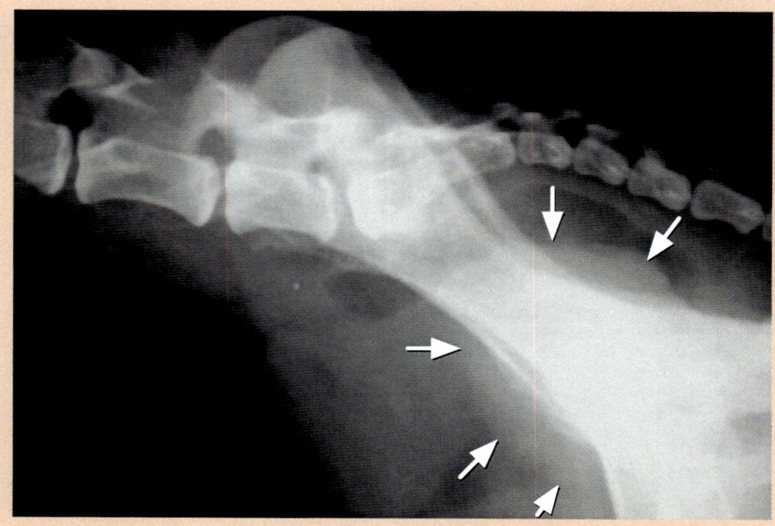

FIGURE 1.86. Enlarged image of the pelvic region on a lateral radiograph of a dog with prostatomegaly. The prostate (arrows) maintains its intrapelvic location. However, a dorsal displacement of the rectum is clearly observed, which is indicative of marked prostatomegaly.

Stomach

Although plain radiography and contrast radiography have traditionally been considered the techniques of choice for the asessment of the stomach and intestine, the now almost daily use of ultrasonography as a diagnostic tool perfectly complements the information provided by plain radiographs and drastically reduces the need to perform other contrast techniques to examine the gastrointestinal tract in small animals.

The stomach is divided into a cardiac part, a fundus, a body and a pyloric part (pyloric antrum and canal). In the dog, the body of the stomach has a central position and the pyloric antrum is located in the right side. In the cat, the stomach is located mainly in the left side, with the pyloric antrum on the median line.

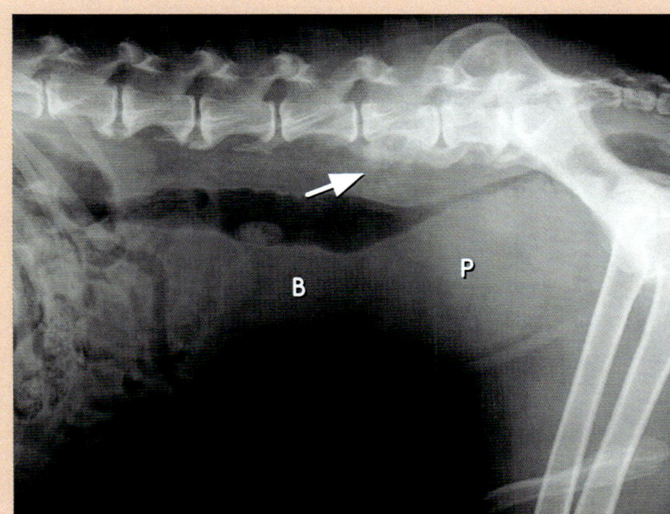

FIGURE 1.87. Lateral radiograph of the abdomen of a dog with a prostatic neoplasm. The prostate (P) is very enlarged in size and occupies a great part of the caudal abdomen, compressing the caudal third of the descending colon. The bladder (B) appears cranial to the prostatic mass. Irregular osteoproliferative lesions (arrow) compatible with bone metastases of the prostatic tumour can be observed in the ventral margin of the L6 and L7 vertebrae.

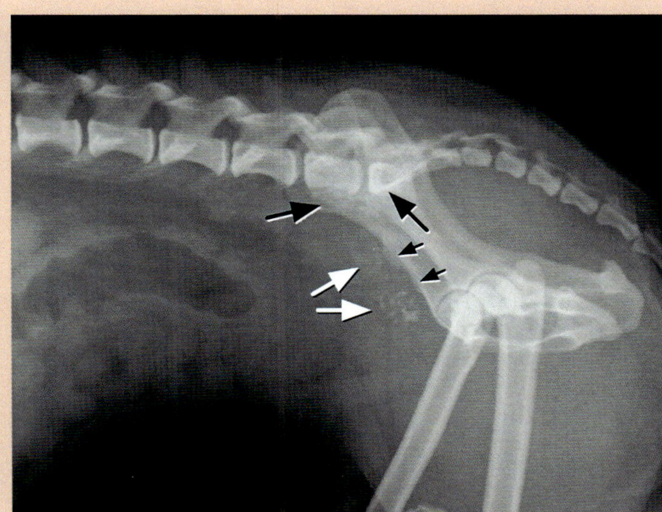

FIGURE 1.88. Lateral radiograph of the abdomen of a dog with a prostatic neoplasm. In the area where the prostate is located, areas of calcification of the soft tissues are observed (white arrows). The outline of the gland is not clearly identified. Irregular bony overgrowths compatible with metastases of the prostatic tumour can be observed in the area ventral to L7, sacrum and cranial margin of one of the wings of the ilium (black arrows).

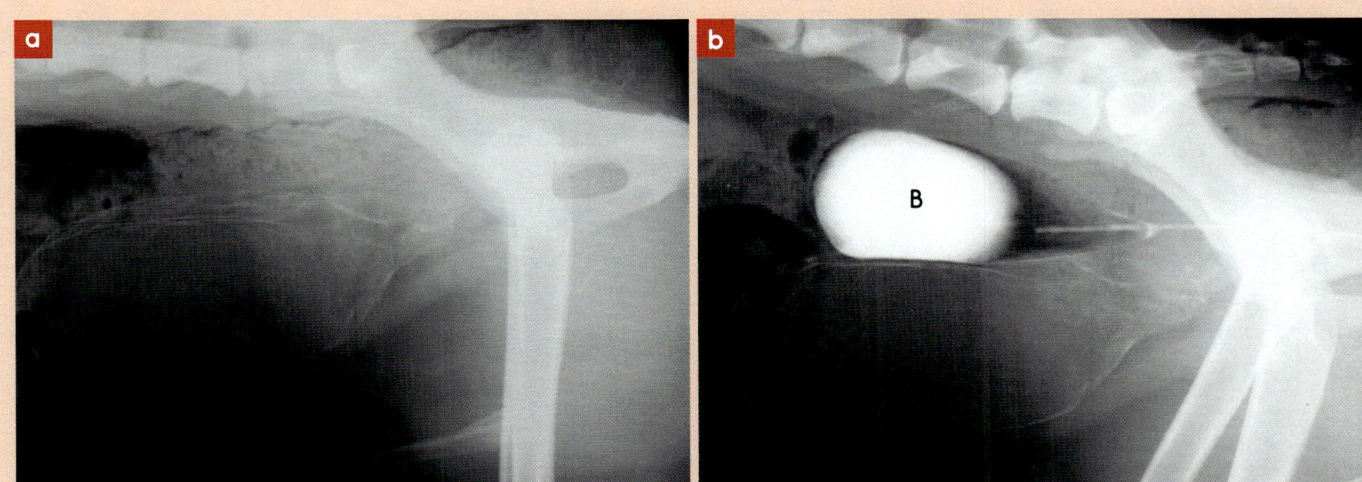

FIGURE 1.89. Enlarged images of the caudal abdomen on lateral radiographs of a dog with a large paraprostatic cyst with calcified walls, before (a) and after (b) introducing a double contrast medium into the bladder to identify its position (B) in relation to this structure.

The image of the stomach depends on its content (fig. 1.93) and on the radiographic projection used. When the patient has not eaten for some time, the stomach usually contains a variable amount of gas and fluid/mucus. In healthy dogs and cats, the stomach with no food usually appears cranial to the last pair of ribs, although it may also extend slightly beyond them, occupying approximately two intercostal spaces. When it contains food, this latter appears as radiopaque material with a granular aspect, and the size of the stomach may double or triple in normal conditions. On lateral radiographs, the axis of the stomach lies perpendicular to the spine, parallel to the ribs or at an intermediate point between these two positions.

One of the most important factors that affect the image of the stomach is the position of the patient when taking the radiograph. The relationship between the

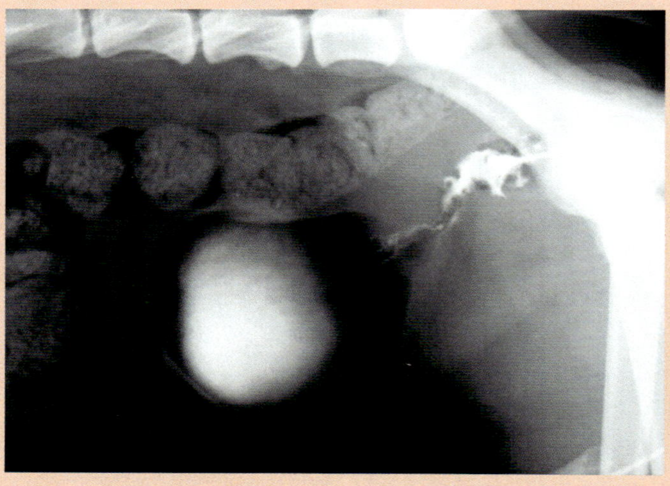

FIGURE 1.90. Enlarged image of a lateral double-contrast cystogram in a dog. It is possible to observe a reflux of positive contrast medium and gas into the prostatic urethra, which has very irregular margins. This indicates aggressive disease of the prostate and urethra. Final diagnosis: prostatic neoplasm.

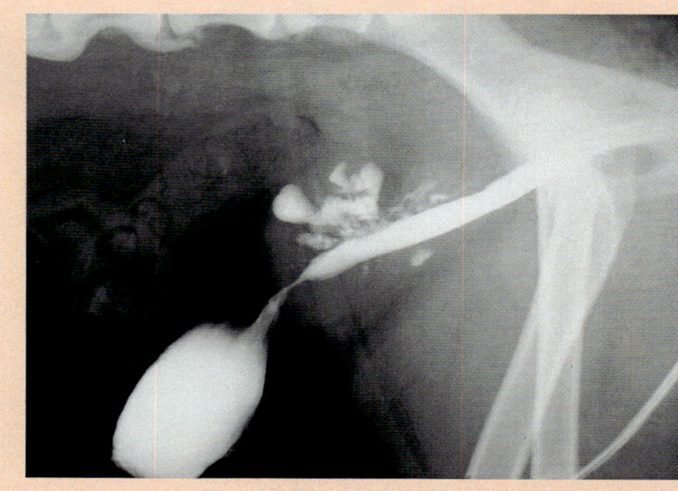

FIGURE 1.91. Enlarged image of a lateral retrograde urethrogram showing the caudal abdomen of a dog. An extravasation of the contrast medium into cavitary areas with an irregular morphology is observed, which is considered indicative of a prostatic neoplasm.

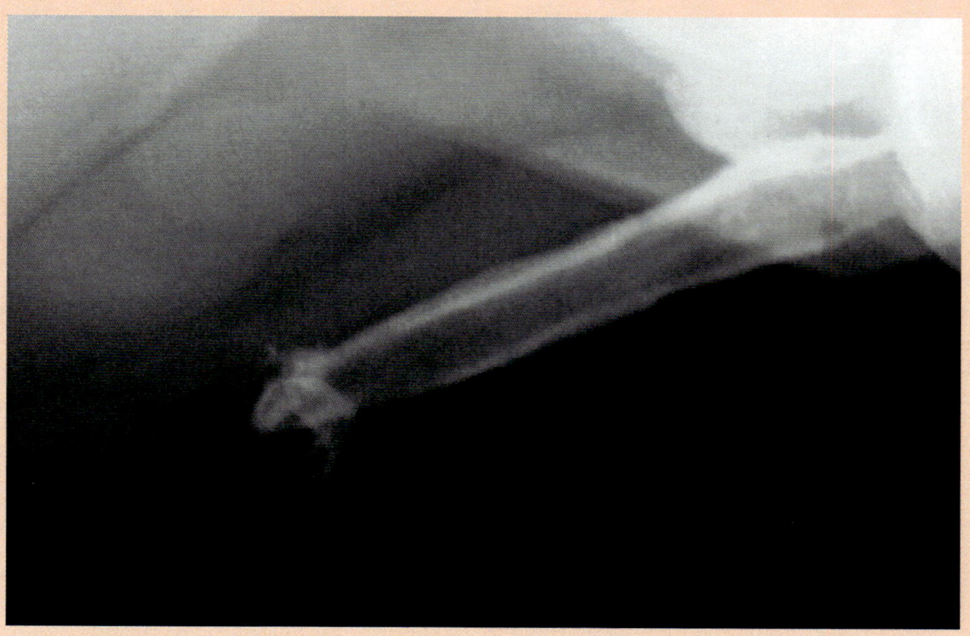

FIGURE 1.92. Enlarged image of the area of the prepuce on a lateral radiograph of a dog with a fracture of the os penis.

position of the stomach and its radiographic image is an important concept that should be borne in mind to interpret radiographs correctly and identify certain gastric lesions. The variation in the image of the stomach is due to changes in the distribution of the fluid and gas that can be found in its lumen: the fluid content is deposited on the inclined area as a result of gravity and the gas is displaced towards the uppermost area of the lumen of the stomach (fig. 1.94).

It is important to know how to make the most of the displacements of fluid and gas in the stomach to visualise some of its parts with more clarity (fig. 1.95).

It is not possible to appropriately evaluate the thickness of the wall or its folds by means of plain radiography, since the wall and the gastric fluid/mucous content have the same radiographic density and cannot be distinguished in the image (that is to say, we can think that a wall is thickened, when in fact what

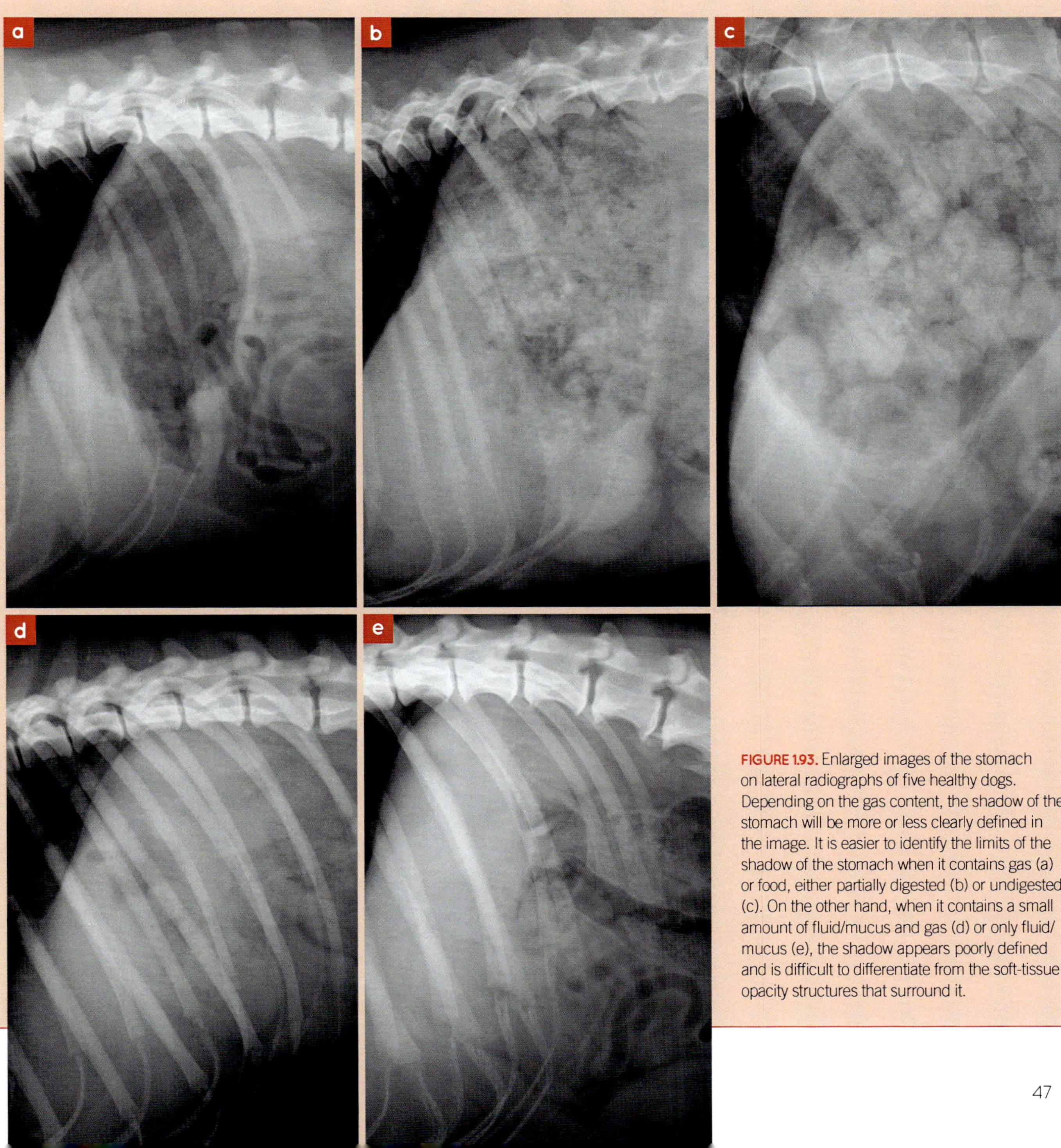

FIGURE 1.93. Enlarged images of the stomach on lateral radiographs of five healthy dogs. Depending on the gas content, the shadow of the stomach will be more or less clearly defined in the image. It is easier to identify the limits of the shadow of the stomach when it contains gas (a) or food, either partially digested (b) or undigested (c). On the other hand, when it contains a small amount of fluid/mucus and gas (d) or only fluid/mucus (e), the shadow appears poorly defined and is difficult to differentiate from the soft-tissue opacity structures that surround it.

we see is the image of the wall plus the fluid in the lumen (fig. 1.96).

Different contrast techniques may be used to assess the stomach:

- Conventional gastrography with barium sulphate.
- Gastrography with iodinated contrast media.
- Pneumogastrography.
- Double-contrast gastrography.
- Gastric emptying studies using food mixed with barium or with radiopaque markers.

Peristalsis and gastric emptying can be observed in real time using fluoroscopy and a positive contrast medium.

Before performing a contrast study of the stomach, the patient must not eat for 12 to 24 hours. The study should start by taking plain radiographs to confirm the need to carry out the examination with a contrast medium, ensure the correct preparation of the patient and adjust the exposure values. If sedation of the animal is necessary, acepromazine or ketamine may be used, since those drugs almost do not affect gastric motility.

Gastrography using barium sulphate

To perform a conventional gastrogram using barium sulphate, this latter is administered in a liquid preparation, preferably at a concentration of 30 % and at doses of 7-15 ml/kg (7-8 ml/kg in large breed dogs and 10-15 ml/kg in small breed dogs and cats). Although it is easier to administer the contrast medium by oral route using a syringe, this method involves some risk of aspirating the contrast medium, which could lead to the development of aspiration pneumonia (fig. 1.97). As an alternative, it is possible to administer the contrast material through an orogastric

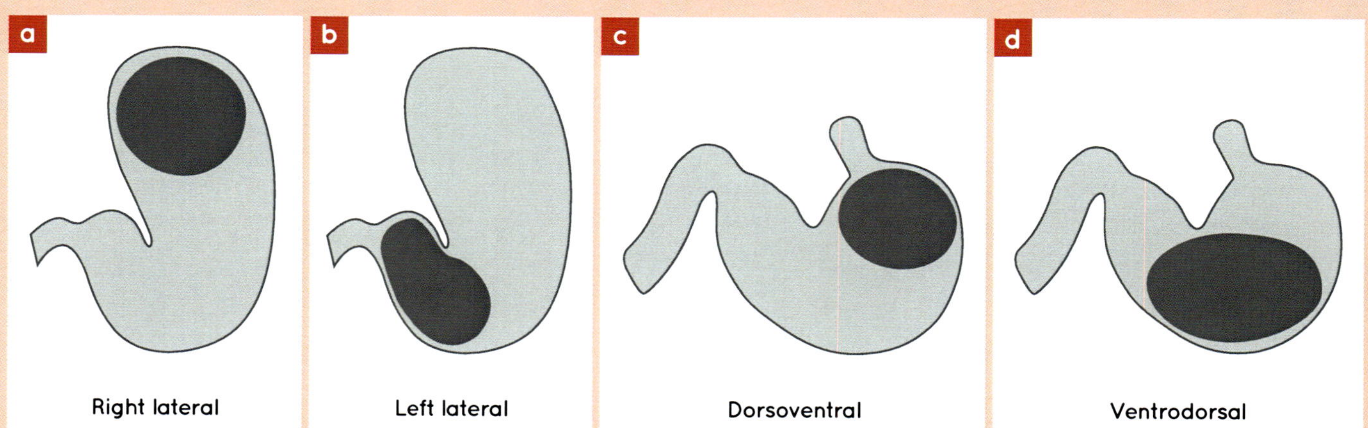

FIGURE 1.94. Representation of the variation of the radiographic image of the stomach due to the changes in the distribution of the fluid content and gas in function of the radiographic projection used. This diagram is only true when the stomach has a moderate amount of gas and fluid/mucus in its lumen.

The differences depending on the projection are:

a On **right lateral views,** the gas is located in the fundus and body of the stomach, since they are located in the left side of the patient and therefore represent the uppermost area in this position. The fluid content is deposited on the inclined area and fills the pyloric part. The fundus and body are identified immediately caudal to the left crus of the diaphragm (in the cranial and dorsal part of the abdomen). The pyloric part appears as a soft-tissue density shadow, located in ventral position immediately caudal to the liver. The shadow of the pyloric part sometimes has a rounded shape and may be mistaken for a mass or a rounded foreign body.

b On **left lateral views**, the gas is displaced to the pyloric part of the stomach, which is located in the right side of the patient and represents the uppermost part of the stomach in this position. The fluid content is deposited in the gastric fundus and body, which makes their identification difficult.

c On **ventrodorsal views**, the gas is located in the cardial part, fundus and part of the body of the stomach, while the fluid content is deposited on the ventral area of the body of the stomach and in the pyloric part.

d On **ventrodorsal views**, the gas is located in the pyloric part and in the ventral area of the body of the stomach. The fluid content fills the fundus and the rest of the body of the stomach. If they are completely empty, the fundus and body may appear as homogeneous soft-tissue density shadows.

tube. Nowadays, this technique is almost only used to carry out gastric emptying studies.

Gastric emptying is a complex phenomenon, which depends on various factors, such as the type of contrast medium used, the volume administered and the use of certain drugs. The greater the volume of intraluminal content, the faster the stomach will empty; it is therefore important to use the standard dose of the contrast medium. In normal conditions, gastric emptying usually starts in the first 15 minutes after the administration of barium, although in nervous animals it may be delayed until 30-45 minutes. The stomach usually completely empties in 1 to 4 hours in the dog. Minimal significance should be given to abnormally fast gastric emptying. On the other hand, a delay in gastric emptying is more significant. If the administered dose of barium is low, a delay in gastric emptying may be observed, which may lead to a false diagnosis of pyloric obstruction. If the administered dose is high, gastric emptying may be faster than normal.

Some gastric emptying studies have been performed using food mixed with barium, but this is not considered useful since the range of normality for the empyting time is very wide (from 7 to 15 hours). Radiopaque barium-impregnated polyethylene spheres (BIPS) have also been used mixed with food. The number and size of the spheres, the type and amount of food with which they are mixed and the amount of time without eating should be strictly adjusted to a standardised protocol, or else the results will be difficult to interpret. A disadvantage of this technique is that the

Normal radiographic anatomy of the abdomen **lateral view**

http://goo.gl/hnl420

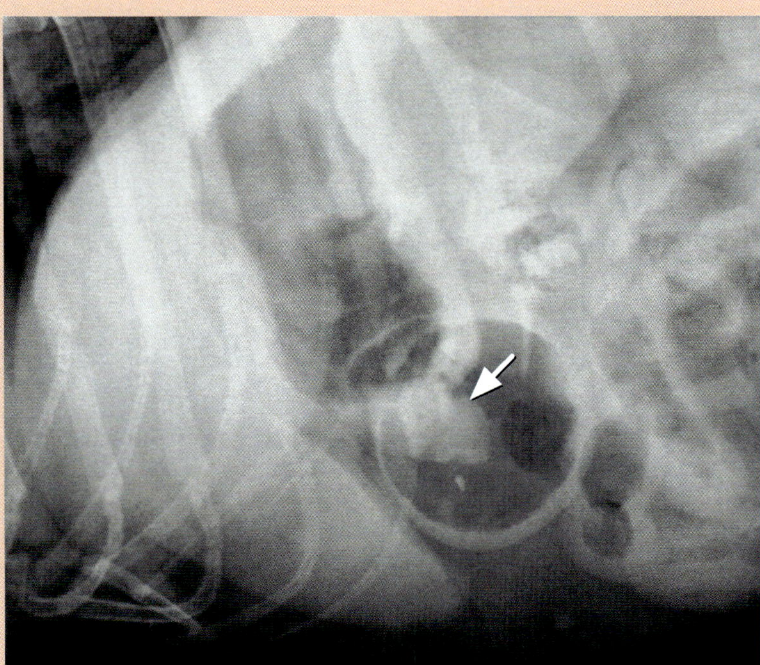

FIGURE 1.95. Enlarged image of the cranial abdomen on a lateral radiograph of a dog with a radiolucent foreign body in the pyloric antrum. When taking a left lateral radiograph, the gas is displaced to the antrum and surrounds the object (arrow), which allows its identification in the image.

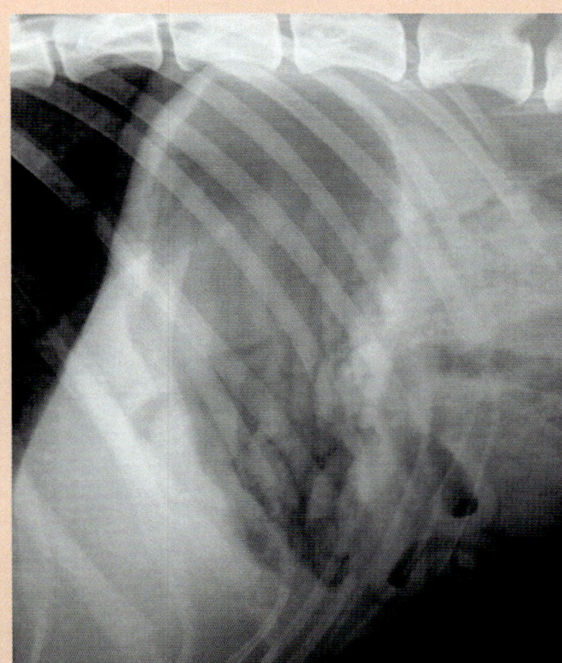

FIGURE 1.96. Enlarged image of the cranial abdomen on a lateral radiograph of a dog, in which prominent gastric folds are observed. This radiological finding may appear in cases of gastritis, but this diagnosis should never be confirmed only by means of radiography, since the presence of fluid or mucus between the folds of a normal gastric wall may create the same image. An ultrasound scan must be performed for a precise assessment of the thickness of the gastric wall.

time of examination may be very long (up to 10 hours), so it is not used in practice.

Positive-contrast gastrography using iodinated contrast media

Positive-contrast gastrography using iodinated contrast media is recommended only when a rupture or perforation of the stomach (or the intestine) is suspected. These contrast media are diluted in the gastrointestinal tract, so the quality of the contrast study is lower in comparison with that of the studies performed with barium, but they will be absorbed in the peritoneal cavity if they extravasate. Their use is contraindicated in dehydrated patients. Although hyperosmotic iodinated contrast media can be used at doses of 7 ml/kg, low-osmolarity nonionic iodinated contrast media such as iohexol and iopamidol, which can be administered diluted at 33 % in doses of 8 ml/kg, are more recommended.

Negative-contrast gastrography

Negative-contrast gastrography is performed by introducing air (20 ml/kg) in the stomach through a gastric tube. It is essential that the animal does not eat for 12-24 hours prior to the study so as to avoid the presence of food in the stomach at the time of examination. It is a relatively simple technique, which can improve the visualisation of certain radiolucent foreign bodies and intraparietal masses. However, it is hardly ever used nowadays, firstly, because double-contrast gastrography would provide more information in these cases and secondly, because the combination of plain radiography and ultrasonography frequently allows the establishment of these diagnoses without the need to sedate the patient or administer contrast media.

Double-contrast gastrography

Double-contrast gastrography would be the most appropriate contrast technique to evaluate the mucosa and folds of the stomach, although we should bear in mind that an ultrasound examination is preferable, since it provides direct information about the thickness, differentiation of the layers and peristalsis of the stomach wall.

In order to perform a double-contrast gastrogram, non-diluted liquid barium sulphate (3-5 ml/kg) is administered first by means of an orogastric tube, followed by air (10-20 ml/kg or simply the sufficient amount to achieve an appropriate distension of the organ). This technique limits the study to the stomach since it is does not allow a correct assessment of gastric emptying or of the intestine.

Pathological alterations

The most common indication for a plain radiograph of the stomach is the suspicion of a **foreign body**. It is easy to visualise objects with a higher radiopacity than that of soft tissues and fluids (radiopaque foreign

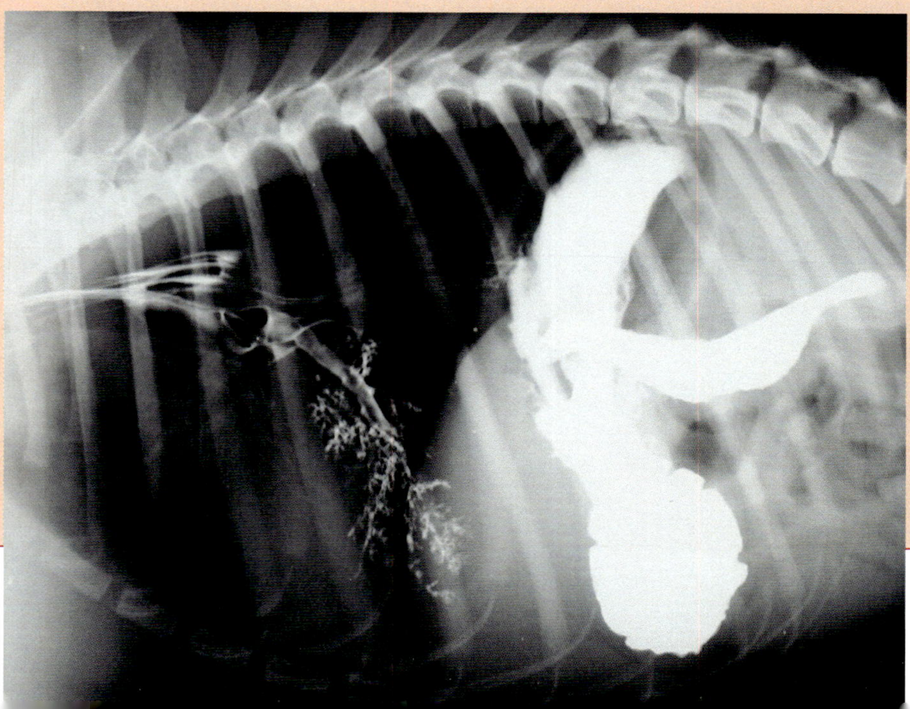

FIGURE 1.97. Lateral radiograph of the thorax and cranial abdomen of a dog with barium aspiration in the airways after its administration by oral route with a syringe. The aspiration of a small or moderate amount of barium is usually well tolerated by the patient, although its reabsorption through the lymphatic system may last months or years, and it may remain visible on radiographs of the thorax during this period of time.

bodies), as there is a clear difference between these and the wall of the stomach and fluid or mucous content in its lumen (fig. 1.98). Diagnostic interpretation may be more difficult when these objects are surrounded by food, which has a heterogeneous opacity that may be confused with that of other objects, especially if these are small.

When foreign bodies have a similar radiopacity to that of soft tissues or fluids (radiolucent foreign bodies), their radiographic identification is much more complicated. Indeed, if they are surrounded by fluid or mucus, or adjacent to the gastric wall, it will often be impossible to distinguish them on plain radiographs (fig. 1.99), unless they have a characteristic morphology (e.g. some types of balls) (fig. 1.100).

Contrast techniques may help to confirm the presence of an object in the stomach, but it is worth trying to identify it by means of an ultrasound examination, although it will provide a limited amount of information when the foreign body is surrounded by gas. If gastrography is used, foreign bodies are usually easier to diagnose when a small amount of barium is administered, or with double-contrast gastrography instead of barium gastrography with the standard dose, since the administration of a large volume of positive contrast agent may lead to the object being masked in the image.

The aspect of foreign bodies on a contrast radiograph of the stomach depends on their characteristics. Some objects such as balls, wood, fruit stones, plastic, etc., produce well-defined and delimited filling defects. On the other hand, objects with an absorbent surface such as fabrics or sponges may not initially create a filling defect image, as they absorb the contrast medium and are better visualised when most of the contrast material has passed from the stomach to the duodenum (fig. 101).

Another diagnosis that is usually made by means of radiographic studies is **pyloric obstruction**, which can be acute or chronic. An acute obstruction may be due to a gastric volvulus or to the presence of foreign bodies. Chronic pyloric obstruction is generally due to a narrowing of the orifice of the pylorus, caused by diseases that affect the wall or block the orifice, such as hypertrophic pyloric stenosis, pyloric spasm, inflammation, fibrosis, neoplasia or hypertrophy of the

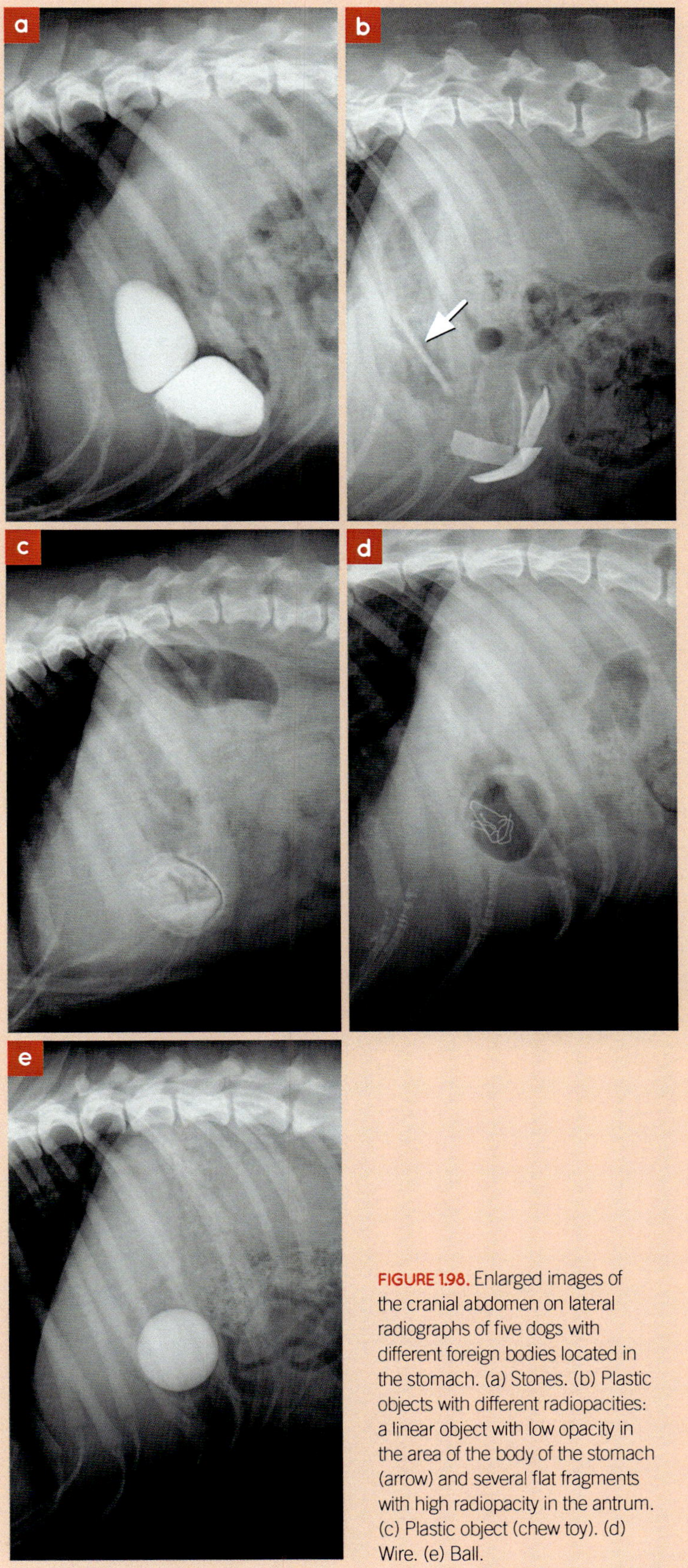

FIGURE 1.98. Enlarged images of the cranial abdomen on lateral radiographs of five dogs with different foreign bodies located in the stomach. (a) Stones. (b) Plastic objects with different radiopacities: a linear object with low opacity in the area of the body of the stomach (arrow) and several flat fragments with high radiopacity in the antrum. (c) Plastic object (chew toy). (d) Wire. (e) Ball.

mucosa of the antrum. On a plain radiograph, obstructive diseases of the pylorus may be visualised as a stomach increased in size, depending on the severity and duration of the obstruction. An accumulation of mineral opacity material located proximal to a point of gastrointestinal obstruction (stomach or intestine), which has been termed "gravel sign", is sometimes observed (fig. 1.102). This sign usually appears associated with chronic digestive obstructions.

In contrast studies, the main finding in cases of pyloric obstructions is delayed gastric emptying. A delayed gastric emptying should be considered significant when only a small amount of contrast material has passed to the duodenum after several hours. The retention of most of the barium in the stomach 3 to 4 hours after its administration is indicative of an obstructive pyloric disease.

A pyloric spasm may occur when the contrast study is performed if the animal is nervous. That is why it is useful to keep the animal in a quiet place for 30 minutes and repeat the radiograph after this period of time. A sedative or spasmolytic drug may also be administered. If the passage of the barium to the duodenum is delayed more than one hour even though the animal has been kept in a quiet place and has been administered a spasmolytic drug, the possibility of a pyloric dysfunction should be considered (1.103).

Gastric dilatation and torsion or volvulus are diagnosed by means of plain radiography. Acute **dilatation** of the stomach may be due to a complex variety of causes. The stomach will maintain its normal position and anatomical relationships, but will appear increased in size and filled mainly with gas in the image (fig. 1.104). The dilatation of the stomach may be caused by an obstruction of the pyloric canal or by atony of the gastric wall, but it may also appear due to aerophagy.

Acute dilatation may or not be followed by a gastric **torsion**. Gastric torsion or volvulus can be differentiated from simple acute dilatation because the stomach is rotated. The radiographic image of the stomach varies depending on the type and degree of rotation, on the one hand, and on the degree of distension, on the other (fig. 105). As the stomach dilates, the greater curvature turns in ventral direction and to the right, and is located along the ventral abdominal wall. The pylorus is displaced in dorsal and cranial direction and to the left. Rotation in the opposite direction is uncommon. In case of doubt, taking radiographs in the four standard radiographic projections (right lateral, left lateral,

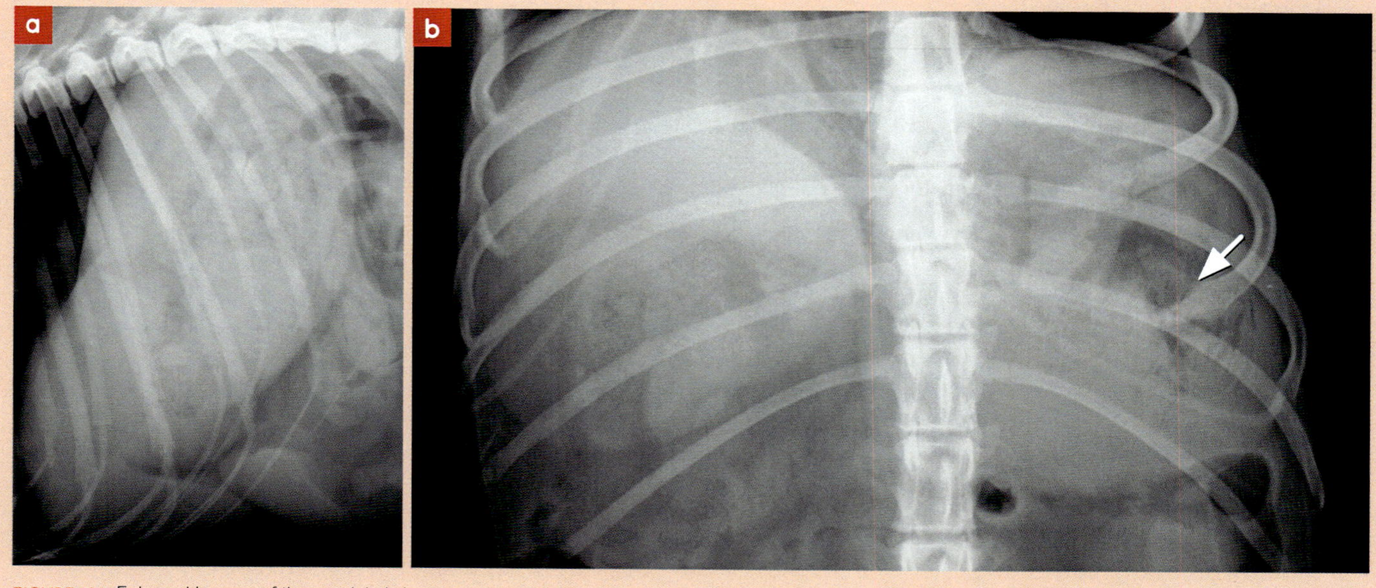

FIGURE 1.99. Enlarged images of the cranial abdomen on lateral (a) and ventrodorsal (b) radiographs of a dog with a radiolucent foreign body in the stomach. On the lateral view, the object (a piece of fabric) may be mistaken for normal gastric content, although on the ventrodorsal projection, the presence of parallel bands of gas density in the fundus (arrow) suggests the presence of a foreign body.

ventrodorsal and dorsoventral) may provide more precise information (fig. 1.106).

Apart from the distension and displacement of the stomach, a typical radiographic finding in case of torsion is the image of compartments, or "double bubble" sign. This image is created by bands of soft -tissue density projected through the stomach lumen, which is filled with gas (they appear because the stomach folds in on itself and the folded wall is projected towards its lumen and is thus outlined by the intraluminal gas that surrounds it).

Gastric torsion can also affect the image of other organs, such as the spleen, which may appear enlarged and displaced from its normal position. Radiographic signs of reflex paralytic ileus, dilatation of the oesophagus due to an obstruction at the level of the

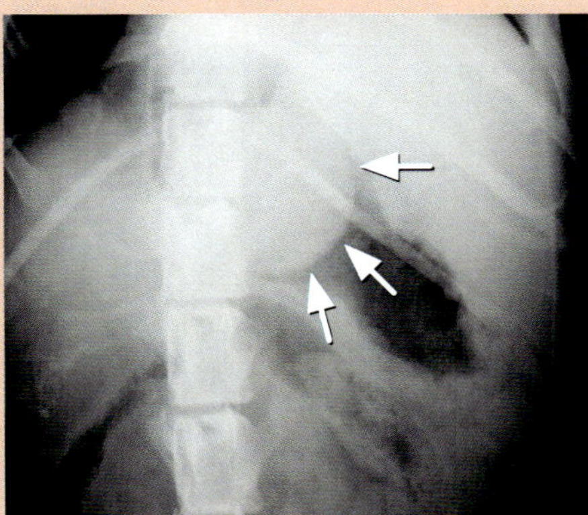

FIGURE 1.100. Enlarged image of the abdomen on a ventrodorsal radiograph of a dog with a ball (arrows) in the body of the stomach. The ball has a very similar radiopacity to that of the gastric wall and fluid/mucous content, but its characteristic round edge allows its identification in the image.

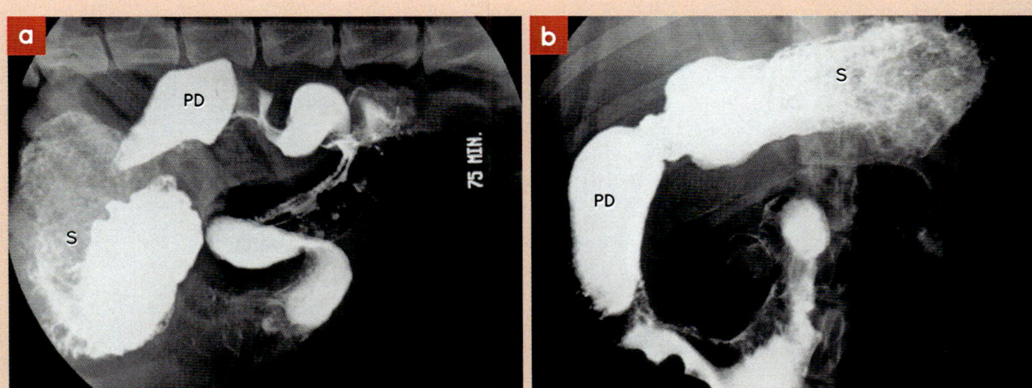

FIGURE 1.101. Enlarged images of the cranial abdomen on lateral (a) and ventrodorsal (b) radiographs of a dog, 75 minutes after the administration of barium. An accumulation of the contrast material can be observed mainly in the stomach (S) and proximal duodenum (PD), due to the presence of a foreign body that retains a great part of the contrast agent (plastic grid).

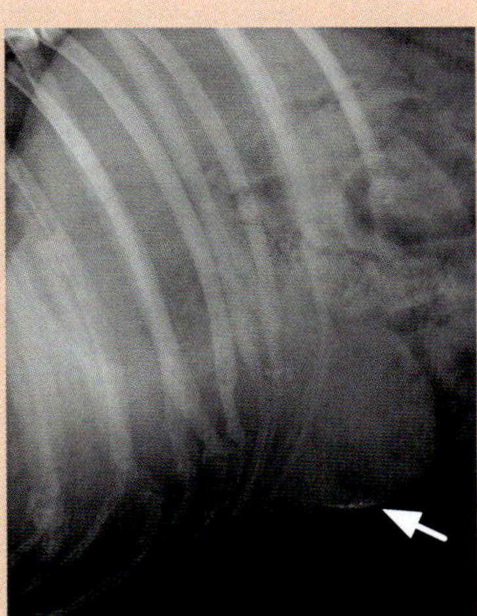

FIGURE 1.102. Enlarged image of the cranial abdomen on a lateral radiograph of a dog with a persistent accumulation of radiopaque material ("gravel sign") in the pyloric antrum (arrow). This finding may be indicative of an obstructive process, in this case in the pylorus.

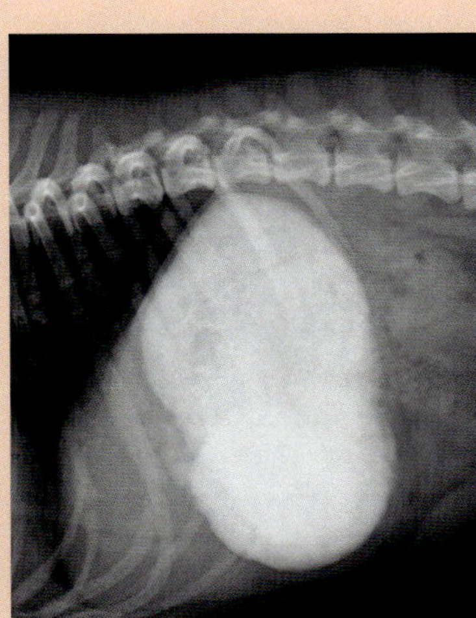

FIGURE 1.103. Enlarged image of the cranial abdomen on a lateral radiograph of a dog after receiving a standard dose of barium 70 minutes before the radiograph was taken. Limited passage of contrast material to the duodenum one hour after the administration of barium is indicative of pyloric dysfunction.

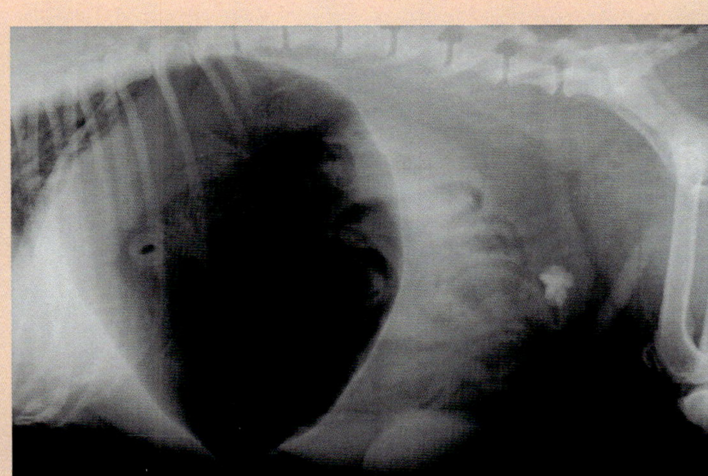

FIGURE 1.104. Lateral radiograph of the abdomen of a dog with severe gastric dilatation. No signs of rotation of the stomach are observed.

gastroesophageal junction and pulmonary hypovolaemia and microcardia may also be visualised.

At the initial stages of **gastric perforation**, the findings on a plain radiograph may be difficult to interpret. Depending on the size of the perforation or rupture, a variable amount of stomach content will pass to the peritoneal cavity. This causes an initially focal peritonitis, which is easily detected with an ultrasound scan, but can be more difficult to detect on radiographs. The most significant radiological finding is the detection of free gas in the peritoneal cavity. When the amount of gas is small, the sign that is easiest to recognise is the visualisation of the diaphragm when gas accumulates between this structure and the liver (fig. 1.107) (see Peritoneal cavity and retroperitoneal space).

It may be difficult to identify the area of perforation or rupture of the gastric wall with an ultrasound examination, which is why in almost all the cases in which a gastric perforation is suspected, the use of positive-contrast gastrography with iodinated contrast media will be recommended, since these latter are absorbed in the peritoneum if they are extravasated, while barium is not.

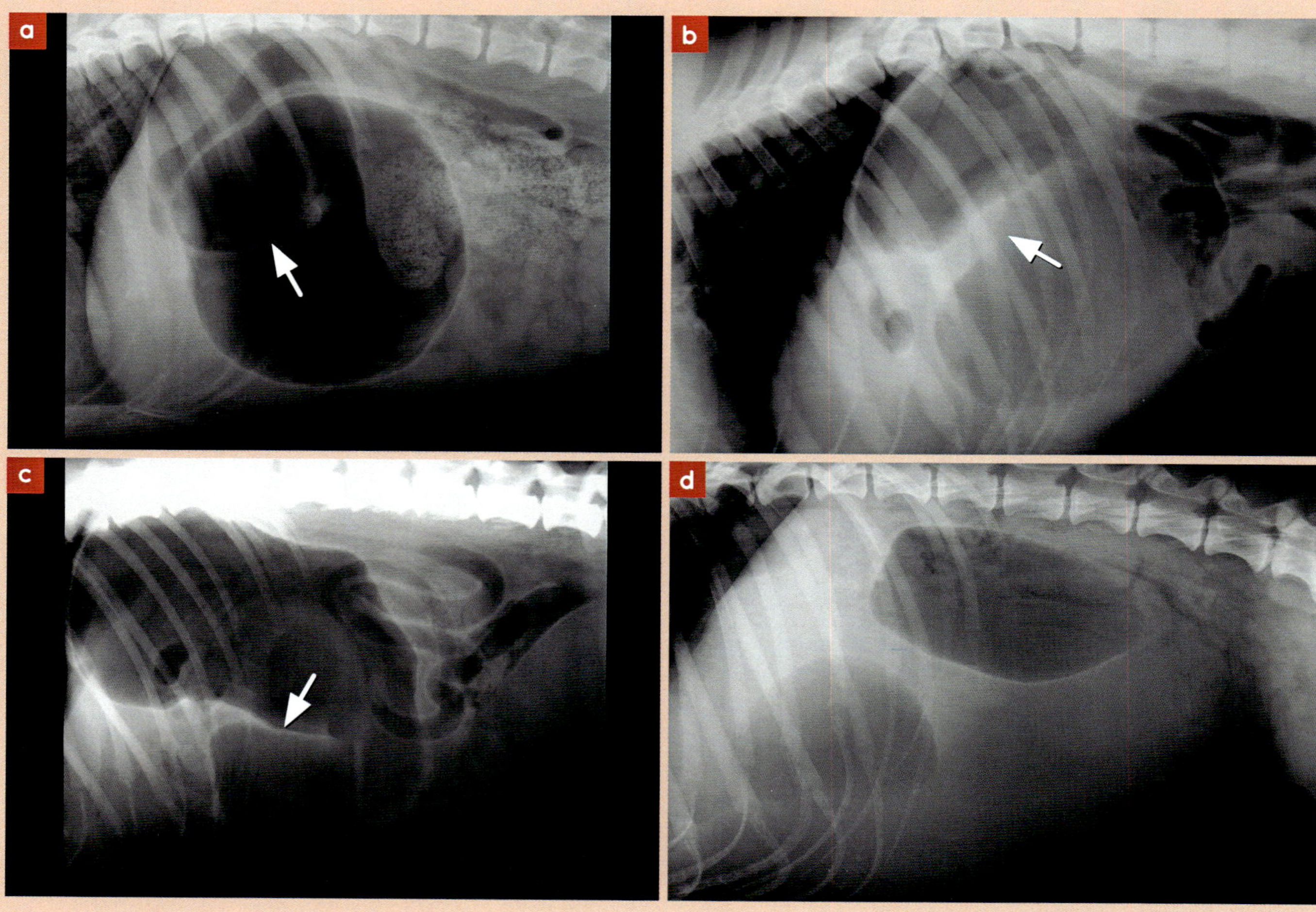

FIGURE 1.105. Lateral radiographs of the abdomen of four dogs with gastric torsion (gastric volvulus). (a) Marked dilatation of the stomach with 180-degree rotation. A soft-tissue density band is projected through the lumen filled with gas, creating an image of compartments or "double bubble" sign (arrows in images a, b and c). (b) Similar image to the previous one, although in this case the radiopacity of the stomach is greater because it contains fluid and gas. (c) Marked gastric dilatation with a rotation of less than 180°, the stomach essentially contains gas. (d) Extreme gastric dilatation with mainly fluid content and a moderate amount of gas, which makes the identification of the rotation of the stomach difficult.

Normal radiographic anatomy of the abdomen **dorsoventral view**

http://goo.gl/yYtSNq

Although an ultrasound scan should always be performed in case of suspicion of a gastric neoplasm, radiography can also provide useful information, especially if no ultrasound scanner is available or we do not have enough experience to establish a precise ultrasound diagnosis. The radiographic image of a gastric neoplasm may vary depending on its size, shape and location. On a plain radiograph, it may be possible or not to observe a more or less evident "mass effect". In contrast studies, the main radiographic finding is the visualisation of a mass-type lesion that is projected towards to the lumen of the stomach, thus creating an image of filling defect on the gastrogram (fig. 1.108). Small masses may be completely masked when a relatively large amount of barium is used.

Diffuses diseases of the stomach include those producing inflammation, hypertrophy or atrophy of

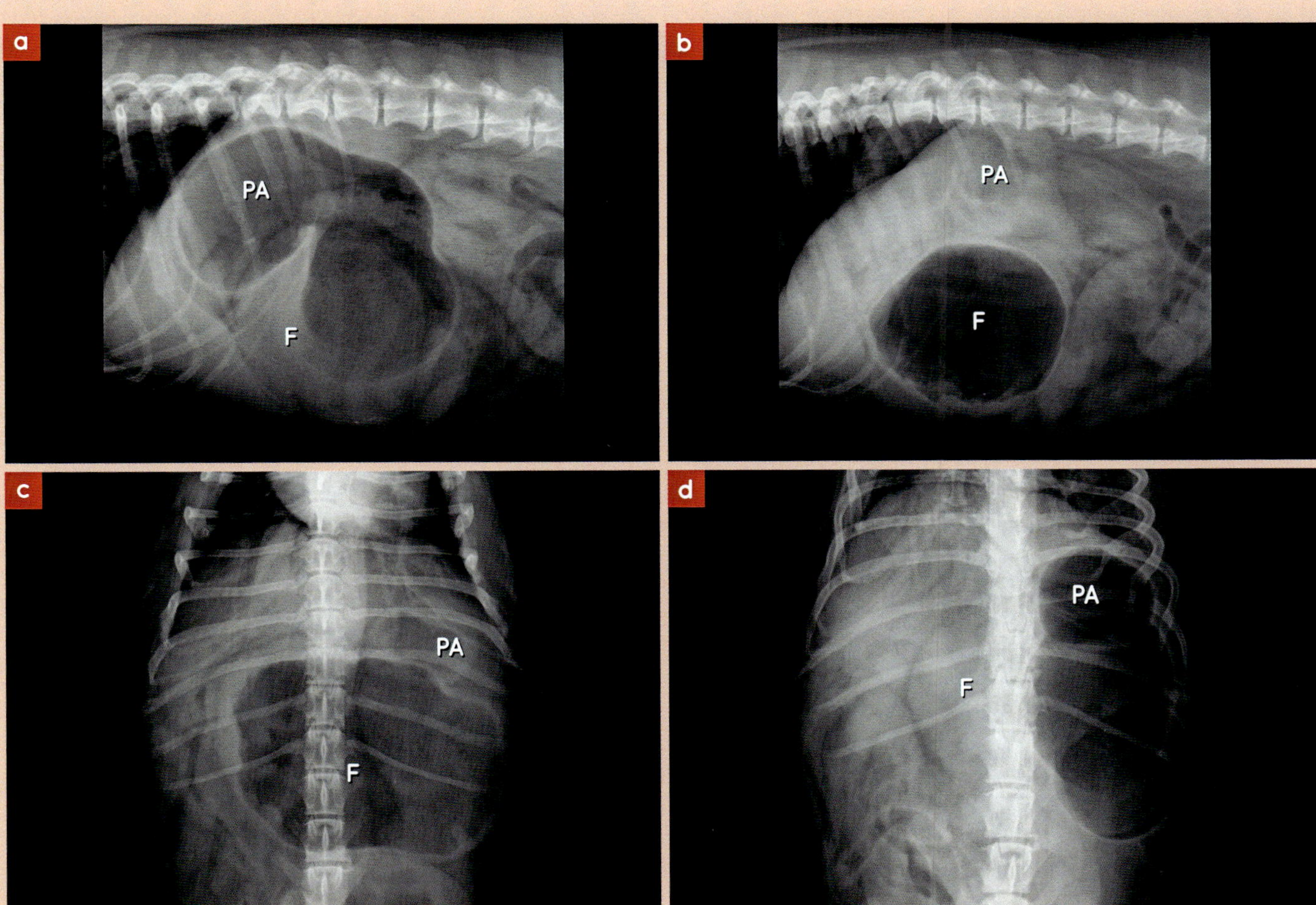

FIGURE 1.106. Enlarged images of the cranial abdomen on right lateral (a), left lateral (b), ventrodorsal (c) and dorsoventral (d) radiographs of a dog with gastric torsion. On the lateral views, the pyloric antrum (PA) is located dorsal and the fundus (F) ventral, and on the ventrodorsal and dorsoventral views the pyloric antrum is located on the left and the fundus on the right, as opposed to what occurs in normal conditions. In a healthy dog, the gas is displaced to the fundus and the fluid content to the pyloric antrum on right lateral views, while on left lateral views the gas accumulates in the antrum and the fluids do so in the fundus. The opposite occurs in this patient due to gastric rotation. In a similar way, when the stomach has a normal position, the gas accumulates in the antrum and part of the body of the stomach and the fluids are displaced towards the fundus on ventrodorsal views, while on dorsoventral views, the gas would be located in the fundus and the fluids in part of the body of the stomach and antrum. In this patient, these relationships are inverted due to the torsion.

the wall. These processes generally do not cause any evident alteration in the radiographic image of the stomach and ultrasonography or endoscopy are more useful diagnostic techniques. We should insist on the fact that an image with prominent gastric folds does not necessarily indicate inflammation of the wall, since the same image may be observed in a healthy animal due to the presence of fluid or mucus between the folds of the stomach. In uraemic gastritis, calcification of the gastric mucosa, which is sometimes radiographically identified, may occur (fig. 1.109).

Small intestine

Plain radiographs allow the assessment of the outline, size, position, shape and radiopacity of the intestine, but contrast studies or ultrasound scans are required to examine the alterations of the wall, as well as peristalsis or abnormal transit times.

Various references for the normal diameter of the small intestine in dogs have been published (fig. 1.10):

- It should not exceed twice the width of a rib.
- It should not exceed the height of the central part of the body of L2.

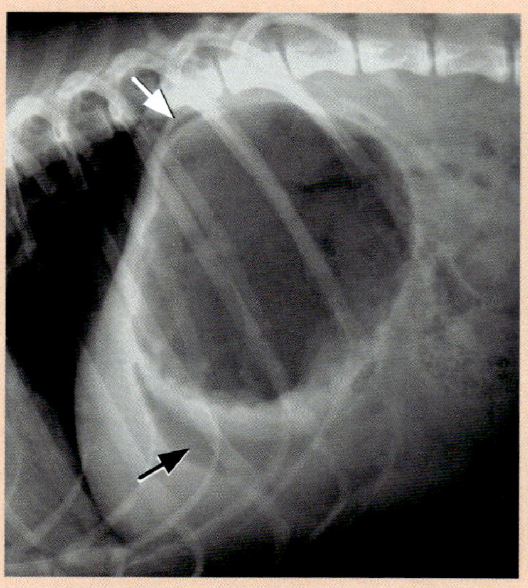

FIGURE 1.107. Enlarged image of the cranial abdomen on a lateral radiograph of a dog with gastric perforation. The amount of free peritoneal gas is small and this essentially accumulates in the area ventral to the stomach (black arrow), which may be mistaken for an accumulation of fat. The identification of the diaphragm (white arrow), which is possible due to the presence of a minimal amount of gas between the diaphragm and the liver, confirms the diagnosis of pneumoperitoneum. A gastrogram with iodinated contrast media is necessary to confirm that this gas comes from the stomach.

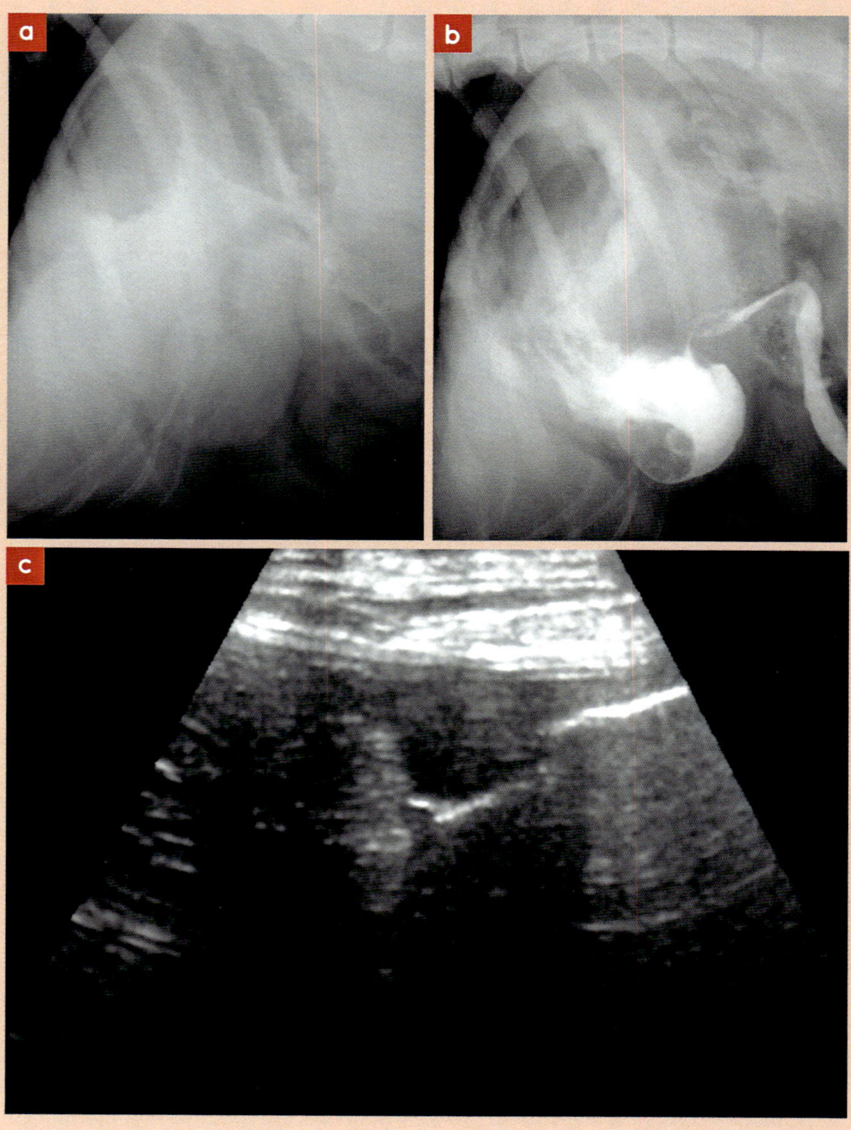

FIGURE 1.108. Enlarged images of the cranial abdomen on lateral radiographs, before (a) and after (b) the administration of barium (lower dose than the standard one so as not to mask the lesion) to a dog with a gastric neoplasm. The mass creates a filling defect in the pyloric antrum. (c) Ultrasound image of the mass.

- The ratio between the maximum diameter of the small intestine and the minimum height of the body of L5 should not exceed 1.6.

Normal radiographic anatomy of the abdomen
lateral view

http://goo.gl/hnl420

In cats, the diameter of the small intestine should not exceed 12 mm or two or three times the height of the central part of the body of L4 (fig. 1.111).

The width of the duodenum may slightly exceed these limits in normal conditions, since its diameter is slightly greater than that of the jejunum and ileum.

It is not possible to appropriately evaluate the thickness of the intestinal wall on a plain radiograph, as we may mistake it for the wall plus intraluminal fluid/mucus (fig. 1.112), which may lead to an incorrect diagnosis of increased thickness (fig. 1.113). The real thickness of the intestinal wall is best observed directly by means of ultrasonography.

Nowadays, the administration of a contrast medium will be necessary to evaluate the intestines only

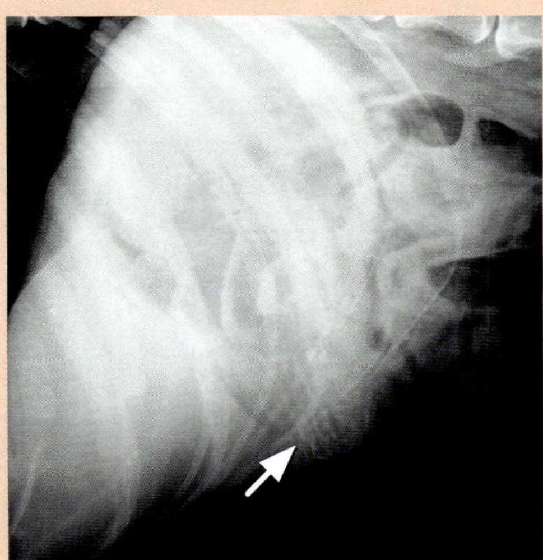

FIGURE 1.109. Enlarged image in lateral projection of the cranial abdomen of a dog with calcification of the gastric mucosa in the area of the pyloric antrum (arrow). This finding often appears associated to uraemic gastritis.

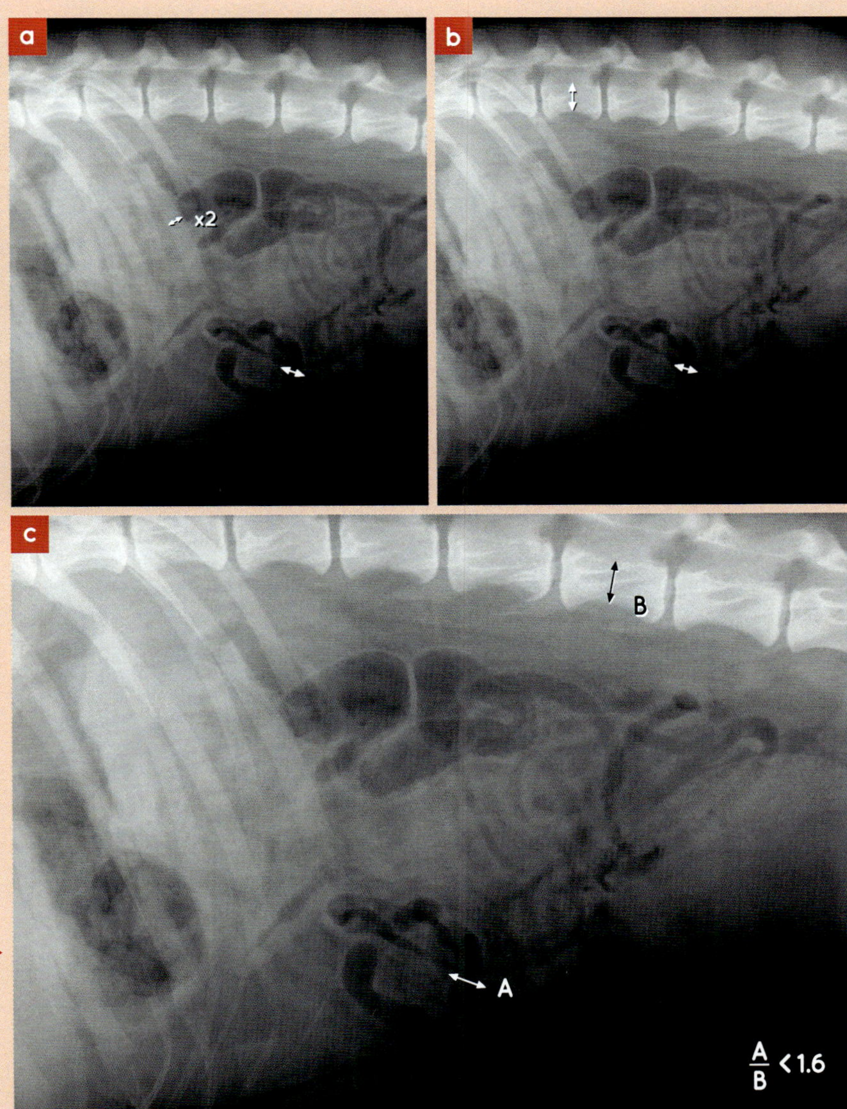

FIGURE 1.110. References of the normal diameter of the small intestine on lateral radiographs of the abdomen in the dog: it should not exceed the width of a rib (a); it should not exceed the height of the central part of the body of L2 (b); the ratio between the maximum diameter of the small intestine (A) and the minimum height of the body of L5 (B) should not exceed 1.6 (c).

on a few occasions. It is recommended to prepare the animal prior to the contrast study (no food for 24 hours and administration of an enema 2 to 4 hours before the test). Barium sulphate in suspension (in the form of micropulverised or liquid preparations) is the contrast medium of choice in most cases. A dose of 6-12 ml/kg at a concentration of 20 % in dogs and 12-16 ml/kg in cats is recommended. The administration of an inappropriate dose is one of the most common cases of non-diagnostic contrast studies.

Lateral and ventrodorsal radiographs are taken every 10 to 30 minutes, depending on the speed of transit of the contrast medium, until this latter reaches the colon. It is convenient to take a radiograph 24 hours later to rule out any abnormal retentions of the contrast material in the small intestine. The normal transit time varies from 2 to 4 hours in dogs and is approximately 1 hour in cats.

Iodinated contrast media are usually used when a perforation is suspected or when a faster transit time is required. Hyperosmotic contrast agents attract fluids towards the lumen of the intestine, are diluted and progress faster than barium, but offer images with a poorer diagnostic quality (fig. 1.114) and may cause transient dehydration of the patient. They are administered in doses of 2-3 ml/kg in dogs and 2 ml/kg in cats. Low-osmolarity iodinated contrast agents, such as iohexol or iopamidol, also progress faster through the intestine, but attract fewer fluids to the lumen. The diagnostic quality of the study is therefore improved (although it cannot be compared to that of barium studies) and their use is more recommended in very sick animals. They may be diluted at 1:2 in water and 10 ml/kg of the mixture may be administered both in dogs and cats.

The use of barium-impregnated polyethylene spheres to detect alterations of the intestinal transit has also been described. They are presented in two sizes: 1.5 mm and 5 mm of diameter. The smaller ones have a similar intestinal transit time to that of food, while the larger ones are designed to remain trapped in the area immediately anterior to an obstructive lesion.

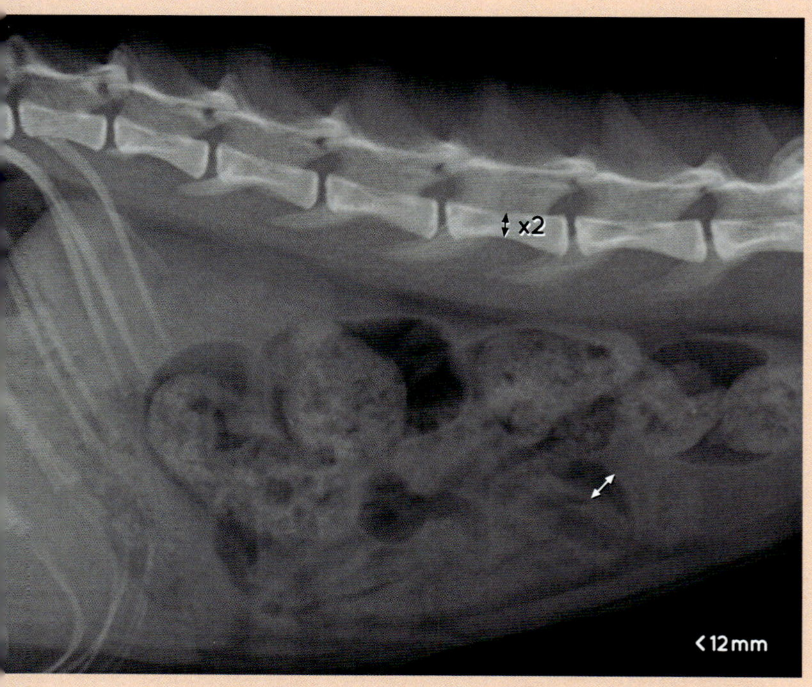

FIGURE 1.111. References of the normal diameter of the small intestine on lateral radiographs of the abdomen in a cat: it should not exceed twice the height of the central part of the body of L4 or it should be less than 12 mm in the image.

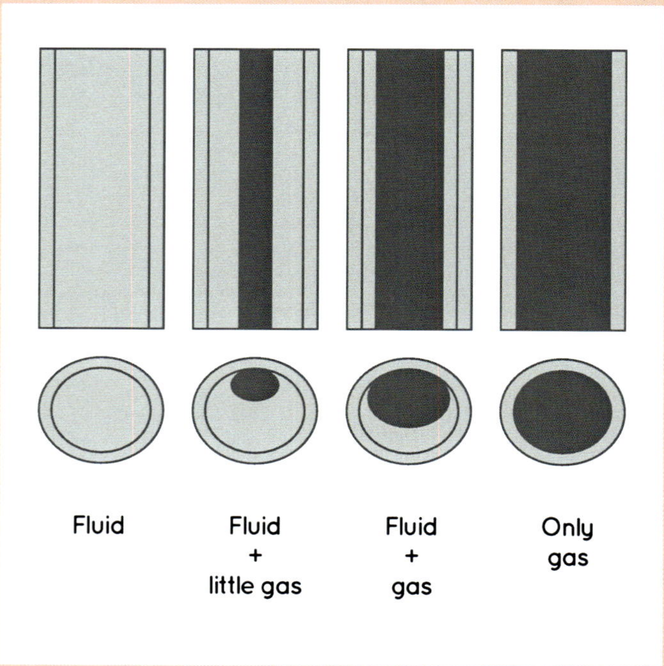

FIGURE 1.112. Diagram representing the radiographic image of the small intestine depending on its intraluminal content. It is not possible to evaluate the thickness of the intestinal wall on a radiograph, since the fluid/mucous content has the same radiopacity and cannot be differentiated from the wall, thus creating a false appearance of increased thickness of the wall.

The lack of passage of luminal content through the intestinal tract is termed **ileus**, and is radiographically characterised by an image of intestinal dilatation. Different patterns of intestinal dilatation may be observed:

- **Mild focal dilatation**: 1 to 3 affected loops and luminal distension of 1.5 to 2 times the normal diameter (fig. 1.115).
- **Severe focal dilatation**: 1 to 3 affected loops and luminal distension greater than twice the normal diameter (fig. 1.116).
- **Mild generalised dilatation**: great number of affected loops and luminal distension of 1.5 to 2 times the normal diameter (fig. 1.117).
- **Severe generalised dilatation:** great number of affected loops and luminal distension greater than twice the normal diameter (fig. 1.118).

An ileus may be mechanical, when it is due to a physical obstruction of the lumen of the intestine, or functional (paralytic ileus), when the peristaltic contractions of the intestine stop due to vascular or neuromuscular anomalies in the intestinal wall.

In a mechanical ileus, the physical obstruction of the intestinal lumen may be complete or partial. The most common causes of obstruction are large foreign bodies, intussusceptions and intestinal masses. A lesion that is extrinsic to the intestine may also cause a mechanical obstruction by external compression of an intestinal loop; adherences due to previous surgeries, hernias of the abdominal wall and, occasionally, masses that originated in other abdominal organs are included in the category.

The most indicative radiographic sign of mechanical obstruction is the dilatation of the intestinal loops anterior to the obstruction. The degree of dilatation of the loops is variable. The more complete an obstruction is, and the longer it lasts, the greater the degree of dilatation of the loops will be (fig. 1.119).

The more distal (along the small intestine) the obstruction is, and the more complete, the greater the number of dilated loops there will be.

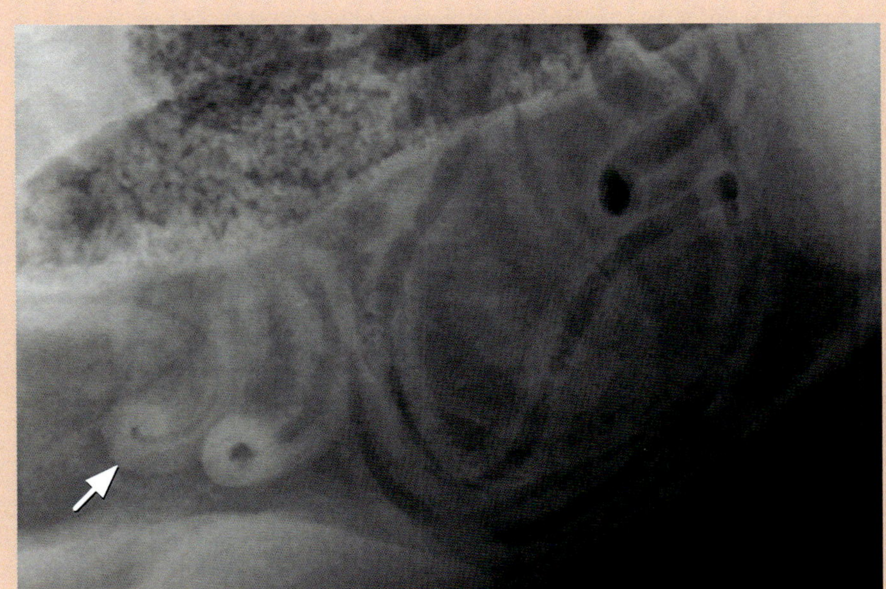

FIGURE 1.113. Very enlarged image of the central area of the abdomen on a lateral radiograph of a healthy dog. The intestinal segments that have a small amount of gas or a large amount of fluid/mucus in the lumen (arrow) have a false appearance of "thickened intestinal wall" on the radiograph. An ultrasound scan, on the other hand, does allow the examination of the real thickness of the wall.

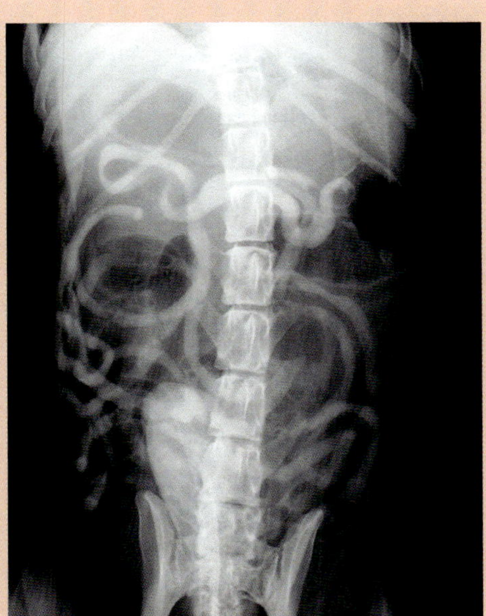

FIGURE 1.114. Ventrodorsal radiograph of the abdomen of a dog 45 minutes after the administration of an iodinated contrast medium by oral route. These contrast media are diluted with the fluid content of the small intestine and progress through it faster than barium. They are therefore only used when a perforation is suspected or when there is a real interest in a faster transit, although a good detailed image of the intestinal mucosa is not obtained.

Thus, partial obstructions create less evident alterations on plain radiographs (fig. 1.120), especially if they are recent or if they are located in proximal segments of the small intestine. The "gravel sign" may appear due to an accumulation of granular material at a site anterior to a point of obstruction. When the obstruction is complete, the segment of small intestine that is distal to the point of obstruction is usually empty.

As a reference to assess a possible obstruction, it is considered that a value above 1.6 times the ratio between the diameter of the intestine and the minimum height of the body of the L5 vertebra is indicative of an intestinal obstruction in dogs.

When the clinical and radiographic findings are indicative of a mechanical obstruction of the intestine, it is recommended to carry out an ultrasound study of

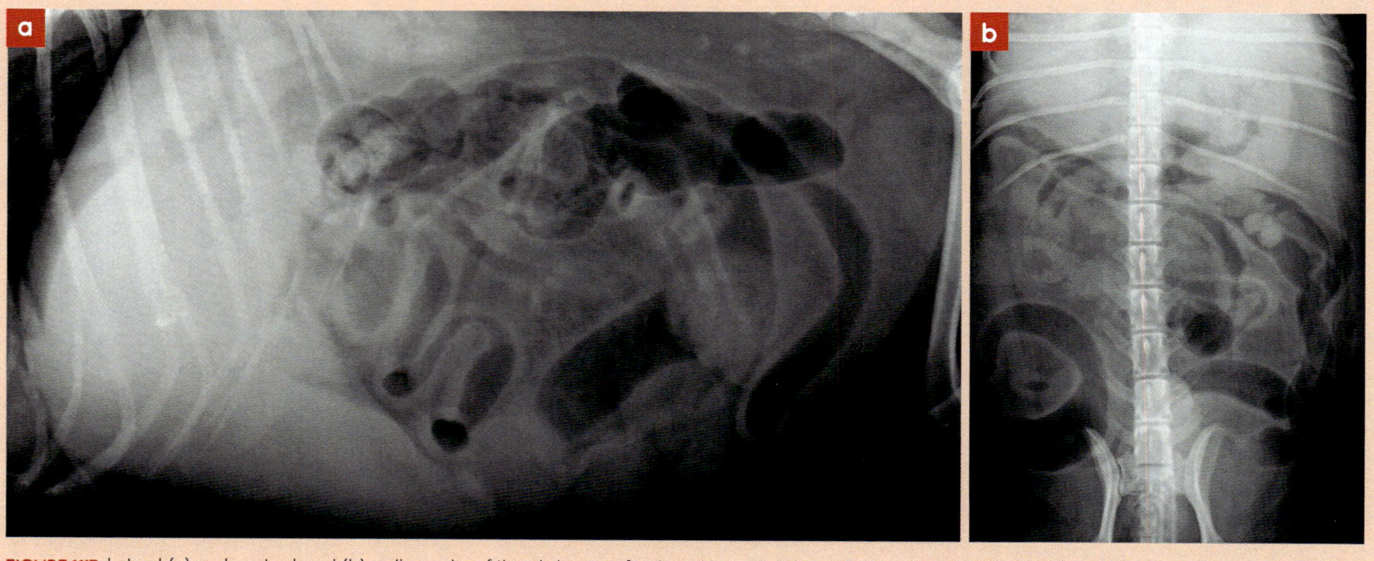

FIGURE 1.115. Lateral (a) and ventrodorsal (b) radiographs of the abdomen of a dog with a mild (1.5 to 2 times the normal diameter) focal intestinal dilatation (1 to 3 dilated loops). This pattern is indicative of a partial obstruction or of a recent complete obstruction in proximal segments of the small intestine.

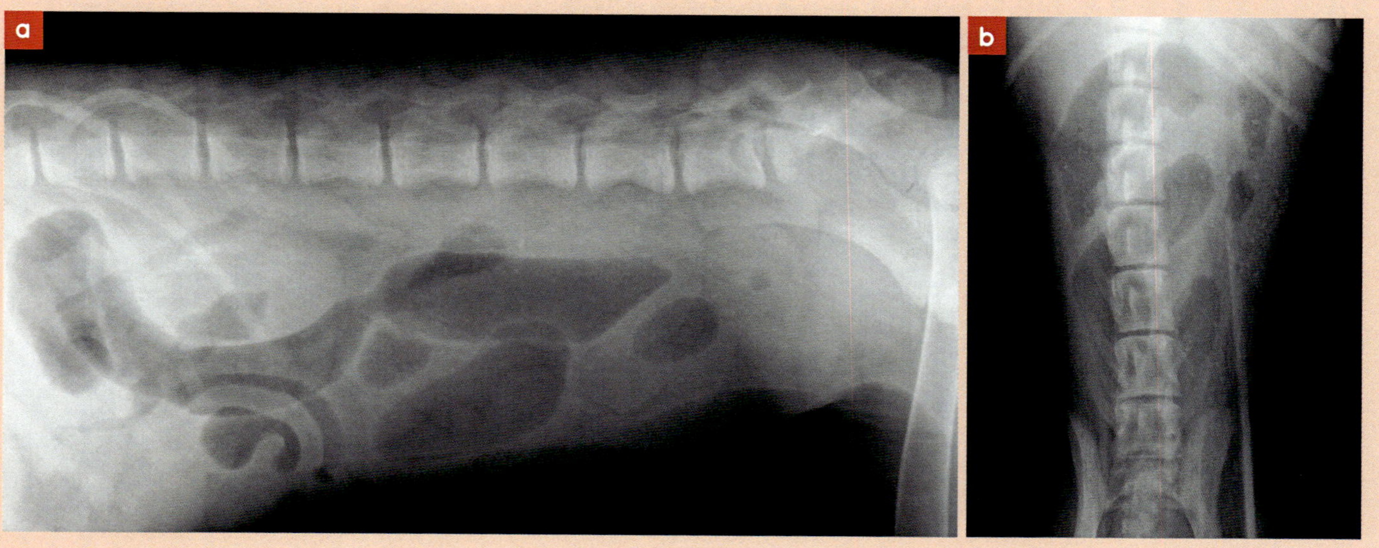

FIGURE 1.116. Lateral (a) and ventrodorsal (b) radiographs of the abdomen of a dog with a severe (more than twice the normal diameter) focal intestinal dilatation (1 to 3 dilated loops). This pattern is indicative of a complete obstruction in proximal segments of the small intestine, recent complete obstruction in any segment of the intestine, or chronic partial obstruction.

the abdomen, since it will often allow the determination of the cause of the obstruction. If the ultrasound scan is not conclusive and the suspicion is maintained, a contrast study or an exploratory laparotomy will then be indicated.

In a functional ileus, the peristaltic contractions of the intestine stop due to vascular or neuromuscular anomalies and the lumen dilates, although it is still permeable.

Normal radiographic anatomy of the abdomen
lateral view

http://goo.gl/hnl420

A functional ileus may be secondary to different processes, such as peritonitis, pancreatitis, a recent abdominal surgery, severe viral enteritis and diseases of the autonomic nervous system, among others (fig. 1.121).

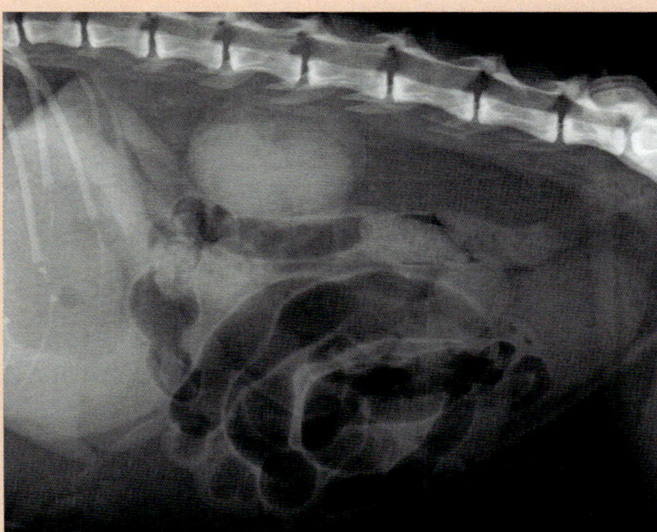

FIGURE 1.117. Lateral radiograph of the abdomen of a cat with mild (1.5 to 2 times the normal diameter) generalised intestinal dilatation (elevated number of dilated loops). This pattern is indicative of a partial or recent complete obstruction in distal segments of the small intestine or functional ileus.

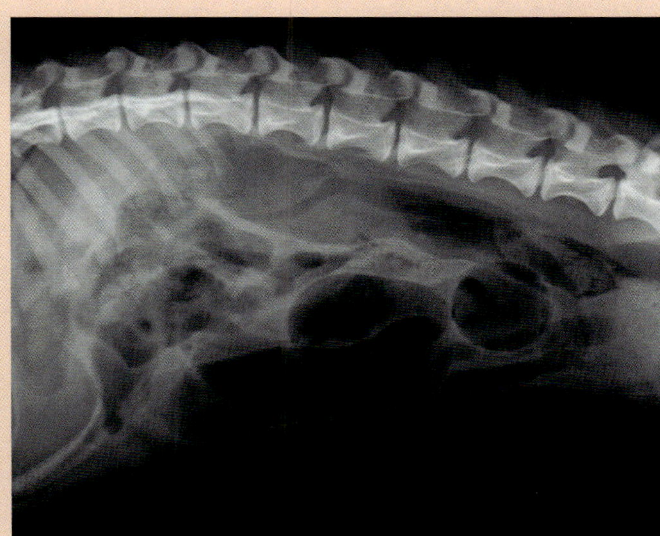

FIGURE 1.118. Lateral radiograph of the abdomen of a dog with severe (more than twice the normal diameter) generalised intestinal dilatation (elevated number of dilated loops). This pattern is indicative of a complete or chronic partial obstruction in distal segments of the small intestine.

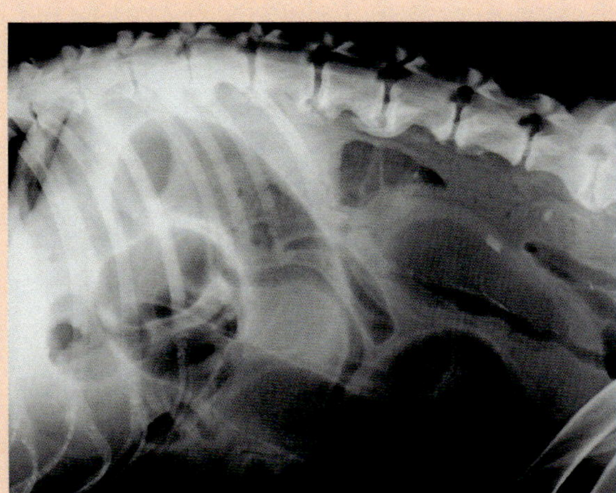

FIGURE 1.119. Lateral radiograph of the abdomen of a dog with a complete obstruction of the small intestine after several days of evolution.

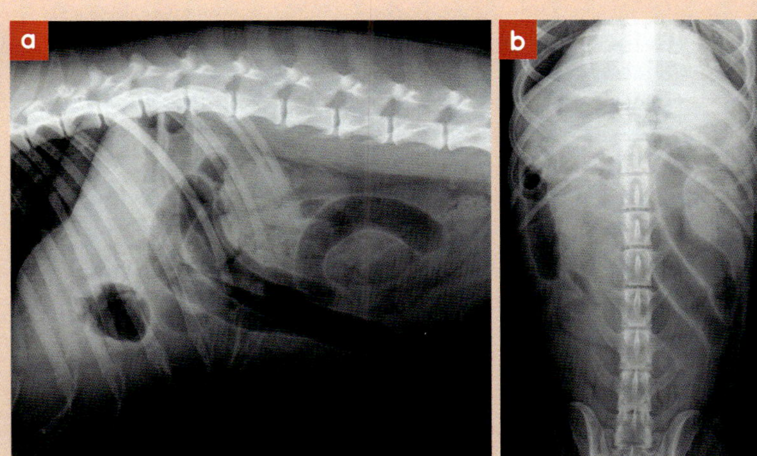

FIGURE 1.120. Lateral (a) and ventrodorsal (b) radiographs of the abdomen of a dog with a chronic partial obstruction in distal segments of the small intestine.

It is often not possible to differentiate intestinal dilatation caused by a functional ileus from that caused by a mechanical ileus on plain radiographs. The affected length of the intestine may provide some information in this sense, since localised dilatations are more likely to be due to mechanical causes while generalised dilatations are more likely to be caused by a functional ileus, although it is not always the case. In fact, moderate to severe chronic mechanical obstructions may lead to a functional ileus.

Radiopaque **foreign bodies** are easily recognised on plain radiographs (fig. 1.122). On the other hand, those objects with a similar radiopacity to that of fluid/mucus and soft tissues (radiolucent) may not be identified on plain radiographs, although intestinal dilatation will be observed depending on the degree of mechanical obstruction they cause. Ultrasound examinations or contrast studies may offer a more precise diagnosis in this aspect. If the foreign body is fenestrated or absorbent, barium may go through it or be retained, thus causing a mottled or linear pattern of opacification (fig. 1.123). If it is not fenestrated or absorbent, the object may stop the transit of barium (fig. 1.124) or create a filling defect in the contrast column.

Linear foreign bodies (e.g. shoelaces, threads, etc.) create a relatively characteristic radiographic image. Part of the object often remains in the stomach (or

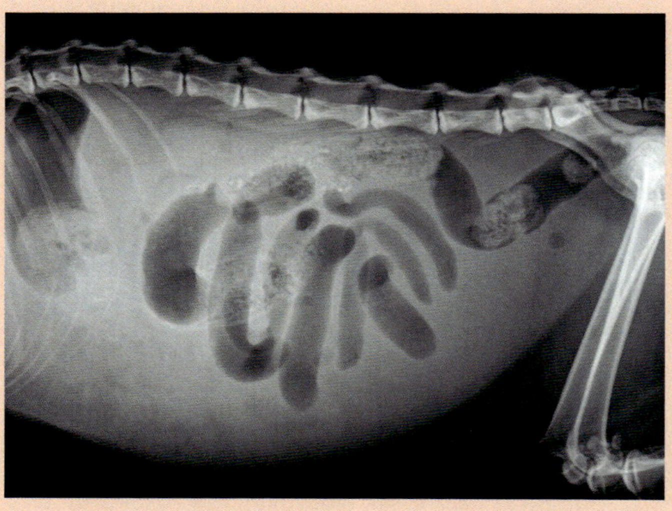

FIGURE 1.121. Lateral radiograph of the abdomen of a cat with a functional ileus secondary to a peritonitis.

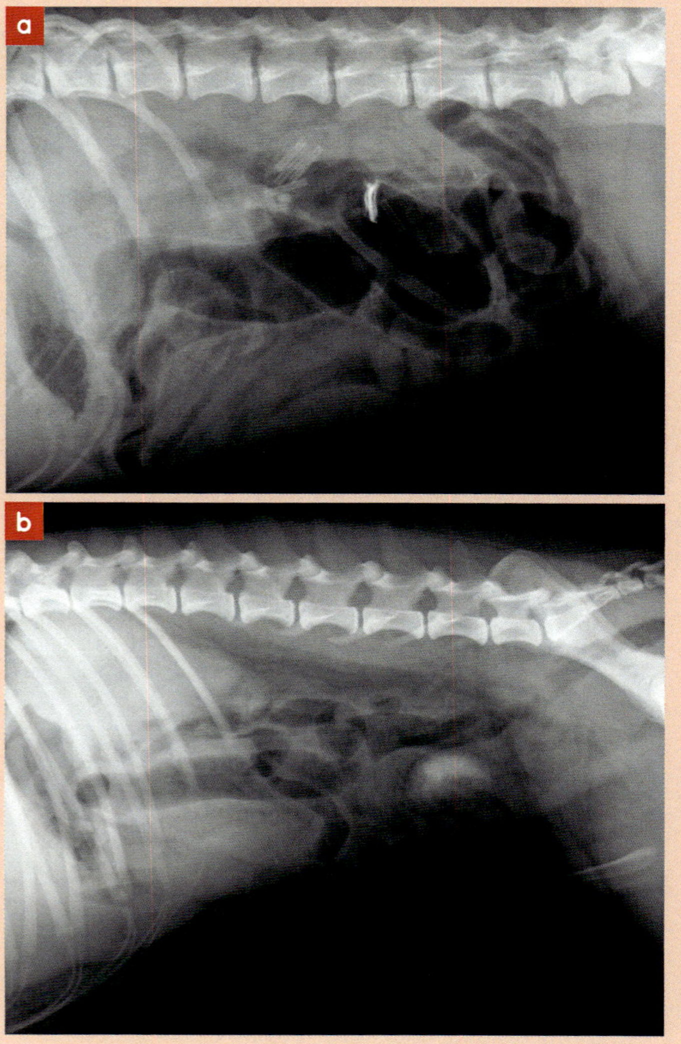

FIGURE 1.122. Lateral radiographs of the abdomen of two dogs with radiopaque foreign bodies in the small intestine. (a) Remnants of plastic tubes. (b) Crushed ball. Signs of intestinal obstruction are observed in both cases.

even in the oesophagus or mouth) while the rest is located in the small intestine. This latter appears pleated in the image, with focal retention of small amounts of gas (gas pockets) between the folds (fig. 1.125). The image of intestinal pleating may be more evident in the contrast study (fig. 1.126) and is also observed by means of ultrasonography.

Invaginations or intussusceptions usually cause severe intestinal dilatation, although in most patients it is not possible to differentiate an invagination from other causes of mechanical obstruction (fig. 1.127) only with plain radiography. The ultrasound diagnosis of an invagination is relatively easy and in most cases, radiographic contrast studies are excluded, as the image may vary in function of the degree of permeability of the *intussusceptum* (invaginated part of the intestine), and of the space between the *intussusceptum* and the *intussuscipiens* (part of the intestine containing the invaginated part).

The **masses** that originate on the intestinal wall include tumours, polyps or granulomatous infiltrates. The development of an obstructive intestinal pattern due to these lesions depends on their size, of whether they grow towards the lumen of the intestine or outside it (fig. 1.128). With time, most of them, which initially do not cause any obstruction, evolve and cause a partial and then complete obstruction. They are usually detected clinically in the phase of partial obstruction,

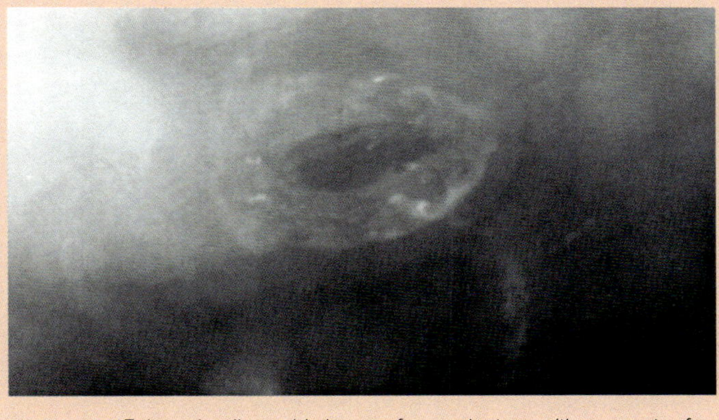

FIGURE 1.123. Enlarged radiographic image of a peach stone with remnants of barium in its structure.

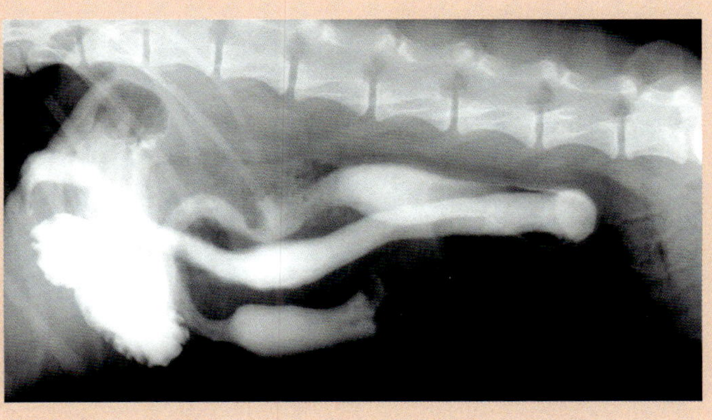

FIGURE 1.124. Lateral abdominal radiograph of a dog with a complete obstruction caused by a foreign body, 30 minutes after the administration of barium. The object causes a sudden interruption of the contrast column.

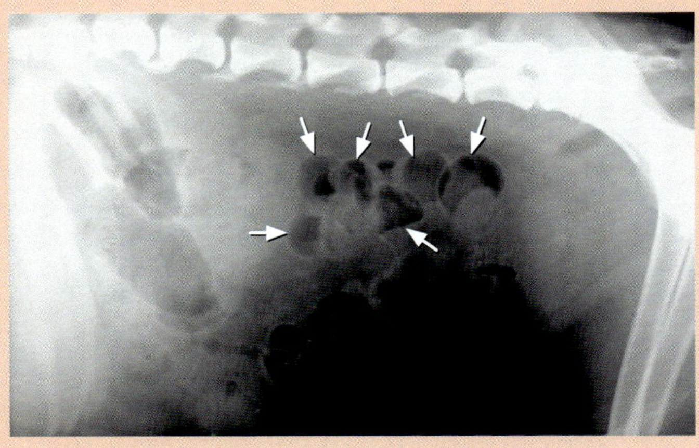

FIGURE 1.125. Lateral abdominal radiograph of a dog with a linear foreign body in the small intestine. The folded intestinal wall causes the retention of gas between the folds (gas pockets, arrows). Bladder lithiasis is also observed.

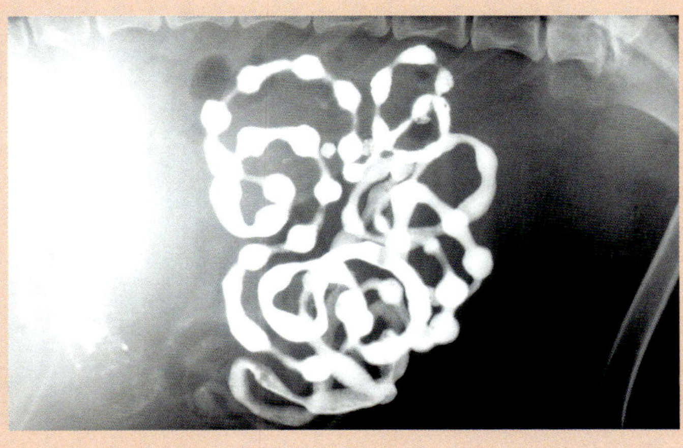

FIGURE 1.126. Lateral abdominal radiograph of a dog, with a linear foreign body in the small intestine, 45 minutes after the administration of barium. The folded intestinal wall causes a "string of pearls" appearance. This type of image may also be found in the duodenum of healthy cats due to peristaltic waves (see chapter Most common diagnostic errors).

Normal radiographic anatomy of the abdomen **ventrodorsal view**

http://goo.gl/6p7452

with mild to severe focal distension. These lesions are better identified if an ultrasound scan is performed or, alternatively, a contrast study, in which an image of a filling defect or luminal narrowing associated or not with multiple marks in the barium column ("apple core" appearance) may appear.

Diffuse infiltrative diseases of the intestinal wall (intestinal inflammatory disease, inflammation of infectious origin and some types of neoplasia) may cause an abnormal gas density pattern with or without intestinal dilatation, although radiography will often not reveal any significant findings. An ultrasound examination is much more appropriate to evaluate this type of disease.

Large intestine

Plain and contrast radiographs have traditionally been used to evaluate the diseases of the large intestine. Nowadays, endoscopy has replaced contrast radiography of the colon to a large extent, especially when a flexible endoscope, which can reach the transverse colon, ascending colon and caecum, is available. Ultrasonography also provides useful diagnostic information, in particular regarding alterations of the wall, excluding the rectum due to its intrapelvic location. Computed tomography and magnetic resonance imaging may have a great interest for the examination of rectal diseases, since they offer images with excellent anatomical detail of the whole pelvic region.

The large intestine is easily identified on plain radiographs because it usually contains faeces and gas, which have a radiographic density that contrasts with the surrounding structures. The colon has a similar shape to that of a question mark (fig. 1.129). The canine caecum is semicircular ("C" or spiral shape), is compartmented and usually contains a certain amount of intraluminal gas. This gas and its characteristic shape make the caecum easy to recognise in the right middle abdomen on most plain radiographs (fig. 1.130). The feline caecum is a short diverticulum, with no compartments, which rarely contains gas, so it is not usually identified on radiographs.

The diameter of the normal colon varies depending on the amount of faeces it contains and on the defecation habits of each individual. As a general rule, the diameter of the normal colon should be smaller than the length of L7 in dogs, while the maximum diameter of the colon does not exceed 2.2 times the diameter of the small intestine or 2.8 times the height of the cranial end of L2 in cats.

A more exhaustive assessment of the large intestine requires a contrast study using barium sulphate in suspension (barium enema), gas (pneumocolon) or a combination of both (double-contrast enema). The most commonly used technique is barium enema. Nowadays, a barium enema would be indicated in the following cases:

- When a narrowing of the lumen hinders the passage of an endoscope.
- If the limitations of the endoscope itself do not allow a complete examination of the colon and caecum.
- When a parietal or extraparietal lesion is suspected and the mucosa has a normal aspect in the endoscopic examination.

The animal that is going to undergo a contrast enema must not eat for 24 to 36 hours and should be administered laxatives by oral route and hot water enemas prior to the study. Plain radiographs will be taken before administering the contrast agent to adjust the exposure values and confirm that the patient has been properly prepared.

After anaesthetising the patient, barium is administered at room temperature through a catheter with an inflatable balloon, which is placed in the distal part of the rectum to avoid leakage of the contrast agent. Doses of 7 to 15 ml/kg of barium sulphate in suspension at a concentration of 20 % are usually used. If a perforation of the colon is suspected, barium should be replaced by an iodinated contrast medium, preferably of low osmolarity, at a concentration of 15 to 20 %, although the amount of detail of the mucosa will be significantly reduced.

The persistence of faecal material in the colon and rectum is termed faecal retention (fig. 131). If there is an accumulation of a great amount of faeces that acquire a very high radiopacity due to the continuous absorption of water from the content of the colon, we are dealing with a case of faecal **impaction** (fig. 1.132). A chronic impaction may cause a generalised increase of the size of the colon.

The presence of **foreign bodies** in the large intestine has a limited significance, since they rarely cause problems if they have not caused any when progressing through the small intestine (fig. 1.133). However, importance should be given to those that are sharp and may seriously damage the wall.

Inflammatory processes do not usually cause any radiographic alterations. They can usually be properly

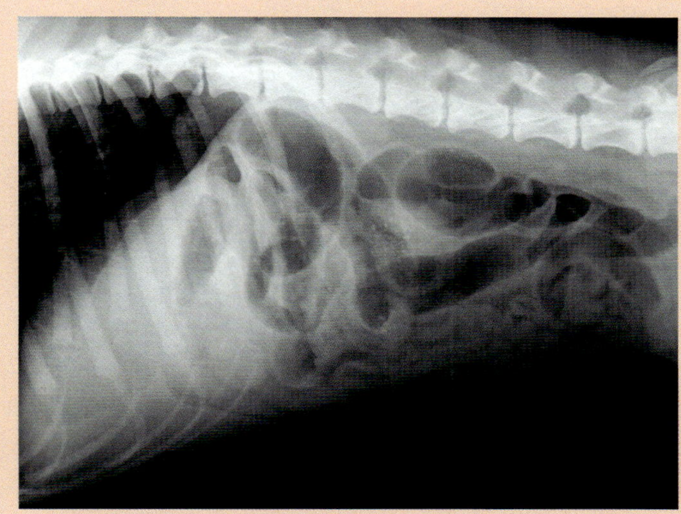

FIGURE 1.127. Lateral radiograph of the abdomen of a dog with an invagination in the small intestine. A pattern of severe focal intestinal dilatation may be observed.

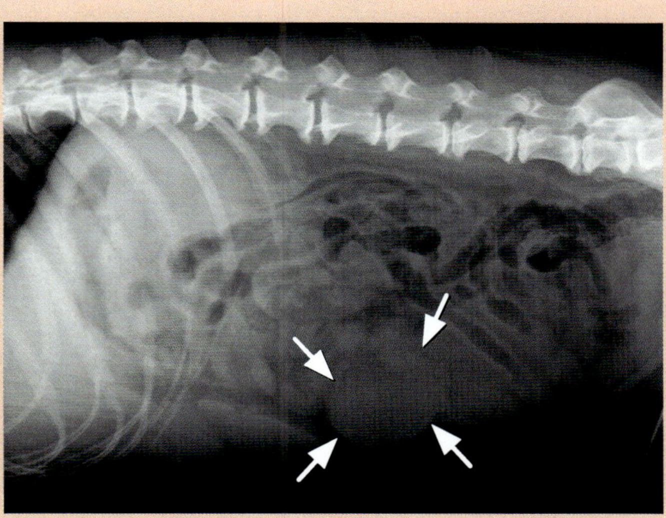

FIGURE 1.128. Lateral radiograph of the abdomen of a dog with a small-intestinal neoplasm (arrows).

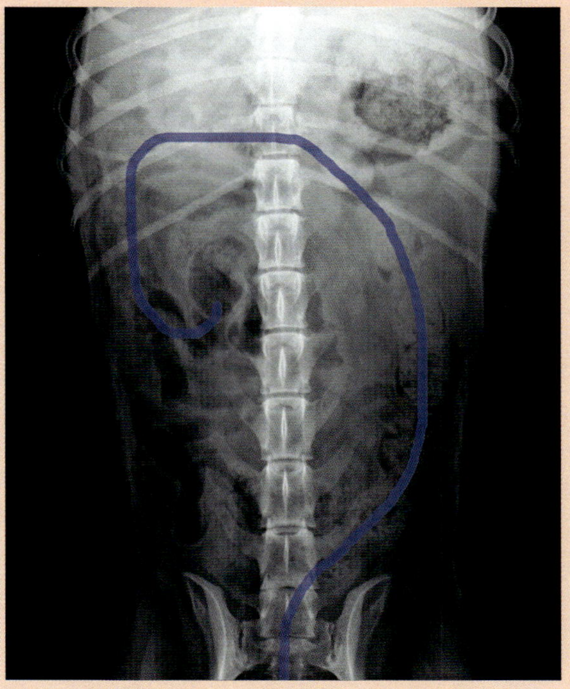

FIGURE 1.129. Ventrodorsal radiograph of the abdomen of a healthy dog. The large intestine has the shape of a question mark on this view.

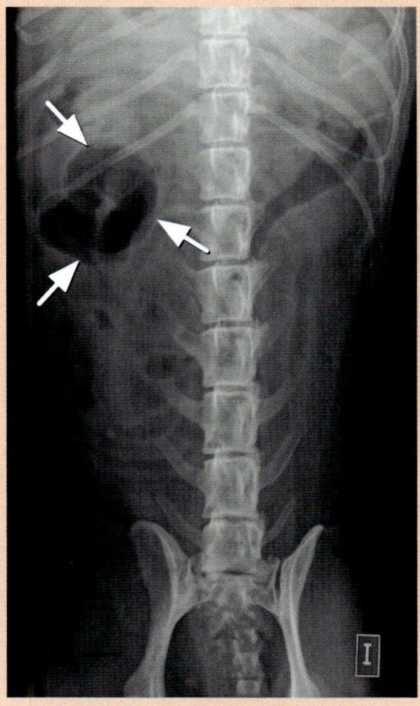

FIGURE 1.130. Ventrodorsal radiograph of the abdomen of a healthy dog. The caecum (arrows) often appears as a curved tubular structure filled with gas in the right cranial abdomen on radiographs. We should not confuse this image with an abnormal dilatation of the small intestine.

Normal radiographic anatomy of the abdomen
lateral view

http://goo.gl/hnl420

evaluated by means of ultrasonography, with the exception of the rectum due to its intrapelvic location.

In case of severe colitis (fig. 1.134), contrast studies may show irregularity and localised or generalised ulceration of the mucosa, narrowing of the lumen, thickening of the folds of the wall, diverticula and adherences.

Localised **dilatations** of the colon are usually due to faecal impactions (fig. 1.135.) or mechanical obstructions, caused for example by caecocolic or ileocolic intussusceptions, narrowing of the pelvic canal due to fractures, tumours of the colon or foreign bodies.

The colon may be generally dilated due to an excess of faecal content. If the dilatation is associated with hypomotility of the wall, it is then called megacolon. The most common causes of megacolon include chronic constipation and alterations of nutritional, metabolic, neurological or mechanical origin (foreign bodies, anorectal anomalies, perineal hernias, intrapelvic masses, etc.). Idiopathic megacolon, which is more frequent in cats (fig. 1.136), has also been described.

A localised **narrowing** of the lumen of the large intestine can be due to a spasm or stenosis caused by a neoplasm, chronic inflammation or scar tissue. As opposed to stenosis, a spasm is transient and is usually caused by an incorrect technique when performing the barium enema. Most cases of stenosis are caused by neoplasms (fig. 1.137), although adenomas, ulcerative colitis and eosinophilic colitis may show similar radiographic findings.

Colorectal **diverticula** are not very frequent and usually appear in senior male dogs with prostatic alteration and chronic constipation, or associated with perineal hernias. A localised accumulation of faeces may be observed on plain radiographs, while in contrast studies the contrast medium accumulates in a structure with a saccular morphology and smooth margin (fig. 1.138).

Vaginorectal, urethrorectal and rectocutaneous **fistulas**, which may have a congenital or acquired origin, have been described. If this type of lesions is suspected, it is recommended to perform the positive-contrast enema with iodinated contrast agents, which may show the communication between the colon and the vagina, urethra or skin.

Congenital anomalies of the large intestine are uncommon in dogs and cats. Anal perforation (fig. 1.139), atresia of the rectum, atresia of the colon, fistulas, diverticula, duplication of the large intestine or rectum, and a short colon and rectum with the caecum in the left hemiabdomen have been described.

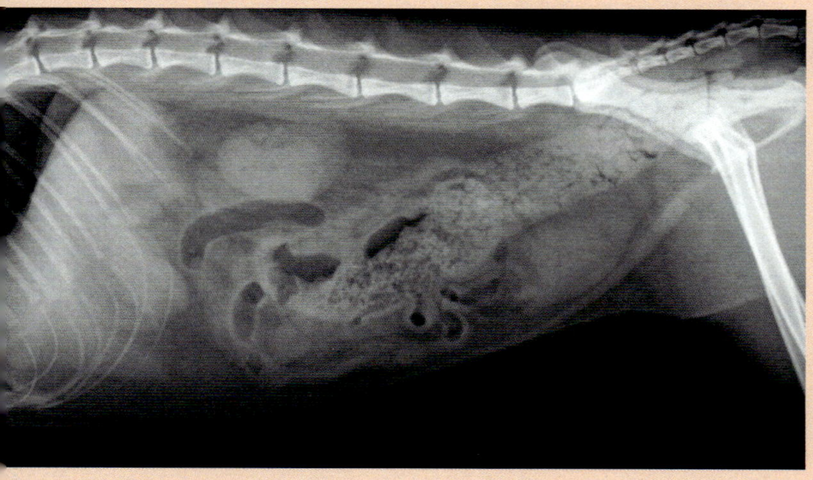

FIGURE 1.131. Lateral radiograph of the abdomen of a cat with faecal retention due to constipation.

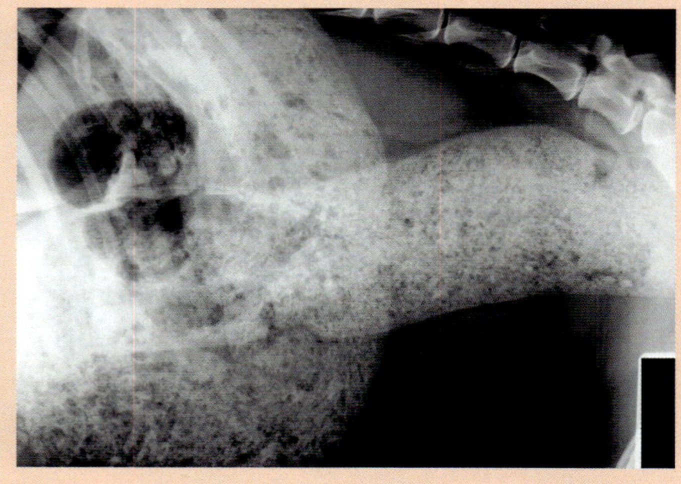

FIGURE 1.132. Lateral radiograph of the abdomen of a dog with faecal impaction. The large intestine appears very dilated (it occupies a great part of the abdomen) and filled with faecal material with a high radiopacity.

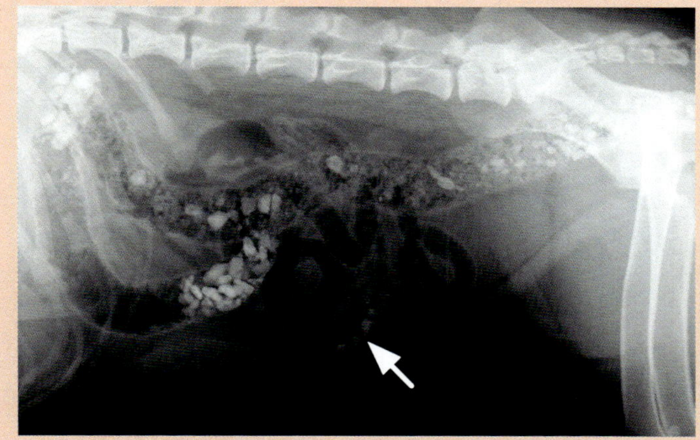

FIGURE 1.133. Lateral radiograph of the abdomen of a dog with foreign bodies (stones) in the large intestine. Most of the stones appear in different segments of the colon and a much more reduced number can be observed in the small intestine (arrow).

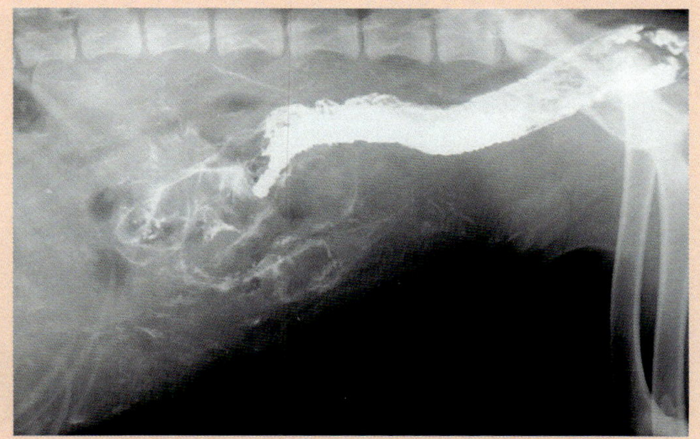

FIGURE 1.134. Lateral radiograph of the abdomen of a dog with severe colitis and peritonitis due to a perforation of the wall of the colon, after an enema with an iodinated contrast medium, which reveals its extravasation to the peritoneal cavity.

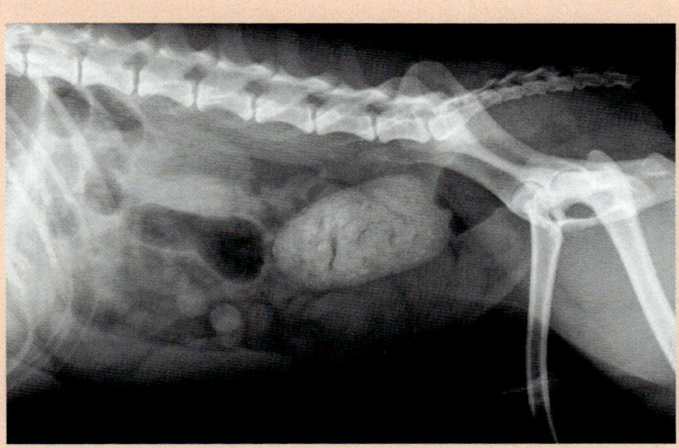

FIGURE 1.135. Lateral radiograph of the abdomen of a dog with focal dilatation of the central area of the descending colon due to the presence of a faecaloma.

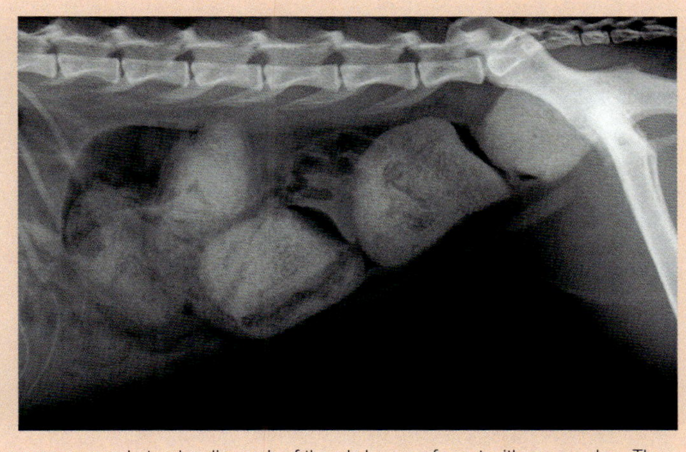

FIGURE 1.136. Lateral radiograph of the abdomen of a cat with megacolon. The colon is very dilated and accumulates a large amount of faeces with high radiopacity.

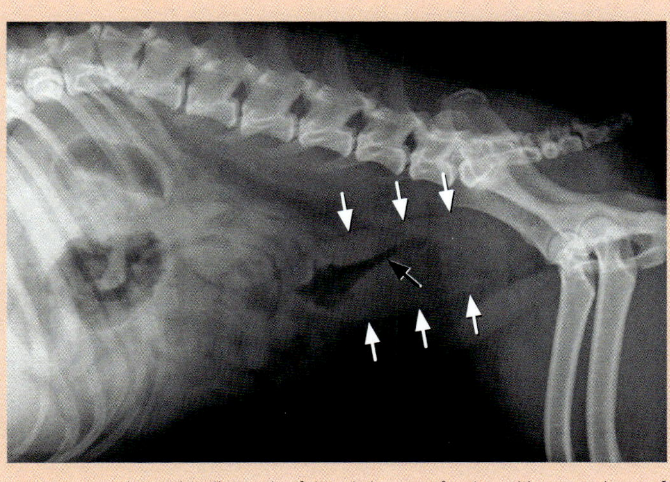

FIGURE 1.137. Lateral radiograph of the abdomen of a dog with a neoplasm of the colon. The external limits of the site of the tumour are marked with white arrows. The pattern of intraluminal gas (back arrow) is indicative of stenosis.

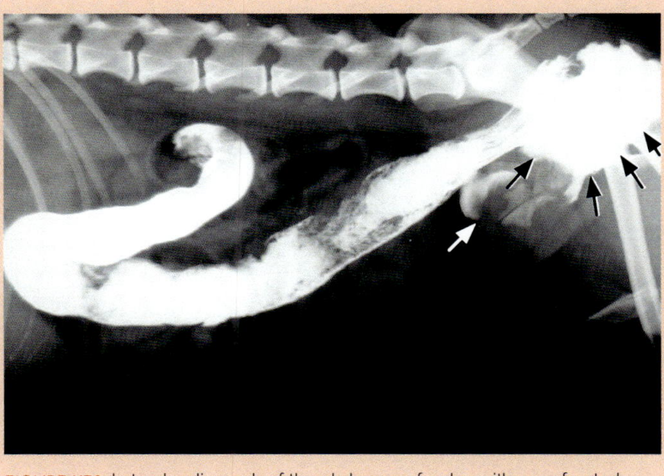

FIGURE 1.138. Lateral radiograph of the abdomen of a dog with a perforated rectal diverticulum (black arrows) after an enema with an iodinated contrast medium, which reveals its extravasation (white arrow) to the peritoneal cavity.

Self-assessment
cases

http://goo.gl/QPo4Zy

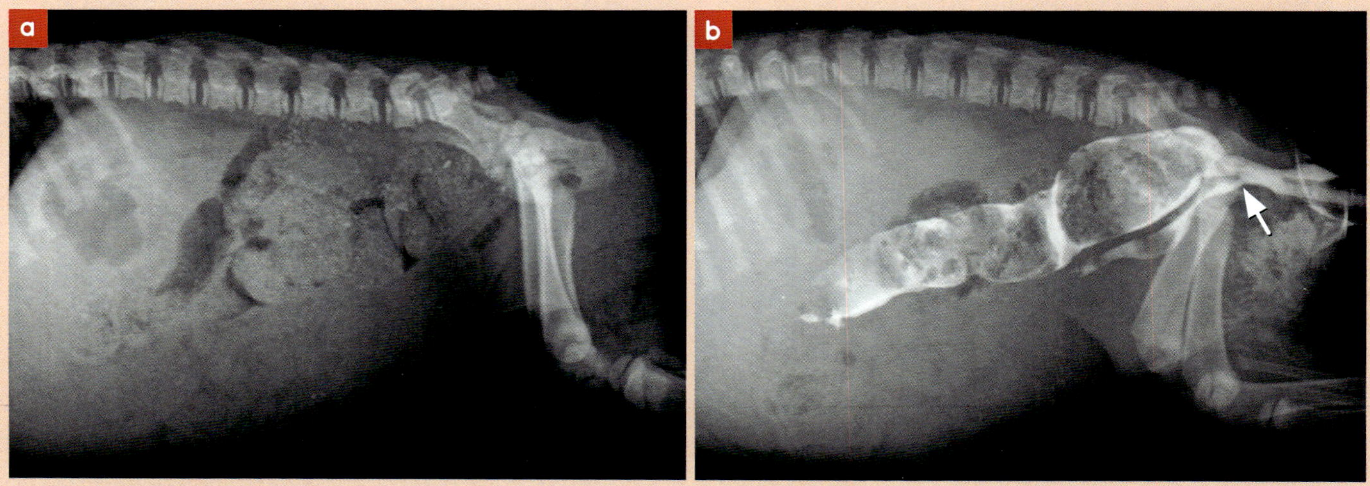

FIGURE 1139. Lateral radiograph of the abdomen of a 1.5 month-old dog with anal atresia and a congenital rectovaginal fistula, before (a) and after (b) an enema with an iodinated contrast agent, which reveals the communication (arrow) between the vagina and the rectum.

Neck and thorax 2

Principles of interpretation

Neck

Except in the case of the cervical spine, which is reviewed in chapter 4, radiographs of the neck provide a limited amount of information on the anatomical structures that form this part of the body. In normal conditions, it is possible identify the pharynx, larynx, cervical trachea, soft palate, epiglottis and hyoid bone. The other soft tissues (oesophagus, blood vessels, lymph nodes, muscles, salivary glands and thyroid and parathyroid glands) are not identified in normal radiographic images. The presence of a very small amount of air in the lumen of the cervical oesophagus is usually an incidental finding associated with aerophagia, although the persistence of this finding in repeated studies may be due to pathological alterations. The partial calcification of the cartilages of the larynx is very common and usually takes place at 2-3 years of age.

Lateral radiographs are most appropriate for the examination of soft tissues in the neck, since most of the identifiable structures are superimposed with the cervical spine on ventrodorsal and dorsoventral radiographs. However, it will sometimes be necessary to take two orthogonal radiographs, for example when a foreign body is identified on the lateral projection, since its exact location cannot be confirmed in any other way.

Other diagnostic techniques may provide much more information about this anatomical region. Ultrasound scans may be very useful for the assessment of the thyroid and parathyroid glands, larynx, salivary glands and masses in general, and they also allow the collection of samples for cytology or biopsy. Computed tomography and magnetic resonance imaging (MRI) are excellent for the examination of this region, although MRI is somewhat better than tomography due to its better definition of soft tissues.

Fluoroscopy, which offers real-time radiographic images, though with little anatomical detail, does not provide any morphological information comparable to that provided by the other diagnostic imaging techniques. Nonetheless, it has an important advantage over them for the assessment of alterations of deglutition, since it allows the direct visualisation of the passage of food from the mouth to the oropharynx and then to the oesophagus.

Thorax

Radiographs of the thorax are essential for the diagnosis of most of the diseases that affect this anatomical region. Although radiographic findings are often sufficient to establish a fairly precise diagnosis, the combination of radiography with other diagnostic imaging techniques, such as ultrasonography or computed tomography, guarantees in most cases an accurate diagnosis of the patient with a thoracic condition.

The main limiting factors in the interpretation of radiographs of the thorax are:

- The loss of information due to the superimposition of structures.
- The wide variety of anatomical conformations and physiological changes that affect the image of the thorax.
- The similarity between physiological and pathological images in some cases.
- The same appearance that very different diseases have on radiographs.

In dogs, the cardiac silhouette and the shadows of the mediastinum and diaphragm may greatly vary depending on the conformation of the thorax. Three types of conformation are basically identified (fig. 2.1):

- Narrow and deep thorax (e.g. Greyhound, Doberman, Collie).
- Intermediate conformation (e.g. German Shepherd, Labrador, Poodle).
- Wide and shallow thorax (e.g. Bulldog, Teckel, Basset Hound).

The conformation of the thorax is quite constant in cats and is similar to the intermediate conformation in dogs.

The thoracic vertebrae, thoracic inlet, sternum and shadow of the diaphragm should be included when taking a radiograph of the thorax. Apart from these structures, the trachea, mediastinum, aorta, caudal vena cava, cardiac silhouette and lung fields may also be visualised in the image. It is recommended to follow a systemic order of assessment and, whenever possible, to carefully examine each of these elements in two orthogonal views, which should include a lateral view and a dorsoventral or ventrodorsal view.

Depending on the reason why the radiographic study is carried out, the projections should be chosen taking the following criteria into account:

- **Assessment of the cardiac silhouette:** the right lateral and dorsoventral projections are used, since they provide a more real image of the silhouette. The silhouette appears falsely round on left lateral radiographs. On ventrodorsal views, the heart is located farther away from the cassette than on a dorsoventral view, so the silhouette appears slightly distorted.
- **Assessment of the lungs:** lateral (generally right) and ventrodorsal projections are used. In order to correctly assess the lung parenchyma, it is better if this is filled with as much air as possible (there will be a greater contrast with the structures that have different radiographic densities), so we will preferably take a ventrodorsal radiograph, as the capacity of distension of the lungs is greater when the animal is placed in dorsal recumbency than in sternal recumbency.
- **Assessment of pulmonary metastases:** the two lateral projections, right and left, are used. When placing the animal in lateral recumbency, the lung that is lower (closer to the cassette) is partially collapsed, as its expansion capacity is limited. On the other hand, the other lung is normally filled with air. If soft-tissue density nodules appear in the lung parenchyma, these would be easier to differentiate in a fully distended lung than in a slightly collapsed lung. That is why the presence of metastases is assessed with a right lateral radiograph, which offers a better image of the left lung, and a left lateral radiograph, which allows a better examination of the right lung. When suspicious images appear on these projections, it is recommended to complete the study with a ventrodorsal radiograph.
- If the animal presents with **severe dyspnoea**, taking standard radiographs may lead to significant respiratory distress. In these cases, it would be recommendable to take radiographs with the animal standing, although not all machines allow the placement of the X-ray tube in horizontal position so as to take this type of radiographs. If this cannot be done, the dorsoventral projection should be chosen ahead of the ventrodorsal and lateral ones, as there is a smaller risk of respiratory distress for the animal.
- Oblique radiographs centred on the lesion may be useful to evaluate **lesions of the thoracic wall**, e.g. rib tumours.

It is very important to pay maximum attention to the technical quality of radiographs of the thoracic wall. The use of incorrect exposure values, a poor positioning of the patients, or a poor developing technique may greatly affect the interpretation of the images.

Generally, a high kilovoltage and low milliamperage should be used so as to reduce the time of exposure and minimise the influence of respiratory movements on the images. If too low exposure values are used (underexposed radiographs), the radiographic image will be clearer than expected, while if the exposure values are too high (overexposed radiograph), the image will be darker. In both cases the image of the lung will be particularly affected and these variations may even be mistaken for pathological alterations. The use of an anti-scatter grid (either stationary or Potter-Bucky) is necessary when the height of the thorax, once placed on the cassette, exceeds 10 cm.

Although it is difficult in practice, chest radiographs should ideally be taken at maximum inspiration. The greater the amount of air in the lungs, the easier it will be to identify small lesions in these organs on the radiograph. If the radiograph is taken in expiration, the cardiac silhouette will look larger and will be in contact or superimposed with the shadow of the diaphragm, and the lungs will have a higher radiographic density.

Normal radiographic anatomy of the thorax
right lateral view

http://goo.gl/otDlnr

As regards the position of the patient, special attention should be paid to the position of the forelimbs, which must be correctly extended so they are not superimposed with the cranial part of the thoracic cavity. In addition, when a radiograph is taken in lateral

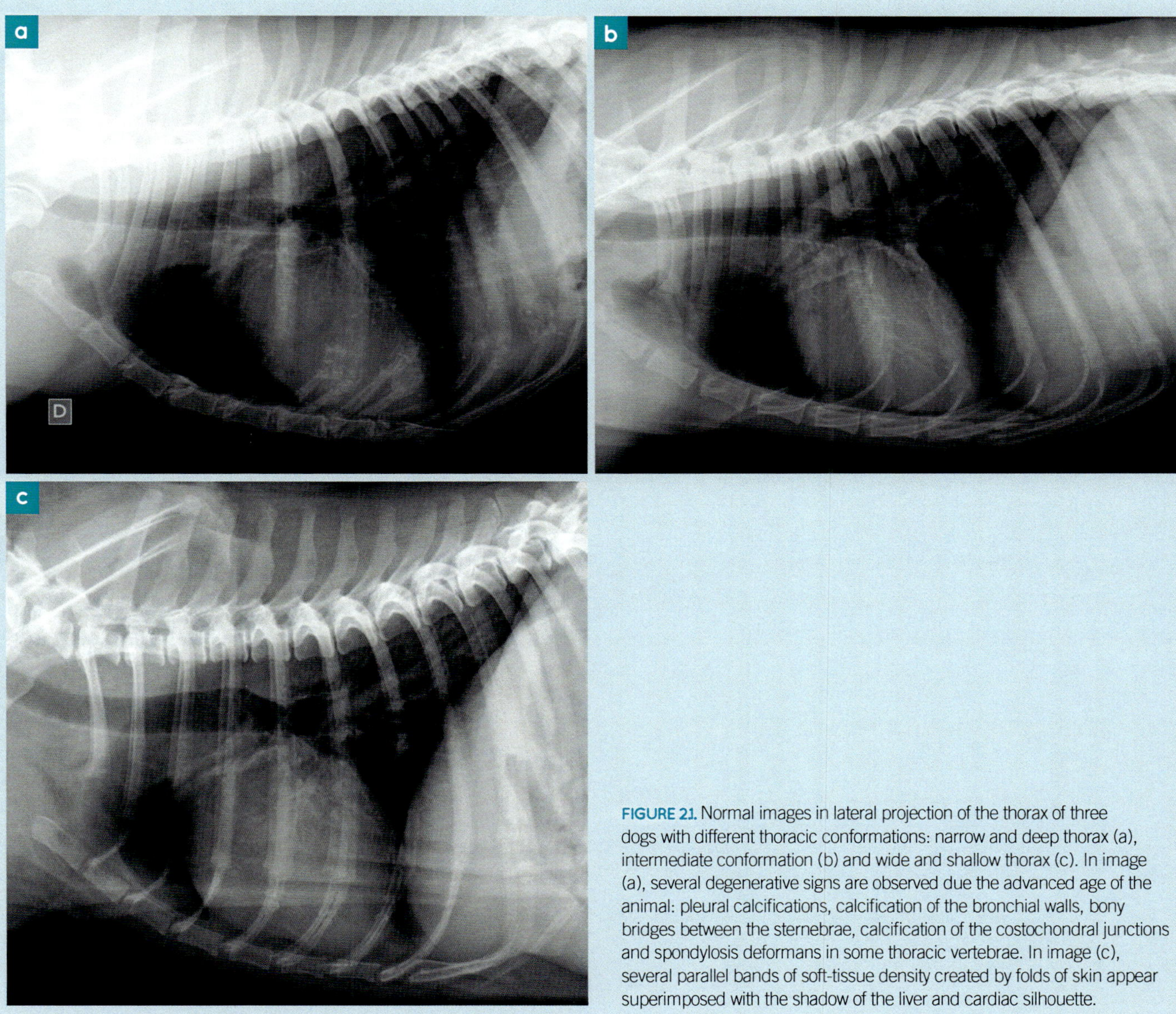

FIGURE 21. Normal images in lateral projection of the thorax of three dogs with different thoracic conformations: narrow and deep thorax (a), intermediate conformation (b) and wide and shallow thorax (c). In image (a), several degenerative signs are observed due the advanced age of the animal: pleural calcifications, calcification of the bronchial walls, bony bridges between the sternebrae, calcification of the costochondral junctions and spondylosis deformans in some thoracic vertebrae. In image (c), several parallel bands of soft-tissue density created by folds of skin appear superimposed with the shadow of the liver and cardiac silhouette.

recumbency, the median plane of the thorax is usually inclined on the cassette instead of being parallel to it, due to the relatively triangular morphology of this anatomical region. A radiolucent block should therefore be placed under the sternum in order to correct the position. When observing a lateral radiograph, we will know that the thorax was correctly placed when the costochondral junctions of both sides appear practically at the same level. If they are very separated in the image, this finding will indicate that the median plane was not parallel to the cassette. This affects the image of the cardiac silhouette and trachea, so that the first one appears to make greater contact with the sternum and the second one appears falsely elevated (fig. 2.2). It is important not to confuse these findings caused by an incorrect positioning with real pathological alterations. The rotation of the thorax at the time of taking a dorsoventral or ventrodorsal radiograph will be identified in the images by the lack of superimposition of the sternum and thoracic spine, and will particularly affect the cardiac silhouette, which will appear falsely deformed (fig. 2.3).

Digital radiography is increasingly used in veterinary medicine. Digital radiographs offer a better contrast resolution than conventional radiographs, which translates into a better definition of some anatomical structures, especially in the thorax, such as the pulmonary vessels or the walls of larger bronchi. Lungs appear less radiolucent than on conventional radiographs and this may lead to an incorrect diagnosis of a pathological increase in lung opacity.

In comparison with dogs, the thorax of cats has a more triangular morphology, their cardiac silhouette has a smaller craniocaudal diameter (2 intercostal spaces compared to 2.5-3.5 intercostal spaces in dogs) and the caudodorsal margin of the caudal pulmonary lobes may appear slightly separated from the spine in normal conditions, a finding that would make us suspect a mild pleural effusion in the case of dogs (fig. 2.4).

In young animals, it is possible to identify the shadow of the thymus until approximately 6 months of age. After that, the shadow cannot be differentiated from the rest of the structures contained in the cranial mediastinal space. Due to the typical organomegaly observed in young animals, the cardiac silhouette may also appear larger in comparison with adult animals.

Degenerative changes can frequently be observed in older animals, such as spondylosis deformans in the thoracic vertebrae, formation of bony bridges between the sternebrae, calcification of the costochondral junctions, calcification of the tracheal rings and bronchial walls, formation of pulmonary osteomas, calcified pleural plaques, thickening of the pleura and a diffuse interstitial lung pattern associated with fibrosis. In older cats, the heart tends to lie more on the sternum due to an elongation of the aorta, which may increase the curvature of the aortic arch and cause a marked undulation of the descending aorta.

The superimposition of subcutaneous fat in obese animals may significantly worsen the quality of the images of the thorax and especially affects the assessment of the lungs. The mediastinum and cardiac silhouette may also appear enlarged in obese patients and the lung margin may be slightly separated from the thoracic wall, which could be confused with a mild pleural effusion.

The combination of radiography and echocardiography offers very complete information about the diseases that affect the heart and great vessels. Non-cardiac thoracic ultrasonography is also useful to obtain complementary information in cases of pleural or mediastinal effusion, assess thoracic masses that are not surrounded by air, pulmonary consolidation and diaphragmatic hernias, and collect samples or perform thoracic drainage under ultrasound guidance.

Fluoroscopy allows real-time evaluation of peristalsis of the oesophagus and of the passage of food or contrast medium through it. It is a very appropriate technique for the diagnosis of tracheal collapse, paralysis of the diaphragm and sliding hiatal hernias. It also allows the collection of samples for cytology and biopsy of thoracic lesions that cannot be detected by means of ultrasonography, as well as angiography studies.

Among advanced imaging techniques, computed tomography is generally more appropriate to examine the thorax than magnetic resonance imaging. A computed tomography examination can be performed in a few seconds, which allows the use of techniques

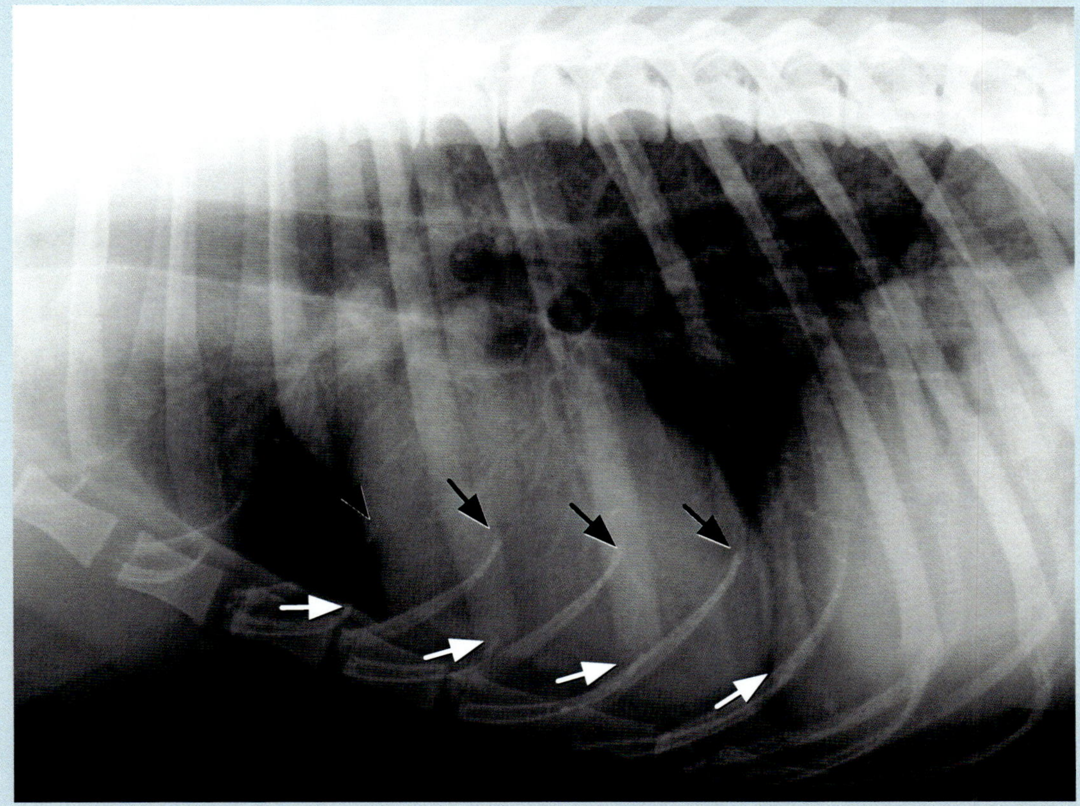

FIGURE 2.2. Lateral radiograph of the thorax of a healthy dog, in which there is a wide separation between the costochondral junctions of both sides (shown by black arrows on one side and white arrows on the other), due to the rotation of the thorax along its longitudinal axis. This rotation is corrected by slightly elevating the sternum with a radiolucent block until the median plane of the thorax is approximately parallel to the cassette. As a consequence of the incorrect position, the contact of the cardiac silhouette on the sternum is falsely increased and the trachea appears falsely elevated.

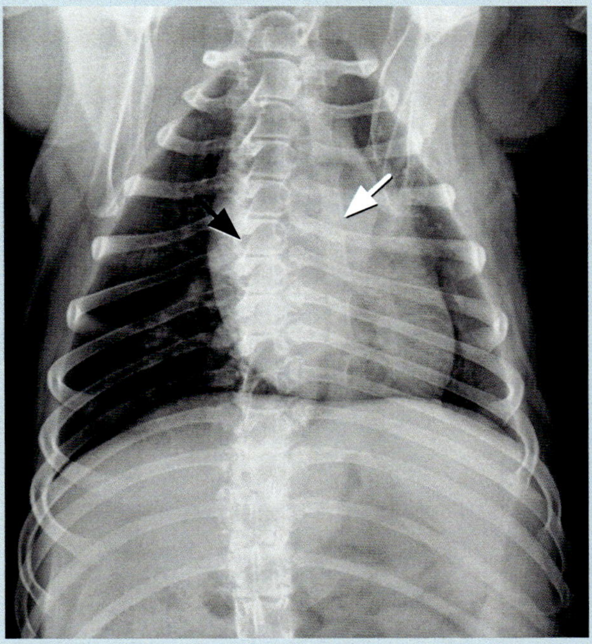

FIGURE 2.3. Dorsoventral radiograph of the thorax of a healthy dog, in which the thoracic spine (black arrow) and the sternum (white arrow) appear separated due to a rotation of the thorax along its longitudinal axis. As a consequence of the incorrect position, most of the cardiac silhouette appears falsely located in the left hemithorax.

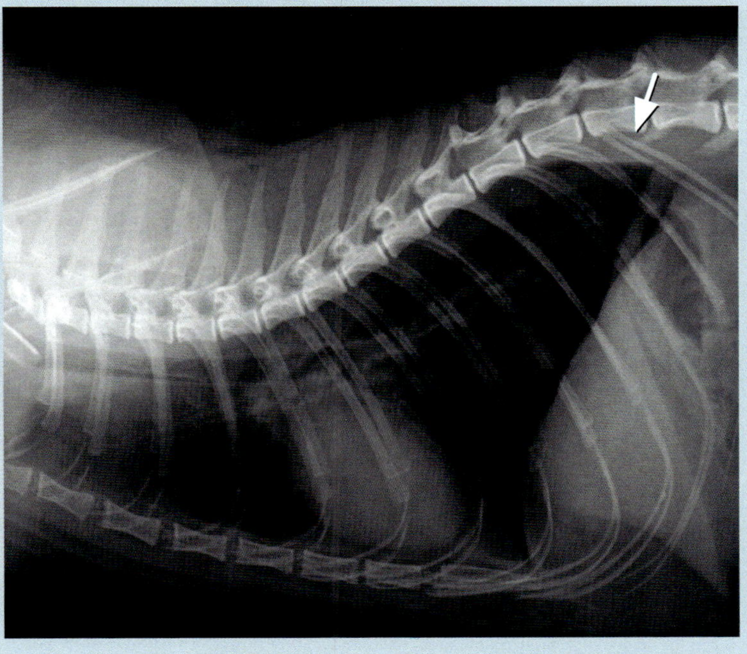

FIGURE 2.4. Lateral radiograph of the thorax of a healthy cat. Compared with that of a dog, the thorax of a cat has a more triangular morphology, the cardiac silhouette has a smaller craniocaudal diameter (2 intercostal spaces) and the caudodorsal margin of the caudal pulmonary lobes may appear slightly separated from the spine in normal conditions (arrows). This latter finding would make us suspect a mild pleural effusion in the case of dogs.

of apnoeic anaesthesia to avoid the influence of respiratory movements on the images. Conversely, several minutes are usually necessary for an examination with conventional magnetic resonance imaging equipment. Such prolonged apnoea cannot be maintained and the artefacts due to respiratory and cardiac movements significantly affect the quality of chest images. Computed tomography is particularly indicated for the assessment of pneumothoraces or persistent and recurrent pleural effusions, localised lesions in the mediastinum, tracheal collapse and bronchial obstruction. It is also useful for the detection of pulmonary metastases and lymphadenopathies, thomboembolism, pulmonary torsion, infiltrative interstitial lung disease, as well as to differentiate between consolidation and atelectasis and assess thoracic masses in general. Magnetic resonance may also be of interest for the pre-surgical examination of the thoracic wall and pleural and mediastinal masses, essentially.

Thoracic wall

The thoracic wall is formed by the thoracic spine (see chapter 4), the sternum, the diaphragm (see chapter 1), the ribs, costal cartilages and intercostal spaces.

Ribs

In normal conditions, the ribs are symmetrical, have a homogeneous density and smooth borders. The space between them must be regular. However, congenital anomalies, hypoplasia or aplasia, which are uni- or bilateral, are often seen in the thirteenth pair of ribs. The C7 and L1 vertebrae may also have rudimentary ribs when they are transitional.

In the first weeks of life, costal cartilages cannot be identified on radiographs as they have soft-tissue opacity. They become apparent as they start calcifying. In older cats, segments of the costal cartilages may appear markedly calcified, thus having an appearance of ruptures. In older dogs and cats, calcifications with an irregular morphology may be observed in the costochondral junctions, and these may even be mistaken for intrathoracic lesions. In chondrodystrophic breeds, especially in the Teckel and Basset Hounds, the ribs have a peculiar curvature, which may create a similar image to that of a mild pleural effusion on dorsoventral and ventrodorsal radiographs.

There may be a generalised increase of the intercostal space in conditions that cause an excessive expansion of the thorax, for example, in severe cases of pleural effusion, pneumothorax or emphysema.

Rib **fractures** are more or less easily identified depending on their location and the degree of displacement of the fragments (fig. 2.5). When dealing with thoracic trauma, a thorough examination of each pair of ribs is advised and should be performed on two orthogonal radiographs whenever possible. The early detection of rib fractures after a trauma is considered to be indicative of possible lung trauma, although the radiographic image of a contusion in the lung may be undetectable until 6 hours after the trauma occurred. A patient with a rib fracture may present with paradoxical motion of the affected region of the thorax: outward motion during expiration and inward motion during inspiration. Fractures are usually transverse and generally affect more than one rib. They are often associated with a pneumothorax or subcutaneous emphysema. Although their most frequent cause is thoracic trauma, pathological fractures may appear secondary to a neoplasm or to conditions that cause severe osteopenia (e.g. secondary renal hyperparathyroidism). They may also be caused by sustained or repetitive stress in cases of feline asthma, chronic bronchial disease or lobular emphysema. Old fractures may appear as incidental findings on chest radiographs.

The most frequent primary **neoplasms** of the ribs are osteosarcomas and chondrosarcomas. Their image is usually that of a mixed aggressive bone lesion, which is both osteolytic and osteoproliferative, with marked inflammation of soft tissues. They may cause a displacement of the adjacent ribs and a secondary involvement of these. They usually originate what is termed the **extrapleural sign**, which refers to a focal displacement of the pleura and lung to the inside of the thorax caused by masses in the thoracic wall, either of costal or soft-tissue origin (it is an adaptation of the general term "mass effect"). Many rib tumours are diagnosed at an advanced stage because their growth is greater towards the inside of the thorax than towards the outside. They are sometimes associated with pleural effusion (fig. 2.6), which may make the radiographic detection of the primary lesion more difficult. In cases of multiple myeloma, ribs and bone metastases in this location may have a multiple osteolytic pattern. Benign neoplasms (osteomas, chondromas and osteochondromatosis) are uncommon and usually appear as osteoproliferative, non-aggressive lesions.

On occasions, we may find soft-tissue tumours that affect the ribs in a secondary manner (e.g. mesotheliomas) and have a similar image to that of primary tumours. In both cases, the differential diagnosis should include osteomyelitis.

Computed tomography and magnetic resonance imaging allow a very accurate assessment of any mass affecting the costal wall, the extension of the lesion and the degree of infiltration in adjacent tissues, although computed tomography is preferred to examine the lung when there is a suspicion of metastasis.

Sternum

Variations in its size, morphology or in the number of sternebrae that have no clinical significance are frequently observed. Cats often have a ventral displacement of the xyphoid process, which sometimes causes pain. In older animals, it is usual to find **bony overgrowths** that originate from the ends

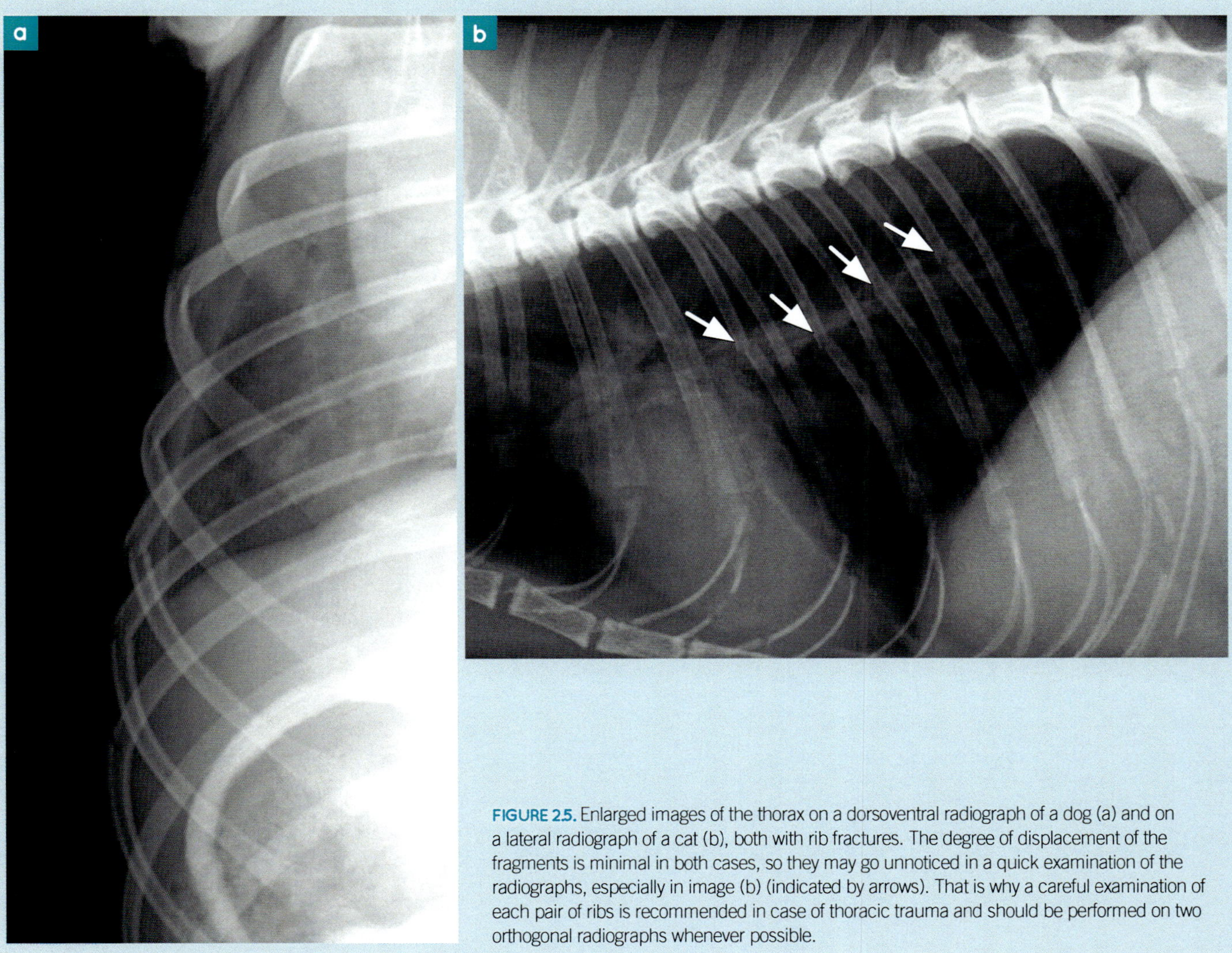

FIGURE 2.5. Enlarged images of the thorax on a dorsoventral radiograph of a dog (a) and on a lateral radiograph of a cat (b), both with rib fractures. The degree of displacement of the fragments is minimal in both cases, so they may go unnoticed in a quick examination of the radiographs, especially in image (b) (indicated by arrows). That is why a careful examination of each pair of ribs is recommended in case of thoracic trauma and should be performed on two orthogonal radiographs whenever possible.

Normal radiographic anatomy of the thorax
dorsoventral view

http://goo.gl/pKMKlb

of the sternebrae and tend to form bridges between each other (fig. 2.7). It is considered to be a degenerative sign associated with age and with no clinical significance.

Fractures of the sternebrae are usually incidental findings and rarely cause clinical signs. A **poor alignment** of the sternum may also be observed, but it should only be considered significant if it is accompanied by inflammation of soft tissues, pleural effusion or associated clinical signs.

It is uncommon to find **neoplasms** affecting the sternum. They usually appear as aggressive osteolytic and osteoproliferative lesions and marked inflammation of the adjacent soft tissues. **Osteomyelitis** may have a similar aspect and is usually caused by penetration of foreign bodies or bites in this region.

Pectus excavatum is a congenital deformity of the sternum, which causes it to have a more or less marked abnormal dorsal curvature (fig. 2.8). The ribs appear deformed and the heart and mediastinum are displaced dorsally, and to one side of the thoracic cavity on some occasions. It does not usually cause any clinical symptoms, but it may make breathing more difficult when the deformity is marked. Although it affects both cats and dogs, it is more common in brachycephalic dog breeds. It is sometimes associated with other congenital deformities such as peritoneopericardial hernia, tracheal hypoplasia or defects of the ventricular septum.

Pharynx, larynx and trachea

Pharynx and larynx

The pharynx is a musculomembranous sac that belongs to the digestive and respiratory system. Its cranial part is connected with the mouth and nasal cavity, while its caudal end communicates with the oesophagus and the larynx. This latter connects the pharynx with the trachea (fig. 2.9).

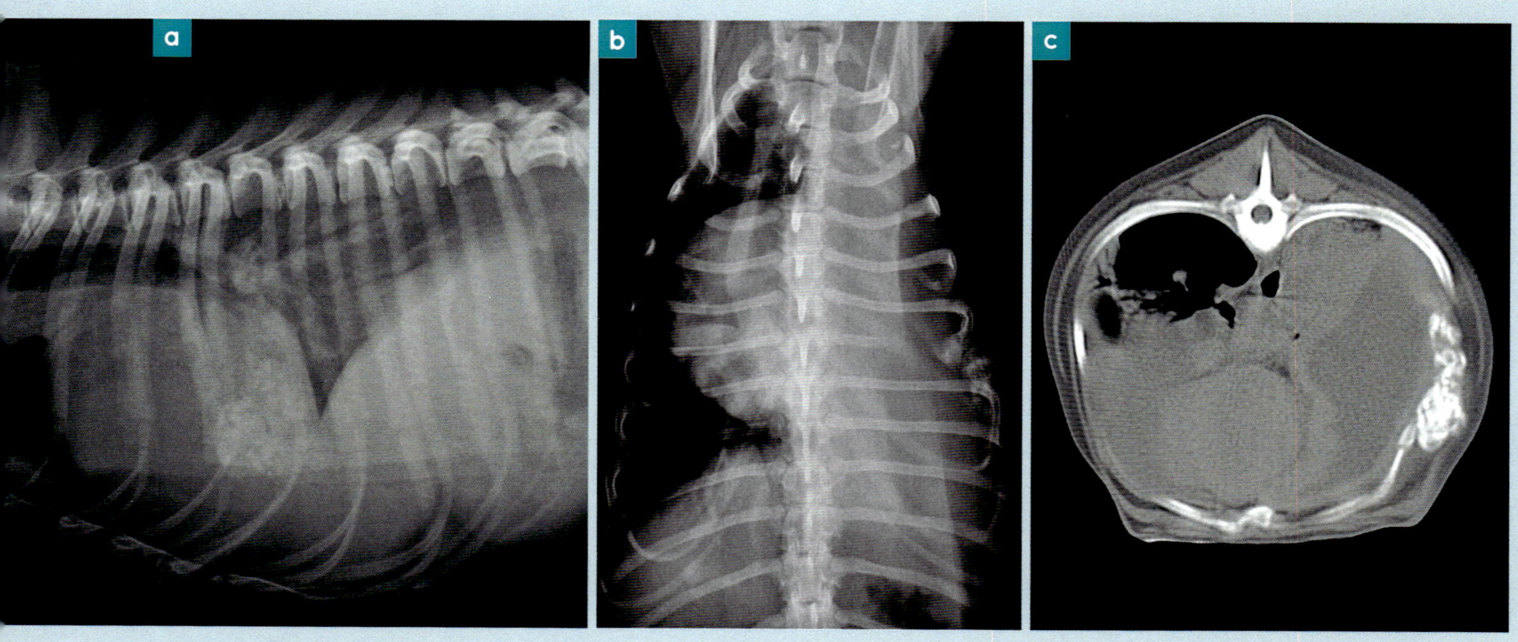

FIGURE 2.6. Lateral (a) and dorsoventral (b) radiographs and computed tomography image of a dog with a primary neoplasm on the seventh left rib. An aggressive osteoproliferative and osteolytic bone lesion is observed, as well as signs of severe pleural effusion in the left hemithorax. In image (b), signs of pleural effusion can be observed in the right hemithorax, while in image (c), obtained several days later, the degree of effusion is moderate.

Radiography provides little information about these structures, but may be useful to detect foreign bodies and soft-tissue masses in this region. Fluoroscopy is required to evaluate functional alterations of the pharynx (pharyngeal and cricopharyngeal dysphagia), since this technique allows real-time examination of swallowing movements in the patient.

Foreign bodies are easily identified when their radiopacity is higher than that of soft tissues (fig. 2.10), or when they are surrounded by gas in the lumen of the pharynx or larynx. If the foreign body is sharp, it may pierce the wall and lead to the formation of abscesses in adjacent areas.

The **masses** that originate in the wall of the pharynx or larynx and grow towards their lumen include nasopharyngeal polyps in cats (fig. 2.11) and some types of neoplasia. It is more frequent to find masses in adjacent tissues, which displace the pharynx and/or larynx from its normal position (fig. 2.12). These masses are most frequently retropharyngeal

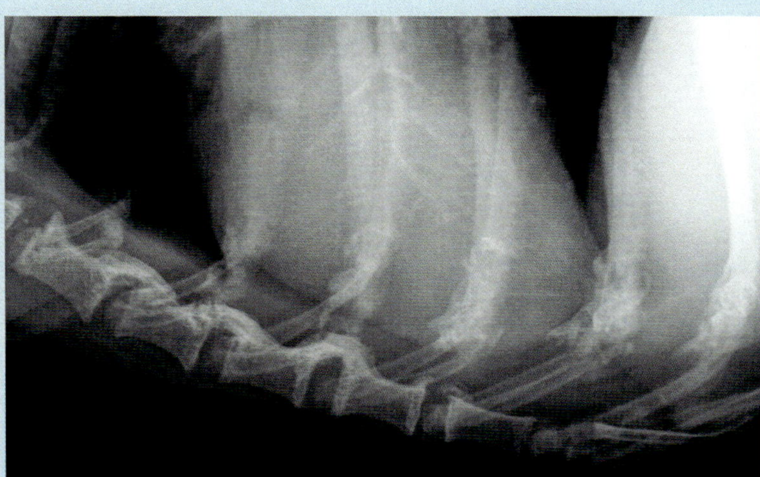

FIGURE 2.7. Enlarged image of the sternal region on a lateral radiograph of an older dog. It is possible to observe bony overgrowths, which tend to connect the ends of the sternebrae, and calcifications with an irregular morphology in the costochondral junctions. Both findings do not have any clinical significance.

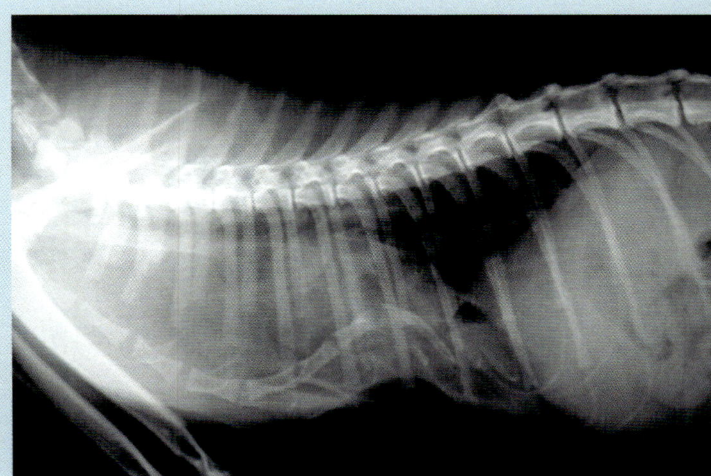

FIGURE 2.8. Lateral radiograph of the thorax of a cat with pectus excavatum. This is a congenital alteration in which the sternum appears deformed and curved in dorsal direction towards the thoracic cavity.

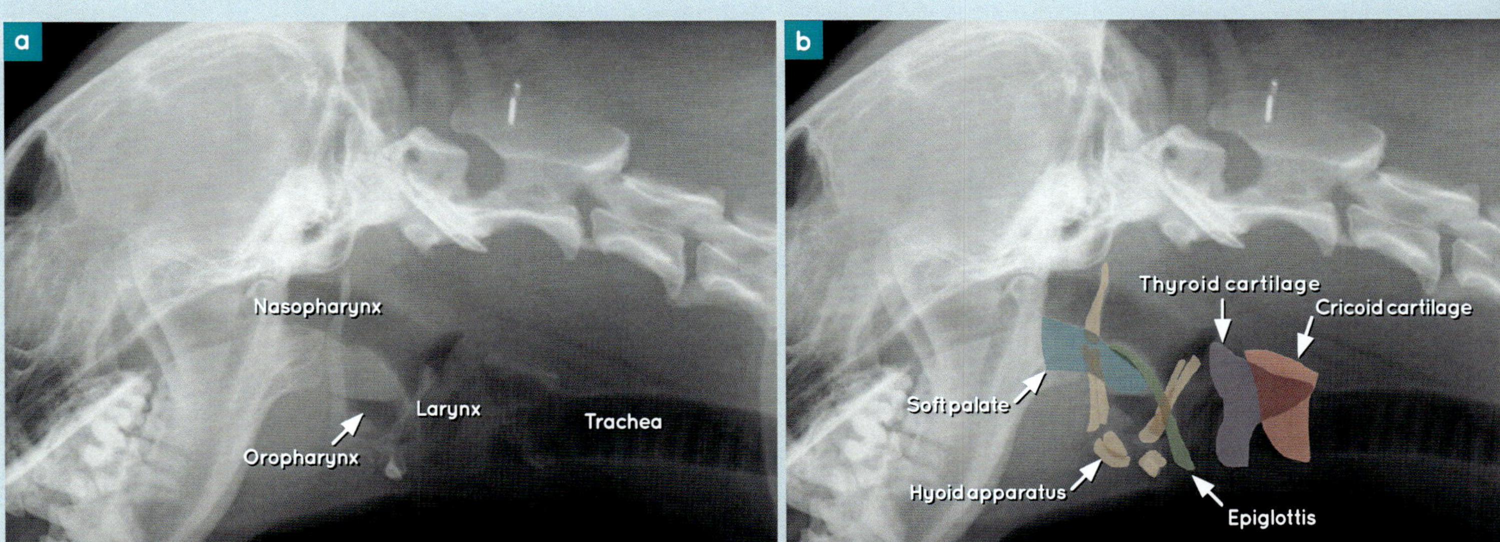

FIGURE 2.9. Normal lateral radiographs of the neck of a healthy dog, where the main anatomical structures related to the pharynx, larynx and cervical trachea are identified.

lymphadenopathies and thyroid tumours. When the retropharyngeal lymph nodes increase considerably in size, they cause a ventral displacement of the pharynx and larynx. This finding is frequently observed in cases of lymphoma or metastatic lymphadenopathy of oral neoplasms, or, on a less frequent basis, of the nasal cavity. Thyroid tumours usually cause a dorsal displacement of the larynx.

Pharyngeal and cricopharyngeal dysphagias may have a congenital origin, especially in Spaniel breeds, or be acquired, generally in older animals, in which they may appear as a sequela of diseases of the central nervous system or neuromuscular diseases. They usually do not cause any significant alterations on radiographs and require a real-time fluoroscopic study of the patient's swallowing movements, in which food mixed with barium is administered to the patient, in order to be diagnosed. In cases of dysphagia, it is possible to observe nasal reflux of barium, its accumulation in the pharynx, a failure in the relaxation of the cricopharyngeal sphincter, aspiration of barium into the larynx and pharynx or uncoordinated movements of the pharyngeal muscle. It is important to take radiographs of the thorax when dysphagia is suspected, since it is very common for the affected patients to suffer from aspiration pneumonia.

In cases of **brachycephalic syndrome**, which is characterised by several anomalies in the upper airways in brachycephalic dog and cat breeds, an anomalous image of the soft palate may be observed in this region. The soft palate may appear fairly elongated (extending beyond the epiglottis) or thickened due to oedema. The affected animals sometimes have laryngeal collapse, but it usually occurs in laterolateral direction and is therefore difficult to identify on lateral radiographs, unless it is very severe. Tracheal hypoplasia also commonly appears in these patients.

In cases of **retroversion of the epiglottis**, caused by its excessive mobility, the epiglottis may have a more vertical position than normal.

Trachea

The trachea is a semi-rigid tubular structure that connects the larynx with the bronchi. The carina can be identified in its distal part. On lateral radiographs, it appears as

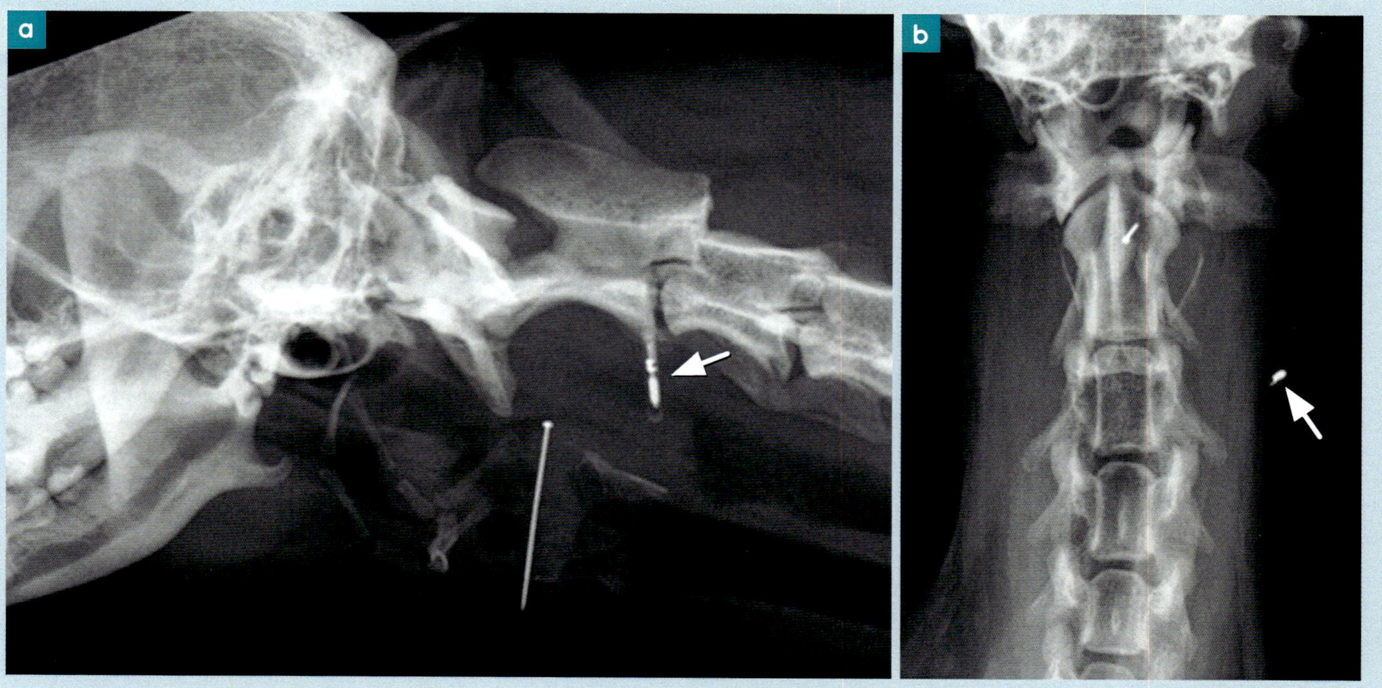

FIGURE 2.10. Lateral (a) and ventrodorsal (b) radiographs of the neck of a dog with a metallic foreign body (nail) in the larynx. It is essential to obtain two orthogonal radiographs to determine the exact location of the object. The identification microchip is shown with an arrow in both images.

a more radiolucent circular or oval area that is located at the level of the 4th or 5th intercostal space. The tracheal rings have a "C" shape and are dorsally connected by the tracheal muscle and connective tissue.

In order to examine the complete trachea, it is necessary to take a radiograph that includes its cervical and thoracic parts (fig. 2.13). In medium or large-sized dogs, it will be necessary to take two radiographs, one of the neck and another of the thorax, to carry out this assessment. On plain radiographs, the internal aspect of the tracheal wall is easily observed because it contrasts with the intraluminal air. On the other hand, in normal conditions, the external aspect of the wall is difficult to differentiate from the structures of the neck or from the mediastinum that surrounds it.

In general, lateral radiographs are more useful, since the trachea is superimposed with the cervical and thoracic spine on dorsoventral and ventrodorsal radiographs. A craniocaudal tangential radiograph of the trachea may be taken to visualise the tracheal lumen at the level of the thoracic inlet, but it is difficult to place the patient correctly and it rarely provides significant additional information.

In cats and dog breeds with an intermediate conformation, the thoracic trachea forms an acute angle with the spine. This angle is greater in dogs with a narrow and deep thoracic conformation, while in those with a wide and shallow thorax, the course of the trachea is almost parallel to the vertebrae.

The diameter of the trachea is assessed by dividing its value by the height of the thoracic inlet, which is measured on a lateral projection. The height of the thoracic inlet is measured from the ventral border of the spine, at the level of the centre of the most cranial rib, to the dorsal border of the manubrium of the sternum, where it is thinnest. The diameter of the trachea is measured between the internal aspect of the dorsal border and the internal aspect of the ventral border of the wall, perpendicularly to the longitudinal axis of the trachea and where the line of measurement of the height of the thoracic inlet crosses the trachea (fig. 2.14). In dogs, the same parameter varies in function of the breed (table 2.1).

A poor position of the neck or head when taking a lateral radiograph may cause the trachea to be flexed,

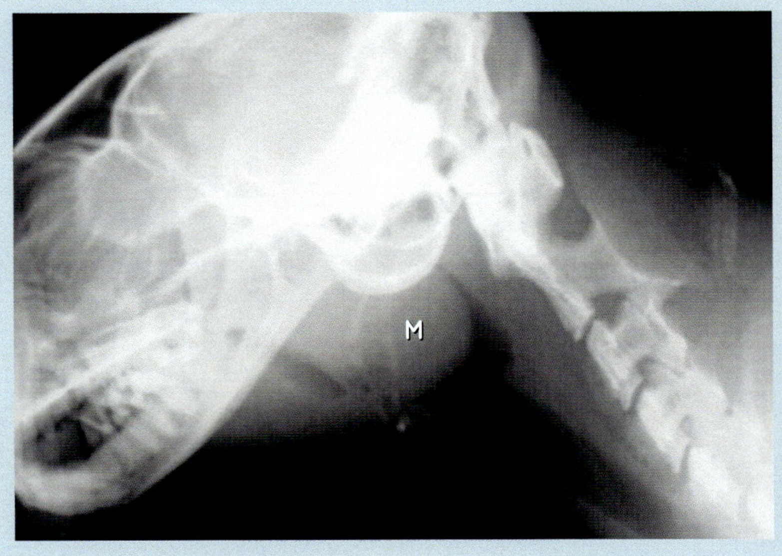

FIGURE 2.11. Lateral radiograph of the neck of a cat with a localised mass in the nasopharynx (M), which causes partial obliteration of its lumen. Pathological diagnosis: nasopharyngeal polyp.

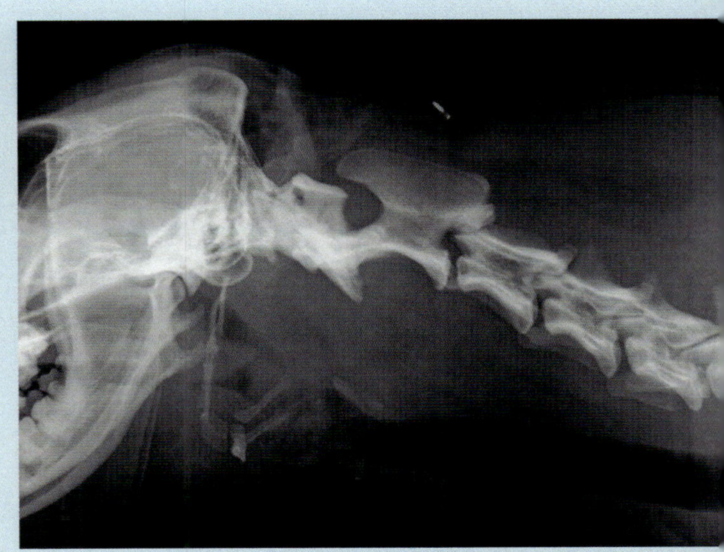

FIGURE 2.12. Lateral radiograph of the neck of a dog with a mass in the retropharyngeal region. Although the margins of the lesion cannot be distinguished, the ventral displacement of the pharynx and larynx indicates a "mass effect" in this location. The presence of a large retropharyngeal lymphadenopahy in this region was confirmed with an ultrasound examination. The identification microchip appears dorsal to C2.

which should not be mistaken for a real displacement of this organ caused by adjacent masses. The trachea will also be falsely elevated if the median plane of the thorax is very inclined on the cassette when the radiograph is taken. This is corrected by placing a radiolucent block under the sternum.

Some animals with no respiratory signs have a narrowing of the tracheal lumen between the central area of the cervical part and the central area of the thoracic part (fig. 2.15). Some authors attribute this image to the superimposition with the ventral muscles of the neck and/or oesophagus, while others consider that the narrowing may be real in these cases and caused by a so-called **redundant dorsal tracheal membrane**, which invaginates towards the lumen in this region of the trachea. The degree of narrowing may even vary with the respiratory cycle, as in cases of tracheal collapse. These two conditions can be differentiated because in cases of redundant dorsal tracheal membrane (or superimposition of structures), the more radiopaque dorsal margin of the tracheal wall maintains its normal position, while in cases of collapse this margin of the wall appears displaced. However, this subject is still controversial today.

An image of apparent tracheal collapse may also be seen in obese animals, due to the accumulation of fat around the trachea, especially at the level of the thoracic inlet. On dorsoventral and ventrodorsal radiographs, the trachea appears superimposed with the spine, perfectly centred or slightly to the right of the median line, but never to its left in normal conditions. In obese animals, the trachea may be clearly located on the right side. The tracheobronchial bifurcation, on the other hand, should always be located on the median line.

Calcification of the tracheal rings is frequently observed in older animals and patients with Cushing's syndrome, but this finding alone has no pathological significance.

Inflammatory processes (tracheitis and tracheobronchitis) do not usually produce any evident radiological signs.

A ventral **displacement** of the trachea may be caused by a megaoesophagus, oesophageal foreign bodies or a significant increase in the size of the tracheobronchial lymph nodes, while the presence of masses in the cranial mediastinum or an increase in the size of the heart causes a dorsal tracheal displacement.

TABLE 2.1. Evaluation of the size of the trachea in function of the breed.

Breed (dogs)	Normal tracheal diameter/ height of the thoracic inlet ratio
Intermediate conformation or deep and narrow thorax	0.21 ± 0.03
Bulldog	0.11 ± 0.03
Other brachycephalic breeds	0.16 ± 0.03

Tracheal **collapse** is defined as a narrowing of the trachea that may affect its cervical part, its thoracic part or both. It occurs in dorsoventral direction, so that only a lateral radiograph is useful for its diagnosis. It is a degenerative and progressive process that essentially affects middle-aged and older small and miniature breed dogs. If the narrowing affects the cervical part, the collapse occurs during inspiration (fig. 2.16), while if it affects the thoracic part, it occurs during expiration (fig 2.17). Since it is a dynamic process, which varies with the respiratory cycle, fluoroscopy is the most appropriate technique for its diagnosis. Alternatively, conventional radiographs that include the cervical and thoracic trachea may be taken in inspiration and expiration, although in practice it is difficult to adjust the exact time when the radiograph should be taken to the respiratory cycle. It is important to bear in mind that some healthy animals, especially small and miniature breed dogs, may have a slacker dorsal tracheal membrane and thinner tracheal rings, which causes a variation in the tracheal diameter that is manifested in the following way: during inspiration, the diameter of the cervical trachea is slightly reduced and that of the thoracic trachea increases, while during expiration, the diameter of the cervical trachea is slightly reduced and that of the cervical part increases. However, in normal conditions, this variation should be minimal. On radiographs, the collapse may be graded according to whether the reduction of the diameter of the trachea reaches 25 %, 50 %, 75 % or from 90 % to 100 %. This grading scale is similar to that used in bronchoscopy, in which the collapse is classified as grade 1 (mild)

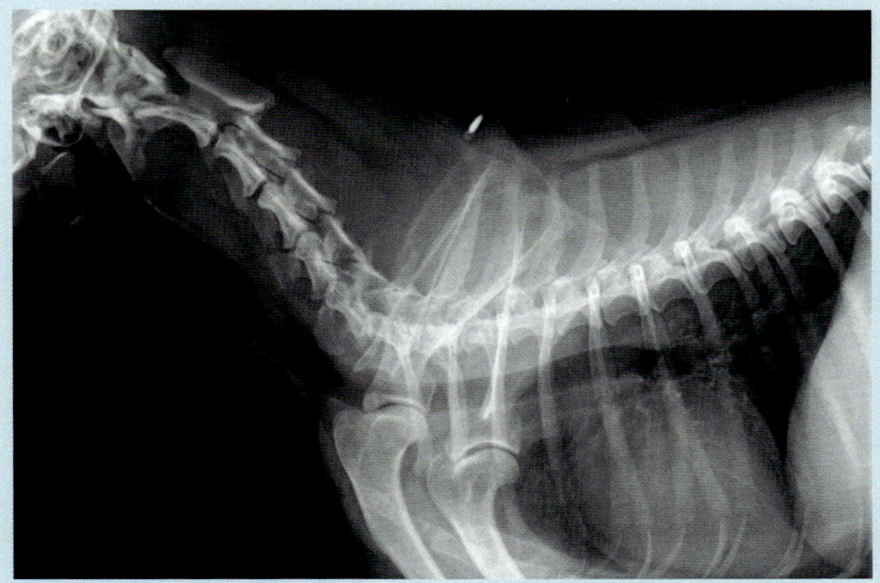

FIGURE 2.13. Normal radiographic image of the trachea of a dog. In order to evaluate its whole course, the cervical and thoracic part should be included in the same image, as long as the size of the patient allows it. In medium and large-sized dogs, radiographs of the two regions have to be taken separately (due to the size of the animal and to differences in exposure values). The identification microchip appears dorsal to the scapulae.

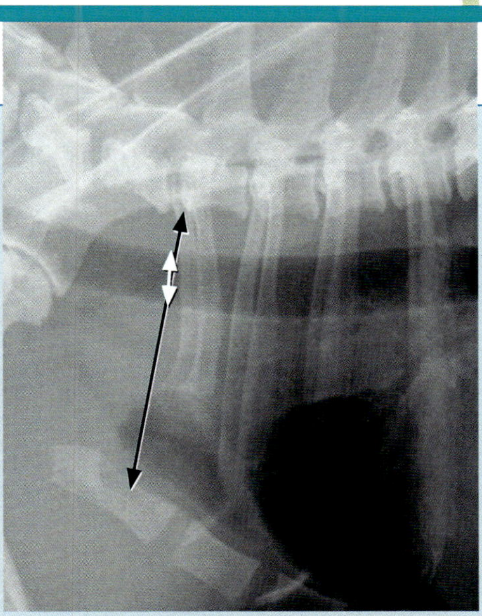

FIGURE 2.14. Enlarged image of the thoracic inlet on a lateral radiograph of a healthy dog. The diameter of the trachea is evaluated using the ratio between the diameter of the trachea (white arrow) and the height of the thoracic inlet (black arrow). The height of the thoracic inlet is measured from the ventral border of the spine at the level of the centre of the most cranial rib, to the dorsal border of the manubrium of the sternum where it is thinnest. The diameter of the trachea is measured between the internal aspect of the dorsal border and the internal aspect of the ventral border of the wall, perpendicularly to the longitudinal axis of the trachea, where the line of measurement of the height of the thoracic inlet crosses the trachea. In dogs, this parameter varies depending on the breed.

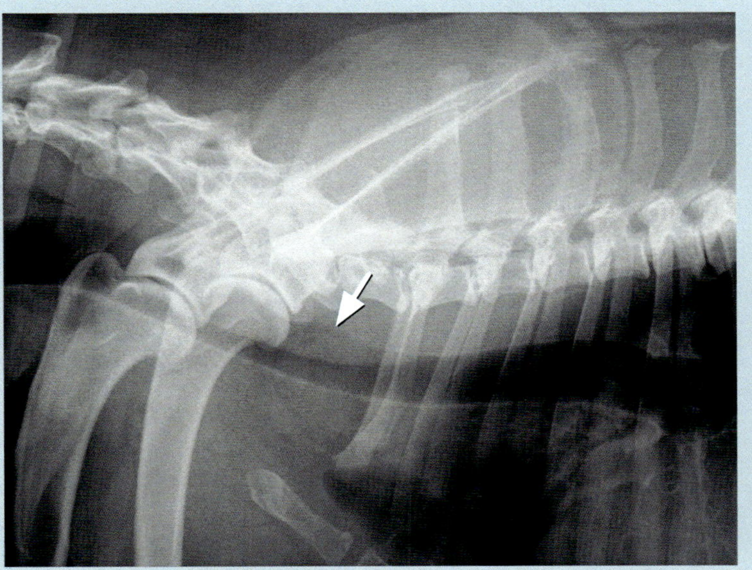

FIGURE 2.15. Enlarged image of the trachea on a lateral radiograph of a dog with clinical signs of respiratory abnormality. A possible narrowing of the lumen of the trachea that extends from the central area of the cervical trachea to the central area of the thoracic trachea is observed, although a dorsal, thin and more radiopaque line that is compatible with the tracheal wall (arrow) can be seen. Some authors attribute this type of image to the superimposition of the muscles and/or oesophagus with the normal trachea, while others consider it is often due to a so-called redundant dorsal tracheal membrane, which can invaginate towards the tracheal lumen to a greater or lesser extent depending on the moment of the respiratory cycle.

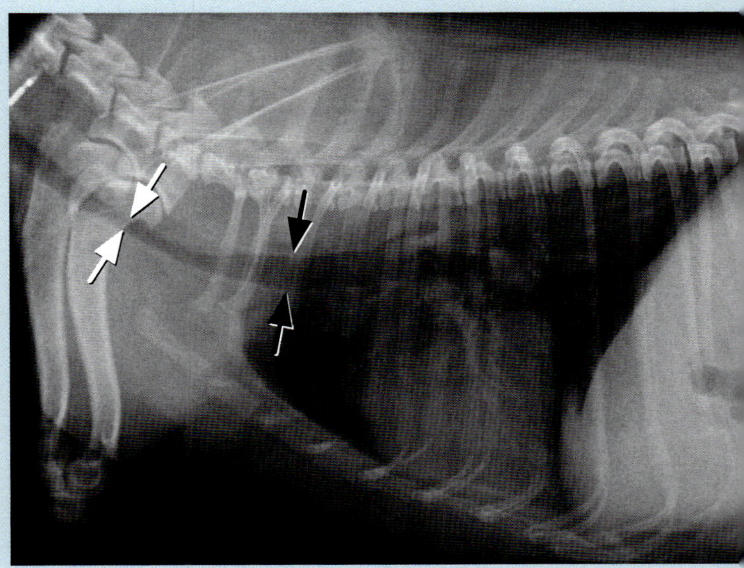

FIGURE 2.16. Lateral radiograph of the thorax and thoracic inlet of a dog with cervical tracheal collapse. The reduction of the diameter reaches 50 %. The diameter in the area of narrowing is indicated with white arrows and the normal diameter of the thoracic trachea is indicated with black arrows.

Normal radiographic
anatomy of the thorax
right lateral view

http://goo.gl/otDInr

when the diameter reduction reaches 25 %, grade 2 (moderate), when it reaches 50 %, grade 3 (severe) with it is reduced by 75 % and grade 4 (total) when it is total. A diameter reduction that is lower than 25 % is not considered significant. A moderate degree of tracheal collapse is frequently observed in small and miniature breed senior dogs with no evidence of significant clinical signs. The bronchi may also be collapsed, in association or not with the tracheal collapse, which is why it is important to examine them too.

Cats rarely suffer from tracheal collapse caused by degeneration of the cartilages. If cervical tracheal collapse is observed in a cat, the possibility of an obstruction in the upper airways should be considered, since it may cause a significant increase of the inspiratory effort and create enough negative intratracheal pressure to collapse the lumen.

Tracheal **hypoplasia** is a congenital alteration that is characterised by a uniform reduction of the tracheal diameter throughout its whole course, from the larynx to the carina (fig. 2.18.). It is due to an incomplete or anomalous development of the tracheal rings. The dorsal membrane may be absent and the tracheal wall thickened. It is more common in brachycephalic breeds (especially in the Bulldog), although it has also been described in the Labrador, German Shepherd, Weimaraner and Basset Hound. Patients with tracheal hypoplasia may also suffer from other congenital anomalies such as megaoesophagus, pulmonary stenosis or aortic stenosis. In some animals, there may be a delay in the development of the trachea, so we must be careful when diagnosing this disease in very young animals. It must be borne in mind that Bulldogs with no signs of disease may have a diameter of the trachea/height of the thoracic inlet ratio of down to 0.09 (fig. 2.19).

Tracheal **stenosis** is defined as a localised and permanent narrowing of the trachea, not associated with the respiratory cycle, which differentiates it from tracheal collapse. It does not usually cause any clinical signs, unless the reduction of the diameter exceeds 80 %. It generally occurs as a result of previous trauma, and the most common causes are injuries of the cervical trachea due to bites or lesions caused by the placement of an endotracheal tube.

A tracheal **rupture** may occur as a result of trauma or due to an incorrect intubation, especially in cats.

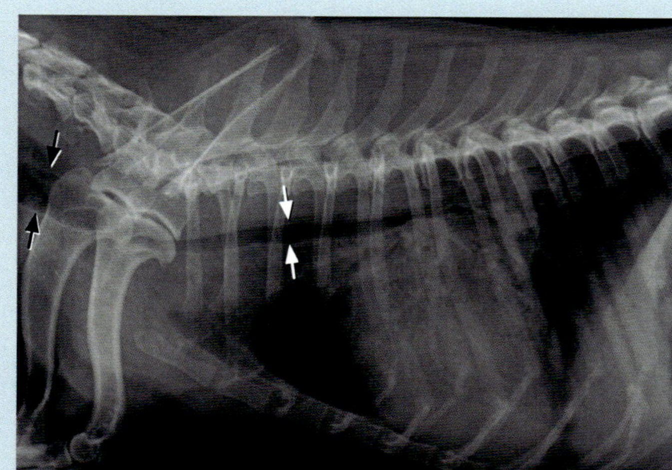

FIGURE 2.17. Lateral radiograph of the thorax and thoracic inlet of a dog with thoracic tracheal collapse. The reduction of the diameter exceeds 50 % (approximately 65 %). The diameter in the area of narrowing is shown with white arrows and the normal diameter of the cervical trachea with black arrows.

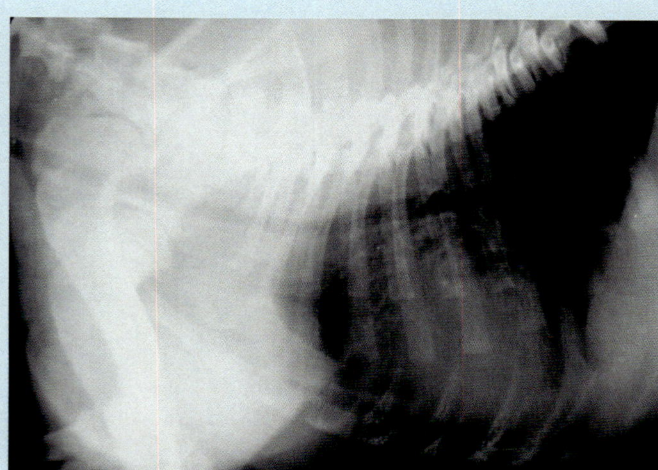

FIGURE 2.18. Lateral radiograph of the thorax of a Bulldog with tracheal hypoplasia. The ratio of the tracheal diameter to the height of the thoracic inlet is 0.07.

The degree of dyspnoea of the patient will depend on the size of the lesion. On radiographs, it is possible to observe an anomalous morphology of the trachea with irregular walls or lumen. It is frequently associated with subcutaneous emphysema or pneumomediastinum, which can extend to the abdomen and cause a pneumoperitoneum or a pneumoretroperitoneum.

In cats, it may cause an **avulsion** of the trachea due to traumas involving a severe extension of the head and neck. Paradoxically, the animal may be taken to the veterinary practice several days or even weeks after the trauma occured, when the subcutaneous emphysema or the pneumomediastinum may have disappeared. On radiographs, it is possible to observe severe focal dilatation of the trachea, which appears delimited by a thin wall formed by the intact adventitia or the surrounding mediastinal tissue.

Intraparietal tracheal **masses** are usually caused by neoplasms, granulomas (e.g. due to *Oslerus osleri*), polyps or haematomas. They are uncommon and difficult to identify on radiographs. Lymphomas may cause a diffuse infiltration of the wall.

Foreign bodies located in the trachea usually cause severe signs of respiratory obstruction. They may be identified or not on radiographs depending on their location, size and radiopacity. Radiopaque foreign bodies are easily identified, while radiolucent ones may or may not be identified depending on their shape. The accumulation of mucus around the foreign body creates focal areas of increased soft-tissue opacity at the site where it is located.

Computed tomography is an appropriate technique to evaluate and confirm cases of collapse, rupture, obstruction and mass in the trachea. Radiographs allow the follow-up of a tracheal stent in order to avoid any possible rupture, displacement or excessive formation of granulation tissue around it. However, computed tomography has the advantage of allowing the differentiation between excessive granulation tissue and accumulations of intraluminal fluid.

Oesophagus

Radiography is a valuable tool to diagnose diseases that affect the oesophagus. Lateral radiographs are usually used, since the oesophagus is superimposed with the spine and sternum on ventrodorsal and dorsoventral radiographs.

The normal oesophagus cannot usually be identified on plain radiographs, since it has the same radiographic density as most of the structures that surround

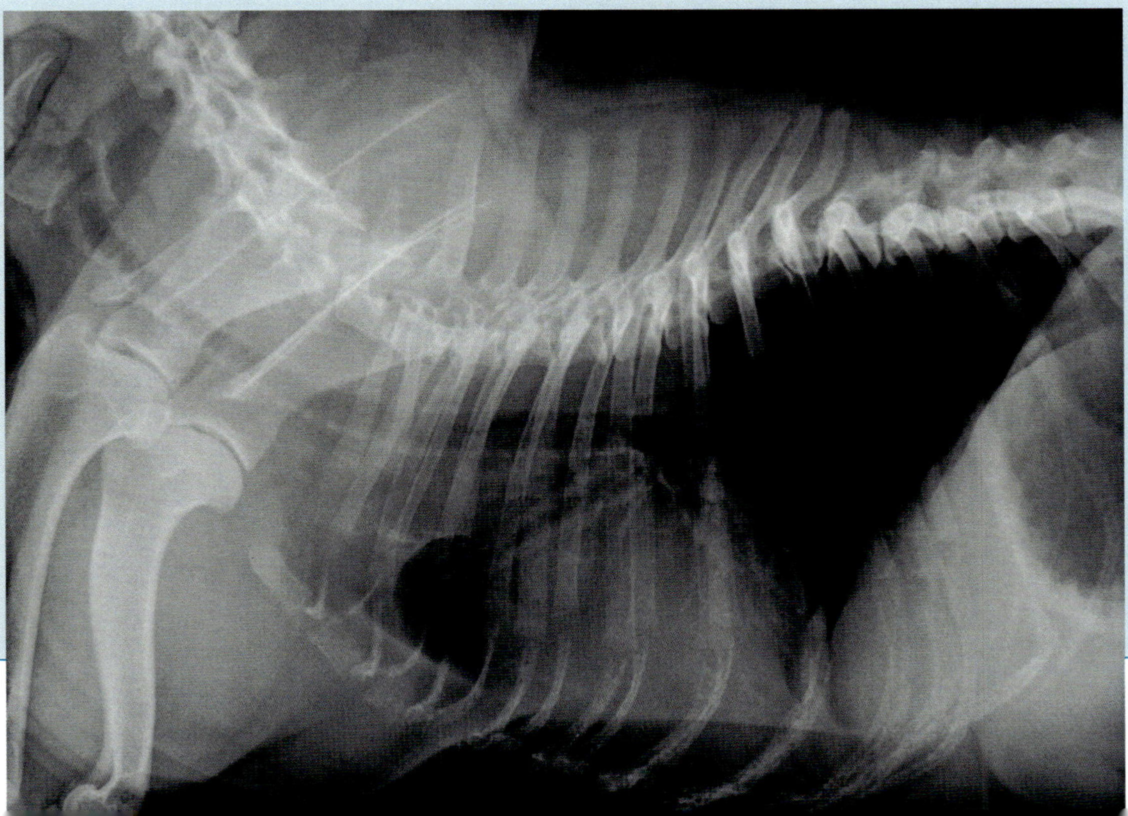

FIGURE 2.19. Lateral radiograph of the thorax of a Bulldog with no respiratory signs. The ratio of the diameter of the trachea to the height of the thoracic inlet is 0.11, which is considered to be within the limits of normality for this breed. The tracheal cartilages appear calcified (with no pathological significance).

it in the neck and mediastinum. Small accumulations of gas are sometimes visualised throughout its course (fig. 2.20), due to the swallowing of air in nervous patients or patients with respiratory difficulties. It is also common to observe, especially on left lateral radiographs, a very small retention of fluid in the distal part of the oesophagus, just before it passes through the oesophageal hiatus of the diaphragm. This creates a long soft-tissue density shadow, which appears centred between the course of the aorta and that of the caudal vena cava on lateral radiographs. Non-significant, moderate oesophageal dilatation may be observed in anaesthetised patients (fig. 2.21) or in those in which an oesophageal catheter was placed.

Since the information provided by plain radiography is limited, contrast studies are often carried out to examine the oesophagus. Barium is usually used in the form of a paste or mixed with food, so as to slow down the passage of the contrast medium through the oesophagus, as it is very fast in normal conditions, especially when it is liquid. The administration of barium in the form of a paste is useful to examine the mucosa, because it adheres to it. It is usually used when oesophagitis or neoplasms are suspected, but it should not be used if the oesophageal study is going to be accompanied by a gastrointestinal study, as the paste does not fill the stomach or the intestine properly, and does not mix well with liquid barium if this is administered at the same time. Liquid suspensions of barium sulphate at a dose of 3 to 5 ml/kg do not adhere to the mucosa as well as the paste, but they easily surround obstructions. It is sometimes necessary to administer an additional amount to delimit the whole oesophagus when this is very dilated.

Barium should not be used when an oesophageal perforation or rupture is suspected, since it may lead to the formation of granulomas if it extravasates. In these cases, hyperosmotic, water-soluble iodinated contrast media may be used, such as meglumine amidotrizoate, or low-osmolarity organic iodinated contrast media,

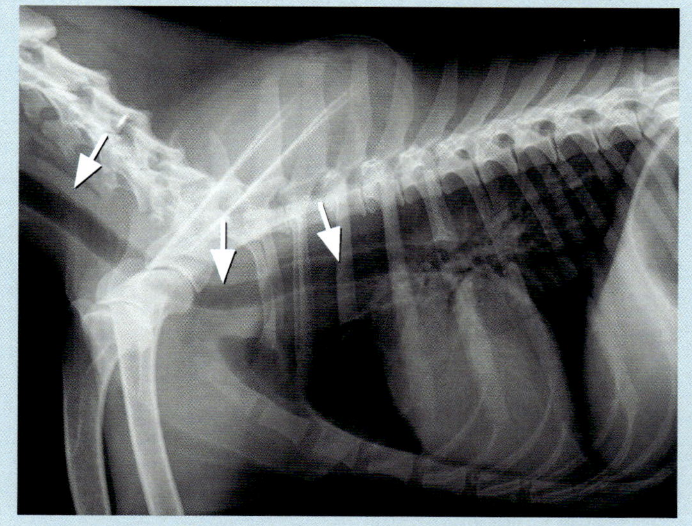

FIGURE 2.20. Lateral radiograph of the thorax and caudal area of the neck of a healthy dog. The normal oesophagus cannot be identified on plain radiographs, since it has the same radiographic density as most of the structures that surround it in the neck and mediastinum, but in this case, some small accumulations of gas in its lumen (arrows) allow the identification of its course. This finding is relatively usual in nervous patients or patients with respiratory difficulties because they swallow air. If the gas retention persists on consecutive radiographs, this may be indicative of a disease (for example, oesophagitis).

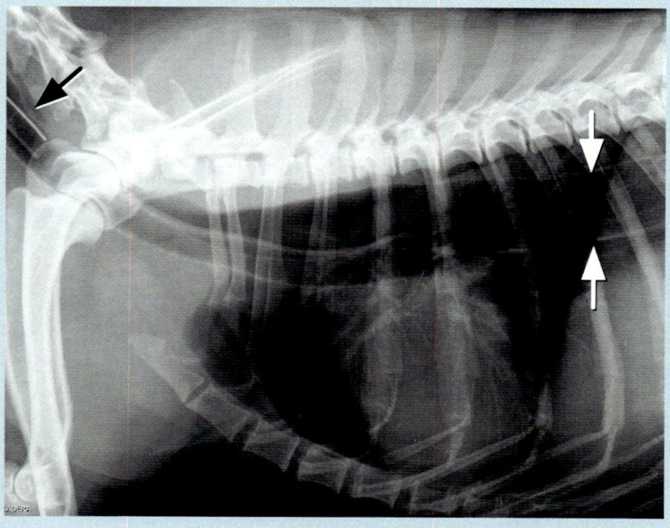

FIGURE 2.21. Lateral radiograph of the thorax of a dog with moderate dilatation of the oesophagus due to the anaesthesia. The dorsal and ventral walls of the oesophagus are indicated by white arrows and the endotracheal tube is shown with a black arrow.

such as iohexol or iopamidol, at a dose of 7 ml/ kg. Although the image of the oesophagus is more poorly defined with these contrast media than with barium, they would be absorbed if they extravasated, while barium would not. Despite their higher cost, it is recommended to use low-osmolarity contrast media. Hypertonic contrast media, due to their osmotic effects, may cause pulmonary oedema if they are aspirated or, if they are used in animals with hypovolaemia, the clinical status of the patient may worsen due to the loss of fluid through the gastrointestinal tract.

After administering barium, a temporary retention of the contrast medium may be observed between the folds of the oesophageal mucosa, which creates an image of parallel longitudinal bands in dogs. In addition to these longitudinal bands, transverse bands are also observed in the caudal third of the thoracic oesophagus in cats, which has been termed "herringbone" pattern. A minimal temporary retention of barium at the level of the pharynx or thoracic inlet may also be observed in normal conditions.

It is possible to examine functional anomalies of the oesophagus by means of fluoroscopy, as it allows real-time observation of the passage of the contrast medium from the oropharynx to the stomach. It is recommended to first administer liquid barium and then solid food mixed with barium. This is particularly useful to diagnose stenosis or regional motility disorders.

The term **megaoesophagus** is used to describe an abnormal dilatation of the oesophagus, generally associated with hypomotility of the wall. The dilatation is usually identified by means of plain radiography, although an oesophagogram may be indicated to confirm the diagnosis in case of doubt, to examine oesophageal motility (using fluoroscopy) or to detect the possible cause of the megaoesophagus. On both plain lateral and ventrodorsal or dorsoventral radiographs, it is possible to identify two thin lines of soft-tissue density in the area of the oesophagus. These lines converge in the diaphragm and correspond to the dilated oesophageal wall (fig. 2.22). These lines are better differentiated when the oesophagus is filled with gas, but may be identified when this latter contains fluid or food. The ventral line is sometimes masked by the superimposed caudal vena cava. When the dilatation is very marked, the trachea and cardiac silhouette may appear ventrally displaced (the ventral displacement of the trachea is sometimes the only evident finding on plain radiographs). On ventrodorsal or dorsoventral views, a moderately dilated oesophagus may be masked by the superimposed spine, although it is common to see a displacement of the trachea to the right. In patients with a megaoesophagus, special attention must be paid to the image of the lungs fields, as aspiration pneumonia can often be detected.

Oesophagitis does not usually cause significant changes on plain radiographs, although a persistent retention of gas in the oesophageal lumen is sometimes observed. The oesophagogram may show an irregular retention of barium between the folds of the mucosa, which is accompanied by diffuse and non-uniform dilatation of the oesophagus.

Foreign bodies located in the lumen of the oesophagus are a common cause of oesophageal dysphagia. The most common sites where oesophageal foreign bodies are observed are:

- Upper oesophageal sphincter.
- Thoracic inlet.
- Base of the heart.
- Area cranial to the diaphragm.

It is easy to recognise radiopaque foreign bodies (fig. 2.23), but the diagnosis may be more complicated in cases of radiolucent ones. On the oesophagogram, an accumulation of contrast medium is often observed cranial to the foreign body, although the contrast medium may also be absorbed if the object is porous. Foreign bodies may also cause a partial or complete obstruction or no obstruction at all. The complications associated with oesophageal foreign bodies are perforation and stenosis due to scarring.

Diverticula are defined as localised dilatations of the oesophagus and are identified on radiographs by the focal accumulation of gas or granular material (food) in the oesophagus. By administrating a contrast medium, it is possible to determine the size and exact location of the lesion. When they are located in the cranial mediastinum, the diverticulum is usually seen ventral to the trachea (fig. 2.24).

Stenoses are localised narrowings of the oesophageal lumen (fig. 2.25). They may appear as a result of the previous presence of a foreign body at the site where the stenosis is located, associated with anomalies of the vascular rings or with tumours, and in cases of oesophagitis due to reflux. An oesophagogram is necessary for their diagnosis. A normal peristaltic oesophageal contraction should not be mistaken for stenosis in static images. They can be differentiated by means of fluoroscopy or, if it is not available, by taking several radiographs at different times to observe whether the narrowing remains in the image.

Congenital anomalies of the vascular rings cause an external compression of the oesophagus. The most common is the persistence of the right aortic arch, which occurs more frequently in dogs than in cats. It is usually diagnosed in young animals with regurgitation. These anomalies usually cause localised dilatation of the oesophagus in the cranial mediastinum, cranially to the heart, which can be confirmed by a contrast study (fig. 2.26). The image of the caudal oesophagus at the base of the heart is usually normal, although it may sometimes appear dilated. Persistent retention of food is often observed in the dilated area.

Oesophageal masses may correspond to benign or malignant neoplasms or to inflammatory masses. Oesophageal masses are rare in small animals. On plain radiographs, it is possible to observe accumulations of food or associated diverticula, and soft-tissue opacity masses in some cases. An area of narrowing of the lumen is usually identified in contrast studies, with irregularity of the mucosa.

An oesophageal **perforation** may be suspected on a plain radiograph if there is subcutaneous emphysema of unknown origin in the neck, or signs of pneumomediastinum in the thorax. It may sometimes be accompanied by a pneumothorax, mediastinal effusion or pleural effusion. The diagnosis is confirmed by administering an iodinated contrast medium, which will be extravasated, although its identification may be difficult if the perforation is small. In case of doubt, fluoroscopy may facilitate the diagnosis.

Fistulae may form between the oesophageal lumen and the respiratory system, although they are uncommon. The origin of the site of communication may be oesophagotracheal, oesophagobronchial or oesophagopulmonary. On oesophagograms, their image may be similar to that created when a contrast medium administrated by oral route is accidentally inhaled.

Hiatal hernias are usually transitory and may be associated with respiratory movements. They are difficult to diagnose on plain radiographs, in which case contrast and fluoroscopy studies are used. In the most evident cases, the stomach (with its characteristic folds) or part of it may be identified in the thorax. In other cases, a less defined soft-tissue density structure is visualised in the caudodorsal part of the thorax, and may disappear on subsequent radiographs. In contrast studies, part of the stomach is identified in the thorax, although it may move in and out of the thoracic cavity with respiratory movements.

Gastrooesophageal invagination or intussusception is an uncommon alteration. The stomach or part of it moves into the lumen of the oesophagus, thus originating an anomalous shadow in the caudodorsal part of the thorax. If a contrast study is performed, the contrast medium may not reach the stomach and may delimit a large intraluminal oesophageal mass instead. In some cases, the intussuception appears intermittently.

Gastrooesophageal reflux occurs when stomach acids enter the oesophagus, which usually causes oesophagitis. Plain radiographs do not usually show any significant findings, although focal dilatation of the distal oesophagus with accumulation of gas or fluid is sometimes detected.

Pleural space

The pleural space is the anatomical space included between the visceral and parietal layers of the pleura (fig. 2.27). The parietal pleura covers the internal aspect of the chest wall, the diaphragm and the mediastinum, and the visceral pleura covers the pulmonary surface and forms the interlobar fissures. It is a potential space, which, in normal conditions, contains a minimal amount of fluid that acts as a lubricant to minimise friction during breathing.

Plain radiography allows us to detect the presence of abnormal contents, which generally consist in fluid (pleural effusion) or gas (pneumothorax), in this anatomical space, as well as to identify masses of pleural origin. Calcifications and minimal pleural thickenings are usual findings in older animals and do not usually have any pathological significance.

Ultrasound examinations may provide diagnostic information of great interest in cases of effusion and pleural masses, but not in cases of pneumothorax, since the air contained in the pleural space is easily mistaken for that contained in the lungs.

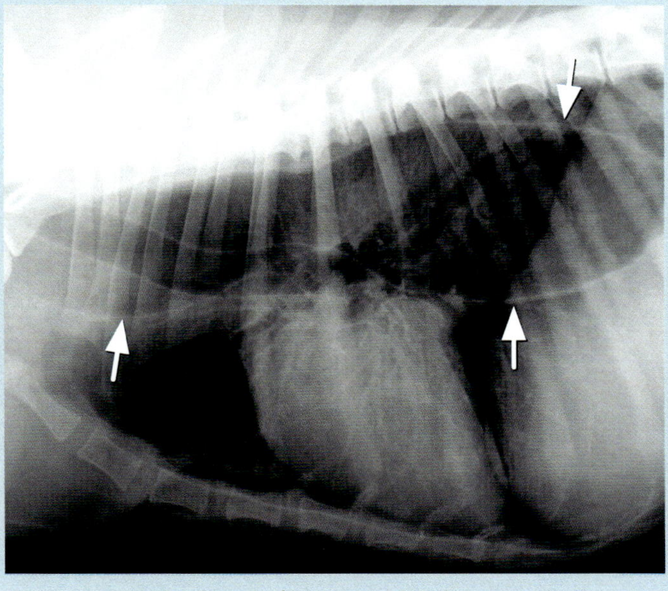

FIGURE 2.22. Lateral radiograph of the thorax a dog with a megaoesophagus. The walls of the oesophagus are shown with white arrows. The trachea appears slightly displaced in ventral direction.

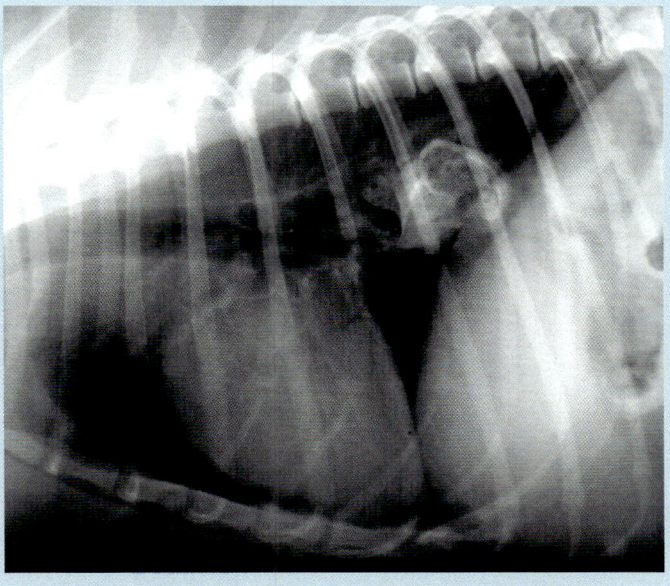

FIGURE 2.23. Lateral radiograph of a dog with a mineral density foreign body (bone) in the oesophagus, cranial to the oesophageal hiatus of the diaphragm.

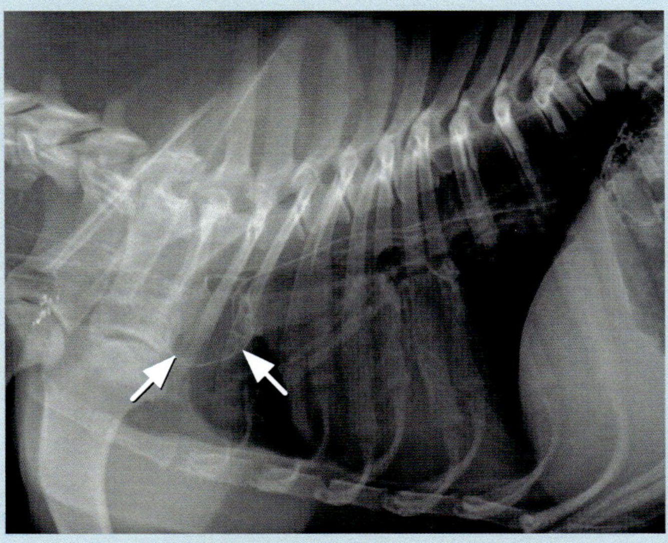

FIGURE 2.24. Lateral oesophagogram of a dog with an oesophageal diverticulum located in the cranial mediastinum, after the administration of barium.

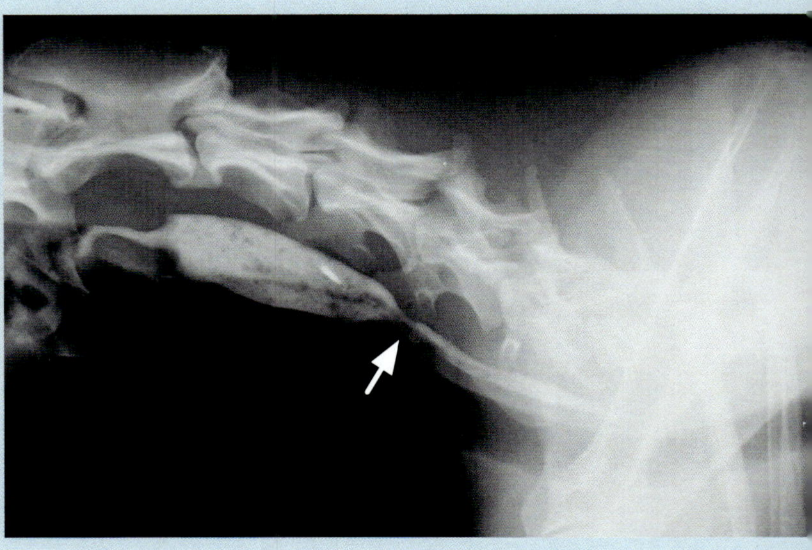

FIGURE 2.25. Lateral oesophagogram showing the neck of a dog with oesophageal stenosis (arrow), after the administration of barium. This image may be confused with that of a peristaltic wave and the persistence of the lesion must therefore be confirmed, either by means of fluoroscopy or by repeating the radiograph at different times.

Normal radiographic
anatomy of the thorax
right lateral view

http://goo.gl/otDInr

Moreover, this technique will facilitate sample collection for cytology or biopsy.

Computed tomography is also an excellent diagnostic alternative to assess the anomalies that affect this anatomical space.

Pleural effusion

In cases of severe pleural effusion, it is convenient to stabilise the patient first, before performing a radiographic study. Radiographs taken with the animal standing may be useful and, alternatively, the dorsoventral projection may be chosen in order not to worsen the state of the patient. If the respiratory involvement is not severe, it is preferable to take a ventrodorsal radiograph instead of a dorsoventral one, since on this latter the fluid accumulates around the heart to a greater extent and makes the visualisation of this organ more difficult (fig. 2.28), in addition to causing an enlargement of the shadow of the mediastinum. On ventrodorsal radiographs, interlobar fissures will be better visualised in cases of mild or moderate effusion, since the fluid tends to enter in the fissures in dorsal recumbency, while it tends to accumulate dorsal to the sternum in sternal recumbency. If the respiratory involvement allows it, in these cases it is recommended to take, in addition, a lateral radiograph.

The radiological signs of a pleural effusion vary in function of the amount of fluid that accumulates. It may be transudate, exudate, blood or lymph, which cannot be identified on a radiograph. It starts to be detectable on radiographs from 50-100 ml. If the amount is very small, radiographs will only show thin bands of fluid density at the site of the interlobar fissures (fig. 2.29). As the amount of fluid increases, it is possible to observe retraction and rounding of the lung margins, which will appear separated from the thoracic wall by bands of fluid density. The cardiac silhouette and shadow of the diaphragm may appear partially or totally masked (fig. 2.30). If there is a very large amount of accumulated fluid, the cardiac silhouette may be elevated and displace the trachea,

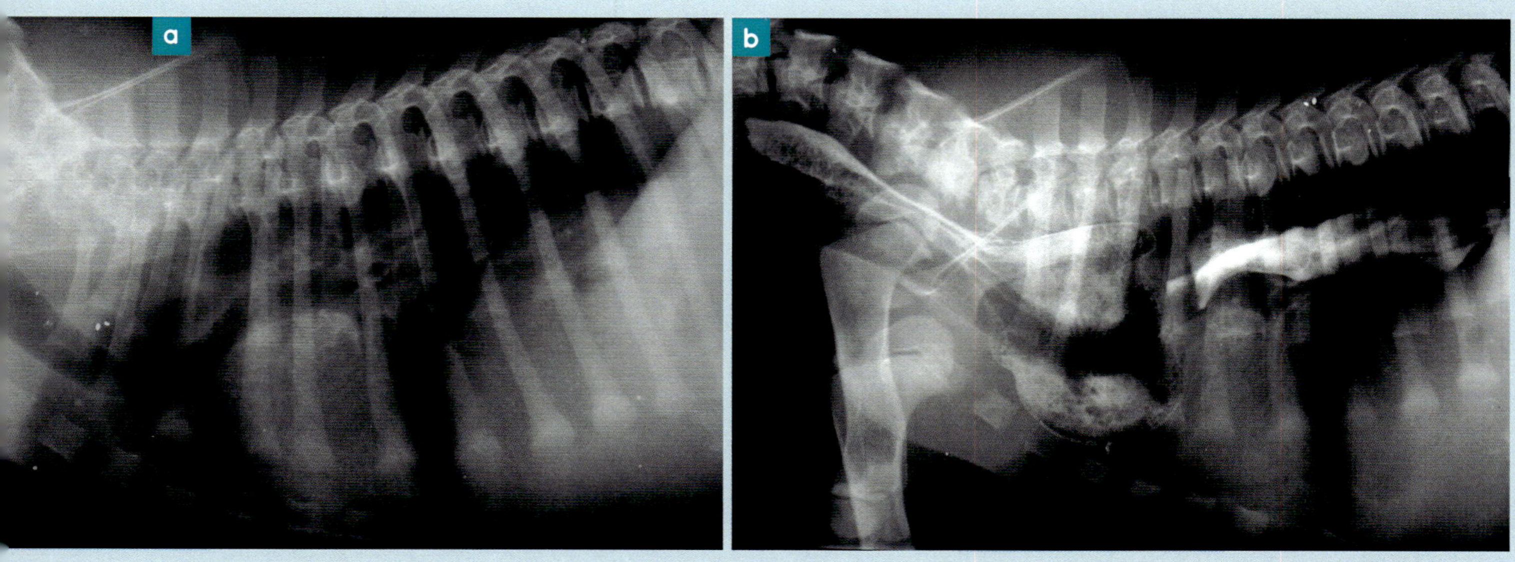

FIGURE 2.26. Lateral radiograph of the thorax of a 2-month-old dog, before (a) and after (b) the administration of barium, with a marked focal dilatation of the oesophagus cranial to the heart. This finding suggests the existence of a congenital anomaly of the vascular rings (the persistence of the right aortic arch is the most frequent anomaly), which causes external compression of the oesophagus at the level of the base of the heart. Note that the only radiographic sign that is indicative of oesophageal dilatation in the image (a) is the marked ventral curvature of the trachea.

which may give a false impression of cardiomegaly or mediastinal mass (fig. 2.31), although we must bear in mind that these conditions may coexist with a pleural effusion in some cases.

Both pleural spaces are interconnected, so the fluid (or gas in cases of pneumothorax) is usually distributed in a relatively uniform manner between both hemithoraces (fig. 2.32). A unilateral effusion means a loss of permeability, which may be due to the formation of fibrin deposits in chronic or reactive effusions (pyothorax, haemothorax, chylothorax) or to an inflammatory or neoplastic process of the pleura. It frequently appears in cats in cases of pyothorax. When the effusion is **unilateral**, the radiographic signs vary to some degree:

- On lateral radiographs, a more diffuse increase in intrathoracic density may be observed instead of lung retraction (this can even be mistaken for a pulmonary infiltrate).
- On ventrodorsal and dorsoventral radiographs, lung retraction is only observed on the affected side (fig. 2.33). In severe cases, the entire hemithorax may have a uniform soft-tissue density, whereas the contralateral one remains normal.
- There may be a displacement of the heart towards the healthy side.

A severe pleural effusion may mask a cardiomegaly, the presence of lung infiltrates, a pulmonary, pleural or mediastinal mass, a diaphragmatic hernia or a lung lobe torsion, so the patient should always be reassessed once the effusion has been drained, so as to rule out the presence of any of these conditions. When fluid rich in fibrin has been removed, the lungs may then not fully expand due to pleural thickening, and their margins may remain rounded until the process is resolved.

Ultrasonography is used to investigate the primary cause of an effusion, for example to assess cardiac function, identify masses and examine possible pleural thickenings, defects in the diaphragm or lung lobe torsion. It also allows the identification of areas of pulmonary atelectasis and the location of small accumulations of fluid in order to take samples and drain the thorax under ultrasound guidance in complicated cases.

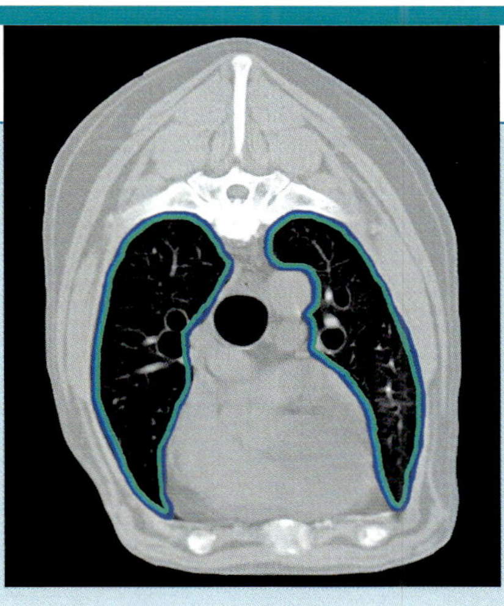

FIGURE 2.27. Representation of the parietal pleura (blue line) and visceral pleura (green line) on a computed tomography image of the thorax of a dog. In normal conditions, the pleural space is a potential anatomical space that only contains a minimal amount of fluid as a lubricant to minimise friction during breathing.

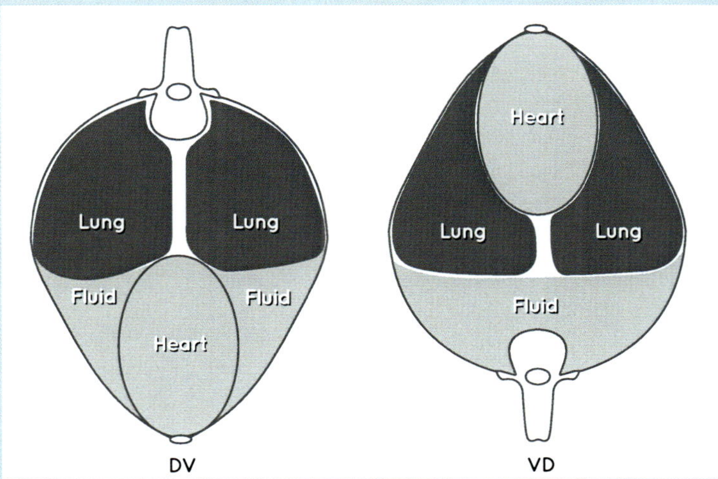

FIGURE 2.28. Schematic representation of the location of a moderate amount of pleural fluid when dorsoventral (DV) and ventrodorsal (VD) radiographs are taken. On the dorsoventral radiograph, the fluid is displaced to the ventral area of the thorax and surrounds the heart, so the cardiac silhouette is less defined. When a ventrodorsal radiograph is taken, the fluid moves to the roof of the thoracic cavity and is separated from the heart, so this latter will be better visualised in the image. In the case of a severe effusion, the cardiac silhouette is masked on both views.

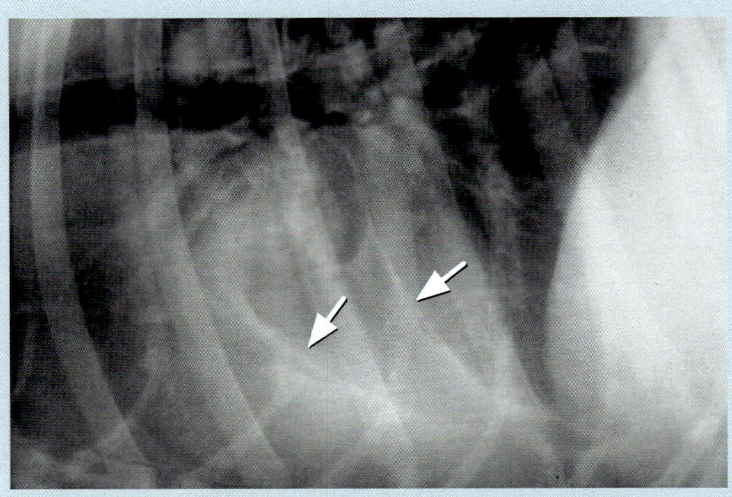

FIGURE 2.29. Enlarged image of the thorax on a lateral radiograph of a dog with mild pleural effusion. Thin bands of fluid/soft-tissue density that delimit the right middle lobe may be observed at the site of the interlobar fissures.

In cases of pyothorax and chylothorax, computed tomography is particularly indicated to assess the extension and distribution of the fluid with more precision, as well as to determine the cause in some cases (e.g.: abscesses, fistulous tracts, thoracic duct leaks, etc.). It provides more complete diagnostic information than an ultrasound examination when the effusion is associated with masses, defects in the diaphragm or lung lobe torsion.

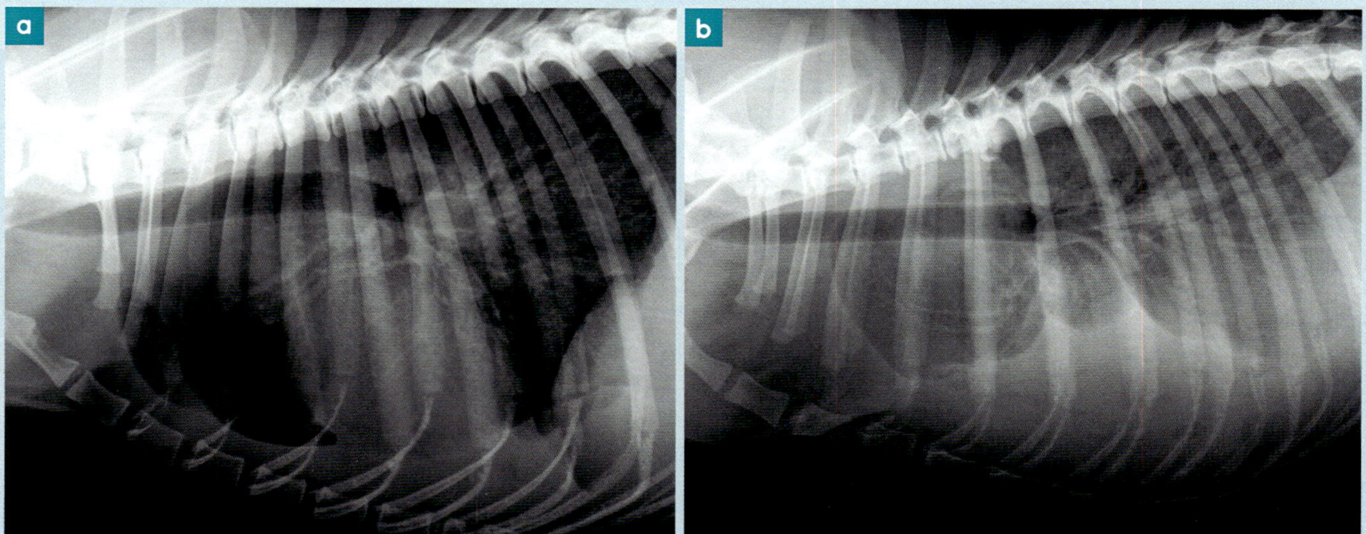

FIGURE 2.30. Lateral radiographs of the thorax of two dogs with pleural effusion, one moderate (a) and the other from moderate to severe (b). In both cases, the lung appears separated from the sternum by areas of fluid/soft-tissue density, but the degree of retraction and rounding of the lung margins is more marked in image (b). In image (a), only the ventral area of the cardiac silhouette and of the dome of the diaphragm is masked by the fluid, while in image (b), neither the cardiac silhouette nor most part of the shadow of the diaphragm can be visualised.

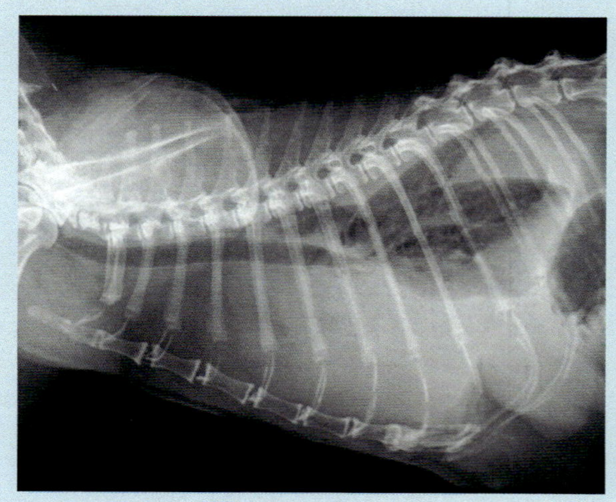

FIGURE 2.31. Lateral radiograph of a cat with a severe pleural effusion. The lungs are slightly distended and the trachea appears elevated. Most of the thoracic cavity has a practically homogeneous fluid/soft-tissue density and neither the cardiac silhouette nor the shadow of the diaphragm can be visualised in the image.

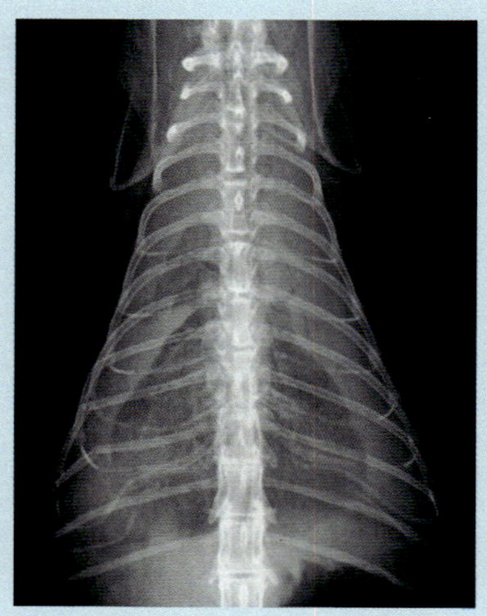

FIGURE 2.32. Dorsoventral radiograph of the thorax of a cat with severe bilateral pleural effusion. The fluid appears distributed in a more or less uniform manner between the two hemithoraces.

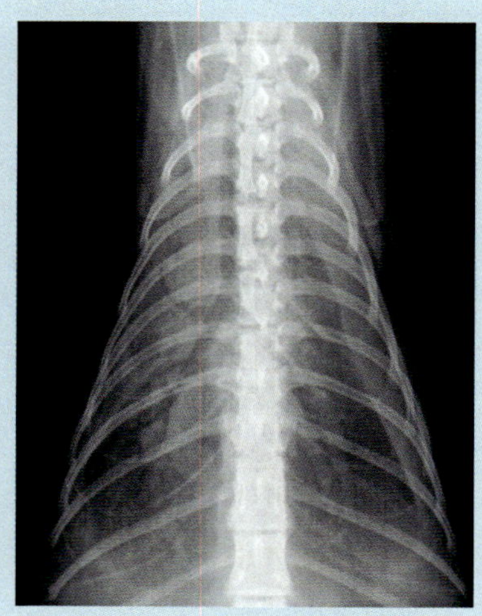

FIGURE 2.33. Dorsoventral radiograph of the thorax of a cat with unilateral left moderate pleural effusion. The right lung has an alveolar interstitial pattern that is mainly compatible with pneumonia, oedema or haemorrhage. The presence of a unilateral pleural effusion in cats suggests the presence of a pyothorax, although it may also appear due to other causes.

In cases of chylothorax, a lymphangiogram is performed by administering an iodinated contrast medium through a mesenteric lymph vessel, or by injecting it in a mesenteric lymph node under ultrasound guidance. This way, leaks in the thoracic duct (or one of its branches) and lymphangiectases may be identified.

Pneumothorax

It is defined as the presence of free gas in the pleural space. This term is sometimes confused with pneumomediastinum, which corresponds to gas in the mediastinal space.

The most frequent cause of pneumothorax is trauma, in which case we should always examine the skeletal structures in the image, particularly the ribs, since rib fractures with minimal displacement of fragments may be difficult to find. A pneumothorax may also appear spontaneously (e.g. by rupture of pulmonary bullae) or due to iatrogenic causes (e.g. due to a puncture of the lung).

In cases of pneumothorax, lateral radiographs will show an elevation of the cardiac silhouette, which appears separated from the sternum by a band of gas density. In fact, the heart is not elevated, but displaced to the centre of the cavity when the patient is placed in lateral recumbency, since it is not supported by the lung as it would normally be, as this latter is partially collapsed (fig. 2.34). As the amount of gas increases in the pleural space, the caudal lung lobes begin to collapse and become separated from the spine and diaphragm (fig. 2.35). In general, lateral views are the most sensitive to detect mild or moderate pneumothoraces, since in these cases it may be difficult to identify lung retraction on dorsoventral or ventrodorsal views. Of these two latter projections, the dorsoventral one is preferred in cases of mild pneumothorax. Lungs may have a variable degree of increased opacity depending on the degree of collapse. This does not allow the correct assessment of the presence of alterations in the parenchyma (they will be ruled out by repeating the radiographs once the cavity has been drained).

If there is a tension pneumothorax, the thorax will appear enlarged, the ribs will be extended to their maximum and the shadow of the diaphragm will be flattened or even curved in the direction opposite to its normal position.

If the pneumothorax is unilateral, it will be possible to observe a displacement of the mediastinal structures to the contralateral hemithorax on dorsoventral and ventrodorsal radiographs. On lateral views, the cardiac silhouette may not appear elevated if the animal is placed with the affected side up.

A hydropneumothorax (presence of fluid and gas in the pleural space) due to trauma, pulmonary abscesses or oesophageal perforation may be detected. The radiographic findings will depend on the amount and proportion of accumulated fluid and gas.

On dorsoventral and ventrodorsal views, folds of skin may create an artefact that may be mistaken for the image of a pneumothorax, which is called **false pneumothorax** or **pseudopneumothorax**. The area medial to the fold has a higher opacity than the area

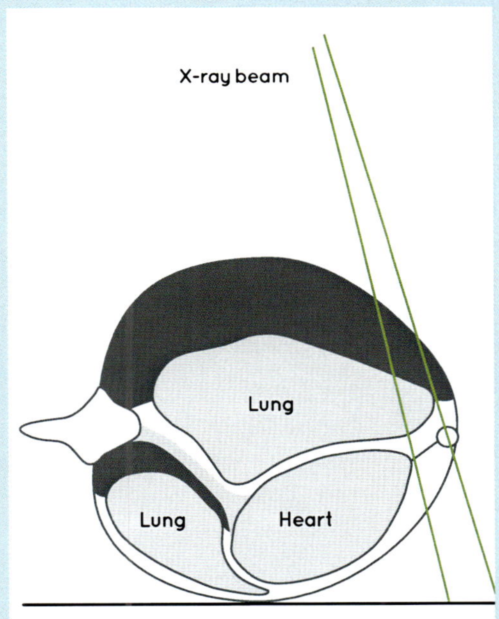

FIGURE 2.34. Schematic representation of the displacement of the heart, which creates an image of "elevation" of the cardiac silhouette on lateral radiographs in cases of pneumothorax. The heart is not supported as it would normally be by a healthy lung. The collapsed lung occupies a smaller volume and as a result, the heart is displaced to the centre of the thoracic cavity, which originates an image of elevation on lateral radiographs.

lateral to it. If there is a high contrast, the lateral area may be mistaken for free gas in the pleural space (fig. 2.36). To differentiate it from a real pneumothorax, we must carefully examine the most radiolucent area and see if the pulmonary vessels can be identified in it. Their presence confirms that the image is due to an artefact. The small vessels are better visualised if we use a bright light source in the case of conventional images, or by significantly increasing image brightness on digital radiographs. An image similar to a pneumothorax may also be observed when lung radiopacity is reduced due to excessive inflation (for example, secondary to asthma or to chronic bronchial disease) or to cases of pulmonary emphysema, hypovascularisation of the lung or hypovolaemia.

It is difficult to distinguish the free gas located in the pleural space from the air contained in the normal lung in an ultrasound image, which is why ultrasonography is not routinely used for the assessment of a pneumothorax. A criterion of differentiation is that the gas contained in the pleural space remains static, while the air contained in the lungs is displaced with inspiration and expiration. An ultrasound examination may be useful to identify foreign bodies or fistulous tracts located in the thoracic wall when these are suspected to be the cause of the pneumothorax.

Computed tomography will provide more complete diagnostic information in cases of recurrent or persistent pneumothorax with no known cause (fig. 2.37).

Pleural masses

Radiologically, pleural tumours, abscesses or haematomas produce an image of localised pleural thickening. Pleural neoplasms may be primary (mesotheliomas) or due to a secondary infiltration of the pleura (pleural carcinomatosis).

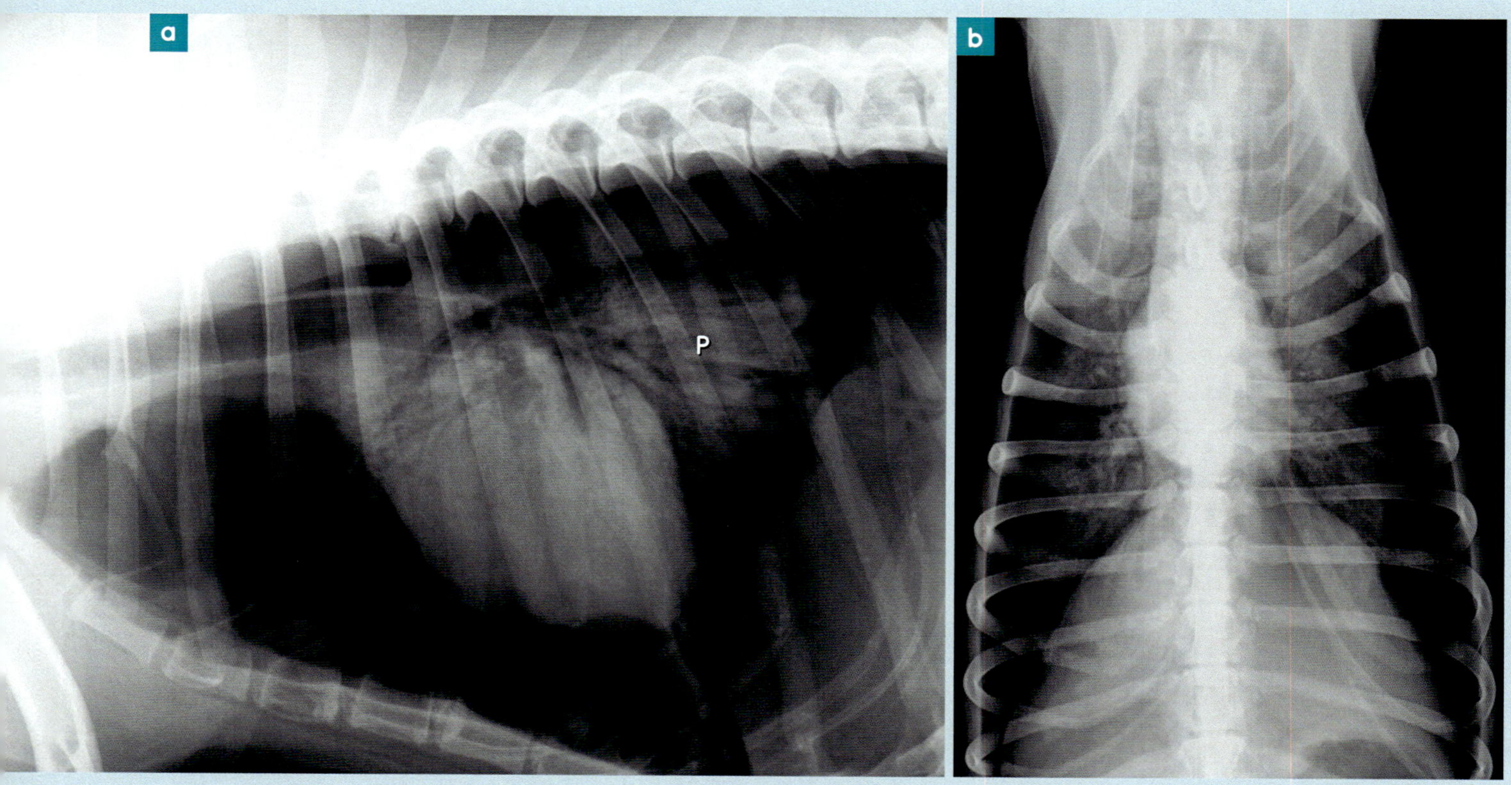

FIGURE 2.35. Lateral (a) and dorsoventral (b) radiographs of the thorax of a dog with a moderate to severe bilateral pneumothorax. In image (a), the cardiac silhouette appears separated from the sternum by a band of gas density and the lung (L) appears collapsed, which is why its radiopacity is increased. In image (b), both lungs are collapsed and separated from the costal wall by bands of gas density, although the degree of lung retraction is greater in the left hemithorax. The cardiac silhouette appears reduced in size, which is a common finding in cases of severe pneumothorax.

Pleural masses are characterised by having relatively wide areas of contact with the thoracic wall, which helps us to identify masses of pulmonary or mediastinal origin on dorsoventral or ventrodorsal radiographs. However, we cannot confirm the pleural origin of a thoracic mass with certainty based only on radiological signs. It is also very common for them to be masked by an associated pleural effusion, and they are therefore more easily identified after draining the thoracic cavity. The displacement of adjacent structures may also help in the diagnosis in cases of effusion associated with the mass (fig. 2.38).

Ultrasonography allows the identification of pleural masses, whether there is a concomitant effusion or not, although it does not clearly differentiate a pleural origin from a possible pulmonary or mediastinal origin. In addition, it facilitates the collection of samples for cytology and biopsies.

Computed tomography will give a better definition of the margins of the mass, although in cases of mesotheliomas the pleural effusion may be the only recognisable finding. It is common to find associated pericardial masses or pericardial effusion in the study.

Pleural thickenings

In older animals, thin lines of soft-tissue or mineral density may be observed at the site of the interlobar fissures. These are normally due to thickenings of the pleura with no clinical significance. Pleural calcifications may also appear as small areas distributed throughout the lung fields on chest radiographs (fig. 2.39).

Pathological pleural thickenings appear as bands of soft-tissue opacity with an irregular morphology (fig. 2.40). They may be the sequela of any type of

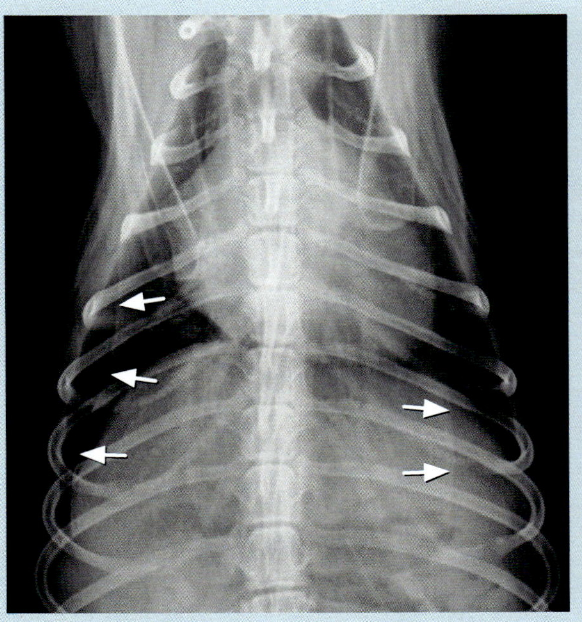

FIGURE 2.36. Dorsoventral view of the thorax of a healthy dog. The folds of skin create bands of soft-tissue density that appear on both sides of the thorax (arrows). In the right hemithorax, the contrast between the area lateral and that medial to the fold is so marked that it may be mistaken for a pneumothorax. This artefact is termed false pneumothorax or pseudopneumothorax. If the most radiolucent area is examined with a bright light source (or brightness is increased in the case of a digital radiograph), the detection of small pulmonary blood vessels will confirm this is due to an artefact and that it is not a real pneumothorax.

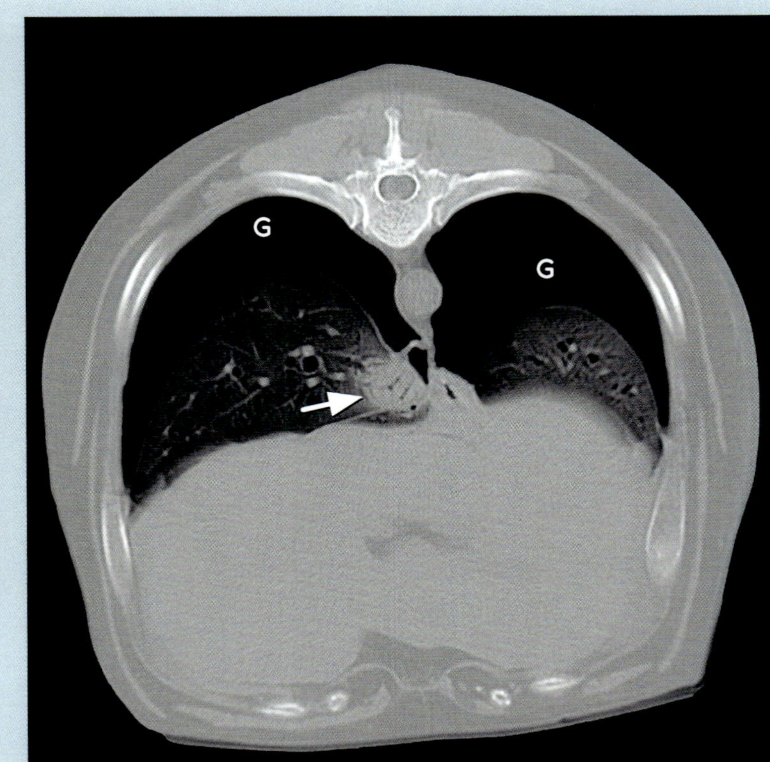

FIGURE 2.37. Computed tomography image of the thorax of a dog with a hydropneumothorax (accumulation of gas and fluid in the pleural space, although in this image it is only possible to observe the gas –G–) associated with a focal area of pulmonary infection (arrow), possible due to the penetration of a foreign body.

Normal radiographic anatomy of the thorax
dorsoventral view

http://goo.gl/pKMKlb

pleural effusion, although they are common and form more rapidly in cases of reactive effusion (pyothorax, haemothorax or chylothorax), in which fibrous adherences that capture and encapsulate small amounts of fluid may form. These focal accumulations of fluid may have a radiographic image similar to that of pleural masses.

Mediastinum

It corresponds to the anatomical space located between the right and left cavities (fig. 2.41). It communicates cranially with the soft tissues of the neck, through the thoracic inlet, and caudally with the retroperitoneum, through the aortic hiatus. The oesophagus, thoracic trachea, lymph nodes, thoracic lymph duct, thymus, some nerves, the heart and great vessels are located in the mediastinum. Of all these structures, only the trachea, cardiac silhouette, aorta and caudal vena cava may be identified on a normal chest radiograph of an adult animal. The remaining structures form a common shadow in the cranial mediastinum, as they cannot be distinguished from one another since they have the same radiographic density (fig. 2.42). The caudoventral mediastinal recess is sometimes identified on dorsoventral and ventrodorsal radiographs as a thin band of soft-tissue density that connects the cardiac silhouette with the diaphragm (fig. 2.43).

On dorsoventral and ventrodorsal radiographs, the shadow of the cranial mediastinum must have approximately the same width as the thoracic vertebrae in cats, while in dogs it should not exceed twice the width of these vertebrae in normal conditions. It should be taken into account that the mediastinum of brachycephalic dogs and obese cats and dogs may be wider, with a displacement of the trachea to the right on dorsoventral and ventrodorsal views, and a significant elevation of the cardiac silhouette due to an accumulation of fat ventral to it (fig. 2.44).

In young animals, it is often possible to visualise the shadow of the thymus, which reaches its maximum size at approximately 4 months of age and is no longer visible at 6 months of age (fig. 2.45). On very rare occasions, a vestige of the thymus is observed in adults.

Most of the diseases that affect the mediastinum are secondary to pulmonary, oesophageal, pleural and lymphatic diseases.

Mediastinal effusion

It corresponds to the presence of free fluid (transudate, exudate, blood, lymph) in the mediastinal space. It may appear associated with mediastinitis, coagulopathies, trauma, feline infectious peritonitis, etc.

The radiographic image of a mediastinal effusion may be confused with that of a pleural effusion on lateral radiographs, but not on dorsoventral or ventrodorsal radiographs. On these views, there will be no retraction of the lateral margins of the lung, but an abnormal enlargement of the shadow of the mediastinum (fig. 2.46). In some cases, triangular or thorn-shaped shadows will appear with their wider base oriented towards the hilum (which differentiates them from interlobar fissures in a pleural effusion). These are called reverse fissure lines. A mediastinal effusion is often accompanied by a mild pleural effusion.

The effusion sometimes masks the presence of localised masses in the mediastinal space, in which case an ultrasound examination will be particularly useful to assess the size and characteristics of the mass, as well as the amount of accumulated fluid. In these cases, ultrasound-guided sampling of the mass and fluid will be indicated. Computed tomography may provide complementary information about the possible origin of the effusion.

Pneumomediastinum

The presence of free gas in the mediastinal space may be indicative of a rupture of the trachea or oesophagus, or less likely of the bronchi or lung, but it may also be due to the presence of subcutaneous emphysema in the neck, since the gas may go from the spaces between the fasciae of the neck to the mediastinal space through the thoracic inlet. If all the possible causes are ruled out, the possibility of an idiopathic pneumomediastimum should be considered.

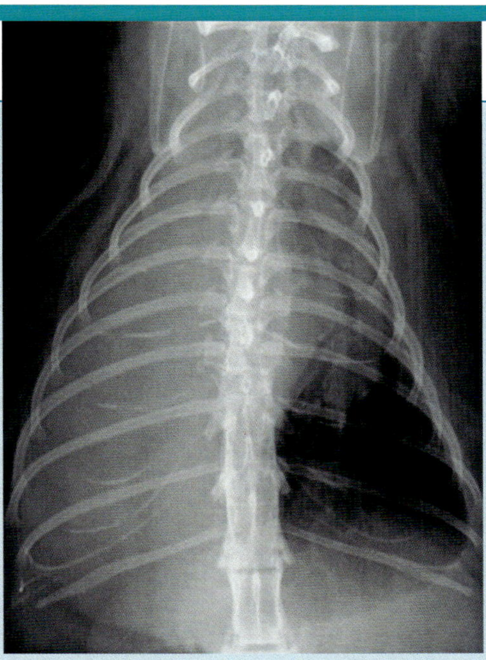

FIGURE 2.38. Dorsoventral radiograph of the thorax of a cat with a pleural haematoma and severe unilateral pleural effusion in the right hemithorax. Although the fluid does not allow the visualisation of the lesion in the image, a marked displacement of the mediastinum towards the left hemithorax may be observed, which indicates the presence of a mass in the contralateral hemithorax. A severe unilateral pleural effusion may slightly displace the mediastinum towards the non-affected side, but the marked displacement in this patient suggests the presence of an additional mass-type lesion, which was confirmed with the subsequent ultrasound study.

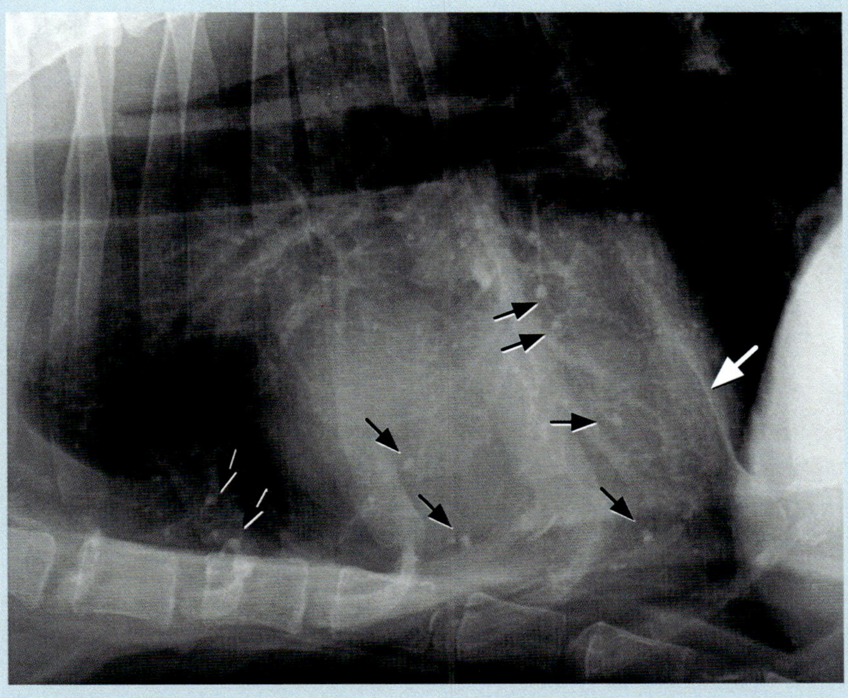

FIGURE 2.39. Enlarged imaged of the thorax on a lateral radiograph of an older dog. In older animals, it is often possible to visualise thin lines of soft-tissue or mineral density at the site of the interlobar fissures (white arrow). These are generally due to thickenings or calcifications of the pleura with no clinical significance. Pleural calcifications may also appear as small areas of mineral density distributed throughout the lung fields, which are visible in this image (some of them are shown with a black arrow).

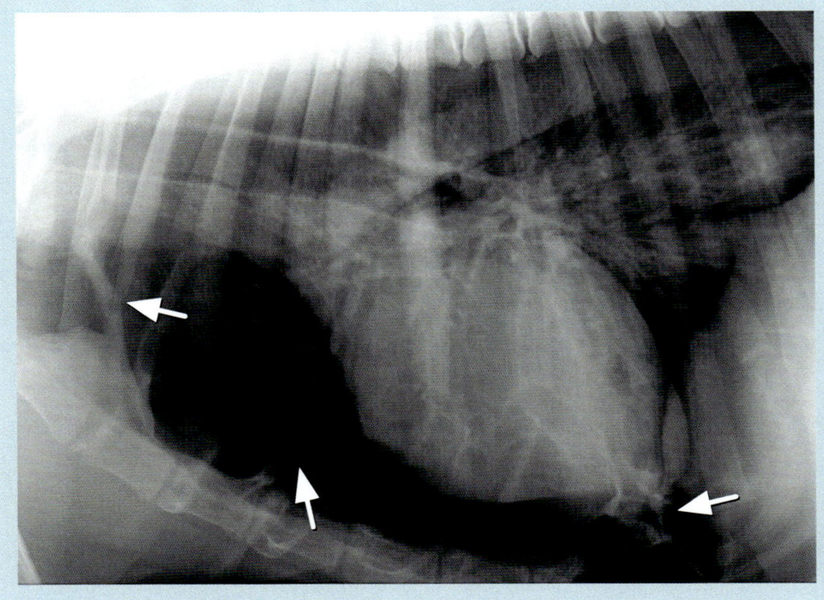

FIGURE 2.40. Lateral radiograph of the thorax of a dog with a hydropneumothorax possibly caused by the penetration of a foreign body, although this latter was not identified during surgery. The pneumothorax causes a displacement of the cardiac silhouette, which appears separated from the sternum by a gas density band. In various locations of the ventral area of the thorax, it is possible to observe soft-tissue density bands with an irregular morphology (arrows), which correspond to pleural thickenings and a focal accumulation of pleural fluid. The sternal lymph node also appears increased in size (dorsal to the manubrium and second sternebra).

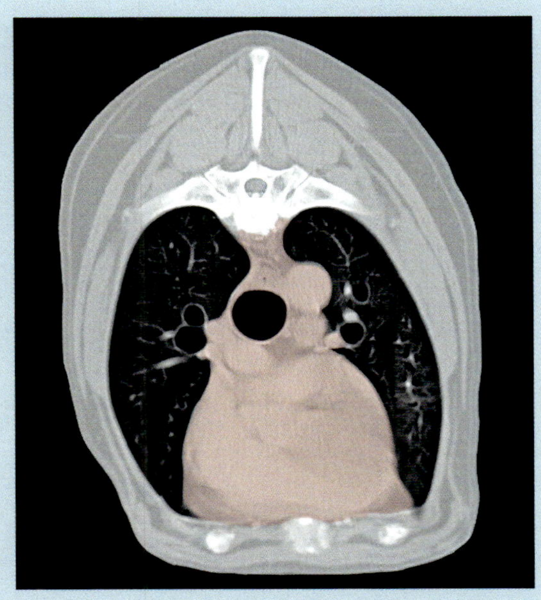

FIGURE 2.41. Representation of the mediastinum (coloured in red) on a computed tomography image of the thorax of a dog. The mediastinal space contains the oesophagus, the thoracic trachea, and lymph nodes, and thoracic lymphatic duct and thymus, some nerves, the heart and the great vessels of the thorax.

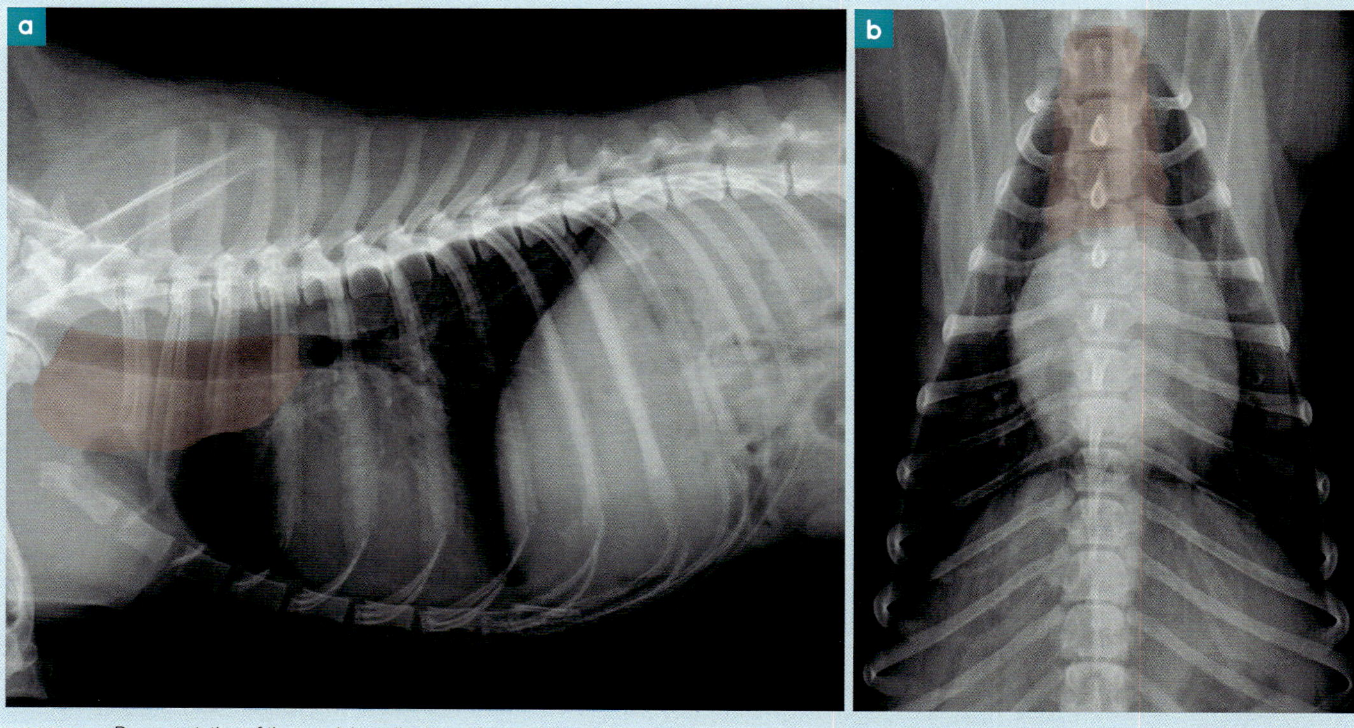

FIGURE 2.42. Representation of the cranial mediastinum (coloured in red) on lateral (a) and dorsoventral (b) radiographs of a healthy dog. Of the anatomical structures it contains, only the trachea can be identified in the image due to its gas content, while the rest (part of the oesophagus, lymph nodes, cranial vena cava, brachiocephalic trunk, left subclavian artery, thoracic duct and thymus) form a global shadow of soft-tissue density, which is referred to as shadow of the cranial mediastinum.

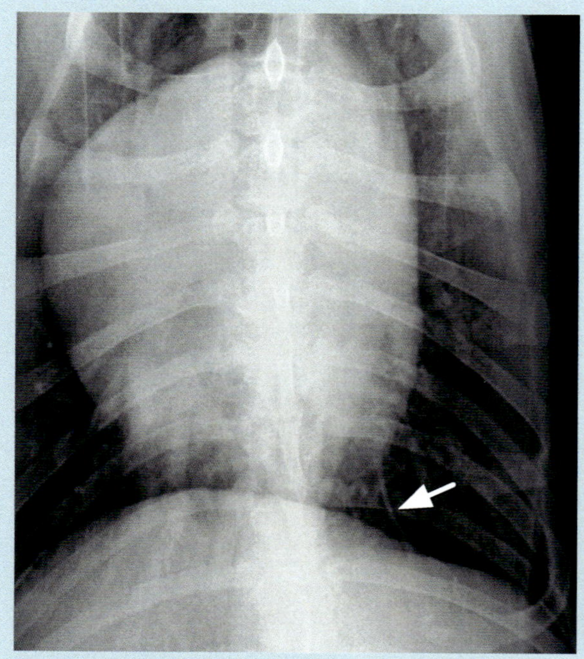

FIGURE 2.43. Enlarged image of the thorax on a ventrodorsal radiograph of a healthy dog. The caudoventral mediastinal recess is sometimes identified on dorsoventral and ventrodorsal radiographs (more often on the latter view) as a thin band of soft-tissue density that connects the cardiac silhouette with the diaphragm (arrow).

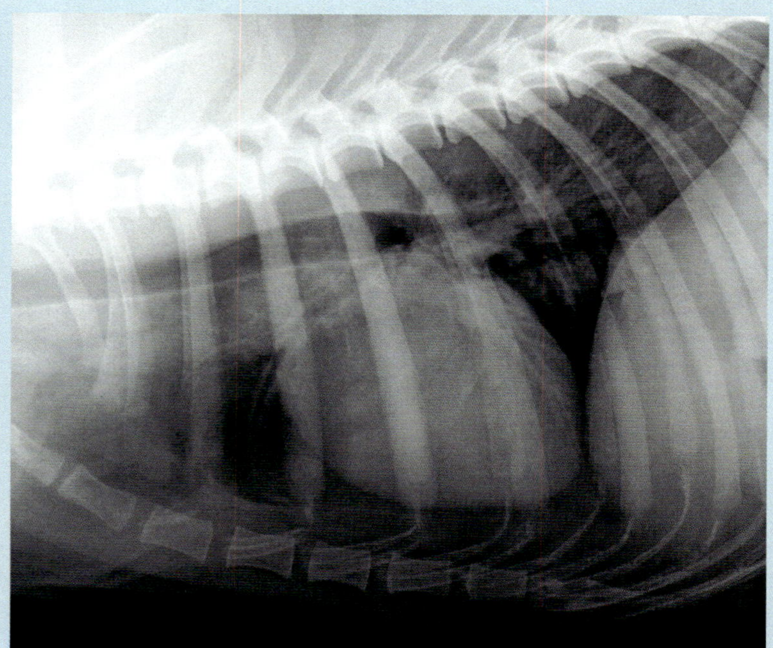

FIGURE 2.44. Lateral radiograph of the thorax of an obese dog. It is possible to observe a marked accumulation of mediastinal fat located ventral to the cardiac silhouette, which causes its elevation. This should not be mistaken for a pleural effusion. An effusion would mask the image of the cardiac apex, while in this case the definition of the whole ventral margin of the heart is improved due to the contrast between the radiographic density of soft tissue and that of fat.

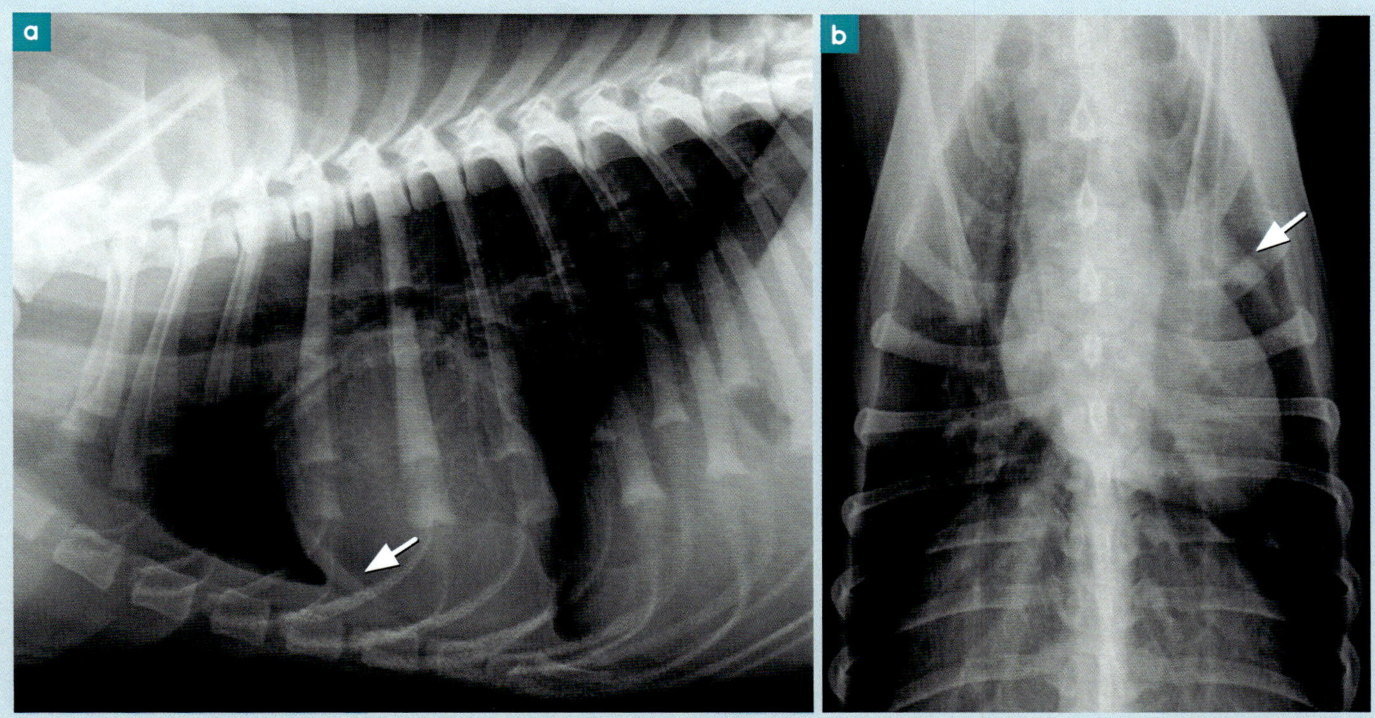

FIGURE 2.45. Lateral (a) and dorsoventral (b) radiographs of the thorax of a young dog, in which the normal shadow of the thymus may be observed. This organ reaches its maximum size at 4 months of age and is usually no longer visible on radiographs from 6 months of age.

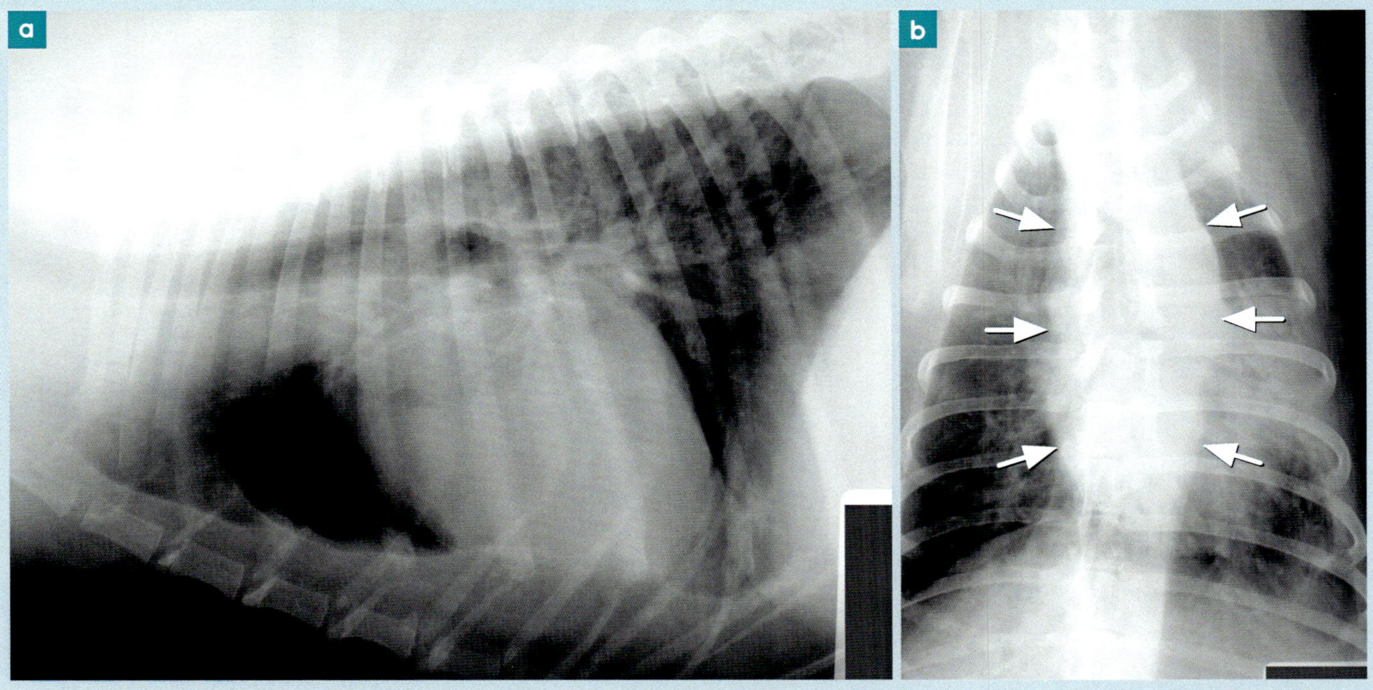

FIGURE 2.46. Lateral (a) and dorsoventral (b) radiographs of the thorax of a dog with a mediastinal effusion. On the lateral view, the findings are similar to those of a pleural effusion, but the dorsoventral view does not show a retraction of the lungs (except a minimal separation between the left caudal lobe and the chest wall, due to a mild pleural effusion) but an enlargement of the mediastinal shadow (arrows). It should be borne in mind that brachycephalic dogs have, in normal conditions, wider mediastinal shadows, as also occurs in obese cats and dogs. This patient has, in addition, a pulmonary infiltrate in the caudal area of the left cranial lobe.

Normal radiographic anatomy of the thorax **right lateral view**

http://goo.gl/otDlnr

Normal radiographic anatomy of the thorax **left lateral view**

http://goo.gl/ipcQxz

In cases of pneumomediastinum, it will be possible to identify the shadows of some mediastinal structures, such as for example, the oesophagus or the blood vessels of the cranial mediastinum. It would not be possible to distinguish these structures from one another if no gas was located between them. When the amount of gas is relatively small, the most significant finding is the improved visualisation of the tracheal wall, which appears internally and externally limited by gas (fig. 2.47).

If air accumulates rapidly in the mediastinum, the mediastinal pleura may rupture and cause a pneumothorax. That is to say, a pneumomediastinum may progress to a pneumothorax. On the other hand, a pneumothorax is never the cause of a pneumomediastinum.

An ultrasound study is not indicated in cases of pneumomediastinum. However, contrast techniques or endoscopy are indicated to rule out a perforation or an oesophageal or tracheal rupture as the causes of the disease. Computed tomography is particularly useful to investigate the cause of a pneumomediastinum.

Mediastinal masses

They appear more frequently in the cranial mediastinum. They usually correspond to neoplasms (heart base tumours, thymomas, tumours of the thyroid gland or parathyroid ectopic tumours) or to mediastinal lymphadenopathies (lymphoma, metastasis, lymphadenitis) (fig. 2.48), although abscesses, granulomas, haematomas and cysts may also appear in this location.

The lymph nodes that can be found in the mediastinum are divided into:

- **Sternal** lymph nodes (there may be one or two): when they considerably increase in size, they appear as a shadow of soft-tissue density dorsal to the second sternebra. They drain lymph from the thoracic wall and abdominal cavity. Therefore, if they are enlarged, the cause may be located in the thorax or in the abdomen.
- **Mediastinal** lymph nodes: they form a chain of lymph nodes that lies adjacent to the great vessels of the cranial mediastinum (cranial vena cava, brachiocephalic trunk and left subclavian artery). When they increase in size they originate an enlargement of the shadow of the cranial mediastinum, as well as a displacement of the trachea in dorsal direction on lateral radiographs, and to the right on dorsoventral and ventrodorsal radiographs.
- **Bronchial** lymph nodes: they are subdivided into pulmonary lymph nodes (often absent, but when present they are distributed throughout the main bronchi) and tracheobronchial lymph nodes (located around the carina). When the tracheobronchial lymph nodes become greatly enlarged, they originate a mass dorsal to the tracheal bifurcation, with a relatively oval morphology on lateral radiographs. The bifurcation of the trachea may be ventrally displaced. This image is similar to that produced by a significant enlargement of the left atrium, but in this case the bifurcation of the trachea appears displaced in the opposite direction –dorsally– and other signs of left cardiomegaly are usually observed. It is more difficult to visualise the mass on dorsoventral or ventrodorsal views, but it may cause a bronchial displacement that is identifiable in the image.

In general, mediastinal masses of non-glandular origin usually cause a more or less marked increase of the width of the cranial mediastinum, as well as a displacement of the trachea in dorsal direction on lateral radiographs (fig. 2.49) and in lateral direction on dorsoventral or ventrodorsal radiographs. The identification of the tracheal displacement helps in the diagnosis of mediastinal masses when these are masked by an associated mediastinal or pleural effusion (fig. 2.50). However, we should remember that a severe pleural effusion may cause an elevation of the trachea, but never its collapse or distortion, which would be more suggestive of a mediastinal mass. Depending on the size of the mass, the cardiac silhouette may also appear caudally displaced and its cranial border may be masked.

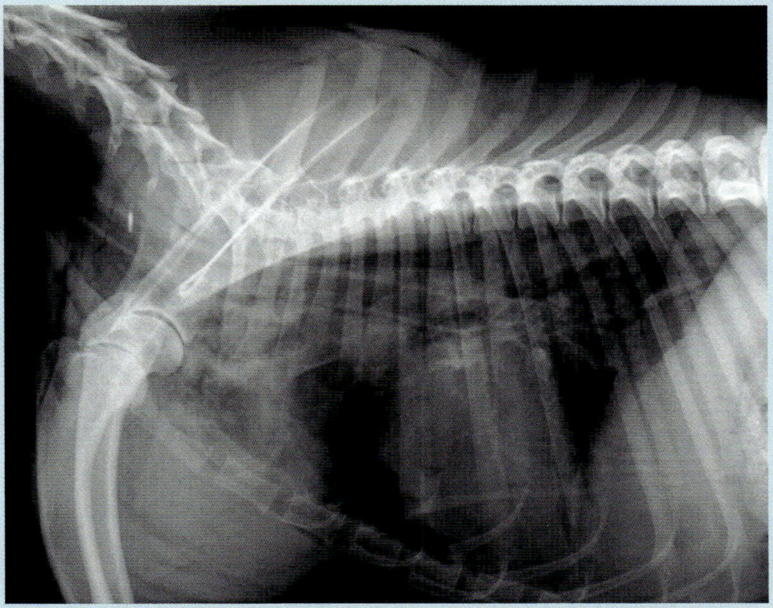

FIGURE 2.47. Lateral radiograph of the thorax of a dog with a pneumomediastinum caused by a bite in the neck. The gas that penetrates between the fasciae of the neck enters in the mediastinal space through the thoracic inlet. The same image may be observed in cases of tracheal or oesophageal perforation or rupture, since the free gas in the mediastinum may move towards the neck.

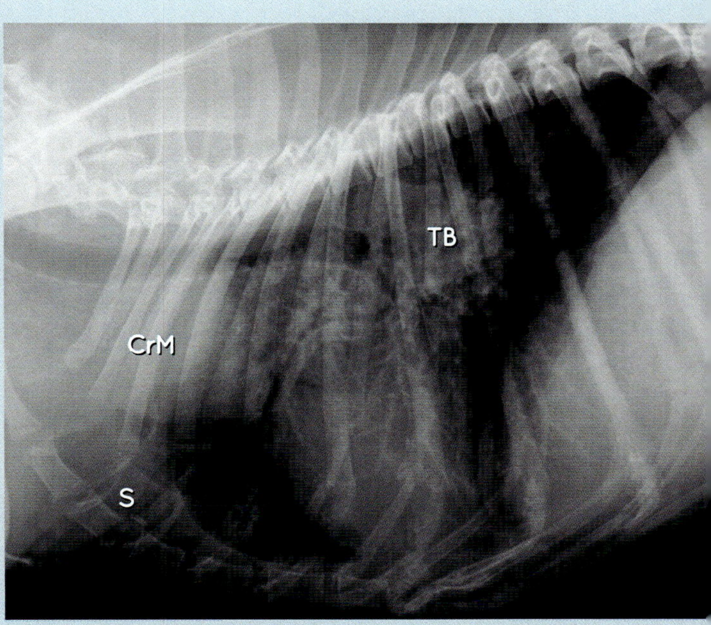

FIGURE 2.48. Lateral radiograph of the thorax of a dog with lymphoma. The enlargement of the sternal lymph node or lymph nodes (S) creates a shadow of soft-tissue density dorsal to the manubrium and most cranial sternebrae. The increase in size of the cranial mediastinal lymph nodes (CrM) causes an enlargement of the cranial mediastinal shadow and elevation of the trachea. Finally, the tracheobronchial lymph nodes (TB), which lie dorsal to the tracheal bifurcation, create an approximately oval shadow dorsal to the main bronchi, next to the carina.

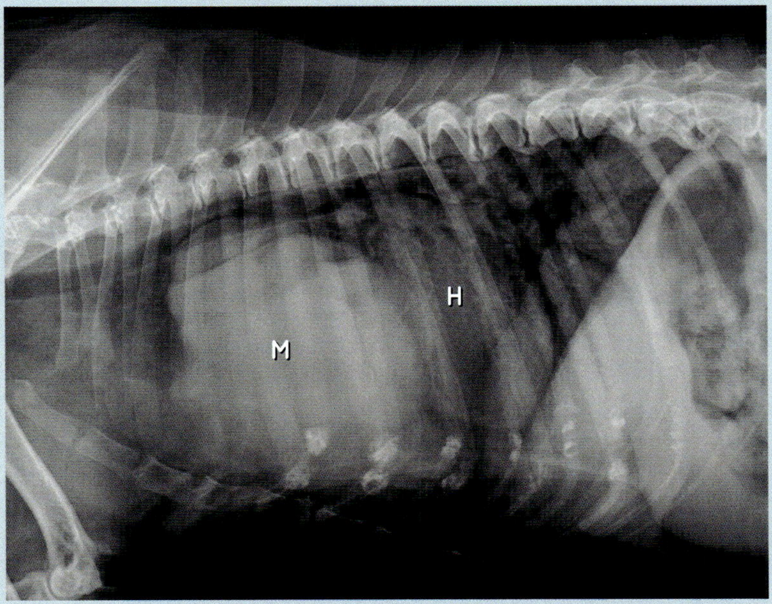

FIGURE 2.49. Lateral radiograph of the thorax of a dog with thymoma. A large mass (M) that causes a marked dorsal displacement of the trachea and a caudodorsal displacement of the heart (H) may be observed in the cranial area of the thorax.

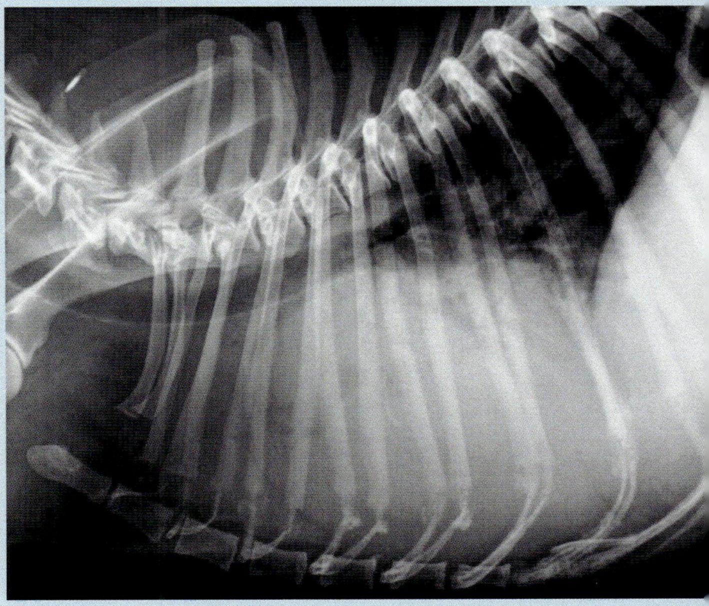

FIGURE 2.50. Lateral radiograph of the thorax of a dog with a cranial mediastinal mass, which is masked in the image due to the associated mediastinal effusion. The marked elevation of the trachea suggests the presence of a mass, although its outline cannot be visualised in the image. Ultrasonography allows the easy identification of the mass.

An ultrasound examination will allow the evaluation of the size and echogenicity of the mass and the presence of an associated effusion, in addition to allowing ultrasound-guided fine-needle aspiration or biopsy.

Computed tomography is an excellent technique to identify mediastinal masses and establish their relationship with the other structures in the mediastinum (fig. 2.51).

Displacement of the mediastinum

The displacement of the structures that form the mediastinum indicates a change of volume in one of the hemithoraces. If the volume of a hemithorax increases, the mediastinum will be displaced to the opposite side, while if the volume of a hemithorax decreases, the mediastinal content will be displaced to the affected side. The most common cause is iatrogenic, due to a partial collapse of the lung, which has a lower position in patients that remain in lateral recumbency for a long period of time, especially if they are anaesthetised. On radiographs, it is possible to observe a displacement of the heart to the side on which the patient was lying and an increase in the density of the lung of the same side caused by temporary atelectasis.

A pathological displacement of the mediastinum may appear due to masses or accumulations located in one of the hemithoraces (unilateral pleural effusion, unilateral pneumothorax), in conditions causing an unequal expansion of the lungs (unilateral emphysema), or when adherences that connect the mediastinum with the thoracic wall remain after a chronic pleural effusion.

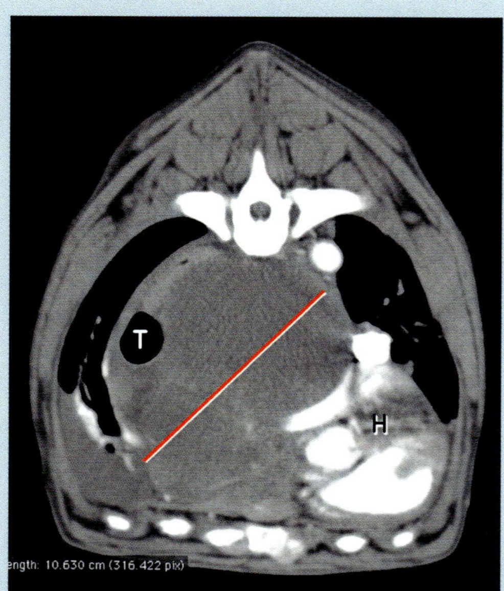

FIGURE 2.51. Computed tomography image of the thorax of a dog with a large mediastinal mass (its diameter is indicated by a red line in the image), which causes an evident displacement of the trachea (T) to the right and of the heart (H) to the left. Tomography allows the assessment of the relationships of the mass with the adjacent anatomical structures and the detection of distant metastases.

Heart

Taking chest radiographs is an essential part of the assessment of patients with a suspected cardiovascular disease. Radiographs allow the assessment of the size and shape of the cardiac silhouette, as well as of the state of the lungs and circulation, thus showing the degree of heart failure of the patient. Thoracic radiographs therefore help to determine the severity of the cardiac disease and allow the evaluation of the efficacy of the treatment.

Contrast studies (angiocardiography) have become less prevalent with the use of echocardiography, which is now an essential routine technique to establish a precise diagnosis of most of the diseases that affect the heart. The diagnostic information obtained by means of radio graphy and echocardiography is often enough for us not to need more advanced diagnostic imaging techniques. Computed tomography is useful for the diagnosis of heart tumours and some diseases of the pericardium.

Right lateral and dorsoventral radiographs are used for the radiological assessment of the cardiac silhouette. On left lateral radiographs, the silhouette appears falsely rounded, while on ventrodorsal radiographs it is more magnified than on dorsoventral ones. We should be particularly careful when positioning the animal before taking a radiograph. On lateral views, the rotation of the thorax causes a false increase of the cardiosternal contact and a false elevation of the trachea. On dorsoventral views, any degree of rotation of the thorax causes a deformation of the cardiac silhouette in the image, which does not allow its appropriate examination.

Size of the cardiac silhouette

The methods to assess the size of the cardiac silhouette are based on the measurement of its height and width on right lateral and dorsoventral radiographs.

According to the traditional method (fig. 2.52), the width of the cardiac silhouette (horizontal craniocaudal diameter) on lateral radiographs should be comprised between 2.5 and 3.5 intercostal spaces in the dog, although this interval varies depending on the conformation of the thorax:

- In dogs with a **narrow and deep thorax** (Greyhound type), the heart has a more vertical position in the thoracic cavity, so the limit of normal will be 2.5 intercostal spaces.
- In dogs with an **intermediate conformation** (German Shepherd type), the normal interval is from 2.5 to 3 intercostal spaces.
- In dogs with a **wide and shallow thorax** (Bulldog type), the normal range extends to 3.5 intercostal spaces, because the heart is anatomically more inclined on the sternum.
- In **cats**, the craniocaudal diameter is not measured horizontally, as in dogs, but perpendicularly to the longitudinal axis of the heart. However, the result obtained is compared to the width of the intercostal spaces horizontally. In normal conditions, its value is 2.

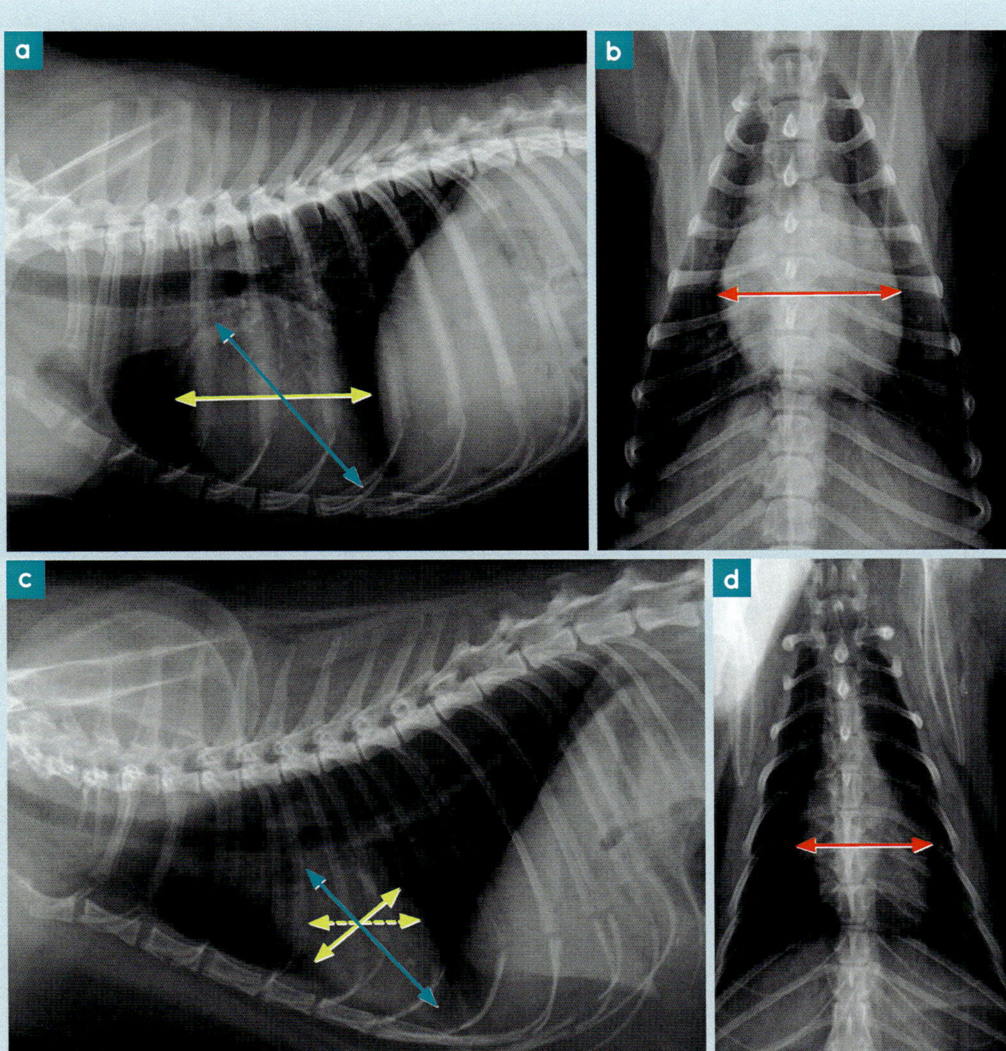

FIGURE 2.52. Normal images of the thorax of a dog in right lateral (a) and dorsoventral (b) projection and of a cat in right lateral (c) and dorsoventral (d) projection, in which the references for the measurement of the cardiac silhouette according to the traditional method are shown. The width of the cardiac silhouette (yellow line) on the lateral view should be between 2.5 and 3.5 intercostal spaces in the dog, although the normal range varies depending on the thoracic conformation. In cats, the width is measured perpendicularly to the longitudinal axis of the heart (to avoid wrong diagnoses of cardiomegaly in old cats, as their heart may be very inclined on the sternum), and the result is then compared to the width of the intercostal spaces (broken yellow line) horizontally. The normal value is 2. Both in dogs and cats, the height of the cardiac silhouette on lateral radiographs –measured from the centre of its base to its apex– corresponds approximately to two thirds of the height of the thoracic cavity at the same level (blue line), while the width of the silhouette (red line) –measured at the level of the 5th intercostal space– should be approximately two thirds of the width of the thoracic cavity on dorsoventral radiographs.

This variation in the measurement system is due to fact that, with age, the feline heart tends to lie closer to the sternum because of a progressive elongation of the aorta (fig. 2.53). If the width is measured horizontally, as in dogs, it will therefore seem increased in older cats.

Both in dogs and cats, the height of the cardiac silhouette on lateral radiographs –measured from the centre of its base to its apex– corresponds approximately to two thirds of the height of the thoracic cavity at the same level. The width of the silhouette –measured at the level of the 5th intercostal space– should be approximately two thirds of the width of the thoracic cavity on dorsoventral radiographs.

The size of the heart in relation to the thoracic cavity is slightly greater in young animals than in adults. The cardiac silhouette also appears slightly larger during expiration when compared to inspiration, and during diastole when compared to systole. However, these changes are minimal and generally do not significantly affect the diagnosis.

Buchanan's vertebral heart scale

It is also possible to evaluate the size of the cardiac silhouette in dogs by means of Buchanan's vertebral heart scale (fig. 2.54). The distance between the ventral margin of the carina and the cardiac apex on lateral radiographs is used as a measure of height and the craniocaudal diameter is then measured perpendicularly to the height axis. In this case, this is done the same way in dogs and cats. The two measurements are then transferred to the thoracic spine to count the corresponding number of vertebrae, always starting from the cranial aspect of T4. The normal range is 9.7 ± 0.5 in dogs and 7.5 ± 0.3 in cats, although some breeds may have slightly different values (for example, Boxer: 11.6 ± 0.8; German Shepherd: 9.7 ± 0.7; Labrador: 10.8 ± 0.6).

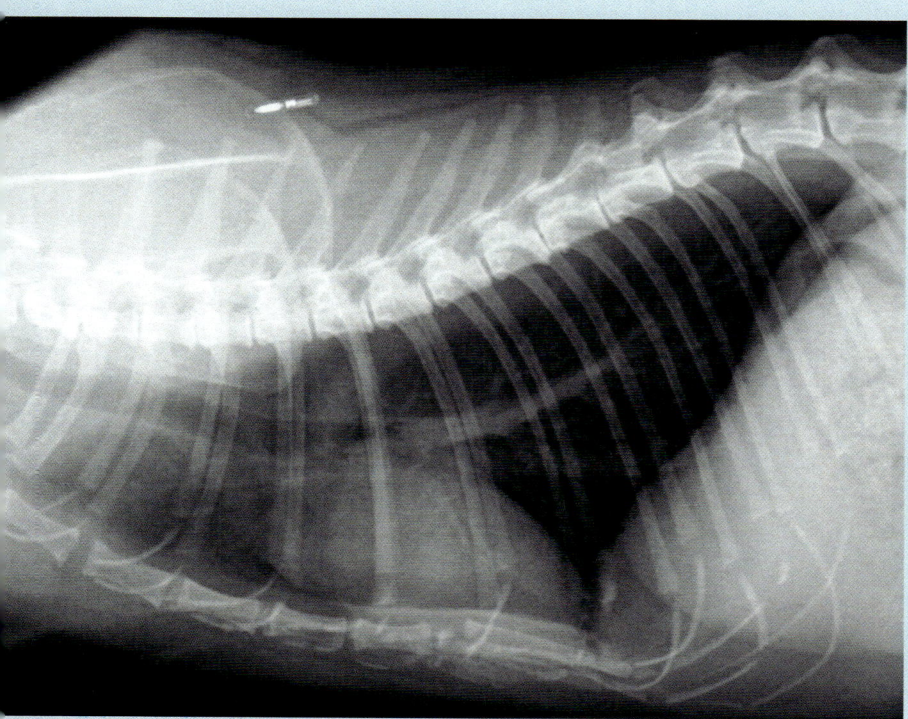

FIGURE 2.53. Lateral radiograph of the thorax of a healthy old cat. The cardiac silhouette appears very inclined on the sternum, which is due to a progressive elongation of the aorta with no clinical significance. This image should not be confused with that of cardiomegaly. The width of the cardiac silhouette, measured perpendicularly to the longitudinal axis of the heart, does not exceed 2 intercostal spaces. The identification microchip appears dorsal to the spinous process of T3.

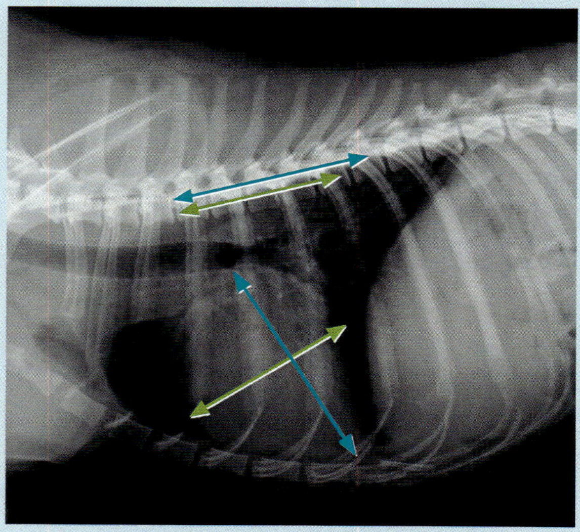

FIGURE 2.54. Normal lateral radiograph of the thorax of a dog, in which the references to measure the cardiac silhouette according to Buchanan's vertebral heart scale are shown. The distance between the ventral margin of the carina and the cardiac apex on lateral radiographs is used as a measure of height (blue line), and the craniocaudal diameter is then measured perpendicularly to the height axis (green line). This is done the same way in dogs and cats. The two measurements are then transferred to the thoracic spine to count the corresponding number of vertebrae, always starting from the cranial aspect of T4. The normal range is 9.7 ± 0.5 in dogs and 7.5 ± 0.3 in cats, although some breeds may have slightly different values. In this case the result is 10.2.

When assessing the size of the cardiac silhouette, it must be taken into account that the exit of the aorta and pulmonary artery, the pericardium and the pericardial space are part of it. In addition, the abnormal presence of fluid or masses in the pericardial space or the enlargement of the great vessels will cause an increase in the size of the cardiac silhouette in the image.

The presence of fat in the mediastinal space may also sometimes create a false impression of increased heart size in obese dogs.

Position of the cardiac chambers and great vessels

The position of the different cardiac chambers, aortic arch and main pulmonary artery on right lateral and dorsoventral radiographs is illustrated with coloured areas in figure 2.55. On lateral views, the cranial border of the silhouette is formed by the outline of the right atrial appendage and right ventricle. The caudal border is formed by the outline of the left atrial appendage and left ventricle. The cardiac silhouette may be compared to that of a clock face (clock-face analogy) and time intervals may be used to locate the cardiac chambers and great vessels.

- **Lateral view** (fig. 2.56):
  - From 12 to 2 o'clock: left atrium.
  - From 2 to 5 o'clock: left ventricle.
  - From 5 to 9 o'clock: right ventricle.
  - From 9 to 10 o'clock: main pulmonary artery and right atrial appendage.
  - From 10 to 11 o'clock: aortic arch.
- **Dorsoventral view** (fig. 2.57):
  - From 11 to 1 o'clock: aortic arch.
  - From 1 to 2 o'clock: main pulmonary artery.
  - From 2 to 3 o'clock: left atrial appendage (the left atrial appendage is located between the two main bronchi, in the central area of the cardiac silhouette on this view).

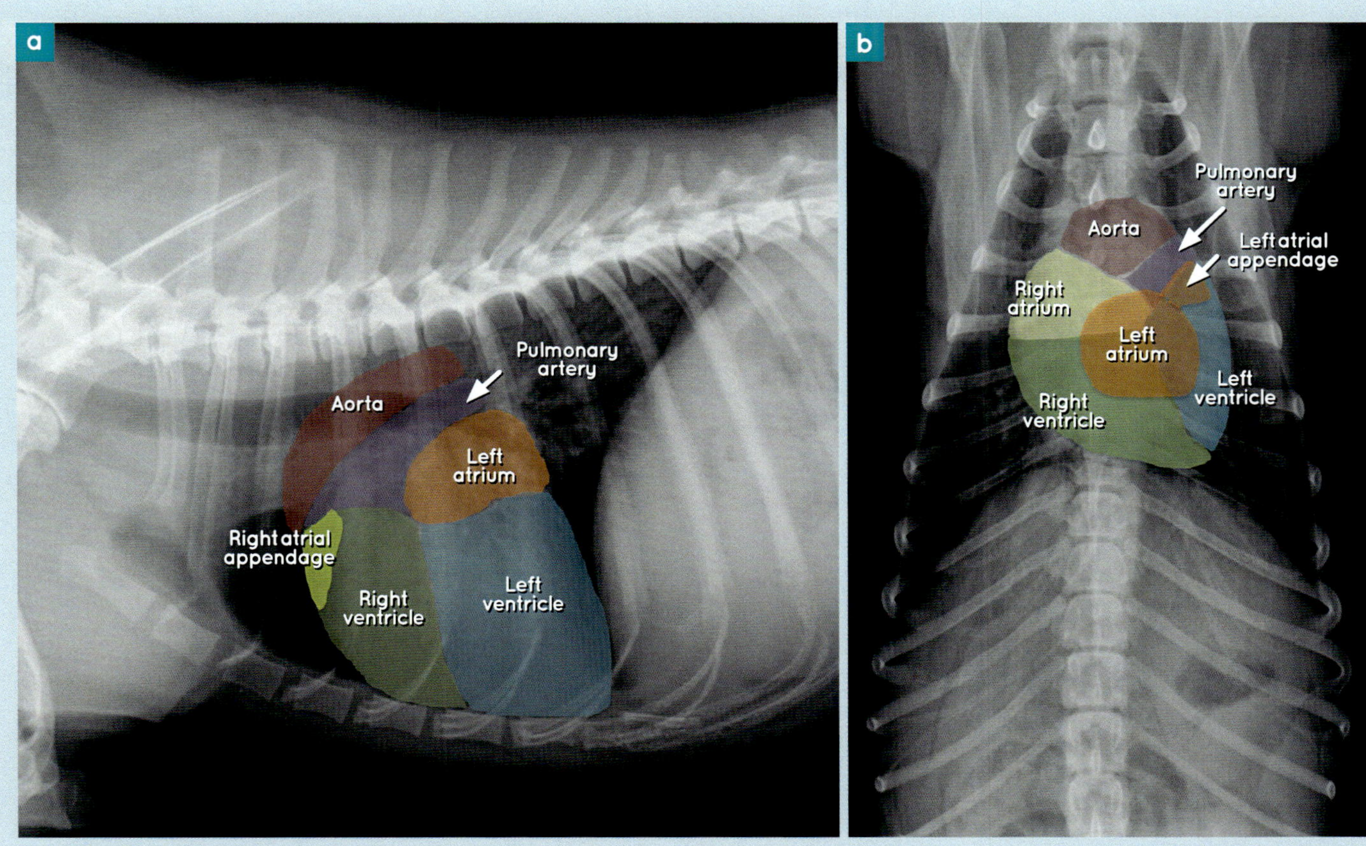

FIGURE 2.55. Normal lateral (a) and dorsoventral (b) radiographs of the thorax of a dog, in which the heart chambers, the aortic arch and the main pulmonary artery are shown with coloured areas.

Normal radiographic anatomy of the thorax
dorsoventral view

http://goo.gl/pKMKlb

- From 2 to 5 o'clock: left ventricle.
- From 5 to 9 o'clock: right ventricle.
- From 9 to 11 o'clock: right atrium.

The identification of prominences of the silhouette in these locations helps to identify a possible enlargement of the different cardiac chambers, as well as of the exit of the aorta and pulmonary artery.

Radiographic signs of enlargement of the heart chambers

From a didactic point of view, it is useful to describe the signs of enlargement of each of the cardiac chambers separately, although in practice it is rare to find a significant increase in the size of only one of them. It will be normal to detect signs of enlargement of the left heart (left atrium and ventricle), as well as global cardiomegaly (with or without predominance of the right or left side of the heart) at different degrees.

The radiographic signs of an increase in size of each of the chambers are summarised in box 2.1 and are illustrated in figures 2.58, 2.59, 2.60 and 2.61.

Radiographic signs of left cardiac failure may be observed when the left heart is enlarged: vascular congestion and pulmonary oedema. Dilatation of the pulmonary veins is the radiological sign that may be detected most early, although it is not always identified. Pulmonary oedema starts in the interstitial tissue, which makes the visualisation of the small pulmonary vessels more difficult. However, these remain visible until the oedema progresses and also affects the alveoli, which is when air bronchograms appear in the affected area. Cardiogenic pulmonary oedema in dogs is typically located in the perihilar area, although it extends to the median and peripheral area of the lung at advanced stages. It usually affects the right lung more than the left one. In cats, cardiogenic pulmonary oedema may appear in any area of the lung and has a patchier pattern. It is also common to observe pleural effusion in cats.

When the right heart is enlarged, it is possible to detect signs of right cardiac failure, which include dilatation of the caudal vena cava, hepatomegaly, ascites and pleural effusion. In cats, a pleural effusion may occur due to left cardiac failure, and can be differentiated from the effusion caused by right cardiac failure because the patient does not also present with hepatomegaly or ascites.

If cardiomegaly is global, the silhouette will appear increased in width and height in the two projections (fig. 2.62). In many cases, the signs of an enlarged left heart predominate; in the other cases it is possible to observe signs of enlargement of the right heart, or a more or less uniform enlargement of both sides of the heart. Depending on which are the most affected chambers, the radiographs may show associated signs of left and/or right cardiac failure.

Moderate or marked cardiomegaly is a quite reliable indicator of cardiac disease, but mild cardiomegaly should be interpreted carefully, and always in correlation with the rest of the patient's clinical data.

On the other hand, a heart that is radiographically normal may not be a healthy heart, since some diseases do not significantly affect its size or shape.

Great vessels

Changes in the image of the great vessels may provide additional information about possible alterations of the heart.

The diameter of the caudal vena cava (CVC), along its course between the cardiac silhouette and the diaphragm, can be compared with the diameter of the aorta (Ao), measured at the same intercostal space and if possible during breathing. A CVC/Ao ratio > 1.5 is very indicative of right cardiac failure. We must bear in mind that the diameter of the caudal vena cava slightly varies with the respiratory cycle, and may be reduced in cases of hypovolaemia.

The diameter of a normal aorta is similar to the height of the adjacent vertebral bodies. It may appear increased in cases of aortic valve stenosis, and occasionally, in patients with patent ductus arteriosus. On dorsoventral radiographs, an increase of the aortic diameter creates a prominence of the cardiac silhouette

BOX 2.1. Signs of enlargement of the cardiac chamber

Left atrium

It is located immediately ventral to the left main bronchus. The enlargement of the atrium leads to its dorsal displacement and to a prominence of the cardiac silhouette at this level, which are both visible on lateral radiographs. On dorsoventral radiographs, it is located between the two main bronchi, caudal to the tracheal bifurcation. An increase in the size of the atrium leads to a greater separation of these two bronchi, although this will only be visible on the radiograph if it is taken with a high kilovoltage so it is intentionally overexposed. In addition, the left atrial appendage is displaced, which originates an image of a prominent cardiac silhouette in the 2 to 3 o'clock position.

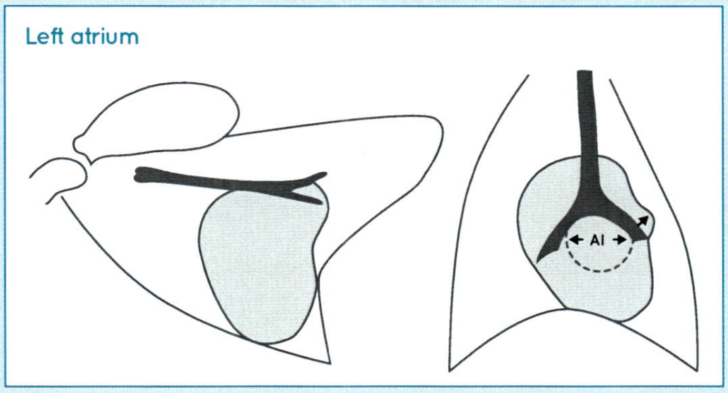

Left ventricle

When this chamber increases in size, it tends to do so in height, which therefore leads to an increase in the height of the cardiac silhouette and to a dorsal elevation of the trachea (along its whole length, from the thoracic inlet to the carina) on lateral radiographs. The caudal vena cava is also displaced dorsally. On dorsoventral radiographs, the left margin in the interval from 2 to 5 o'clock becomes rounded and lies closer to the thoracic wall.

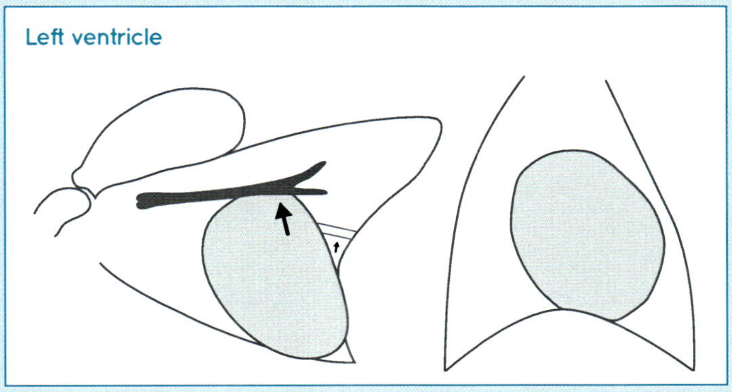

Right atrium

On lateral radiographs, the increase in size of the atrium causes a dorsal displacement of the caudal part of the trachea (on the cranial part of the base of the heart), while the carina tends to maintain its normal position. It is difficult to assess on dorsoventral radiographs, although it may give rise to a prominence of the margin of the cardiac silhouette in the 9 to 11 o'clock position.

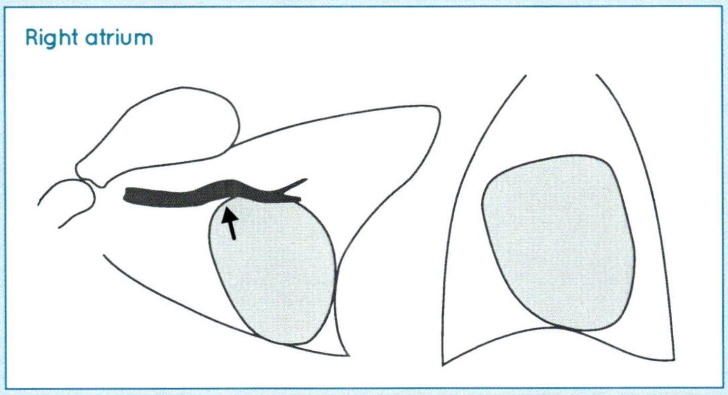

Right ventricle

When this chamber increases in size, it tends to do so in width, which therefore leads to an increase in the width of the cardiac silhouette and to a greater cardiosternal contact on lateral radiographs. On dorsoventral radiographs, the margin of the cardiac silhouette becomes rounded in the 5 to 9 o'clock position, and even acquires a "inverted D" shape when the enlargement is significant.

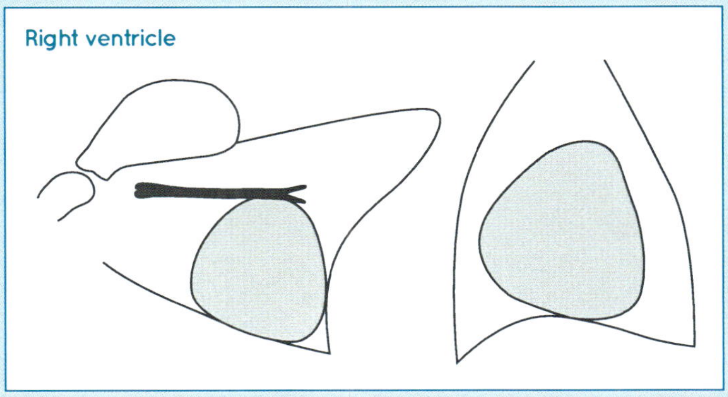

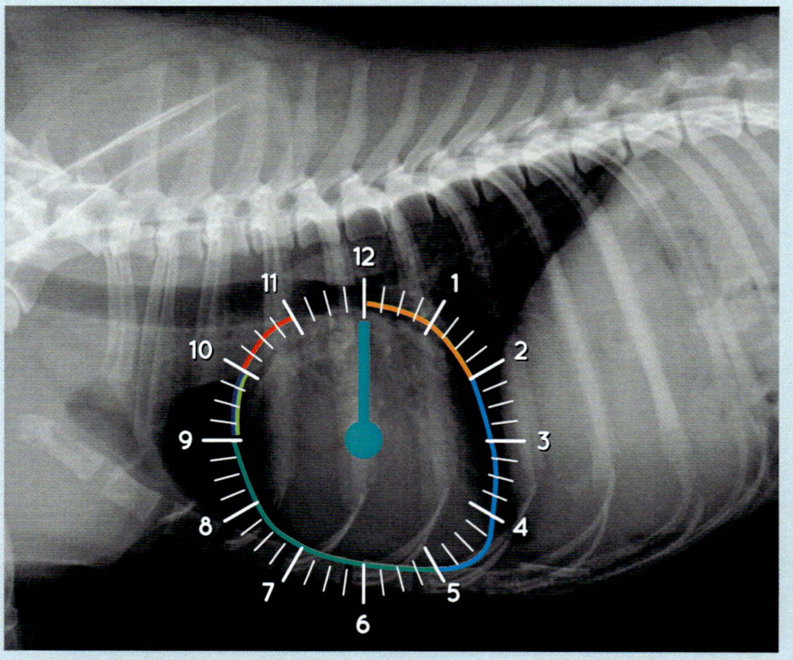

FIGURE 2.56. Normal lateral radiograph of the thorax of a dog, in which the position of the cardiac chambers and great vessels is shown according to the clock-face analogy. Left atrium: from 12 to 2 o'clock (orange line); left ventricle: from 2 to 5 o'clock (blue line); right ventricle: from 5 to 9 o'clock (dark green line); right atrial appendage (light green line) and pulmonary artery (purple line): from 9 to 10 o'clock; aortic arch: from 10 to 11 o'clock (red line).

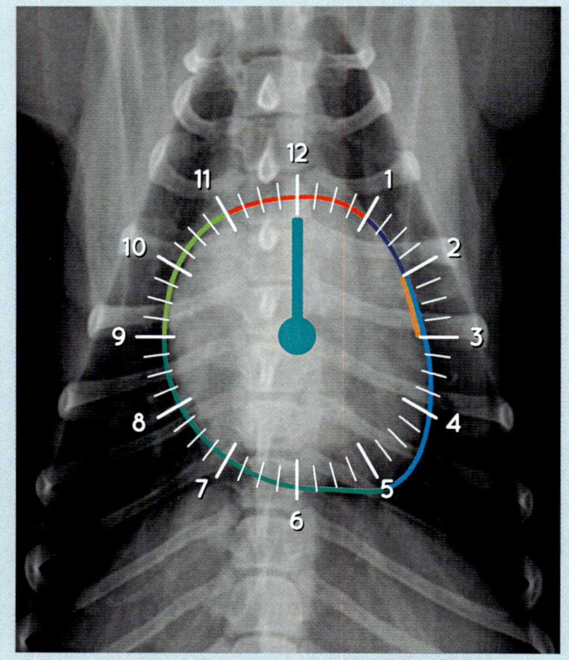

FIGURE 2.57. Normal dorsoventral radiograph of the thorax of a dog, in which the position of the cardiac chambers and great vessels is shown according to the clock-face analogy. Aortic arch: from 11 to 1 o'clock (red line); main pulmonary artery: from 1 to 2 o'clock (purple line); left atrial appendage: from 2 to 3 o'clock (orange line); left ventricle: from 2 to 5 o'clock (blue line); right ventricle: from 5 to 9 o'clock (dark green line); right atrium: from 9 to 11 o'clock (light green line).

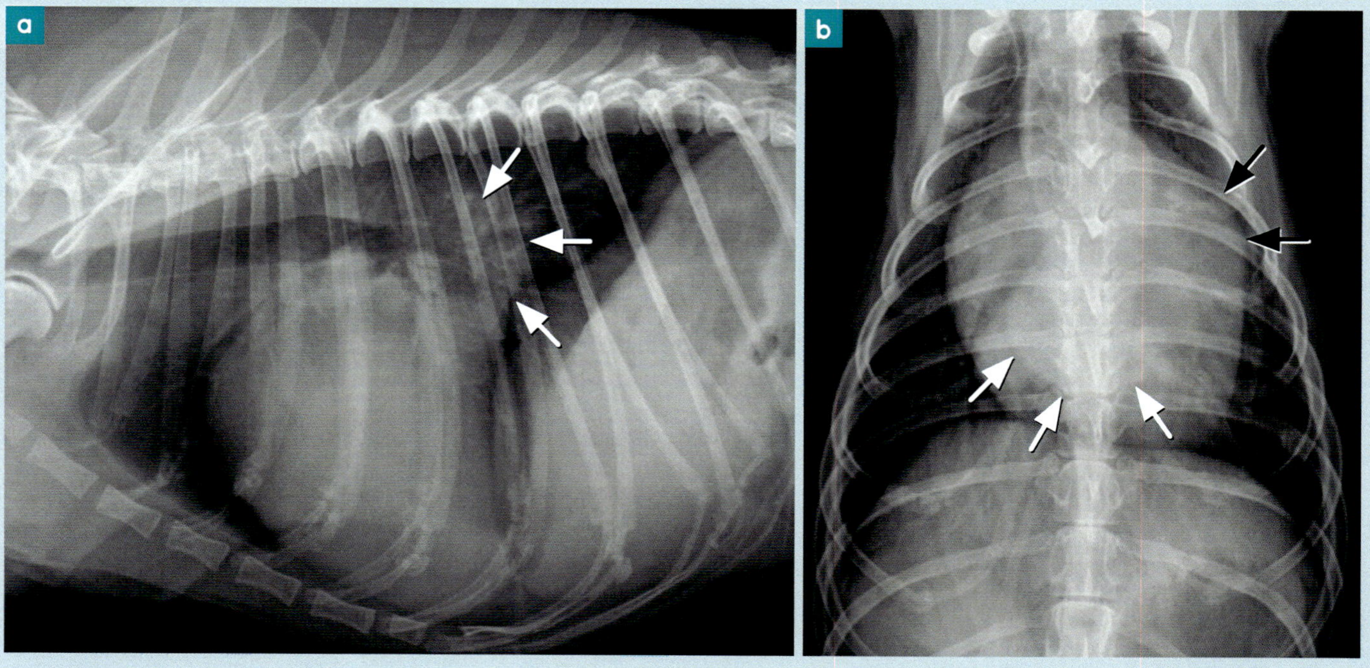

FIGURE 2.58. Lateral (a) and dorsoventral (b) radiographs of the thorax of a dog with signs of enlargement of the left atrium. In image (a), the left atrium is prominent in the caudodorsal margin of cardiac silhouette (white arrows). In image (b), the left atrium appears in the central area of the silhouette, where only part of its contour can be visualised (white arrows), and laterally displaces the left atrial appendage, thus causing a prominence in the 2 to 3 o'clock position (black arrows) according to the clock-face analogy.

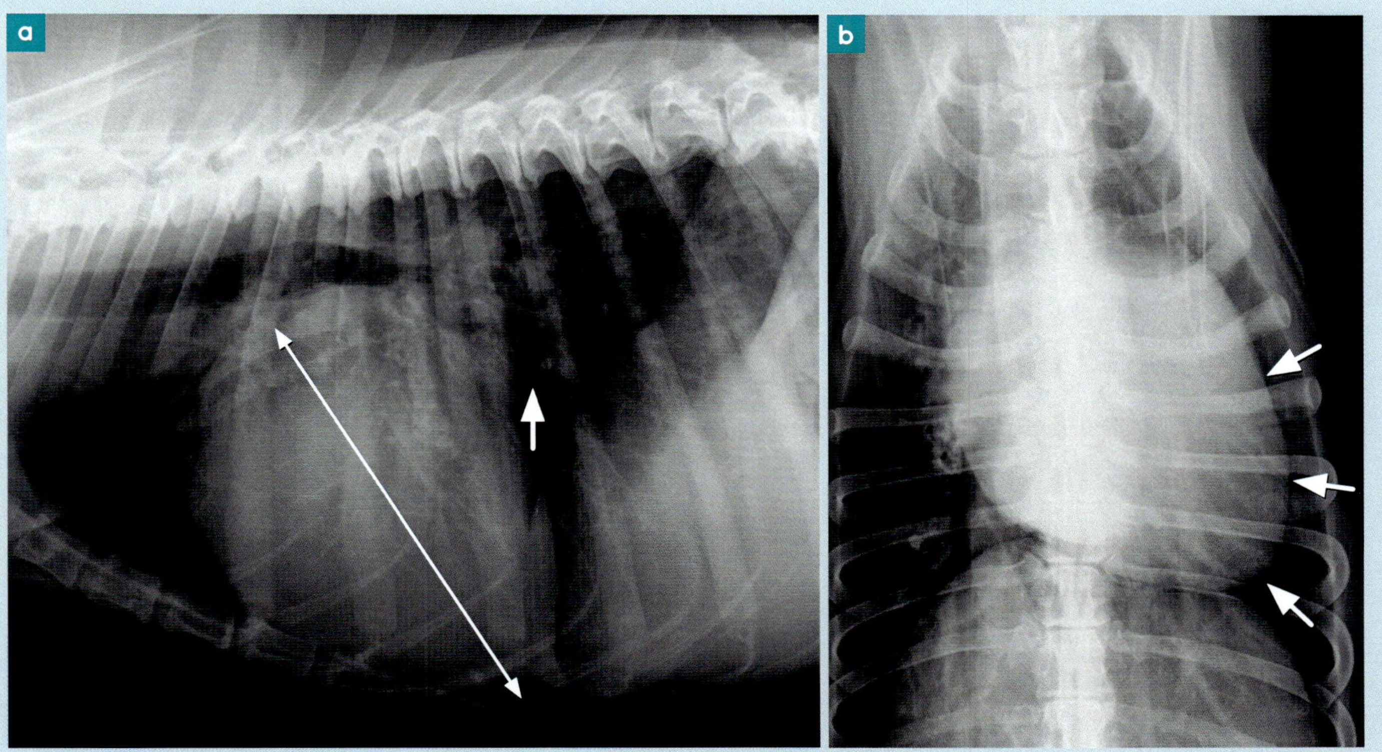

FIGURE 2.59. Lateral (a) and dorsoventral (b) radiographs of the thorax of a dog with signs of enlargement of the left ventricle. In image (a), the silhouette appears increased in height (white arrow), and the trachea and caudal vena cava (short white arrow) are displaced in dorsal direction. In image (b), the margin of the silhouette in the 2 to 5 o'clock position (white arrows) according to the clock-analogy lies closer to the thoracic wall. The left atrium is also moderately prominent on the lateral radiograph and venous congestion may be observed (initial sign of left cardiac failure).

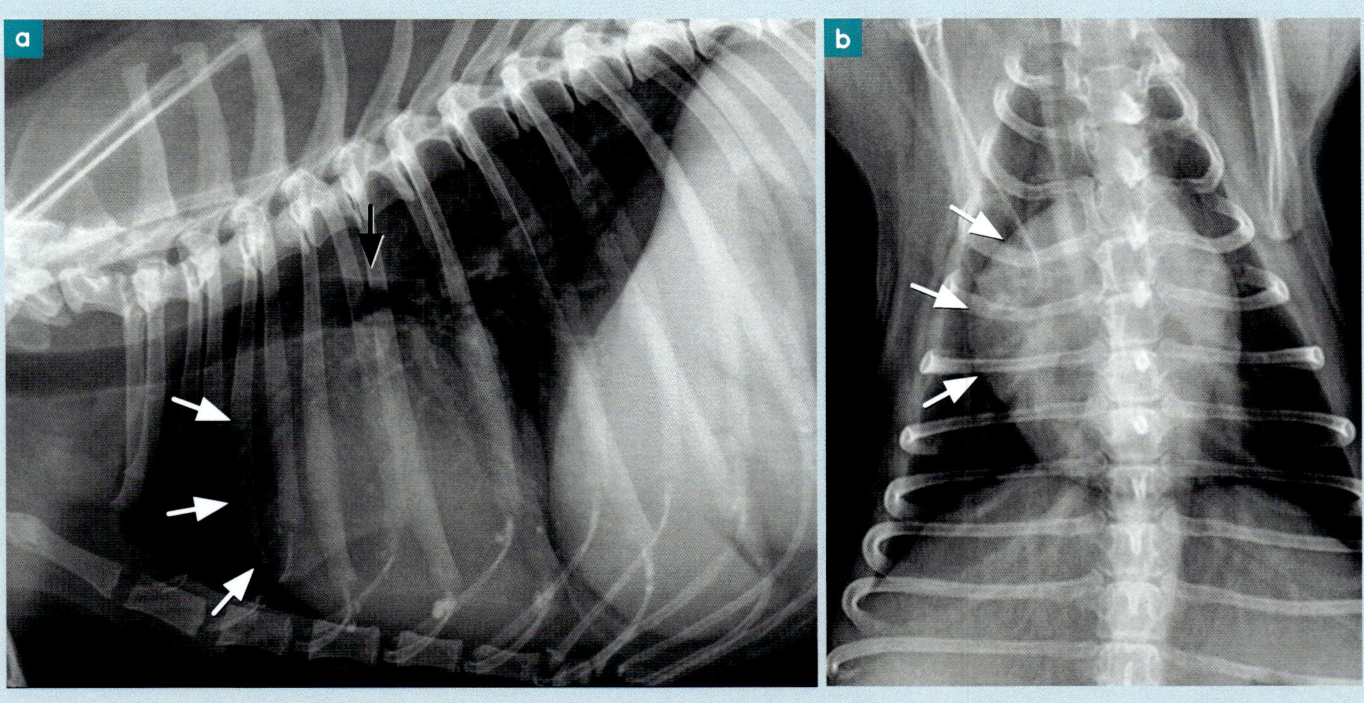

FIGURE 2.60. Lateral (a) and dorsoventral (b) radiographs of the thorax of a dog with signs of enlargement of the right atrium. In image (a), the craniodorsal margin of the silhouette is prominent (white arrows) and the trachea appears elevated on the base of the heart, while the carina (black arrow) tends to maintain a lower position. In image (b), the cardiac silhouette is prominent in the 9 to 11 o'clock position (white arrows) according to the clock-face analogy.

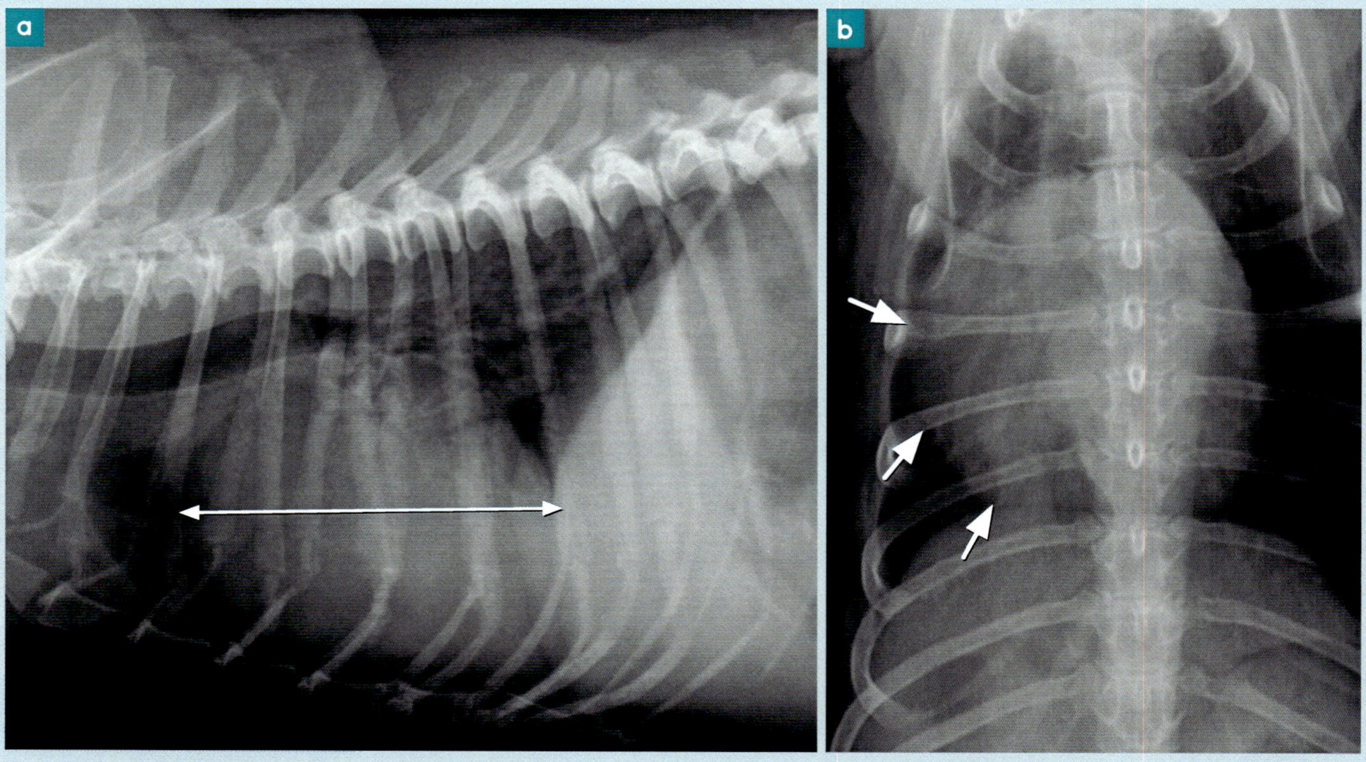

FIGURE 2.61. Lateral (a) and dorsoventral (b) radiographs of the thorax of a dog with signs of enlargement of the right ventricle. In image (a), the width of the cardiac silhouette appears enlarged (white line), thus leading to increased cardiosternal contact. In image (b), the cardiac silhouette is prominent in the 5 to 9 o'clock position (white arrows) according to the clock-face analogy, and the whole right margin of the cardiac silhouette has a more rounded shape ("inverted-D" shape).

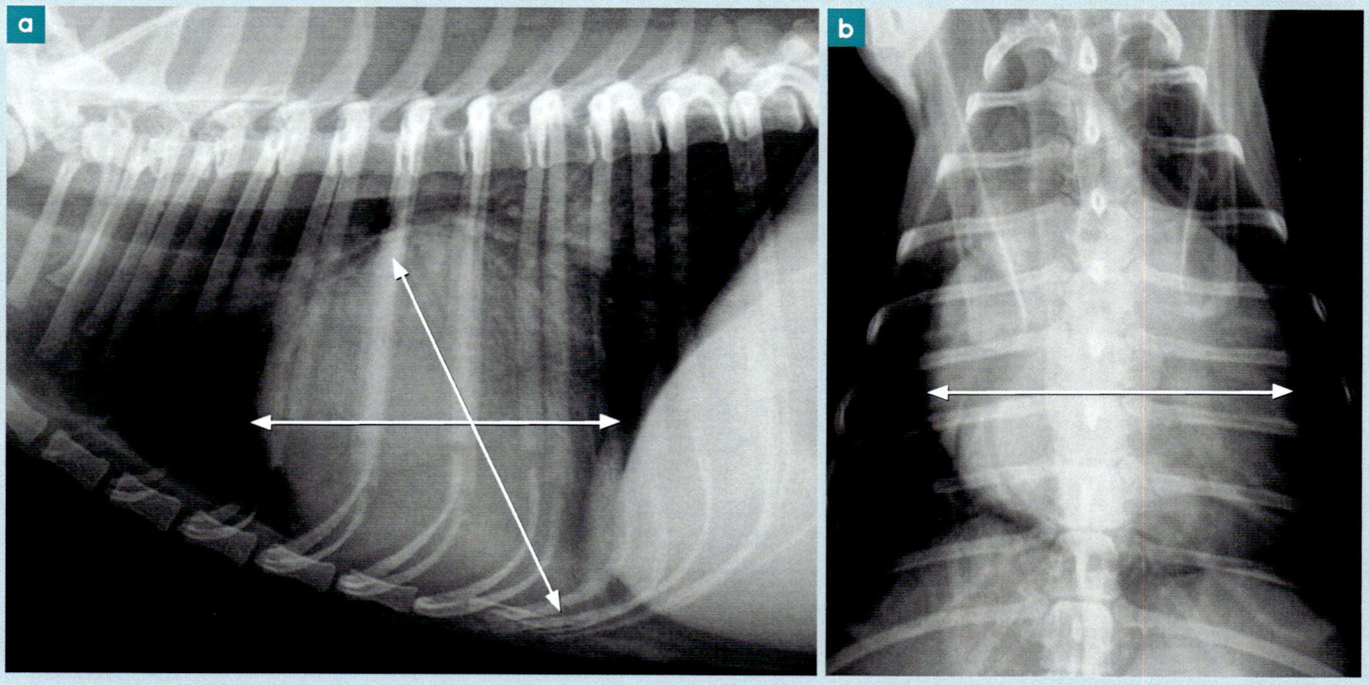

FIGURE 2.62. Lateral (a) and dorsoventral (b) radiographs of the thorax of a dog with global cardiomegaly. Signs of enlargement of all the heart chambers may be observed and the height and width of the cardiac silhouette are increased on the lateral view, as well as its width on the dorsoventral view.

in the 11 to 1 o'clock position according to the clock-face analogy, while on lateral radiographs the aortic arch is more marked. In older cats, the aorta may be elongated and its curvature may be more marked and even have an undulatting course, which has been termed "redundant aorta".

The main pulmonary artery (pulmonary trunk) may appear enlarged in cases of pulmonary stenosis, patent ductus ateriosus, pulmonary hypertension or dirofilariasis, essentially. On ventrodorsal radiographs, its enlargement gives rise to a prominence of the cardiac silhouette in the 1 to 2 o'clock position according to the clock-face analogy in dogs. In cats, its location is more medial. On lateral views, it is more difficult to identify its enlargement, although the superimposition with the trachea may facilitate its visualisation.

Acquired heart diseases

Acquired valvular disease

Primary acquired valvular disease in cats and dogs is usually degenerative (endocardiosis) or, on a less frequent basis, infectious (bacterial endocarditis).

Myxomatous degeneration of the mitral valve is the most common heart disease in dogs. Clinical signs are generally observed in old animals, especially in small breeds. The incompetence of the mitral valve caused by valvular degeneration leads to the backflow of blood to the left atrium, which initially originates its dilatation, and will be followed by an enlargement of the left ventricle. The clinical signs of the disease, particularly cough due to the compression of the main bronchi by the enlarged left atrium (sometimes visible on radiographs), seem to precede the development of signs of heart failure.

Degeneration of the tricuspid valve is uncommon as an isolated lesion. It usually appears associated with degeneration of the mitral valve. It causes signs of enlargement of the right atrium and ventricle, and may be accompanied by signs of right heart failure (dilatation of the caudal vena cava, hepatomegaly, ascites and pleural effusion).

Bacterial endocarditis is rare in cats and dogs. Radiography does not provide any significant information. The cardiac silhouette may appear normal, or show signs of enlargement of the left atrium and pulmonary oedema.

Cardiomyopathies

Dilated cardiomyopathy is one of the most frequent heart diseases in dogs. It generally causes signs of global cardiomegaly, and secondary signs of left and right heart failure may appear. In the Doberman, dilated cardiomyopathy may cause a very remarkable enlargement of the left atrium only.

Hypertrophic cardiomyopathy is the most common acquired heart disease in cats and is usually manifested as a significant enlargement of the left atrium (fig. 2.63), which creates the so-called "Valentine's heart" shape of the cardiac silhouette. Associated signs of left and/or right cardiac failure may appear.

Dilated cardiomyopathy is much less frequent in cats, and usually causes global cardiomegaly with rounding of the apex. The cardiac silhouette is often masked by pleural effusion in these cases.

The diagnosis of cardiomyopathy is always confirmed by means of echocardiography.

Dirofilariasis

Adult parasites live in the right ventricle and in the pulmonary arteries. On chest radiographs, it is possible to visualise the enlargement of the right ventricle, as well as the dilatation and tortuous course of the pulmonary arteries. The enlarged main pulmonary artery creates a prominence of the cardiac silhouette in the 1 to 2 o'clock position according to the clock-face analogy (fig. 2.64). Poorly defined pulmonary infiltrates may appear around the lobar arteries due to lung inflammation.

Congenital cardiac diseases

The value of plain radiography in the diagnosis of congenital diseases of the heart and great vessels is limited. Nowadays, contrast techniques have been almost totally replaced by echocardiography, which is the method of choice for the diagnosis and assessment of these diseases.

The most common congenital heart defects in dogs are patent ductus arteriosus, pulmonary stenosis, aortic stenosis, ventricular septal defect and tetralogy of Fallot. Mitral valve dysplasia, atrial septal defect, tricuspid valve dysplasia, *cor triatatum dexter* and mitral valve stenosis are diagnosed on a less frequent basis. Persistent truncus arteriosus, tricuspid

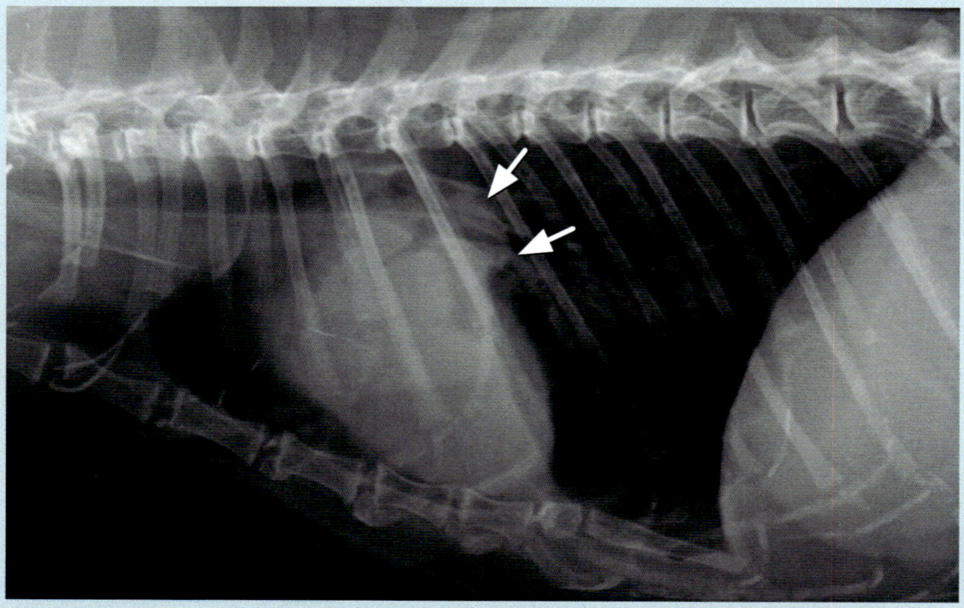

FIGURE 2.63. Lateral radiograph of the thorax of a cat with hypertrophic cardiomyopathy. It is possible to observe an increase in the height of the cardiac silhouette, an elevation of the trachea and caudal vena cava and a marked prominence of the left atrium (arrows).

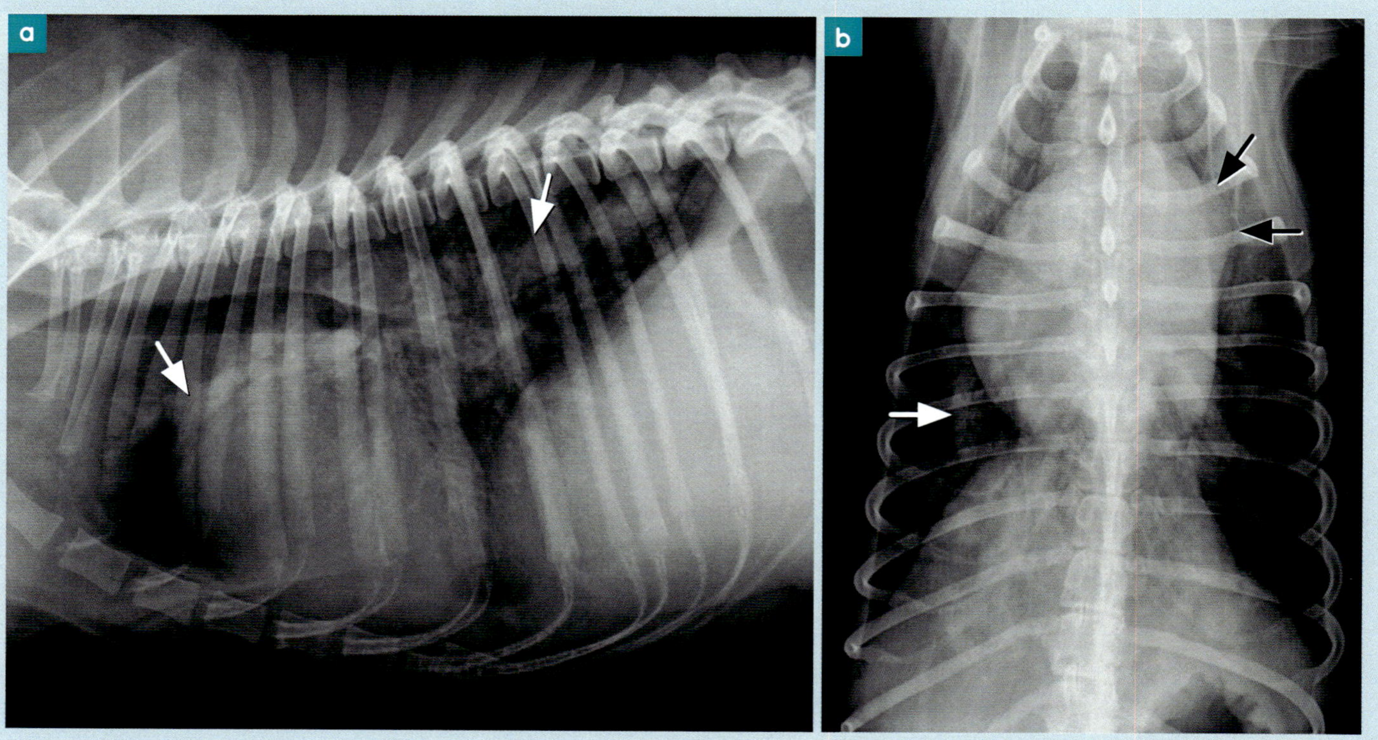

FIGURE 2.64. Lateral (a) and ventrodorsal (b) radiographs of the thorax of a dog with dirofilariosis. It is possible to observe signs of enlargement of the right ventricle and dilatation and tortuous course of the pulmonary arteries (indicated by white arrows). In image (b), the enlarged main pulmonary artery creates a prominence of the cardiac silhouette in the 1 to 2 o'clock position (black arrows) according to the clock-face analogy.

valve stenosis, right ventricular hypoplasia, double outlet right ventricle and transposition of the great vessels are rarer. In cats, the most frequent defects are mitral valve or tricuspid valve dysplasia, patent ductus arteriosus, tetralogy of Fallot, ventricular septal defect, aortic valve stenosis, tetralogy of Fallot, persistent common atrioventricular canal or endocardial fibroelastosis.

In some cases, plain radiography provides data that may help or guide us in case of a clinical suspicion of a congenital heart or vascular disease.

Patent ductus arteriosus

In the foetal circulation, the ductus arteriosus shunts the oxygenated maternal blood to the aorta. The permanent closure of this duct occurs soon after birth, thus forming the ligamentum arteriosum. A failure in the closure of the duct maintains a communication between the aorta and the main pulmonary artery, and is called patent ductus arteriosus. The consequences of this failure to close will depend on the diameter of the duct and on the pulmonary vascular resistance. When the pulmonary vascular resistance is normal, there is a continuous shunt flow from the aorta (high resistance) to the pulmonary circulation (low resistance). This type of flow (systemic to pulmonary) is termed left-to-right shunt and is the most common pattern. Reverse or right-to-left patent ductus arteriosus refers to those cases in which blood flows back from the pulmonary artery to the aorta (pulmonary to systemic), and occurs because the pulmonary vascular resistance is higher than the systemic vascular resistance.

The radiographic signs of a patent ductus arteriosus considerably vary depending on the volume of blood being shunted, the age of the animal and the degree of cardiac decompensation. In left-to-right shunts, it is possible to observe a mild to moderate enlargement of the left atrium and ventricle due to volume overload and vascular congestion. It is common to observe three prominences in the margin of the cardiac silhouette on dorsoventral radiographs: in the 11 to 1 o'clock position, due to an enlargement of the aortic arch; in the 1 to 2 o'clock position, due to an enlargement of the outflow tract of the pulmonary artery; and in the 2 to 3 o'clock position, due to a

Normal radiographic
anatomy of the thorax
right lateral view

http://goo.gl/otDlnr

lateral displacement of the left atrial appendage. In animals with severe pulmonary hypertension, caused by a right-to-left patent ductus arteriosus, an enlargement of the right ventricle and tortuous pulmonary arteries (fig. 2.65) are observed.

Pulmonary stenosis

It is a narrowing of the outflow tract of the right ventricle at the valvular (pulmonary valve dysplasia), subvalvular or supravalvular level. The most common type is the first one. When blood passes through the area of narrowing, the flow accelerates and poststenotic turbulences that cause dilatation of the main pulmonary artery appear. The pressure overload in the right ventricle leads to its enlargement.

The radiographic signs of this condition depend on the degree of narrowing, although it is often possible to see signs of enlargement of the right heart and main pulmonary artery in the two projections. It is easier to see the prominence of the pulmonary artery on dorsoventral radiographs, in the 1 to 2 o'clock position according to the clock-face analogy (fig. 2.66), although its shadow may be seen superimposed with the trachea on lateral radiographs (as a kind of "hat"). The pulmonary arteries may appear normal or have a reduced diameter.

Aortic stenosis

It is a narrowing of the outflow tract of the left ventricle at the subvalvular (fibrous or muscular ring), valvular or supravalvular level. The subvalvular type is the most common type in dogs (subaortic stenosis). When blood passes through the area of narrowing, the flow accelerates and poststenotic turbulences that cause dilatation of the aortic arch appear. Secondarily, the left ventricle dilates due to pressure overload.

The radiographic signs of this disease depend on the degree of the narrowing. An enlargement of the aortic arch and signs of increased height of the left ventricle may be observed on lateral radiographs (fig. 2.67), as well as a prominence of the cardiac silhouette in the 1 to 1 o'clock position, and in the 2 to 5 o'clock position on dorsoventral radiographs. Signs of enlargement of the left atrium will appear at advanced stages.

Ventricular septal defect

Interventricular septal defects may occur in any area of the septum, but they are more frequent in its membranous part, in its most dorsal area. They may be isolated defects or be associated with other congenital anomalies, such as atrial septal defects or patent ductus arteriosus. If the right and left ventricular pressures are normal, the blood flow will be shunted from left to right because the left ventricular systolic pressure is higher than the right one. However, if the defect is very dorsal, the blood will flow directly into the pulmonary artery, which causes almost no effects on the right ventricle. The blood that is shunted to the pulmonary circulation returns to the left atrium and ventricle, which causes pulmonary (arteries and veins) congestion and enlargement of the left heart. If the defect has a more ventral location, a large volume of blood may enter the right ventricle, so this latter may also appear enlarged in these cases.

Small defects do not usually cause any alterations on chest radiographs. If the defect is large, there will be signs of enlargement of the left ventricle and atrium, although this will be less marked in the later, as well as signs of enlargement of the right ventricle on some occasions (if the defect is ventral) and pulmonary congestion.

Tetralogy of Fallot

Tetralogy of Fallot is the congenital defect that most often causes cyanosis. It is the result of the combination of pulmonary stenosis, ventricular septal defects,

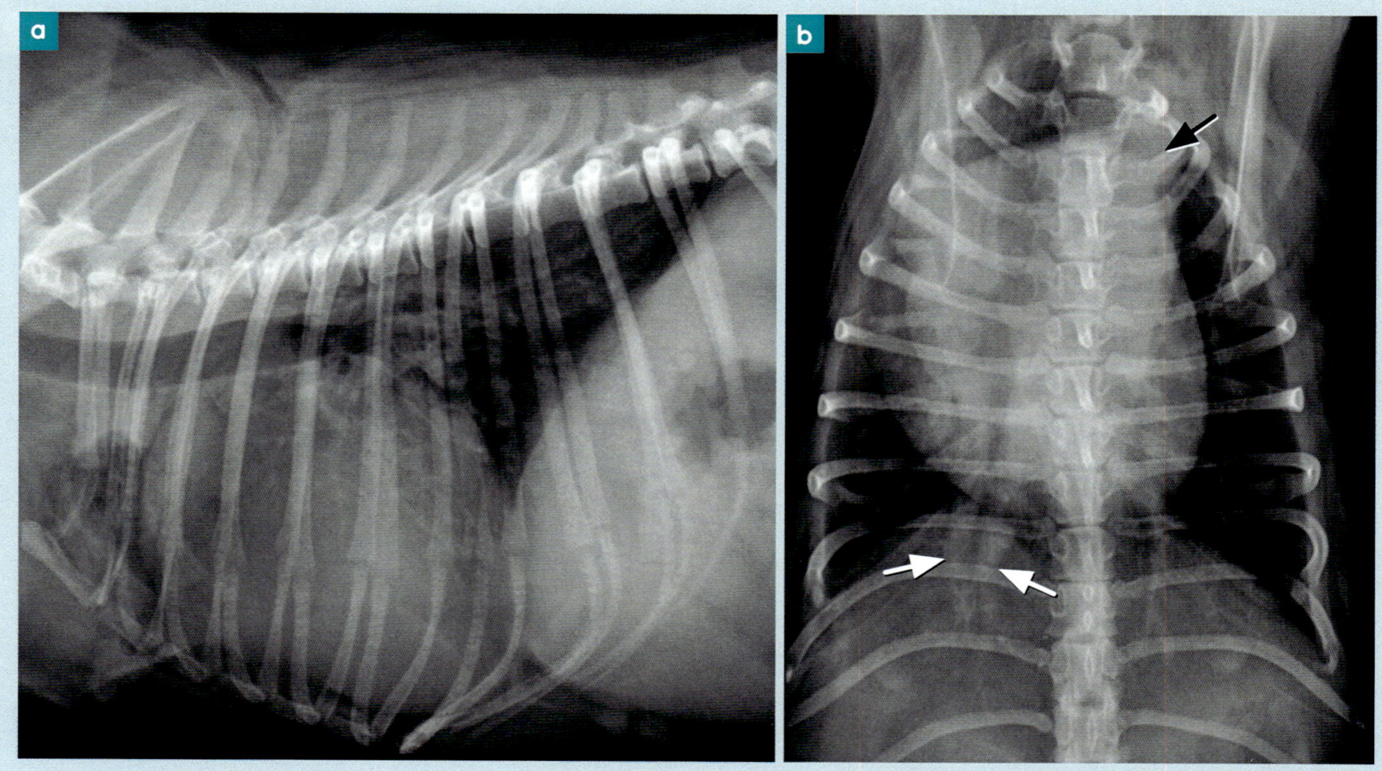

FIGURE 2.65. Lateral (a) and ventrodorsal (b) radiographs of the thorax of a dog with patent ductus arteriosus. These images show marked global cardiomegaly with a prominence of the cardiac silhouette in the 12 to 2 o'clock position (black arrow) according to the clock-face analogy, which indicates an enlargement of the main pulmonary artery, and, to a lesser extent, of the aortic arch. Dilatation of the pulmonary arteries and veins may also be observed (white arrows).

secondary hypertrophy of the right ventricle and several degrees of dextroposition and overload of the aorta.

The radiographic signs of this disease may greatly vary depending on the severity of the pulmonary stenosis and size of the ventricular septal defect. An enlarged right heart and reduced pulmonary vessels are usually observed.

Diseases of the pericardium

The disease that most frequently affects the pericardium is pericardial effusion. It causes a generalised enlargement of the cardiac silhouette, which acquires the aspect of a water bottle when the volume of fluid that has accumulated in the pericardial sac is very large (fig. 2.68). When the amount of fluid is minimal or moderate, the cardiac silhouette does not necessarily acquire a characteristic water-bottle shape and its enlargement is variable. On radiographs, the globally rounded shape of the cardiac silhouette in the two projections and the fact that the heart chambers cannot be identified help us to differentiate this image from that of global cardiomegaly. Even so, it is necessary to perform an echocardiogram to establish a differential diagnosis between both conditions. In many cases, this will also allow us to detect the presence of tumours as a cause of the effusion.

Peritoneopericardial hernias may have a congenital origin and are characterised by a communication between the peritoneal space and the pericardial space through a defect in the diaphragm. The identification of clumped abdominal structures that mask the image of the normal cardiac silhouette in the centre of the thorax is a typical radiological finding in this anomaly (fig. 2.69). The liver is the most frequently herniated organ, followed by the gallbladder, the stomach, the intestine and the omentum. If there is a communication,

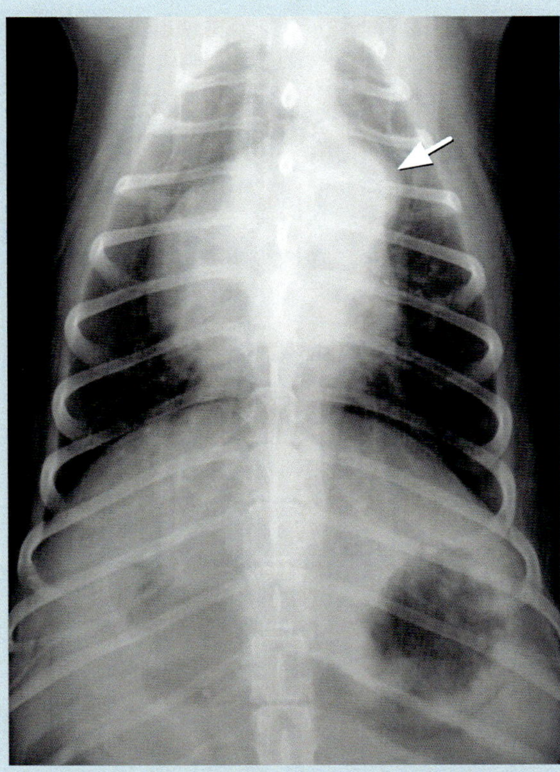

FIGURE 2.66. Dorsoventral radiograph of the thorax of a dog with pulmonary stenosis. The right margin of the cardiac silhouette appears rounded and it is possible to observe a prominence in the 1 to 2 o'clock position, according to the clock-face analogy, due to the enlargement of the main pulmonary artery.

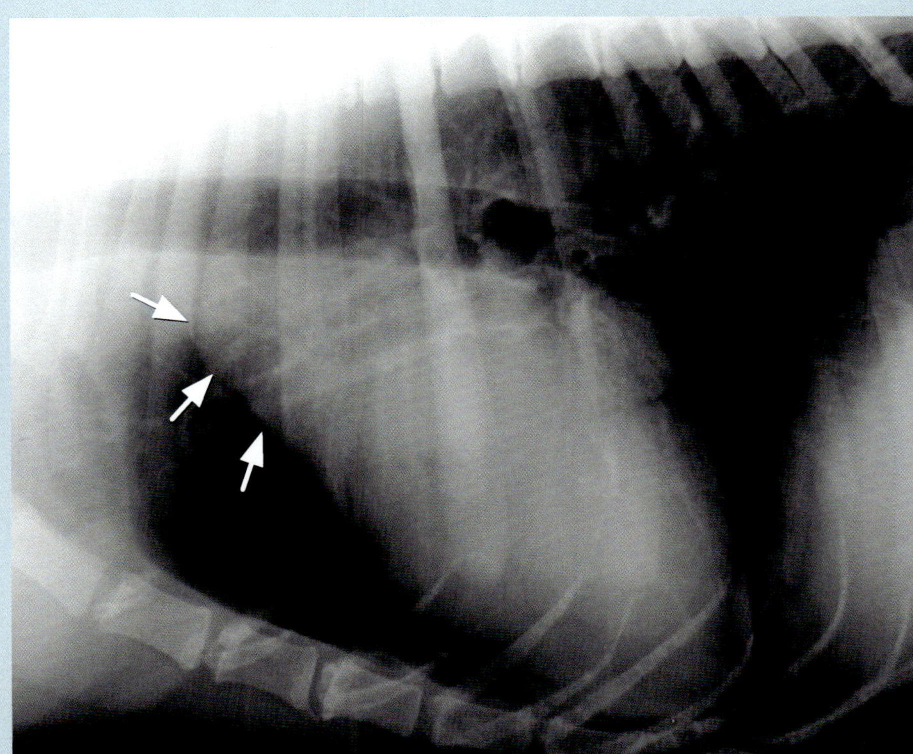

FIGURE 2.67. Lateral radiograph of the thorax of a dog with aortic valve stenosis. The shadow of the aortic arch appears enlarged.

but the passage of abdominal contents to the pericardial sac is minimal, the cardiac silhouette may appear enlarged and have an asymmetric morphology, although the diagnosis is more difficult to reach. In these cases, an echocardiogram will allow the identification of abnormal contents in the pericardial space. The oral administration of barium may confirm the anomalous position of the stomach and intestine if these are herniated.

Cardiac tumours

Most cardiac tumours are associated with a pericardial effusion. Haemangiosarcoma is the most frequent tumour in dogs, while lymphoma is the most frequent type in cats. Haemangiosarcomas originate in endothelial cells and may appear in any part of the heart, although their most common location is the wall of the right atrium. Chemodectomas originate in neuroepithelial cells and are typically located at the base of the heart, where they create a more or less defined "mass effect" on radiographs depending on their size (fig. 2.70). Other tumours (myxomas, ectopic thyroid carcinomas, fibrosarcomas, etc.) are less frequent.

Microcardia

The term microcardia is used to describe the reduction of the size of the heart. The decrease in the size of the cardiac silhouette may be real or apparent on radiographs. An increase of the amount of air in the lungs (emphysema) or in the pleural space (pneumothorax) may create a false image of microcardia. When hypovolaemic shock occurs, either due to haemorrhage or to severe dehydration, and in cases of hypoadrenocorticism (Addison's disease), the heart really decreases in size. In Addison's disease the image may be particularly remarkable because hypovolaemia is accompanied by atrophy of the muscular mass of the heart. The size of the pulmonary vessels is usually reduced as an associated finding in cases of microcardia (fig. 2.71).

Cor pulmonale and pulmonary thomboebolism

The radiological identification of an enlargement of the right ventricle in a patient with a pulmonary or vascular disease is very indicative of cor pulmonale, which is defined as a right heart failure caused by a pulmonary or thoracic disease. By definition, there must be pulmonary hypertension in cor pulmonale for right heart failure to happen. In dogs, the most common cause of cor pulmonale is dirofilariasis, although any obstruction of the pulmonary vessels may cause hypertension and, therefore, cor pulmonale. The obstruction of the pulmonary arteries may occur as a result of the presence of blood clots (pulmonary thromboembolism) or by embolisation of fat, septic material, neoplastic cells or nematodes of the genus *Dirofilaria*. Although they are difficult to identify, in cases of thromboembolism it is possible to observe signs such as dilatation of the pulmonary arteries in the perihilar area and their abrupt narrowing or interruption in more peripheral areas, more radiolucent areas in the lung due to a focal reduction of perfusion, atelectasis of a pulmonary lobe, pleural effusion around the affected lobe and, occasionally, peripheral triangular areas of pulmonary consolidation (especially in the caudal lobes). The chest radiographs of up to 27 % of cats and dogs with a confirmed pulmonary thromboembolism at necropsy do not show any anomalies. In an animal with tachypnoea that does not respond to the administration of oxygen, a normal chest radiograph will be very indicative of thromboembolism.

Computed tomography may be very useful to identify grade 1 and 2 thrombi in arteries, although very small thrombi may not be detectable in the images.

Lung

In cats and dogs, the right lung is divided into four (cranial, middle, caudal and accessory) lobes and the left lung is divided into two (cranial and caudal) lobes. The approximate areas occupied by each pulmonary lobe are shown with coloured areas in figure 2.72.

The lungs contain air in the alveoli and in the lumen of the bronchi and bronchioles, and are formed by structures of soft-tissue density, which include the alveolar walls, the interstitial tissue, the blood vessels and the walls of the bronchi and bronchioles. Of these latter, only the blood vessels and walls of the bronchi

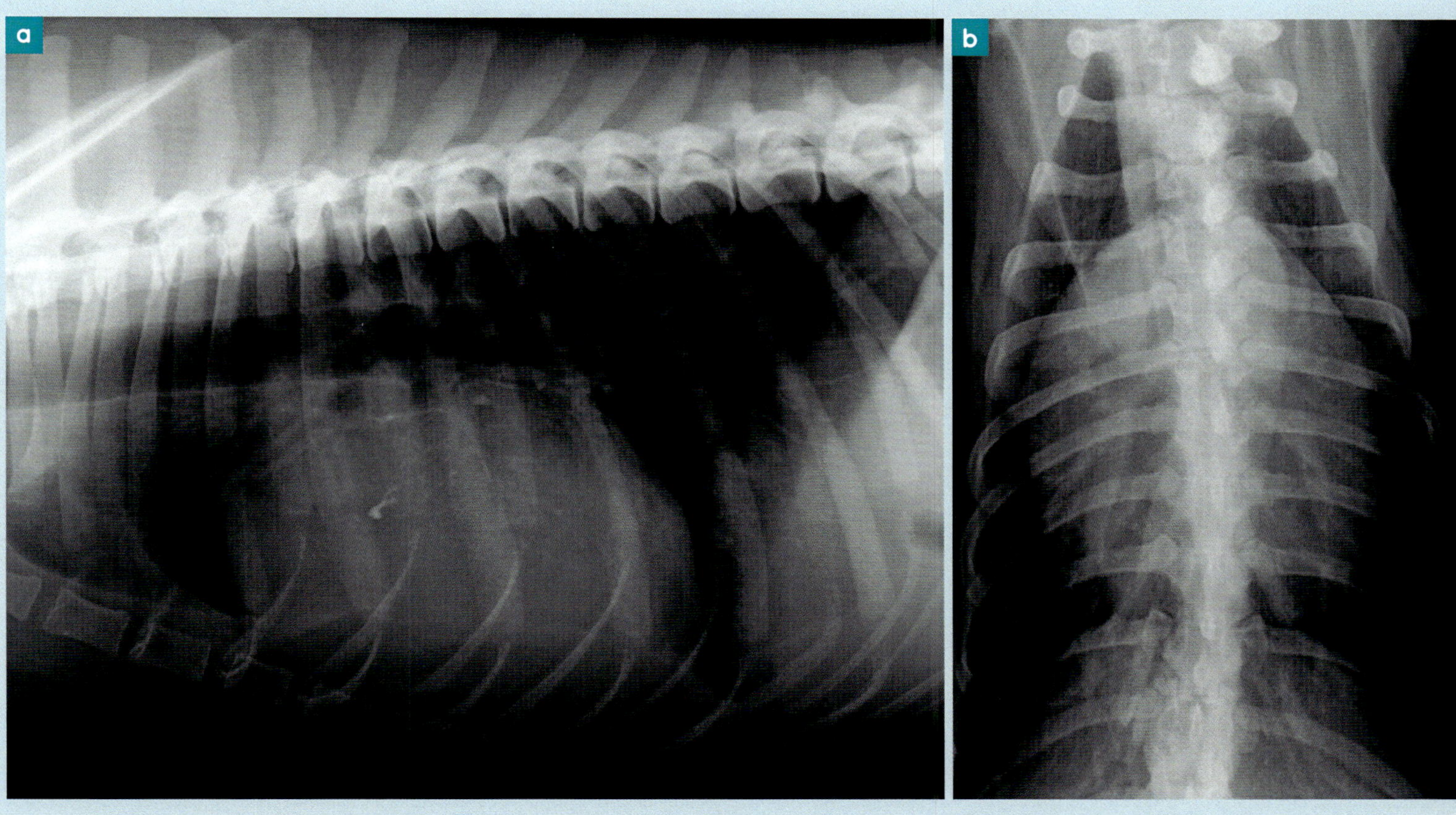

FIGURE 2.68. Lateral (a) and dorsoventral (b) radiographs of the thorax of a dog with a pericardial effusion. The cardiac silhouette appears enlarged and with a "water-bottle" shape. A dilated cardiomyopathy may give rise to a similar image, although it is usually possible to distinguish the cardiac chambers to some extent, while in the image of a pericardial effusion it is not. However, an echocardiogram is necessary to confirm the diagnosis with certainty.

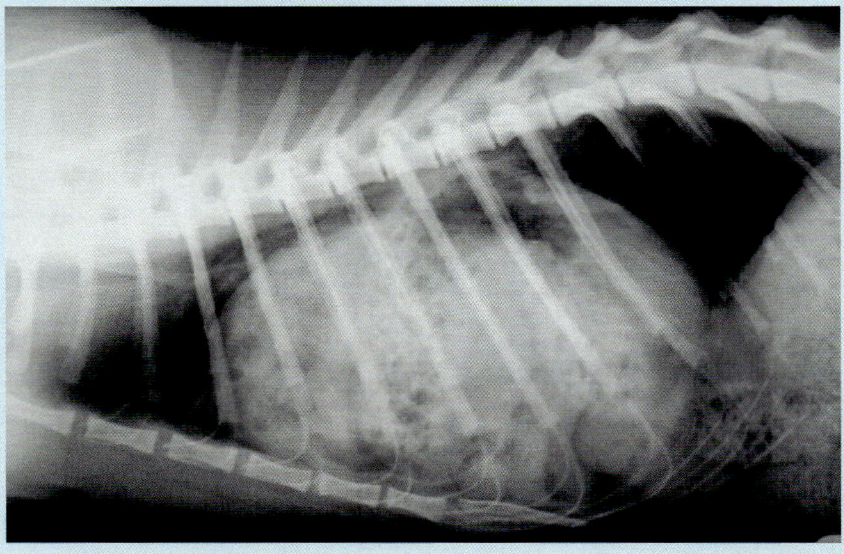

FIGURE 2.69. Lateral radiograph of a cat with a peritoneopericardial hernia. It is possible to identify the presence of the small and large intestines in the pericardial sac, which probably contains other abdominal organs, such as the liver or stomach. Their presence may be confirmed by means of echocardiography.

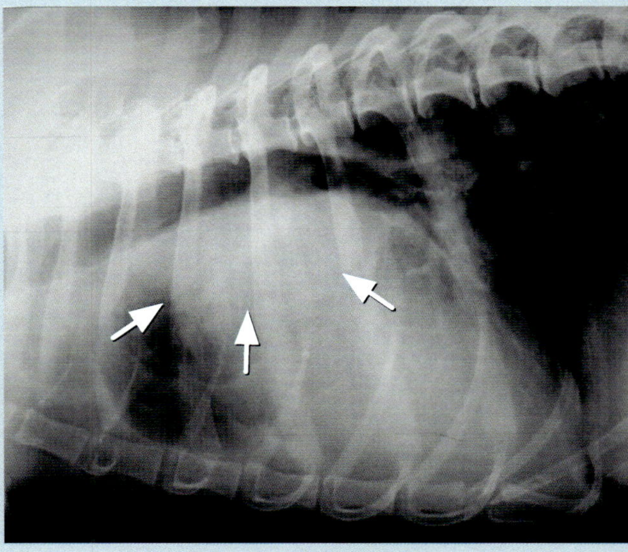

FIGURE 2.70. Lateral radiograph of a dog with a tumour at the base of the heart (chemodectoma). The white arrows indicate its approximate location, although it is not possible to observe its exact outline in the image. However, it creates a "mass effect" that is obvious due to the marked dorsal displacement of the trachea.

Normal radiographic
anatomy of the thorax
ventrodorsal view

http://goo.gl/MECQmD

with a larger diameter can be identified on a radiograph of a normal thorax.

If we divided the radiograph in three concentric areas –perihilar area, middle area and peripheral area of the lung–, in normal conditions it would only be possible to visualise the walls of the bronchi in the area most proximal to the pulmonary hilum, since these are usually too thin to be identified in the image in the middle and peripheral areas. The blood vessels, however, are visible in the three areas as they have soft-tissue density walls and content. They appear as structures with a linear morphology that branch out and become narrower as they run from the hilum to the periphery of the lung. Following this criterion, we will talk about a **normal lung pattern** when the lung appears essentially radiolucent (due to its air content) and when the pulmonary vessels –with a normal size and morphology– and larger bronchi can be identified in it (fig. 2.73).

The pulmonary vessels and bronchi have a parallel course: the arteries appear dorsal to the veins on lateral radiographs and are lateral to the veins on dorsoventral and ventrodorsal radiographs. The bronchi appear as radiolucent bands located between the arteries and veins (the distance between the artery and vein does not necessarily coincide with the diameter of the bronchus). The diameter of the arteries and veins must be approximately equal in normal conditions.

Although they have already been dealt with in this chapter in the section "Principles of interpretation", the factors that most affect the radiographic image of the lungs are:

- **Exposure values:** on underexposed radiographs, the lung has a higher radiopacity, which may be mistaken for an interstitial infiltrate of the parenchyma, while on overexposed radiographs all the structures in the image appear darker, which may be confused with emphysema.
- **Moment of the respiratory cycle:** if the radiograph is taken during expiration, the lungs contain a lesser amount of air, which slightly increases their radiopacity.
- **Obesity:** An excess amount of subcutaneous fat leads to a slight increase in pulmonary radiopacity, as the density of fat is added to that of the lungs. In addition, the accumulation of intrathoracic fat somewhat limits lung expansion, which also contributes to the increase in pulmonary radiopacity.
- **Age:** The lungs of young animals may be more radiopaque than those of adults because they contain more water. The lungs of old animals may be slightly more radiopaque due to interstitial fibrosis, as well as to calcification or fibrosis of the bronchial walls, which make these more visible on radiographs (it will also be possible to visualise them in the middle area of the lungs).
- **Prolonged lateral recumbency:** the animals that remain in a recumbent position for a relatively long period of time, especially if they are anaesthetised, will have a partial collapse of the lung that corresponds to the side on which they had been lying. This causes a focal increase in the density of the atelectasic lung, which helps to differentiate atelectasis caused by a recumbent position from a real pulmonary infiltration.
- **Digital radiographs:** digital radiographs have a much higher contrast resolution than conventional radiographs and make the lungs appear less radiolucent. They also improve the visualisation of soft-tissue density structures, such as the pulmonary vessels and walls of the bronchi, which will sometimes be identified in the middle area of the lungs despite having no anomalies.

Lateral and ventrodorsal radiographs are recommended for a general assessment of the lungs. If ventrodorsal and dorsoventral views are compared, the capacity of the lungs to expand is greater with the first one, which improves the definition of the lung in the image. On a lateral radiograph, the lung that is higher will be better visualised, since its capacity of expansion is at its maximum, while the lung that is lower will always have some degree of partial collapse, which may limit its radiological examination. The right lateral projection is usually used as the standard view. However, in the specific case of an assessment of pulmonary metastases, the combination of the two lateral projections, right and left, is used, since if there are small lesions, these will be better viewed in the most distended lung (higher position). In case of doubt, a ventrodorsal radiograph is added in order to obtain complementary information, although small lesions that are visible on

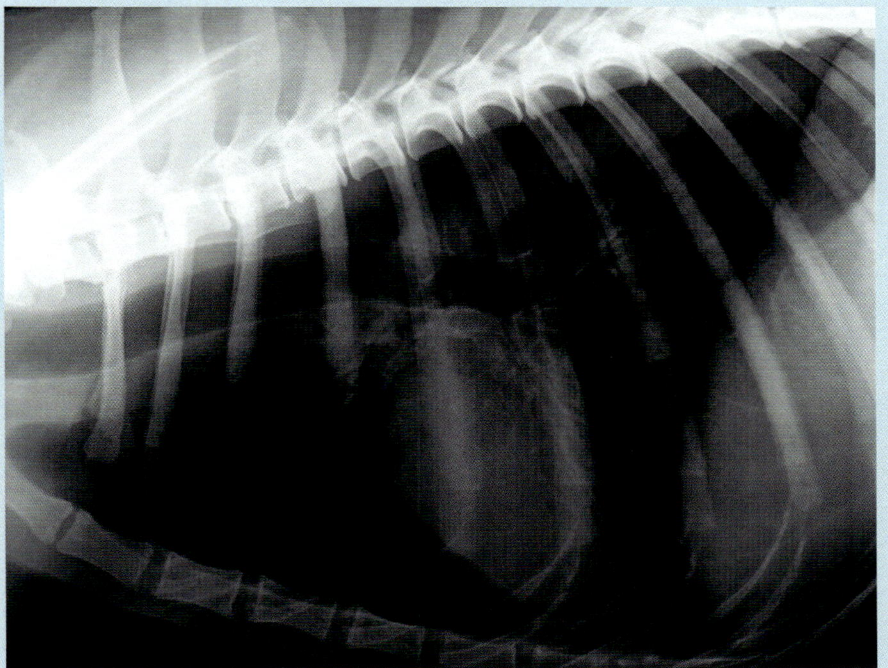

FIGURE 2.71. Lateral radiograph of the thorax of a dog with microcardia and hypovascularisation. The cardiac silhouette and pulmonary lungs appear smaller, which leads to the lung fields appearing wider and more radiolucent. This may be mistaken for pulmonary emphysema.

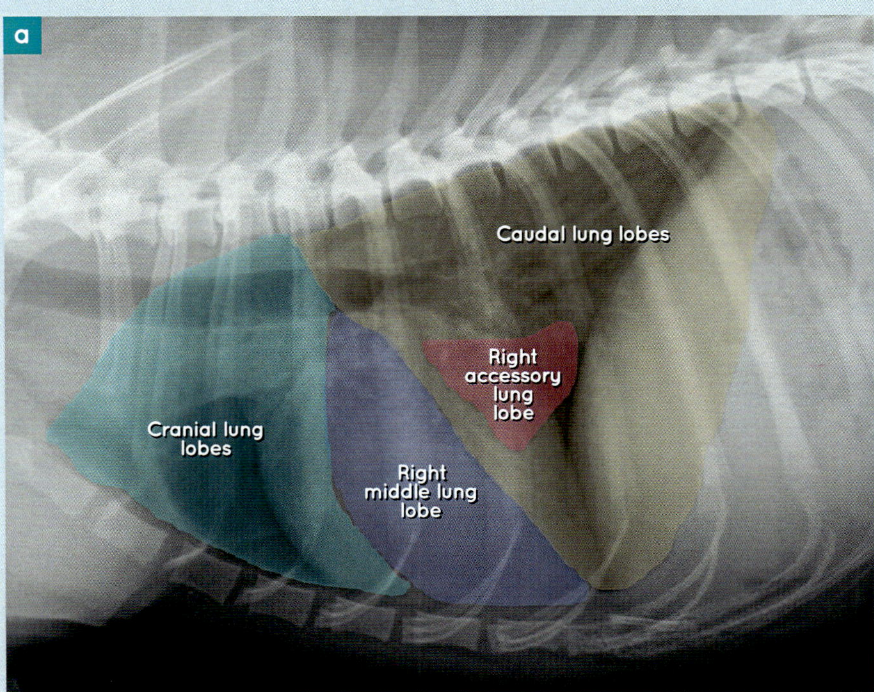

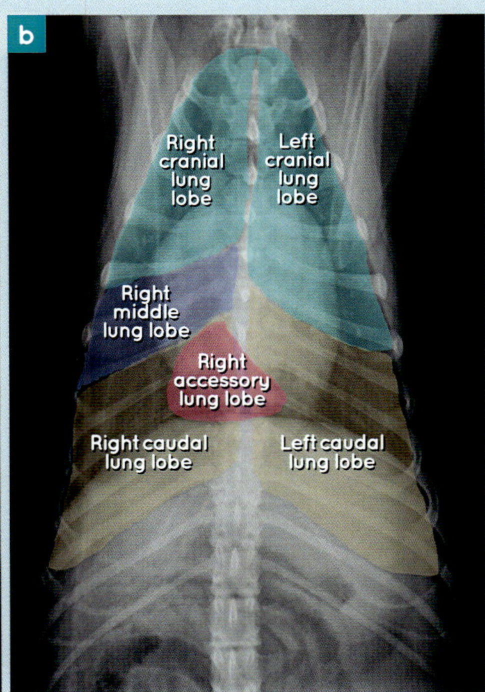

FIGURE 2.72. Normal lateral (a) and ventrodorsal (b) radiographs of the thorax of a dog, in which the location of the different lung lobes is shown with coloured areas.

one or the two lateral views often cannot be identified on the ventrodorsal view.

Ultrasound examinations of the lungs have important limitations. It will only be possible to visualise areas of the lungs that do not contain air and are in contact with the thoracic wall, since the presence of air will hinder the examination in other locations. In cases of pleural effusion, the fluid facilitates the visualisation of the pulmonary content. Ultrasonography is indicated in the study of pulmonary masses and consolidation, since it provides information about the internal structure of the lesion, its vascularisation may be examined with Doppler ultrasound and it allows the collection of samples for cytology or biopsies under ultrasound guidance.

As opposed to magnetic resonance imaging, which provides low-quality lung images with conventional equipment, computed tomography will be indicated whenever the findings on the radiographs are suspicious, when a torsion is suspected, in cases of bronchial foreign body or pulmonary thromboembolism, for a thorough examination of metastases and for the assessment of masses (it allows the determination of its exact location and examination of the rest of the lung to rule out any associated lesions), as well as for guided punctures or biopsies of lesions that are not identifiable by means of ultrasonography.

Abnormal lung patterns

The radiological assessment of the lungs is based on the identification of abnormal lung patterns, which have been classified in function of the affected components of the lung:

- Bronchial.
- Vascular.
- Alveolar.
- Interstitial.
- Mixed (combination of two or more of the previous patterns).

The identification of the pattern may be more or less difficult depending on the location and extension of the lesions. Once it is identified, a differential diagnosis is made for each abnormal lung pattern.

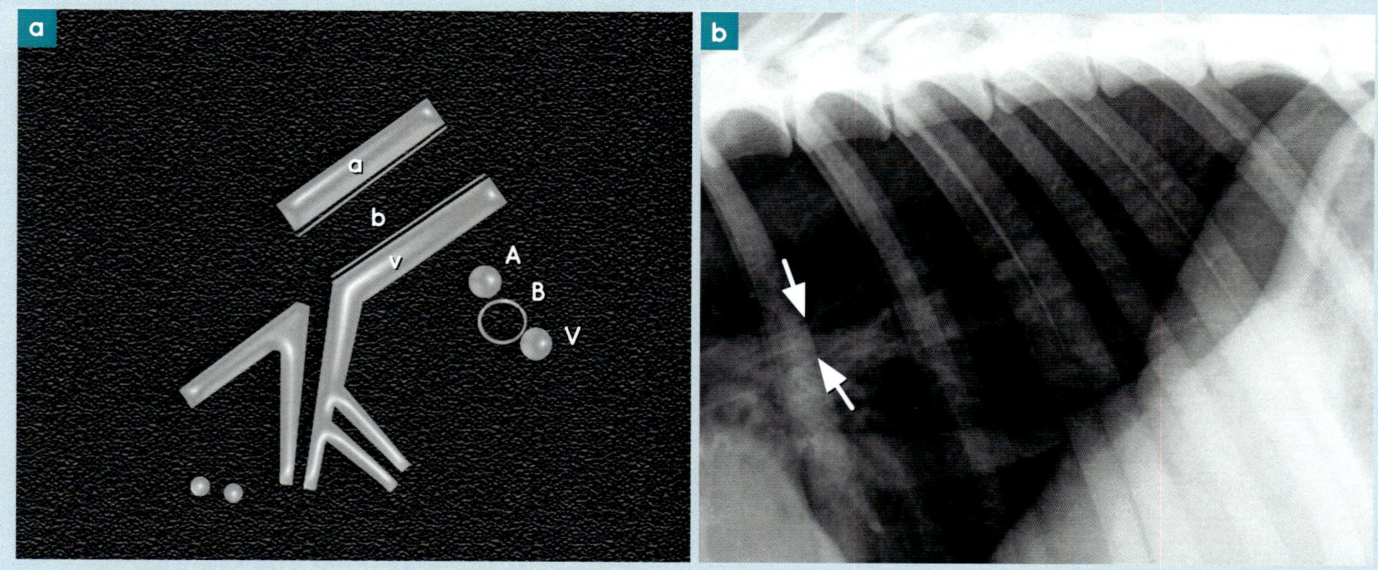

FIGURE 2.73. Schematic representation of the normal (a) pulmonary pattern and enlarged image of the caudodorsal area on a lateral radiograph of the thorax of a healthy dog. Image (a) represents the normal lung parenchyma, which is mainly radiolucent (dark grey background), with parallel pulmonary vessels (arteries and veins with a similar diameter) that branch out as they run towards the peripheral area, and bronchial walls that are only visible in the area where the diameter is larger; the vessels and bronchi are represented longitudinally (a: artery, b: bronchus, v: vein) and transversally (A: artery, B: bronchus, V: vein). In image (b), the soft-tissue density structures with a linear morphology that branch out and extend to the peripheral lung correspond to vessels, while the bronchial walls (arrows) can only be observed as thin parallel lines in the perihilar area.

The length of the list of diseases may vary depending on the correlation of the radiological findings with the rest of the patient's clinical data (anamnesis, examination, laboratory tests, etc.). The main limitation in the interpretation of lung radiographs lies in this fact: very different diseases may have a similar radiographic image.

Bronchial pattern

A bronchial pattern is identified when bronchial walls that could not be observed become visible in normal conditions, in general in the middle or peripheral area of the lung, although we must remember that digital radiography can allow the visualisation of walls of normal bronchi in the middle area.

The typical radiological sign is the visualisation of "ring-" or "donut-"shaped images, which correspond to transverse shadows of bronchial walls (of those bronchial branches with a course that is parallel to the X-ray beam), and "train track" images, which correspond to the longitudinal shadows of these branches (bronchial branches with a course that is perpendicular to the X-ray beam).

The visualisation of the bronchial walls may be due to an increase in their radiographic density (calcification), to their thickening or to the presence of peribronchial infiltrates.

The calcification of the walls is a common finding in middle-aged and older animals (especially in brachycephalic breeds), and is usually not considered pathological, although it may also appear as a sequela of chronic bronchitis or in cases of hyperadrenocorticism. The walls appear as very thin and well-defined lines of mineral density (fig. 2.74).

The thickening of the wall or presence of peribronchial infiltrates generally occurs in cases of chronic bronchitis (of inflammatory, infectious, allergic or irritative origin) and, on a less frequent basis, due to a neoplastic infiltration. In these cases, the bronchial walls appear in the image as thin and poorly defined bands of soft-tissue density (fig. 2.75).

We must bear in mind that, in cases of acute bronchitis and tracheobronchitis, no obvious alterations of the bronchi are usually observed in the radiographic image. However, radiography is indicated to rule out the presence of bronchopneumonia.

The typical lung pattern of feline asthma is bronchial (fig. 2.76), although it may be associated with other lung patterns. The severity of the clinical signs often does not directly correlate with the magnitude of the radiological findings. In patients with feline asthma, it is common to observe secondary atelectasis of the right middle lobe and emphysema.

In chronic or severe bronchial diseases, the bronchi may have irreversible sac-like dilatations, which are termed bronchiectases. These may also be caused by obstructions of the airway or smoke inhalation.

Computed tomography is of great interest in the study of the diseases of the bronchi. It allows the visualisation of bronchi and bronchioles with a small diameter, bronchiectases that are not detectable by means of radiography or bronchial ruptures, and the differentiation between foreign bodies, presence of intraluminal mucus and bronchial masses (fig 2.77). In the case of bronchial neoplasms, it also facilitates the identification of pulmonary metastases and lymphadenopathies. With CT virtual bronchoscopy, it is possible to follow the course of the trachea and large bronchi (fig. 2.78).

Vascular pattern

A vascular pattern is identified when there are alterations in the size, morphology or number of pulmonary vessels.

Although the size and number of peripheral vessels may be evaluated subjectively, it is more advisable to evaluate the diameter and shape of those vessels with a larger diameter: cranial lobar arteries and veins on lateral radiographs (fig. 2.79) and caudal lobar arteries and veins on dorsoventral radiographs (fig. 2.80). On lateral views, the cranial lobar arteries and veins appear as two pairs of vessels located in the cranioventral lung field, which run cranially. In normal conditions, the diameter of the artery and that of the vein must be approximately the same, and these values at the level of the 4th intercostal space should not exceed the width of the 4th rib at its proximal third. The caudal lobar arteries and veins are better visualised on dorsoventral radiographs than on ventrodorsal ones and should not exceed the width of the 9th rib at the point where they are superimposed. In cats, it is easier to visualise the cranial lobar arteries and veins than the caudal ones.

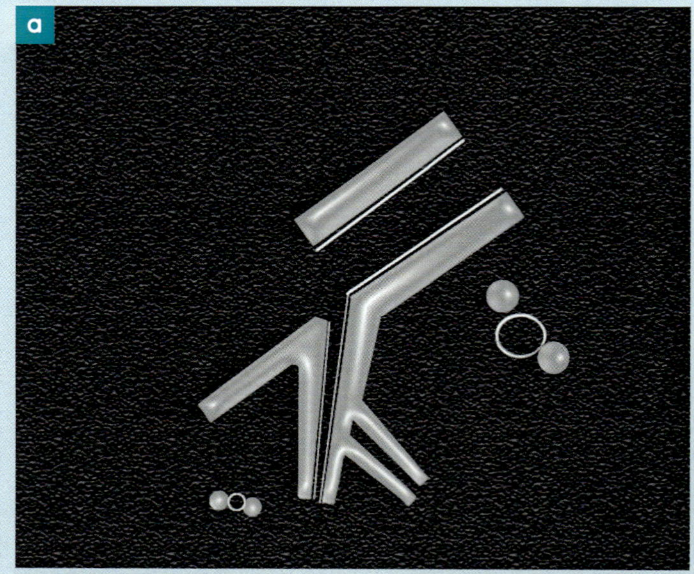

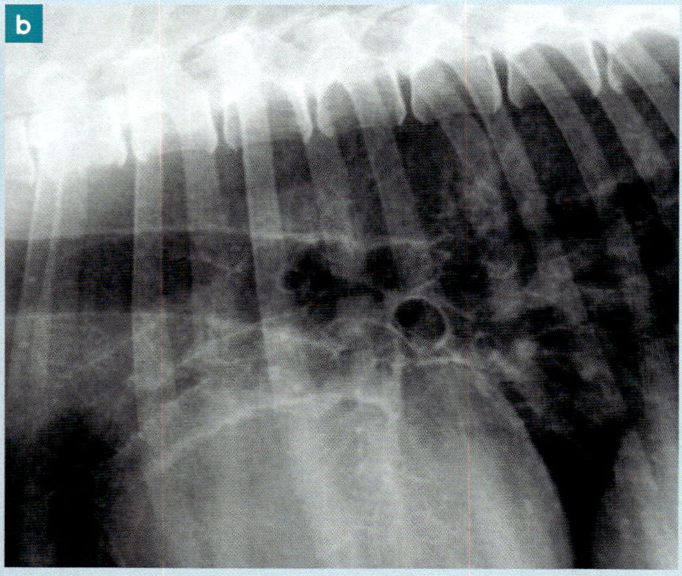

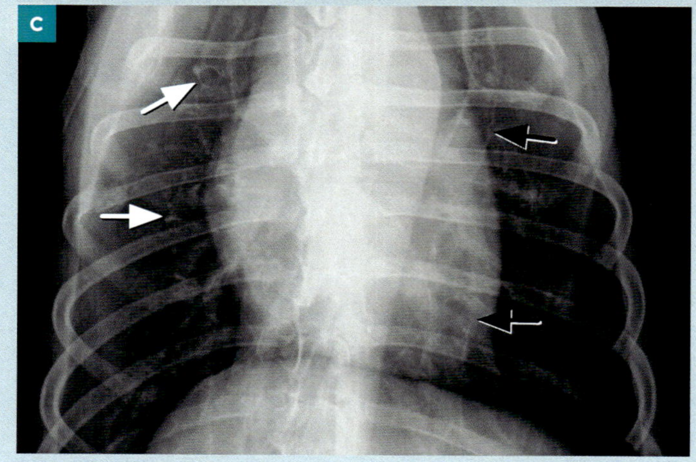

▲ FIGURE 2.74. Schematic representation of the bronchial lung pattern due to calcification (a) and enlarged image in lateral (b) and ventrodorsal (c) projection of the central area of the thorax of a dog with calcified bronchial walls, with no clinical significance. The black arrows show longitudinal ("train track") images of the bronchi and the white arrows show transverse ("ring" or "donut" shaped) images of smaller bronchial branches.

▼ FIGURE 2.75. Schematic representation of the bronchial lung pattern caused by thickened walls or peribronchial infiltrates (a) and radiographic image in ventrodorsal projection of the thorax of a dog with eosinophilic bronchitis (b). The black arrow shows a longitudinal ("train track") image of a bronchus and the white arrows show transverse ("ring-" or "donut-" shaped) images of bronchial branches with different diameters.

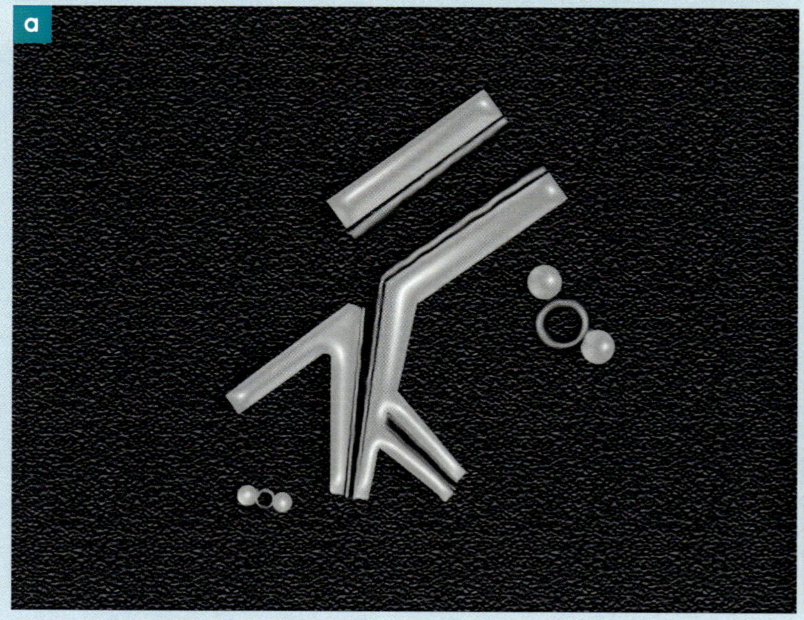

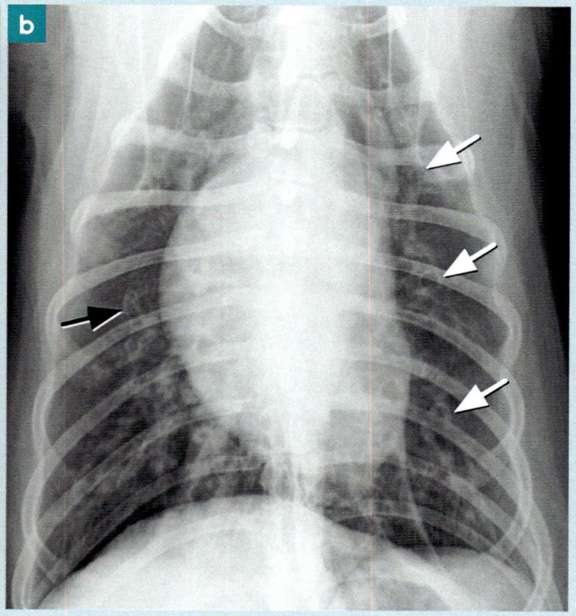

If the diameter of the arteries is greater than that of the veins, this indicates the presence of arterial congestion in the lung (fig. 2.81). It may be observed in cases of pulmonary hypertension, in which it is usually accompanied by an enlargement of the right lung (cor pulmonale). The most frequent cause is dirofilariasis, in which the vessels may have an undulated or tortuous course and be so dilated that their transverse shadow may be confused with pulmonary nodules. Arterial congestion may also appear in congenital diseases with a left-to-right shunt (patent ductus arteriosus, atrial or ventricular septal defects, etc.).

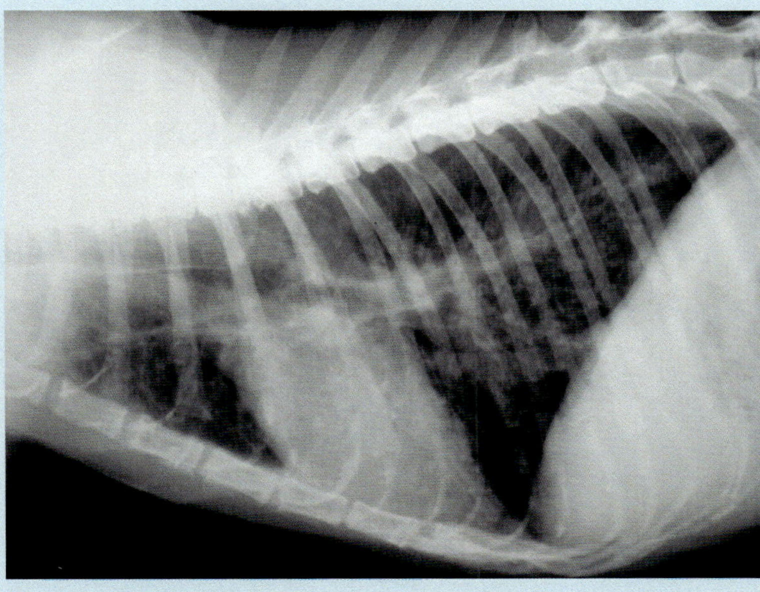

FIGURE 2.76. Lateral radiograph of the thorax of a cat with a bronchial pattern due to feline asthma.

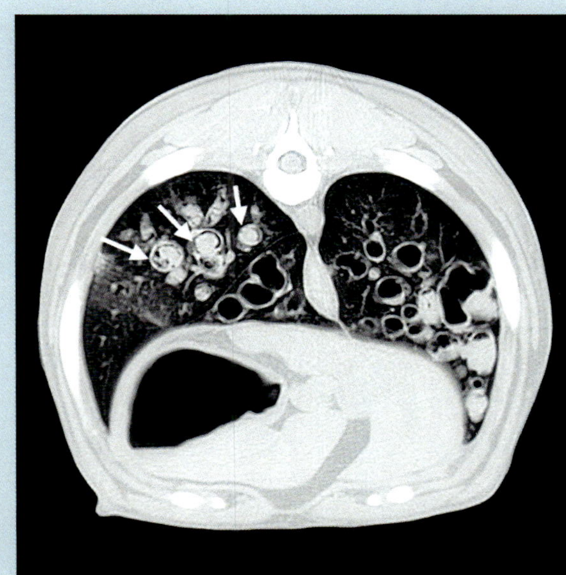

FIGURE 2.77. Computed tomography image of the thorax of a dog with bronchiectases and presence of multiple masses in the lumen of numerous bronchial branches (arrows), which may correspond to parasite granulomas or neoplastic nodules.

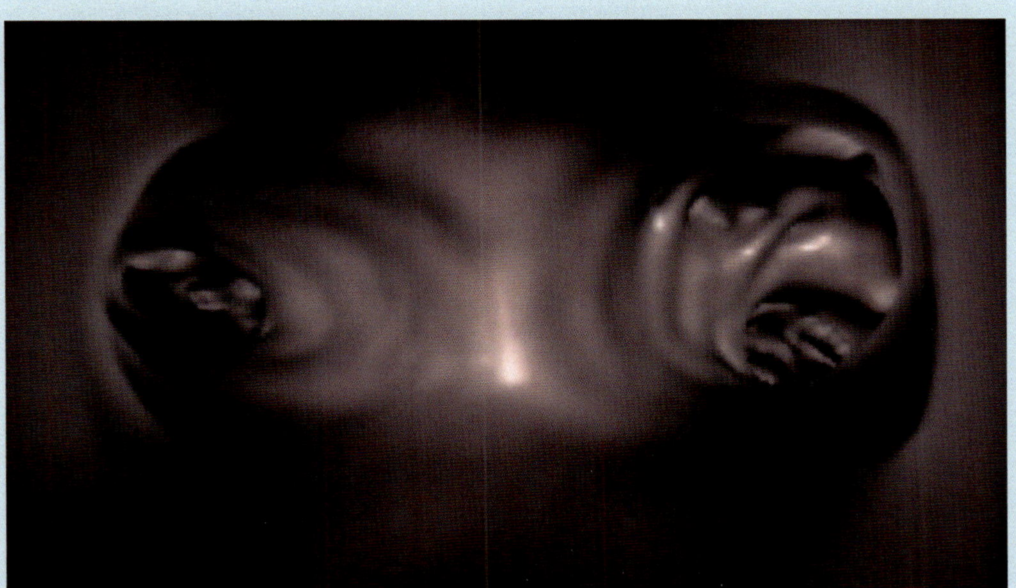

FIGURE 2.78. Image of a CT virtual bronchoscopy of a healthy dog, in which the bifurcation of the trachea in the two main bronchi may be observed. Subdivisions into smaller branches may be identified in the lumen of these latter.

If the diameter of the veins exceeds that of the arteries, this indicates venous pulmonary congestion (fig. 2.82). The main cause is left cardiac failure due to acquired or congenital diseases (with a right-to-left shunt essentially, although in some cases with a left-to-right shunt too).

In a mixed congestion, the arteries and veins will appear enlarged (fig. 2.83). It will therefore be necessary to compare their diameter with that of the ribs and follow the criteria previously explained. An increased number of visible vessels in the peripheral areas may be observed. Apart from pathological causes (left heart failure and congenital defects with left-to-right shunts), mixed congestion may also appear if an excessive volume of fluids has been administered to the patient (iatrogenic overhydration).

A reduction of the size of the pulmonary vessels (**pulmonary hypovascularisation**) (fig. 2.84) may occur in cases of hypovolaemia (dehydration, haemorrhage, Addison's disease), in some congenital diseases with a right-to-left shunt and in severe cases of pulmonary stenosis. As the size and number of vessels that are visible on the radiograph decrease, the lung fields appear darker and it may be difficult to identify vessels in the peripheral area. This should not be mistaken for overexposure of the radiograph (with a bright light source it will be possible to identify those peripheral vessels with a normal diameter on an overexposed radiograph). In cases of thromboembolism, it is possible to observe a focal or lobar hypovascularisation pattern, with a reduction of the diameter of the vessels or their abrupt interruption in the affected area.

According to some authors, the loss of definition of the vessels that takes place when radiopacity of the pulmonary interstitium significantly increases is also an abnormal vascular pattern.

Alveolar pattern

An alveolar pattern is identified when fluid (transudate, exudate or blood) or cells (e.g. neoplastic cells) accumulate in the alveolar space, or, when the alveoli lose their normal air content (atelectasis).

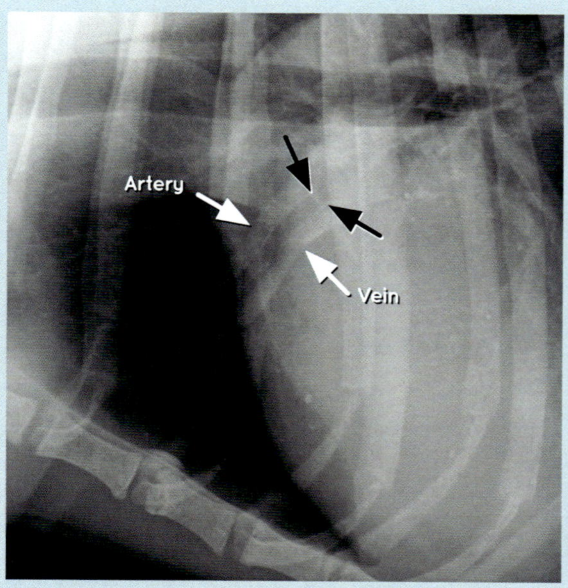

FIGURE 2.79. Enlarged image of the cranioventral area on a lateral radiograph of the thorax of a healthy dog, in which the left cranial lobar artery and vein are shown with white arrows, and the calcified walls of the bronchus that runs between these two vessels are shown with black arrows. On lateral radiographs, the arteries are dorsal to the veins, which allows them to be identified.

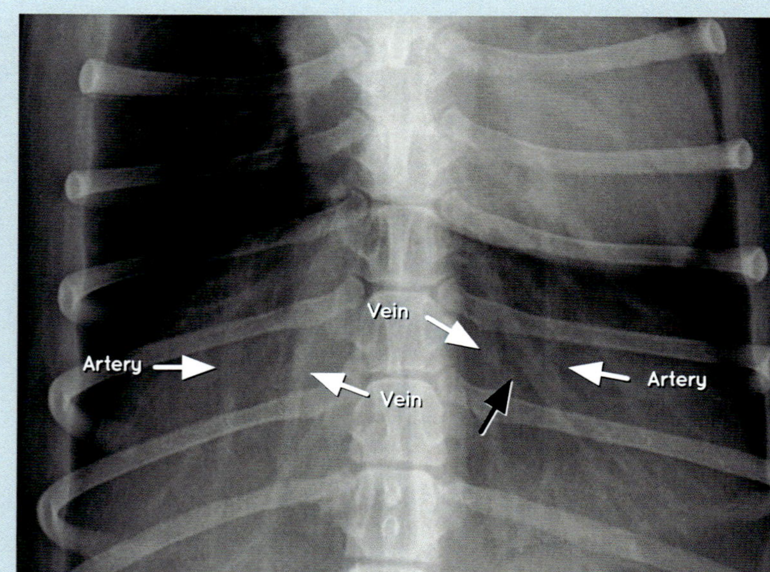

FIGURE 2.80. Enlarged image in dorsoventral projection of the medial and caudal areas of the thorax of a healthy dog, in which the caudal lobar arteries and veins of both lungs are shown with white arrows. The black arrow shows the wall of the bronchus that runs between the left caudal lobar artery and vein. On dorsoventral and ventrodorsal radiographs, the arteries are lateral to the veins, which allows them to be identified.

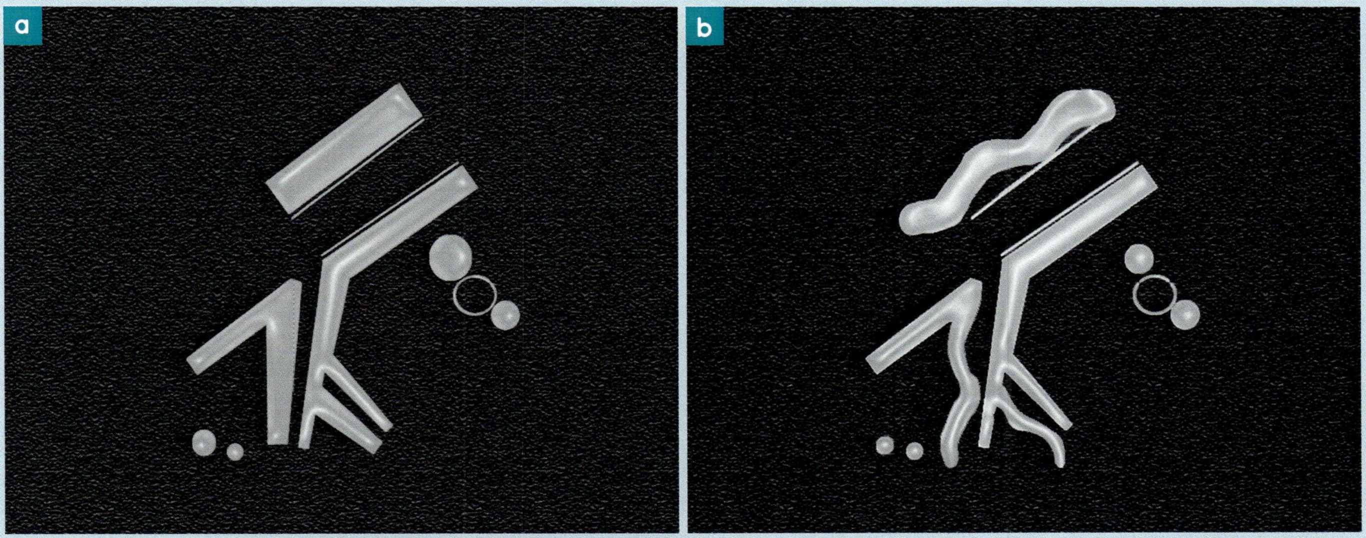

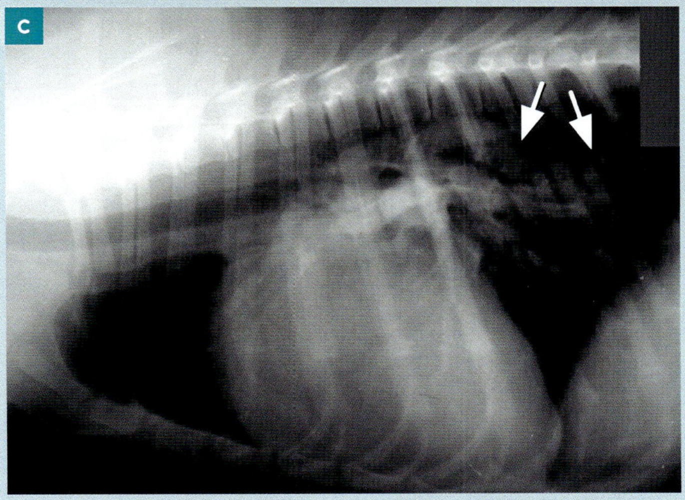

◀ FIGURE 2.81. Schematic representation of the vascular lung pattern due to an increase in size (a) and tortuosity (b) of the pulmonary arteries, and lateral radiograph of the thorax of a dog with dirofilariasis (c). The left cranial lobar artery has a larger diameter than the vein (visible in the cranioventral area of the thorax) and very dilated pulmonary arteries with a tortuous course (arrows) can be identified in the caudodorsal lung field.

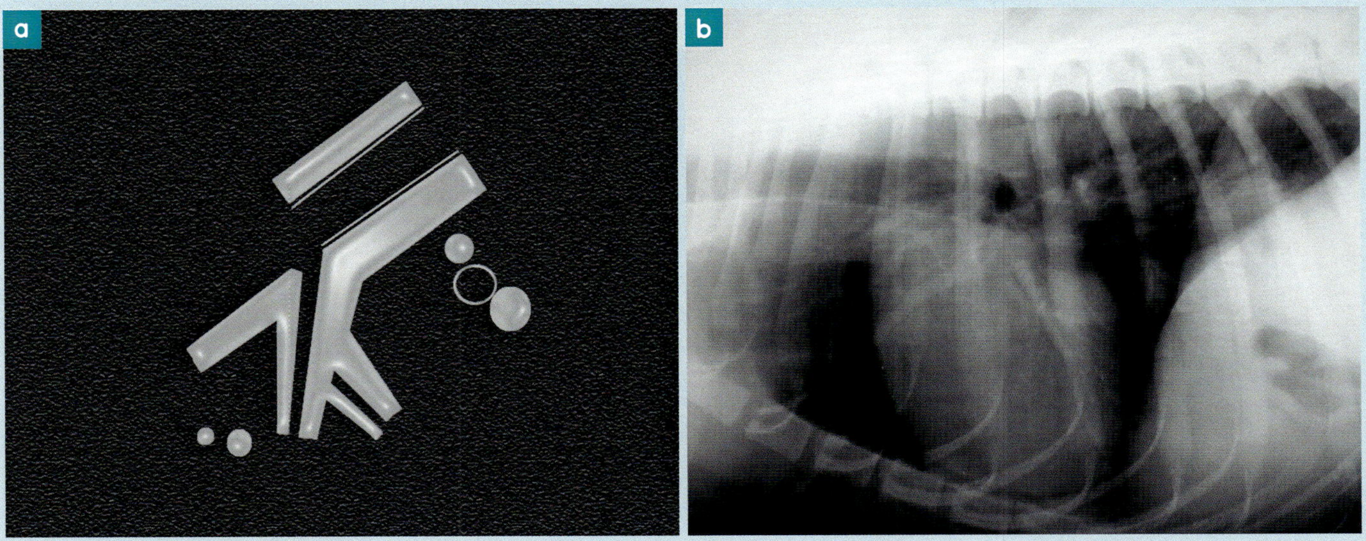

FIGURE 2.82. Schematic representation of the vascular lung pattern caused by an enlargement of the pulmonary veins (a), and lateral radiograph of the thorax of a dog with venous congestion due to left heart insufficiency (b). The left cranial lobar vein has a larger diameter than the artery (they are visible in the cranioventral area of the thorax).

On radiographs, it is possible to visualise areas of fluid density with an irregular content and ill-defined limits ("cloudy" or "cotton-like" appearance). These areas tend to increase in size and converge as the process progresses, that is to say, as the number of affected alveoli increases. There may be small areas of normal radiopacity between the areas in which radiopacity is increased. These are termed **air alveolograms**. At more advanced stages, the affected area or areas of the lung acquire homogeneous fluid/soft-tissue density (**pulmonary consolidation**) and only the lumen of the bronchi that are filled with air

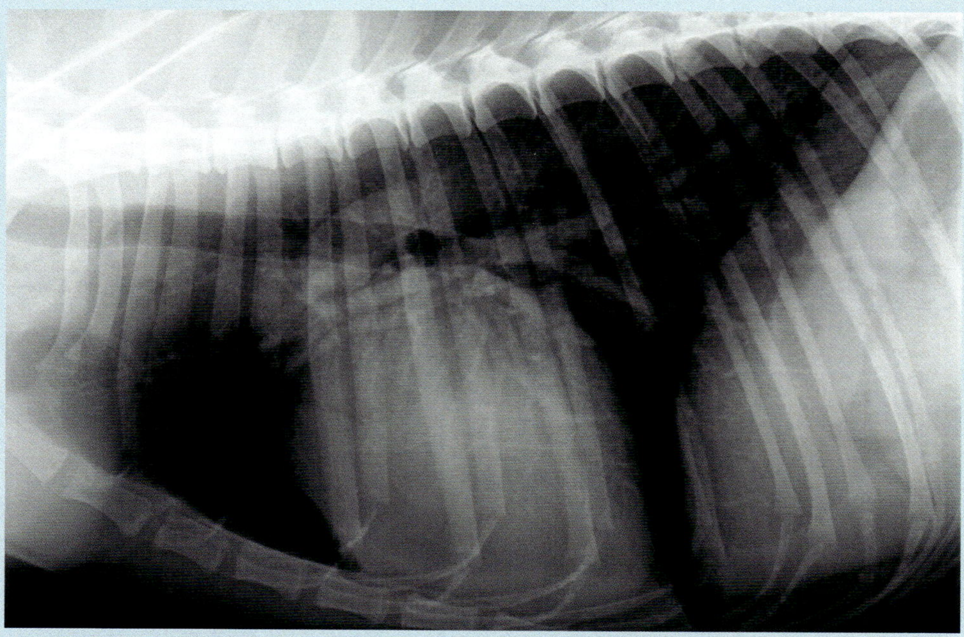

FIGURE 2.83. Lateral radiograph of the thorax of dog with mixed vascular congestion. The width of the cranial arteries and veins at the level of the 4th intercostal space exceeds the width of the 4th rib in its proximal third.

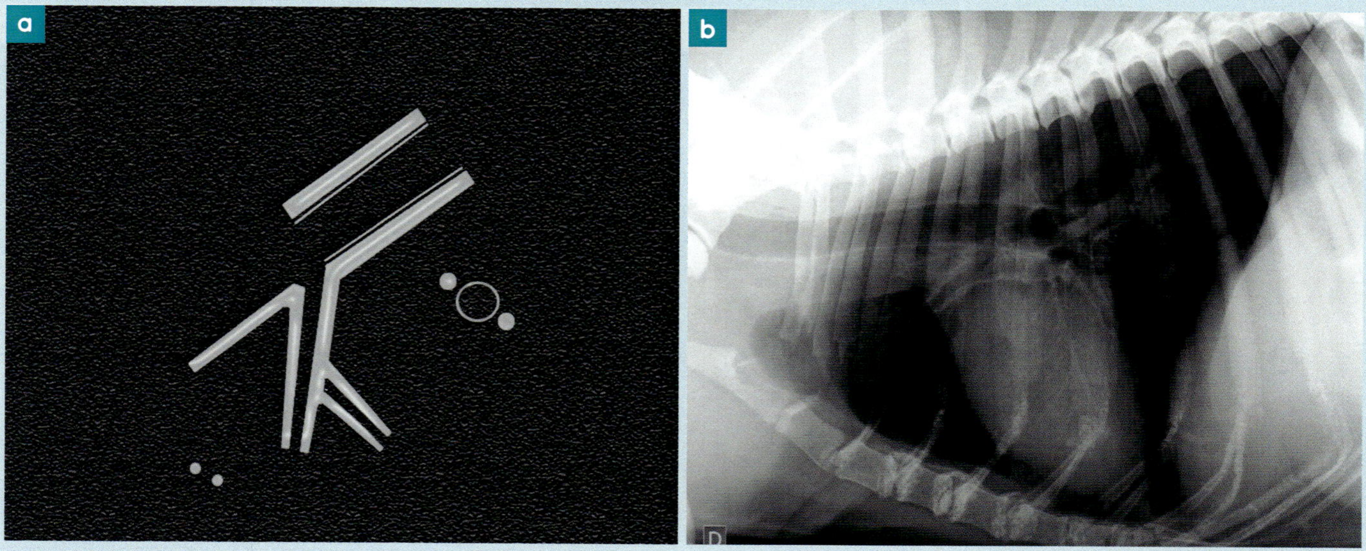

FIGURE 2.84. Schematic representation of the vascular lung pattern caused by a decrease in the size of the pulmonary vessels (a), and lateral radiograph of the thorax of a dog with hypovascularisation and microcardia (b).

Normal radiographic anatomy of the thorax **right lateral view**

http://goo.gl/otDlnr

may be identified. These visible bronchi are called air **bronchograms**. When the lumen of the bronchi is collapsed or filled with fluids, the air bronchograms are no longer visible and there is a complete consolidation of the affected lung area (figs. 2.85-2.90). Air bronchograms may not be visible in every case of alveolar infiltration, but when they are identified, this is considered a pathognomonic finding of alveolar pattern.

If the alveolar pattern affects a complete lobe, it will be possible to identify the limit between the affected and the adjacent lobes. This is termed **lobar sign**. If the affected area is in contact with the heart or diaphragm, the outline of these structures will be lost as they have the same radiopacity. In radiology, this is generally termed **silhouette sign** (fig. 2.91).

Most of the lung diseases in which the alveolar pattern predominates also affect other components of the lung, usually the interstitium or bronchi. The location of the lesions and the speed at which they develop and then disappear may guide our differential diagnosis. For example, oedema may develop and disappear in a few hours if the appropriate treatment is administered (fig. 2.92). However, a haemorrhage or aspiration pneumonia may appear in a few minutes, but it may take days before they disappear. Bacterial pneumonia develops in a few days or hours, but disappears after several days or weeks when treated.

Alveolar oedema is characterised by the accumulation of transudate in the alveoli. Oedemas of cardiogenic origin are interstitial at first and then progress to alveolar involvement. Their typical location is the perihilar area in dogs, but they may affect any area of the lungs in cats. Acute non-cardiogenic pulmonary oedema may occur in any location, although it often appears in the caudodorsal area of the lungs. The causes of non-cardiogenic oedema include neurogenic causes (electrocution, cranial trauma, post-convulsion), hyperdynamic causes (due to excessive negative intrathoracic pressure; asphyxia, strangulation, obstruction of the upper airways), fluid overload (overhydration), toxicity, hypovolaemic shock, hypersensitivity or suffocation.

Alveolar pneumonia is characterised by the accumulation of exudate in the alveoli. The distribution of the affected areas may guide the diagnosis to some extent. For example, it is common for bacterial bronchopneumonias to be located cranioventrally, while aspiration pneumonias usually appear in the ventral area of the lungs, especially in the right middle lobe (fig. 2.93). Aspirated foreign bodies (e.g. foxtails) are often located in the right caudal lobe, where inflammatory changes will appear (fig. 2.94).

In an alveolar haemorrhage, blood accumulates in the alveoli (fig. 2.95). It is usually caused by trauma, but may also appear in cases of coagulopathies, intoxications or be associated with neoplasms. A pulmonary contusion due to trauma is usually observed as an image of consolidation of the affected area, which is generally ipsilateral to the area of impact (fig. 2.96).

The accumulation of cells in the alveoli is uncommon, although it may occur in some types of neoplasia (e.g. bronchoalveolar carcinoma).

The term atelectasis indicates incomplete expansion or collapse of a lung or of part of it. As said previously, prolonged lateral recumbency leads to temporary atelectasis of the lung that is in lower position, and can be solved by changing the patient's position (fig. 2.97). The pathological causes of atelectasis include the obstruction of the airways (fig. 2.98), a limitation of the expansion capacity of the lungs (e.g. pneumothorax, pleural effusion) or their compression due to the presence of adjacent masses. When it is not associated with a mass, the reduction of the volume of the atelectatic lung area causes a more or less marked displacement of the mediastinum towards the affected side. It should be highlighted that in many cases, the diseases that cause the alveoli to be filled with fluid also have an atelectatic component, which contributes to a greater or lesser extent to the alveolar pattern that is visible on the radiograph.

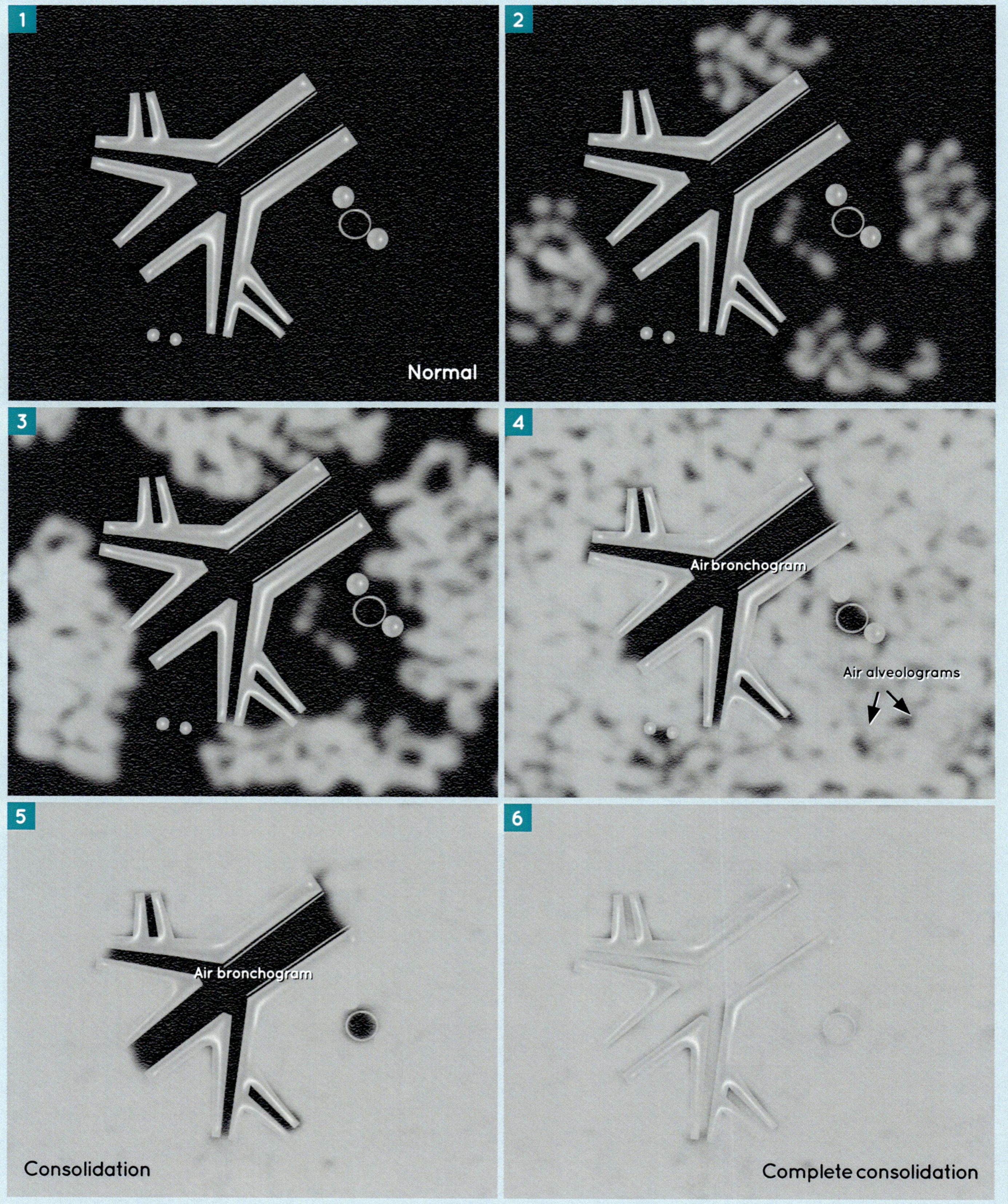

FIGURE 2.85. Schematic representation of the different phases (1-6) in the evolution of an alveolar pattern.

The image of atelectasis may be similar to that of lung consolidation, although in this latter there is no reduction of the volume of the affected area or lobe and it therefore does not cause any displacement of the mediastinum.

Interstitial pattern

An interstitial pattern is identified when the pulmonary interstitium appears infiltrated by fibrous tissue, fluid or cells (e.g. neoplastic cells).

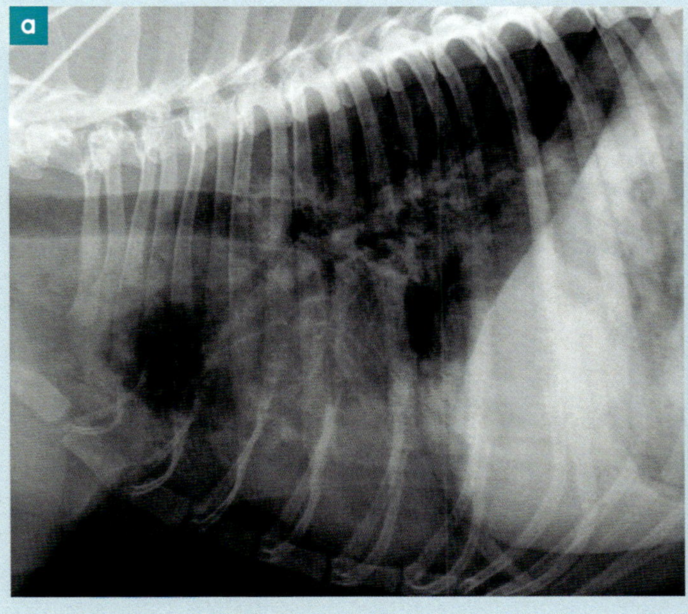

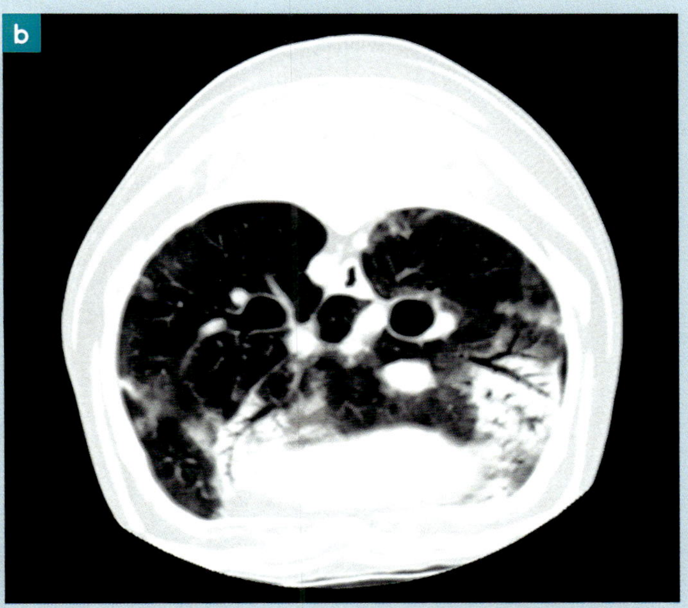

FIGURE 2.86. Lateral radiograph (a) and computed tomography image (b) of the thorax of a dog with an alveolar pattern due to pneumonia. In image (a), areas of soft-tissue density with an irregular morphology may be observed in the peripheral areas of the lung, where some air bronchograms can be identified, though with difficulty. The affected areas and air bronchograms are much more evident in the computed tomography image.

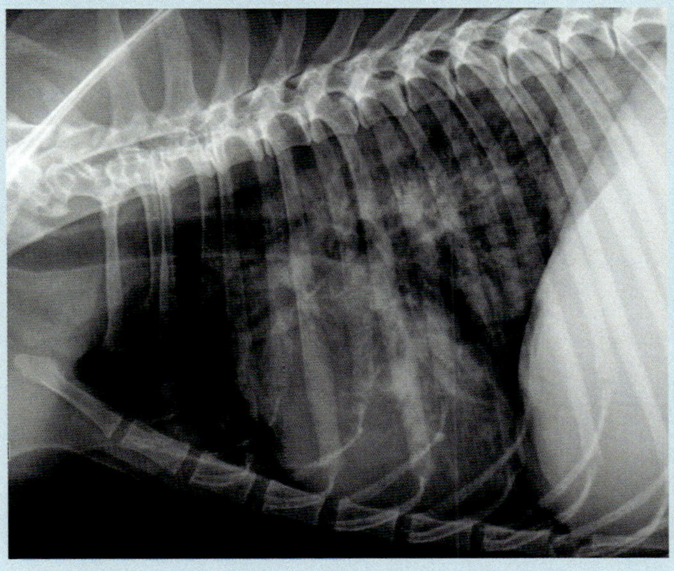

FIGURE 2.87. Lateral radiograph of the thorax of a dog with an alveolar pattern due to bronchopneumonia. The pattern is essentially observed in the caudodorsal lung field, where it is possible to identify small lung areas with normal radiopacity (air alveolograms) and the lumen of some air-filled bronchi surrounded by lung parenchyma with increased radiopacity (air bronchograms).

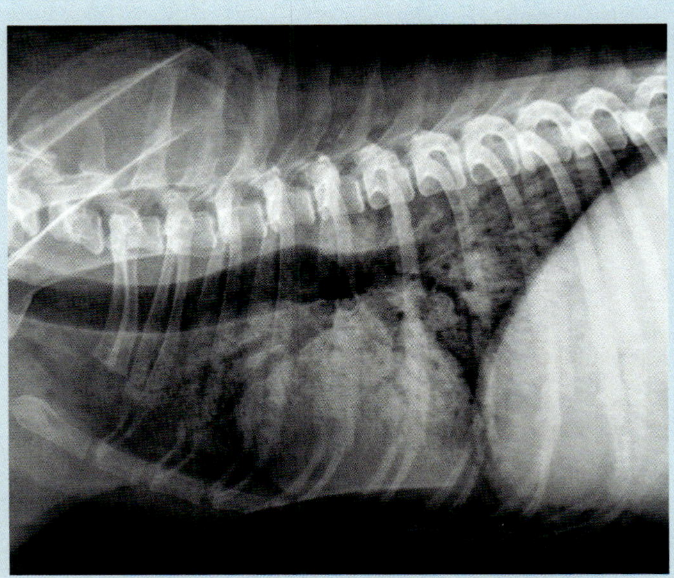

FIGURE 2.88. Lateral radiograph of the thorax of a dog with an alveolar pattern due to bronchopneumonia, which affects all the lung lobes. Large air bronchograms and numerous small air alveolograms, which give the lung the appearance of a "sponge", can be observed.

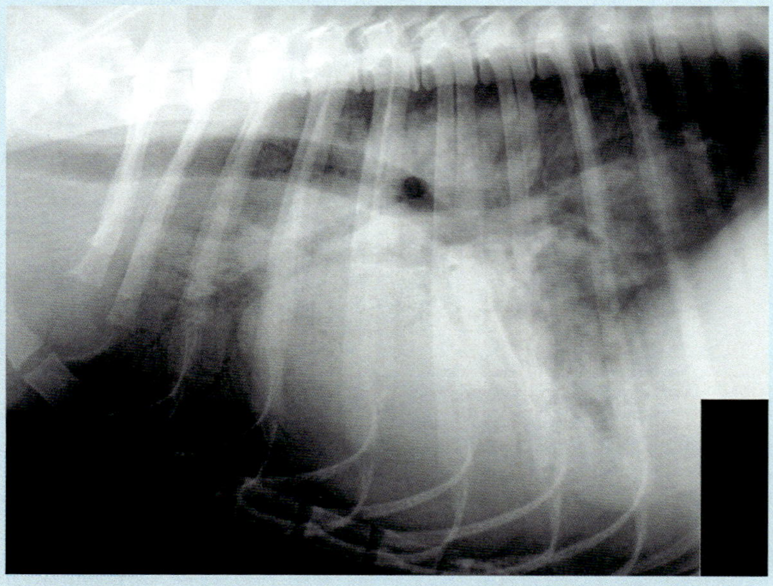

FIGURE 2.89. Lateral radiograph of the thorax of a dog with an alveolar pattern due to a bronchopneumonia, which affects all the lung lobes, but particularly the cranial and right middle lobes, where air bronchograms surrounded by consolidated lung parenchyma can be identified (with homogeneous soft-tissue density).

Normal radiographic anatomy of the thorax **ventrodorsal view**

http://goo.gl/MECQmD

Normal radiographic anatomy of the thorax **dorsoventral view**

http://goo.gl/pKMKlb

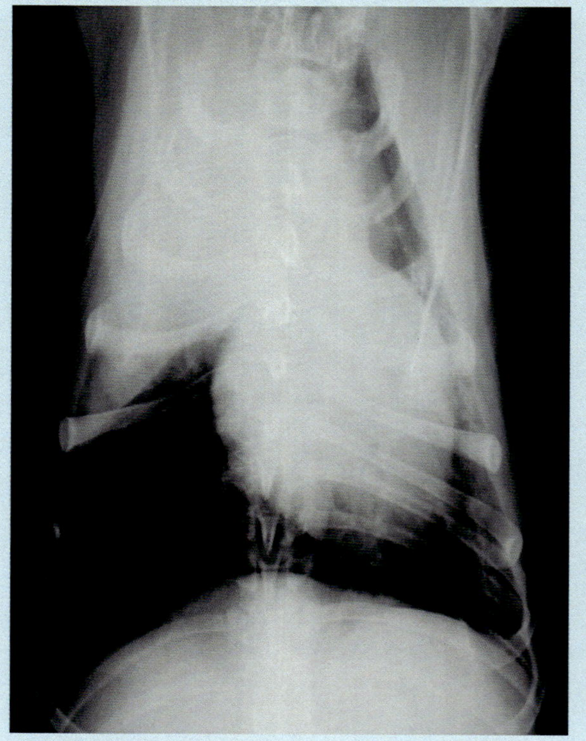

FIGURE 2.90. Ventrodorsal radiograph of the thorax of a dog with complete consolidation of the right cranial lobe, which has homogeneous soft-tissue density with no air bronchograms. This indicates that the lumen of the bronchi is filled with fluid or no longer contains air. A severe pneumonia or haemorrhage may cause the complete opacification of the lobe, but its volume would not change. Atelectasis of the lobe would cause the displacement of the mediastinum towards the affected side. However, in this case the mediastinum appears displaced to the left. This indicates an increase in the volume of the opacified lobe, which suggests a primary lung neoplasm or torsion as the most probable causes.

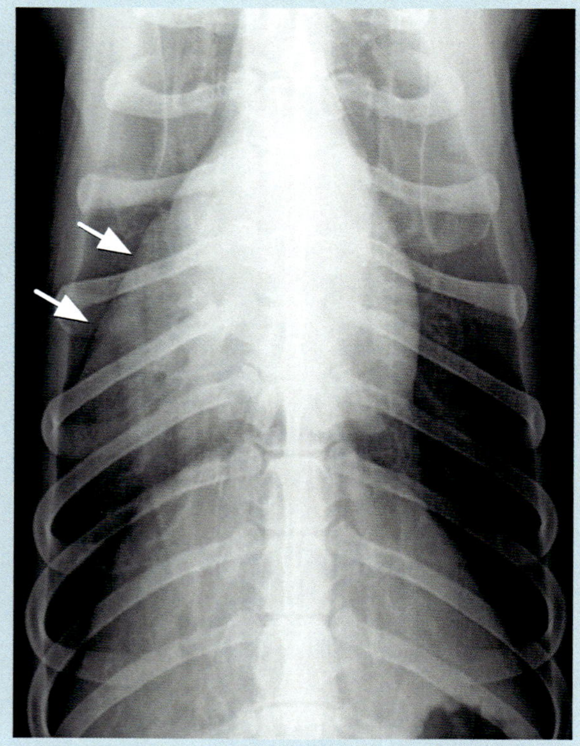

FIGURE 2.91. Dorsoventral radiograph of the thorax of a dog with localised pneumonia in the right middle lobe. The opacification of the lobe allows the clear identification of the margin of the cranial lobe (arrows). This is termed lobar sign and causes a loss of the cardiac border that is adjacent to the lesion, which is referred to as silhouette sign.

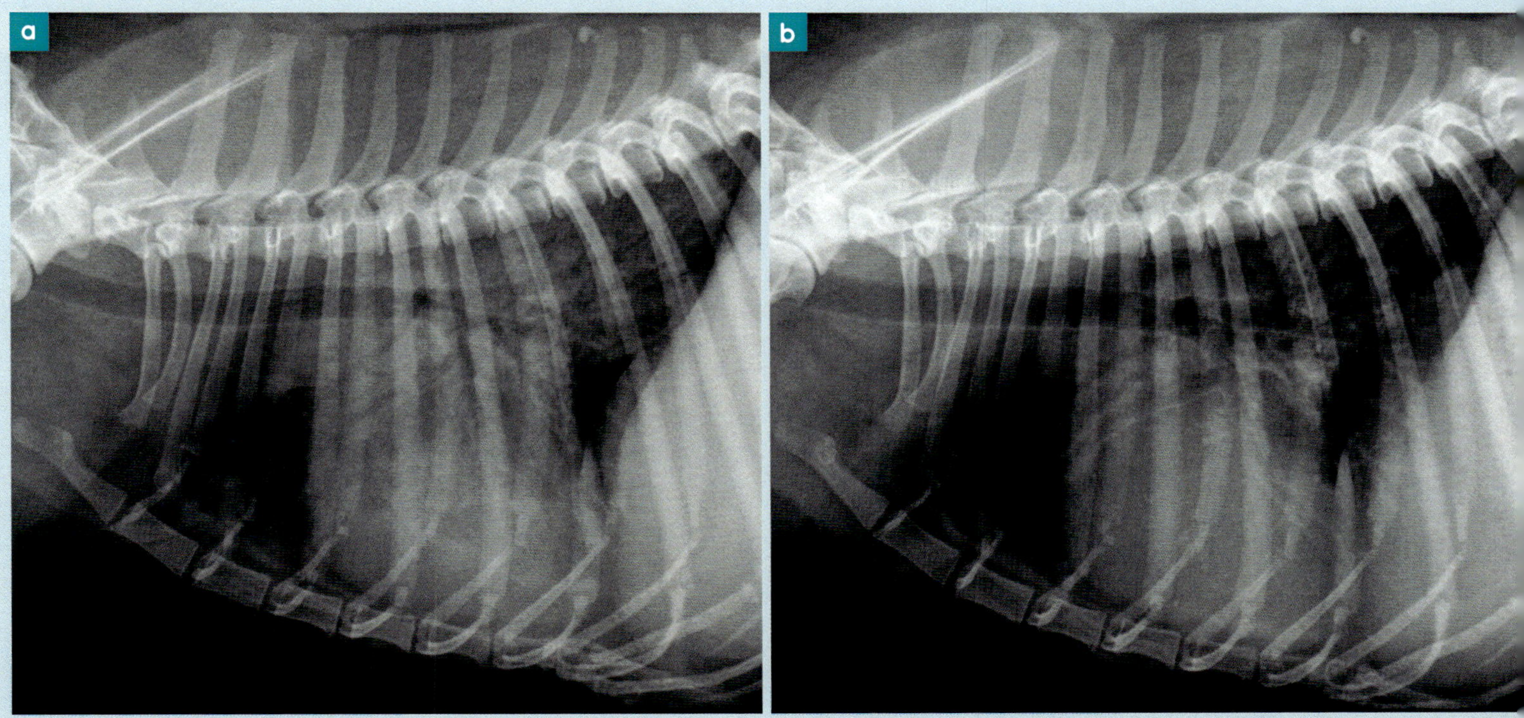

FIGURE 2.92. Lateral radiographs of the thorax of a dog with an alveolar pattern in the caudodorsal area of the lung due to cardiogenic oedema, before (a) and a few hours after (b) the treatment. The time an alveolar pattern takes to appear and disappear may be of help to establish a differential diagnosis. An oedema takes several hours to disappear or reduce with the appropriate treatment, while a haemorrhage or pneumonia will take days to do so.

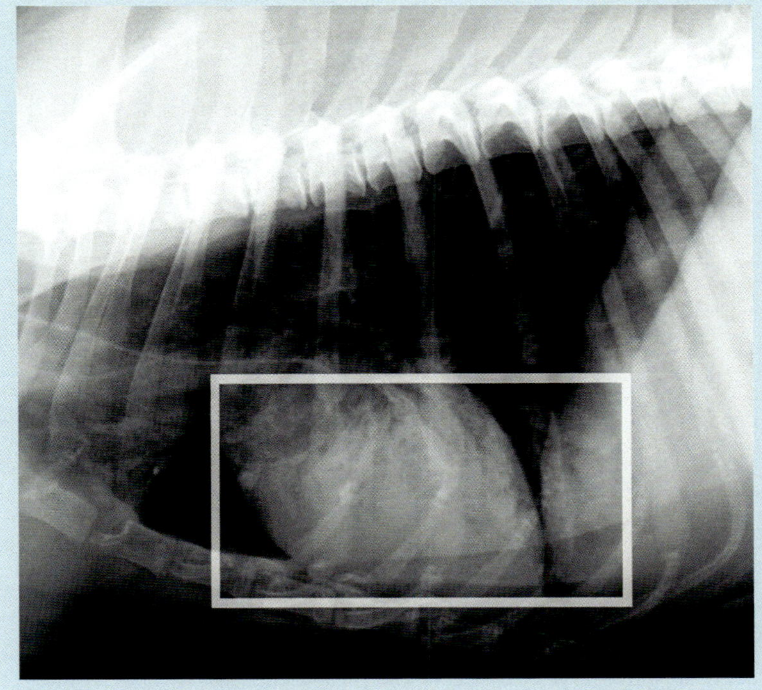

FIGURE 2.93. Lateral radiograph of the thorax of a dog with an alveolar pattern in the area of the right middle lobe and ventral area of the caudal lobes (shown in the rectangle) due to aspiration pneumonia. The additional findings in the image may be of help to establish a differential diagnosis. In this case, it is possible to identify the dilated walls of the oesophagus and a slight ventral displacement of the trachea and cardiac silhouette caused by the megaoesophagus.

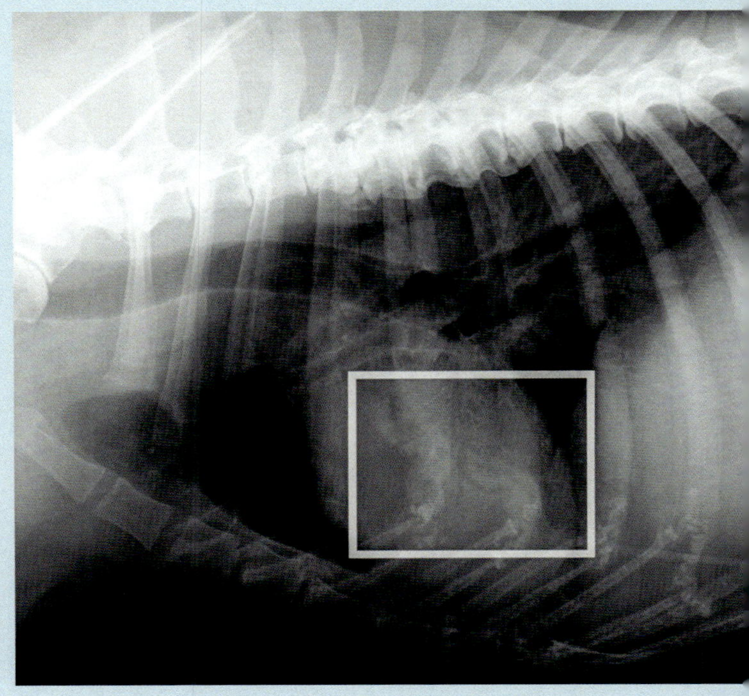

FIGURE 2.94. Lateral radiograph of the thorax of a dog with an alveolar pattern in the area of the right middle lobe (shown in the rectangle) due to focal pneumonia caused by the penetration of a plant awn in the lung. The affected area is very small, but the identification of an air bronchogram in it confirms the diagnosis of alveolar pattern.

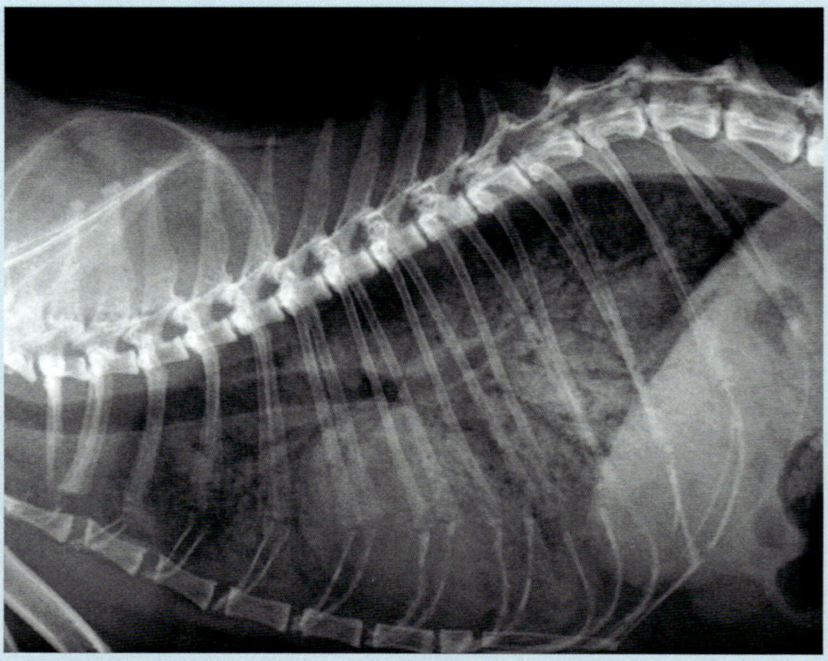

FIGURE 2.95. Lateral radiograph of the thorax of a cat with a generalised alveolar pattern due to a pulmonary haemorrhage.

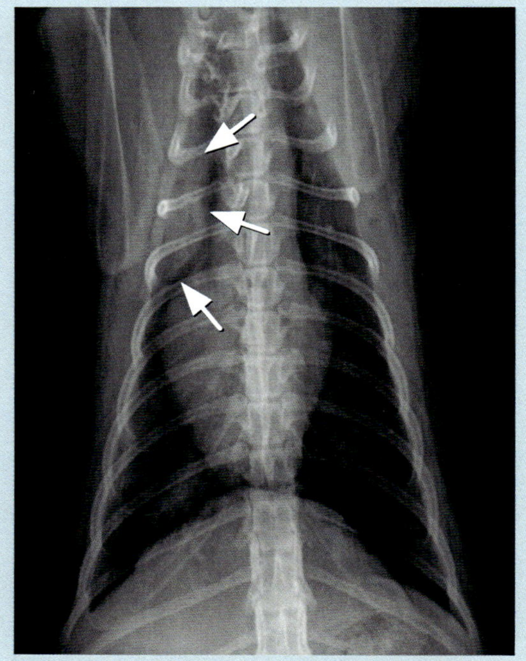

FIGURE 2.96. Ventrodorsal radiograph of the thorax of a cat with a pulmonary contusion, which appears as an area of focal consolidation (arrows) in the same side as that of the trauma that caused it.

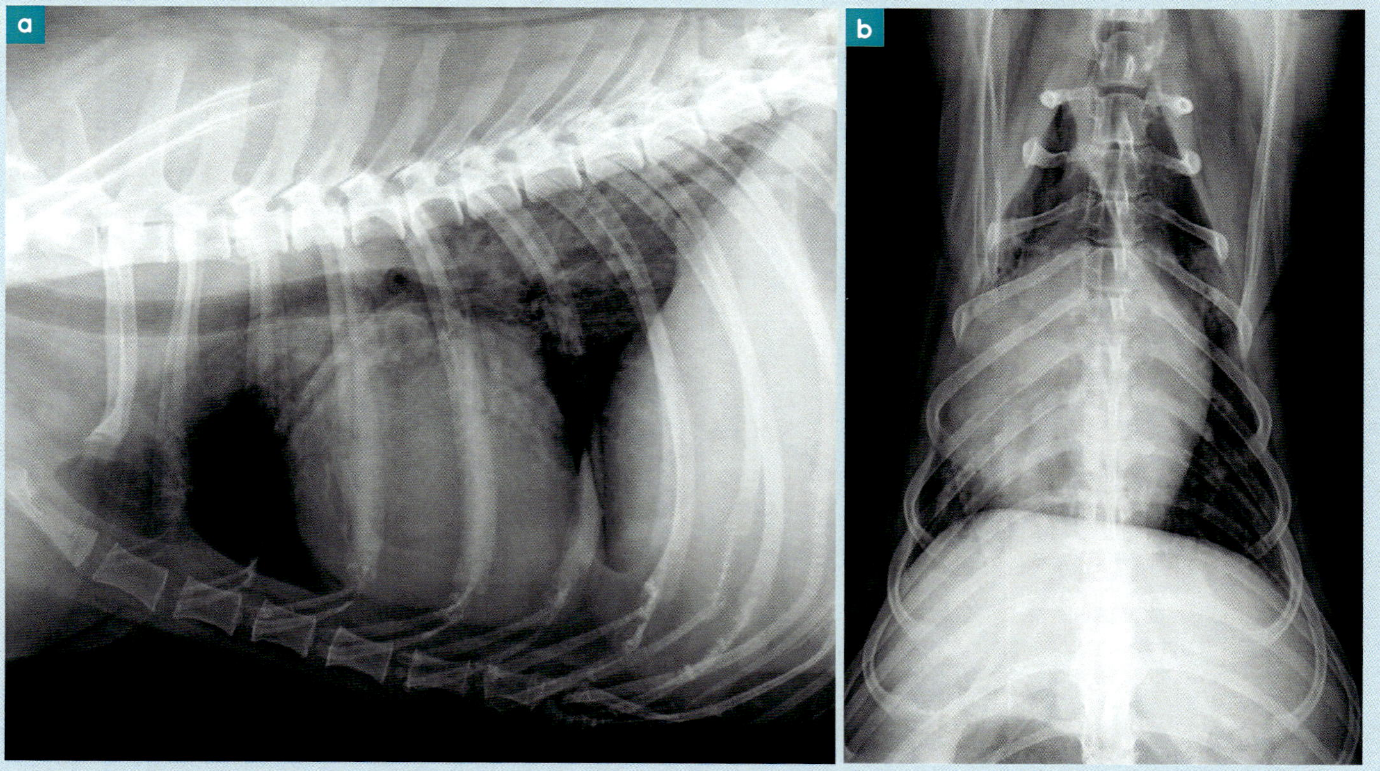

FIGURE 2.97. Lateral (a) and dorsoventral (b) radiographs of the thorax of a dog with atelectasis of the right caudal and medial lobes caused by prolonged lateral (right) recumbency. On the lateral view, the alveolar pattern is more evident in the caudodorsal area of the lung. On the dorsoventral view, the slight displacement of the cardiac silhouette to the right hemithorax indicates a loss of volume in the affected area of the lung. In order to rule out pathological causes of atelectasis, the radiographic study should be repeated after placing the animal in sternal recumbency or in standing position for some time.

There are two types of perfectly differentiated interstitial patterns:

- Unstructured interstitial pattern: it is characterised by the accumulation of fluid (transudate, exudate, blood), cells (e.g. lymphoma) or fibrous tissue in the pulmonary interstitium.
- Nodular interstitial pattern: due to a focal accumulation of cells in the interstitium, which gives rise to nodular lesions in the lung.

Unstructured interstitial pattern

The diffuse infiltration of the interstitium, either by fluid or cells, causes compression of the alveoli and a decrease in the amount of air they contain, which leads to a diffuse increase of lung radiopacity in the affected area (fig. 2.99). The blood vessels are less defined, since they contrast less with the lung parenchyma that surrounds them, but their image is not lost, as would occur with an area of alveolar infiltration. In some cases, the unstructured interstitial pattern acquires a reticular aspect (as in a "honeycomb") (fig. 2.100).

The unstructured interstitial pattern is the most difficult pattern to diagnose, and is often mistaken for an increase in lung radiopacity caused by obesity, underexposure or radiographs taken during expiration. In addition, it usually appears associated with other lung patterns, more than alone.

Many diseases cause infiltration of the interstitium and alveoli, in which case an alveolar pattern will be predominant on the radiograph. If a condition affects only the interstitium and not the alveoli (much less frequent), a diffuse increase of lung density with no evidence of air alveolograms or air bronchograms will be observed in the affected area.

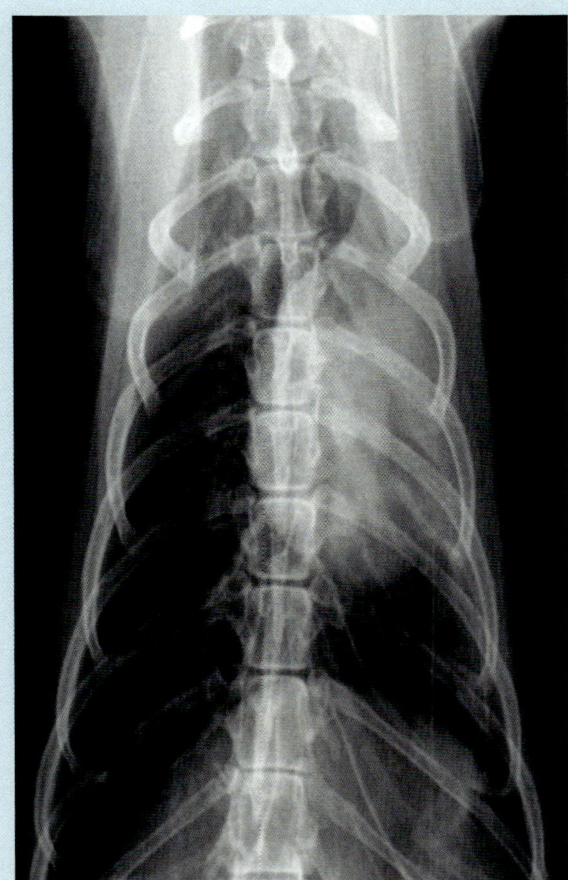

FIGURE 2.98. Dorsoventral radiograph of the thorax of a cat with atelectasis of the caudal segment of the left cranial lung lobe. The displacement of the cardiac silhouette (displacement of the mediastinum) to the left hemithorax indicates a loss of volume in the affected lung lobe. A mass was detected by means of bronchoscopy in the bronchus of the caudal segment of the left cranial lobe.

FIGURE 2.99. Schematic representation of the unstructured interstitial pattern, which is characterised by a diffuse increase of lung radiopacity, which reduces the visibility of the pulmonary vessels.

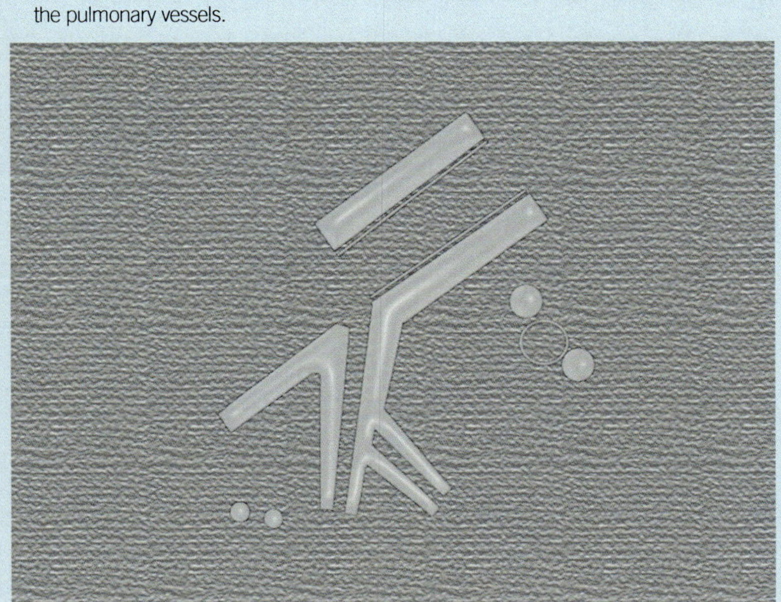

As explained previously, an oedema may be interstitial at first and then extend to the alveoli. Oedemas with an exclusively interstitial component mainly affect cats. Viral pneumonias (e.g. canine distemper) may also result in a significant interstitial pattern, but are nearly always associated with an alveolar component. Haemorrhages may have a more or less marked interstitial component.

Pulmonary fibrosis may appear as a degenerative sign associated with age in older animals and causes a slight increase in interstitial radiopacity. It may also appear as the final consequence of a great variety of lung diseases leading to an irreversible alteration of the support tissue of the interstitium. The initial cause may be inflammatory, infectious or idiopathic. Idiopathic pulmonary fibrosis mainly affects senior dogs of the Terrier breeds, especially the West Highland White Terrier and Cairn Terrier.

The involvement of the lung in cases of multicentric lymphoma usually causes an unstructured interstitial pattern in dogs or, on a less frequent basis, a miliary pattern or masses. The simultaneous presence of mediastinal lymphadenopathies guides the diagnosis (fig. 2.101). In cats with lymphoma, no significant findings can usually be observed in the image of the lung.

Computed tomography is very sensitive to detect or confirm this type of lung pattern (fig. 2.102).

Nodular interstitial pattern

The differential diagnosis of a nodular pattern varies in function of the number and size of the lesions. A nodular lesion may be distinguished from an area of alveolar infiltration because a nodule has a regular shape (generally round or oval) and well-defined borders, while an area of alveolar infiltration has an irregular morphology and poorly defined limits (fig. 2.103). Nodular lesions may be identified on radiographs from 5 mm of diameter. With smaller diameters, they may be confused with transverse images of the pulmonary blood vessels. However, if the lung has an elevated number of nodular lesions of less 5 mm (this is called **miliary nodular interstitial pattern**), these will no longer be mistaken for vessels.

The differential diagnosis of a nodular interstitial pattern with lesions of more than 5 mm (fig. 2.104) includes: pulmonary metastases (the most common

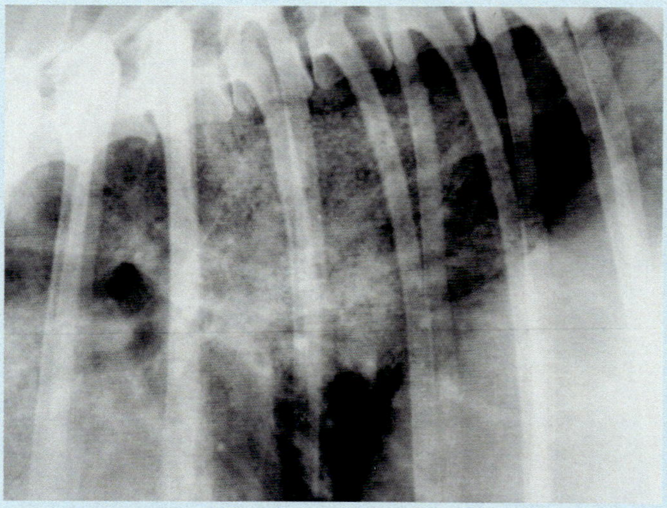

FIGURE 2.100. Enlarged image in lateral projection of the caudodorsal area of the lung of a dog with an unstructured interstitial pattern with a reticular aspect ("honeycomb" aspect) due to a pneumonia caused by *Aspergillus*.

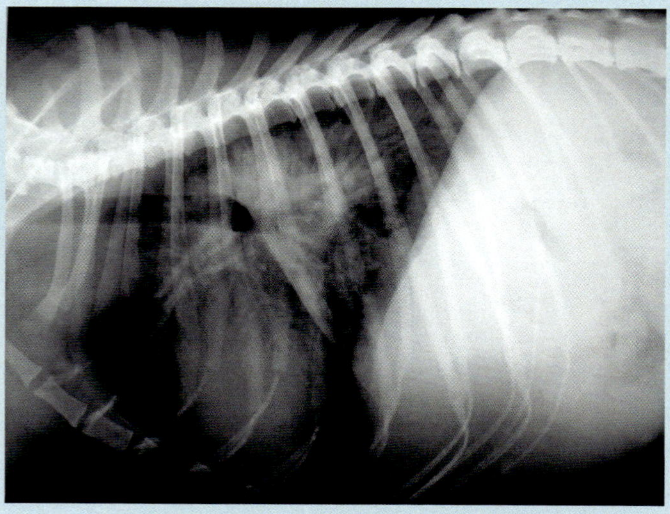

FIGURE 2.101. Lateral radiograph of the thorax of a dog with an unstructured interstitial pattern in the area of the caudal lobes, due to a lung infiltration caused by a multicentric lymphoma. Signs of enlargement of the sternal lymph node (shadow dorsal to the second sternebra), cranial mediastinal lymph nodes (enlargement of the shadow of the cranial mediastinum) and tracheobronchial lymph nodes ("mass effect" around the carina, in this case partially masked by the increased radiopacity of the lung) may also be observed on the radiograph.

diagnosis), primary lung neoplasms, abscesses and pulmonary granulomas (not frequent). A miliary interstitial pattern (fig. 2.105) may be due to metastases or mycotic pneumonia as the most probably diagnoses, followed by primary lung neoplasia and lymphoma.

The use of the terms pulmonary "nodule" or "mass" depends on the size of the lesion: if its diameter is less than 3 cm, it is called nodule, and if it exceeds this value, the term "mass" is used. It is important not to confuse nodules with transverse images of pulmonary vessels, images created by the superimposition of the ribs and other structures, or with calcified pulmonary or pleural plaques.

The most probable cause of a single pulmonary mass (fig. 2.106) is primary lung neoplasia, although the differential diagnosis should also include abscess, granuloma, haematoma or cyst. Pulmonary masses may occasionally be calcified in the centre due to dystrophic calcification, or have a more or less irregular central area with gas density (**cavitary mass**). The most probable causes of a cavitary lung mass are tumours with a necrotic centre and abscesses (fig. 2.107).

Normal radiographic anatomy of the thorax
right lateral view

http://goo.gl/otDlnr

We should not mistake a cavitary mass for a pulmonary bulla (also called **pneumatocele**), which often appears as an incidental finding. A pulmonary bulla is due to a focal accumulation of gas in the lung caused by loss or rupture of the alveolar walls, which may be of congenital, traumatic or idiopathic origin. The wall of the bulla is usually thin and is formed by pulmonary connective tissue and the visceral pleura (fig. 2.108).

When a large lung mass is observed next to others with a smaller diameter, these latter usually correspond to metastases of the first mass. In dogs, lung metastases usually appear as well-defined, round lesions, while in cats they often have a more irregular shape and a more poorly defined outline. The metastases of haemangiosarcomas may also appear less defined because they are usually accompanied by haemorrhage.

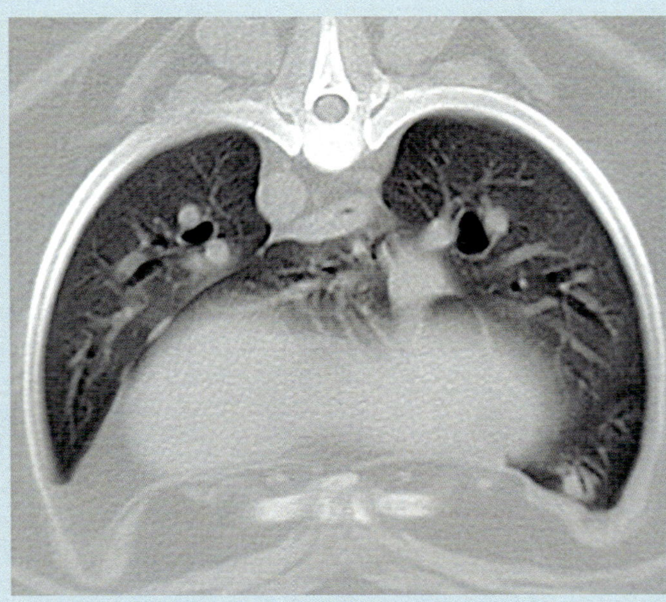

FIGURE 2.102. Computed tomography image of the thorax of a dog with a generalised unstructured interstitial pattern.

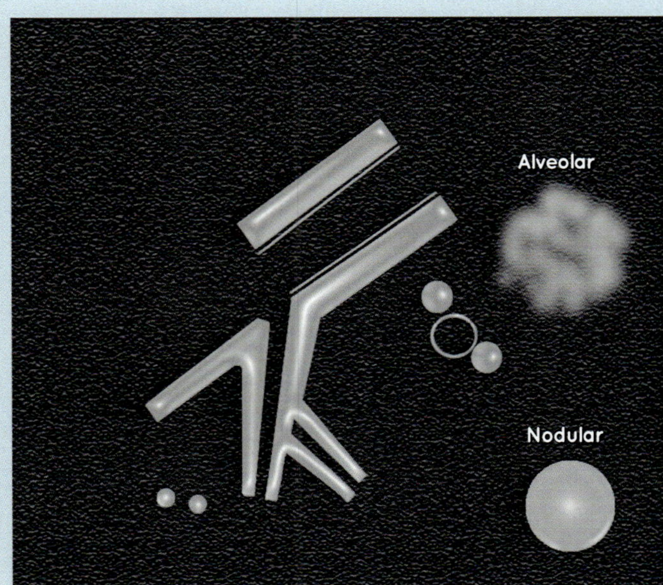

FIGURE 2.103. Schematic representation of a nodular interstitial pattern in comparison with an area of alveolar infiltration. A nodular lesion has a regular shape (generally round or oval) and well-defined limits, while the area of infiltration has an irregular morphology and ill-defined borders.

When a mass is located adjacent to the thoracic wall, it is possible to assess it by means of an ultrasound examination, and thus to determine whether it is solid or cystic, to examine its vascularisation and to perform an ultrasound-guided fine-needle aspiration or biopsy.

Computed tomography is particularly indicated to look for metastases (nodules smaller than 2 mm can be detected) and for the study of lung masses, since it allows us to determine their exact location for a possible surgical treatment, assess their extension to adjacent structures (fig. 2.109) and perform a guided biopsy if this cannot be done by means of ultrasonography.

Mixed pattern

It is the result of the combination of two or more of the patterns that have already been described, due to the simultaneous involvement of several components of the lung. Mixed patterns are more often visualised than each of the four patterns alone, although there is usually dominant a one, which is considered to be the most significant. Lung neoplasms often have a mixed pattern (fig. 2.110), in which a nodular interstitial pattern (miliary or not) usually predominates. Oedemas and pneumonias usually have a more alveolar and often bronchial unstructured pattern. Dirofilariosis may have a more bronchial, alveolar and interstitial pattern.

Performing a tracheobronchial lavage to obtain samples may often be useful to establish the differential diagnosis of diseases with similar lung patterns.

Lung hypertranslucency

Generalised hypertranslucency may appear due to an increase in the volume of air contained in the lungs (due to an obstruction of the intrathoracic airways or emphysema) or due to a reduction in the size of the pulmonary vessels. Real hypertranslucency should not be confused with an overexposed radiograph.

Pulmonary emphysema occurs due to an abnormal increase in the size of the alveolar spaces caused by the destruction of the alveolar walls. It may appear associated with an obstructive bronchiolar disease (chronic bronchitis, feline asthma, bronchial neoplasia or bronchial foreign body), where compensatory excessive lung inflation may lead to emphysema. Radiographic changes are usually moderate in cats with asthma and marked signs rarely appear in dogs and cats. On radiographs, it is possible to observe

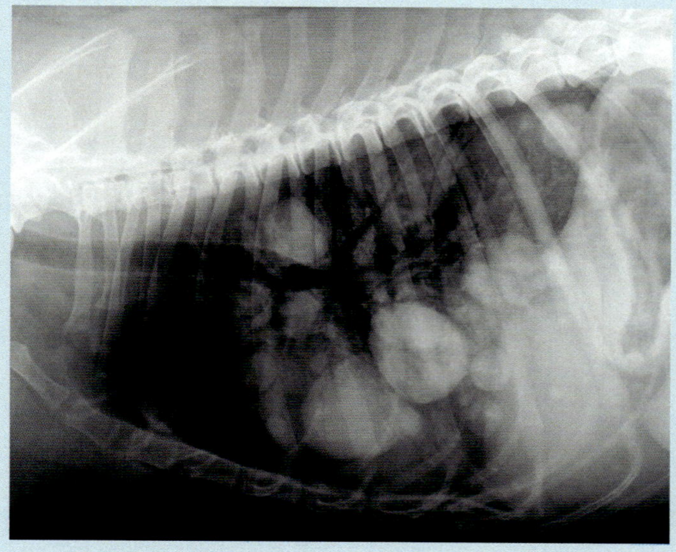

FIGURE 2.104. Lateral radiograph of the thorax of a dog with a nodular interstitial pattern caused by pulmonary metastases. This image could also be due to primary neoplasia of the lung, abscesses or multiple pulmonary granulomas, although this latter disease is unlikely.

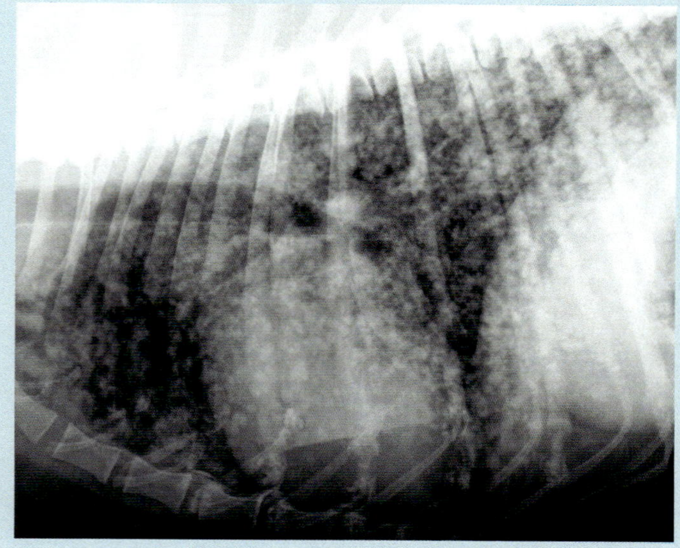

FIGURE 2.105. Lateral radiograph of the thorax of a dog with a miliary nodular interstitial pattern (nodules smaller than 5 mm) caused by pulmonary metastases. The second most probable disease in the differential diagnosis would be mycotic pneumonia, followed by primary neoplasia of the lung and lymphoma.

hypertranslucency and enlargement of the lungs, the shadow of the diaphragm is flattened and caudally displaced (fig. 2.111), and spontaneous costal fractures may even occur.

Emphysema is confirmed if, when comparing an inspiratory radiograph with an expiratory one, no changes in the position of the diaphragm or in the radiopacity of the lung are observed.

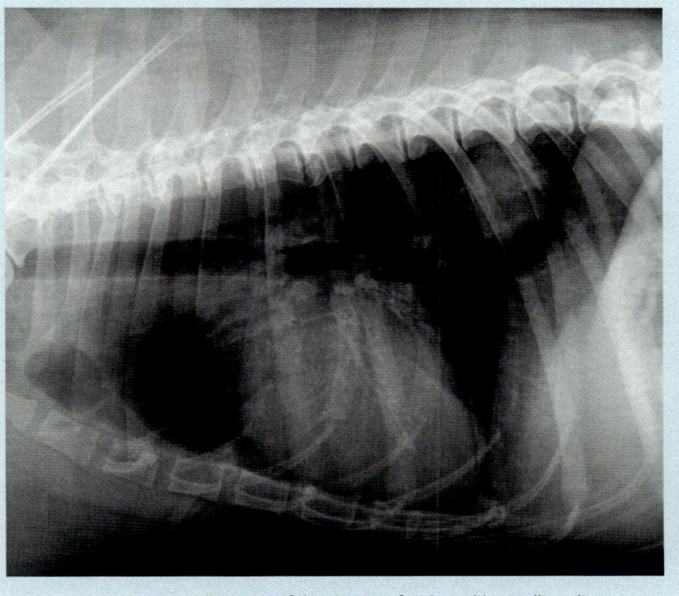

FIGURE 2.106. Lateral radiograph of the thorax of a dog with a solitary lung mass. The most probable cause is a primary lung neoplasm, although an abscess, granuloma, haematoma or pulmonary cyst should be included in the differential diagnosis.

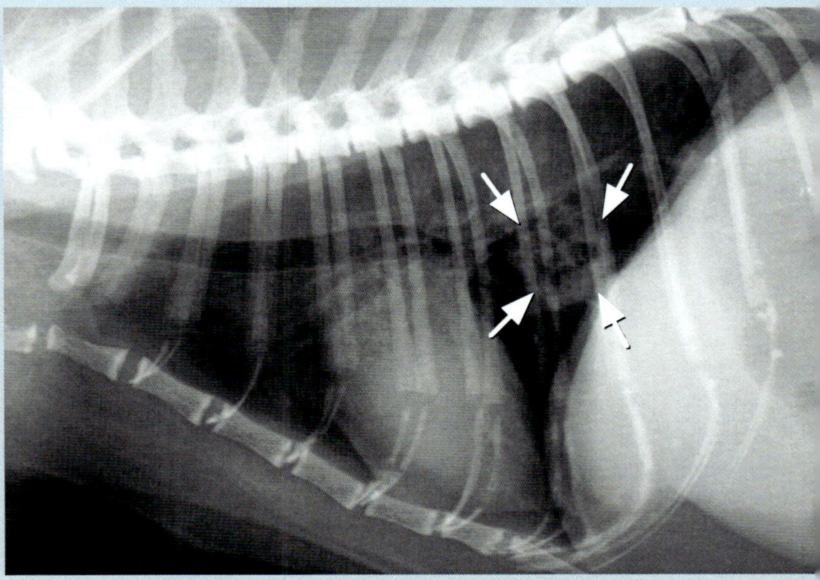

FIGURE 2.107. Lateral radiograph of the thorax of a cat with a cavitary lung mass (arrows). It is possible to observe areas of gas density with an irregular morphology in the central area of the mass. The most probable diseases to include in the differential diagnosis are neoplasms with a necrotic centre and abscesses.

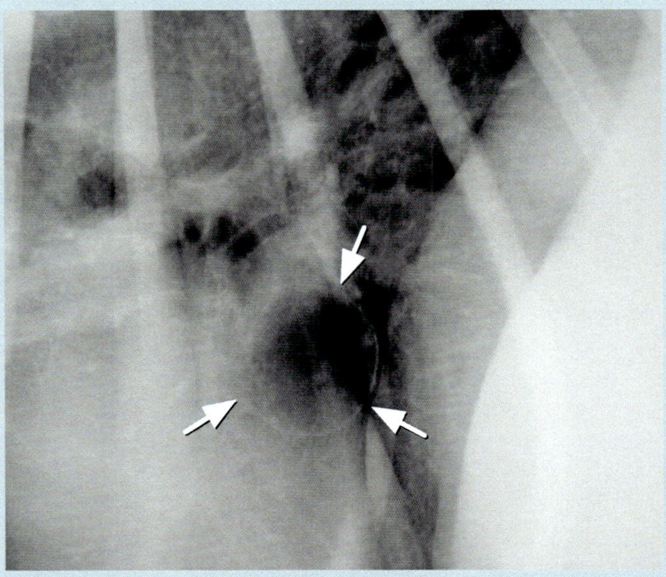

FIGURE 2.108. Enlarged image of the perihilar region on a lateral radiograph of the thorax of a dog with a pulmonary bulla (arrows). As opposed to cavitary lung masses, bullae usually have a very thin wall and are incidental findings.

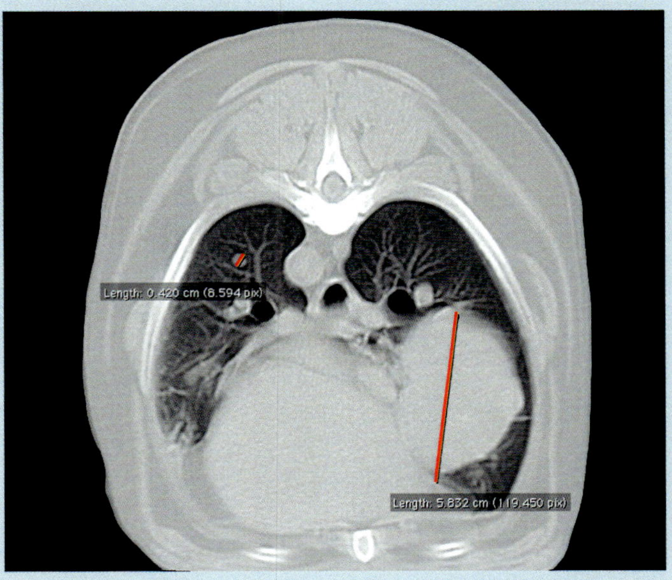

FIGURE 2.109. Computed tomography image of the thorax of a dog with a 6-cm mass in the left lung (long red line), previously diagnosed by means of radiography. Computed tomography allowed the determination of the exact location of the mass and the detection of small metastases (short red line) that had not been identified in the right lung.

Self-assessment cases

http://goo.gl/av1O5B

Lung lobe torsion

It is unusual in small animals. Torsion causes an occlusion of the bronchi and pulmonary vessels. However, the arterial flow may be preserved in a first phase as arteries have stronger walls than veins. Congestion and oedema may initially be observed in the affected lobe, and necrosis may appear at advanced stages. Lung lobe torsion affects more frequently the right middle lobe in breeds with a deep thorax and the left cranial lobe in breeds with a wide and shallow thorax.

The ideal technique for its diagnosis is computed tomography, although it is possible to observe indicative signs of torsion on radiographs:

- Consolidation of the affected lobe, which initially appears enlarged and with round margins due to vascular congestion. Small air bronchograms or air alveolograms, which give the affected area the aspect of a "sponge" (vesicular pattern), may sometimes be identified.
- The presence of a pleural effusion is very common as a result of the torsion. It may be bilateral or unilateral, symmetric or asymmetric, although in many cases it is concentrated around the affected lobe.
- At advanced stages, necrosis of the parenchyma will lead to a reduction of the volume of the affected lobe.
- It is possible to see that the bronchi have an abnormal direction and a sudden interruption of the vessels.
- If a bronchus ruptures, a pneumothorax or pneumomediastinum may develop.

Doppler ultrasonography may be of great help in the diagnosis as it allows the detection of the absence of venous flow and of the reduction or absence of arterial flow in the affected lobe. However, in practice, good quality images may not be obtained due to the breathing difficulties of patients with torsion.

It is easier to detect an anomalous position of the bronchial and vascular structures and to assess their permeability by means of computed tomography. The administration of an intravenous contrast medium allows the differentiation between the vascularised collapsed lung and the necrotic lobe with torsion.

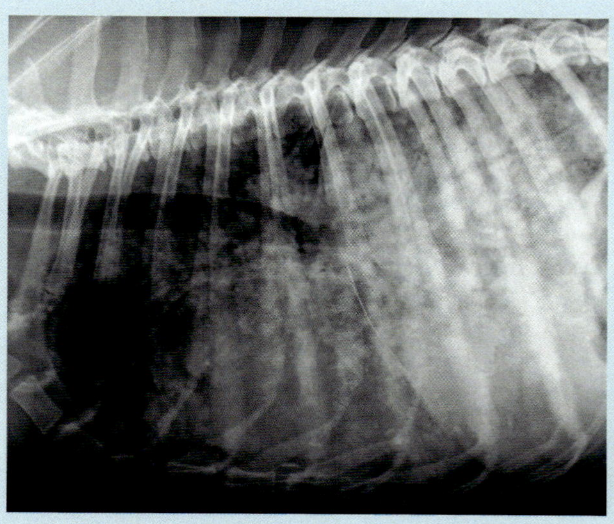

FIGURE 2.110. Lateral radiograph of the thorax of a dog with a mixed pattern (alveolar, bronchial and miliary nodular interstitial patterns) due to a primary lung neoplasm. As an incidental finding, a pleural calcification is observed at the level of the fissure between the right middle and caudal lobes.

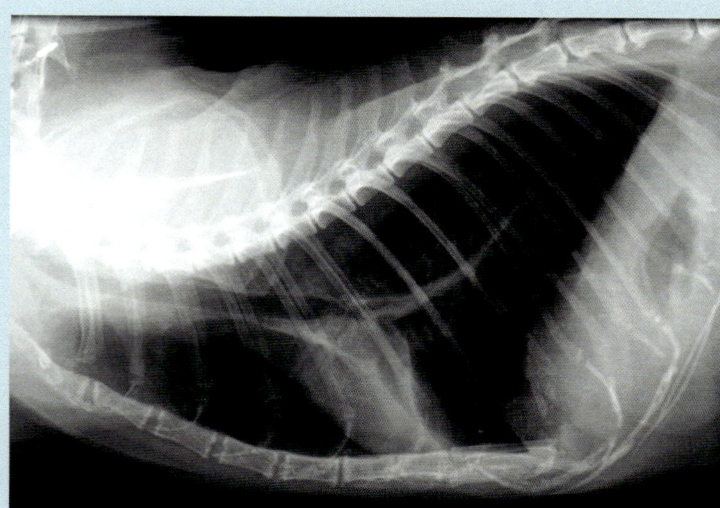

FIGURE 2.111. Lateral radiograph of the thorax of a cat with hyperlucency and increase of the lung volume due to emphysema. The cardiac silhouette appears reduced in size and the diaphragm is flattened and caudally displaced. Emphysema is a common complication of feline asthma.

Appendicular skeleton

3

Principles of interpretation

Radiography is an excellent technique for skeleton assessment. As with other anatomical regions, the main difficulty in the radiological diagnosis of some appendicular diseases is that the same radiological findings are shared by different diseases. In such cases, it is essential to correlate findings with other clinical data (history, examination, laboratory data, etc.) from the patient. Useful information for the diagnosis can be obtained in some cases by assessing the evolution in time of the radiographic image of a lesion. This is why serial radiographs are often performed.

When studying the appendicular skeleton, a comparison of the obtained images with those from radiographic atlases is of special interest, especially when examining complex anatomical joints, such as the tarsus or the carpus. When an animal has a lesion only in one limb, we can obtain a better reference of normality by radiographing the contralateral limb.

A few technical tips to optimise appendicular skeleton images are summarised below:

- **Projections:** In general, two radiographic projections should be always taken at a 90° angle, although in some cases it can also be useful to obtain oblique radiographs or radiographs with flexion or forced extension of a joint. When radiographing a large bone, the corresponding proximal and distal joints should be included.
- **Positioning:** In order to avoid image distortions caused by obliquity, it is important to correctly centre the anatomical region that is to be radiographed. In addition, the median plane of the bone structures should be parallel to the cassette, if possible.
- **Collimation:** It is very important to correctly collimate the anatomical region that is to be radiographed. Thus, the image quality will be optimised, unnecessary radiation to other anatomical regions of the animal can be avoided, and the amount of diffuse radiation that can affect the operator who holds the patient can be reduced.
- **Anti-scatter grid use:** Only needed when radiographing anatomical regions over 10-cm thick, which generally correspond to the scapula, the scapulohumeral joint and the humerus in the forelimb, and the hip and femur in the hind limb. The rest of limbs are radiographed without the grid.
- **Image observation:** on a conventional radiograph, small-sized lesions can be better observed using an intense focal source of light (e.g.: placing the film next to a halogen lamp). On a digital radiograph, the same effect can be achieved using image post-processing tools.

A good appendicular skeleton radiograph should provide good detail of the trabeculae of bone and the cortex. At the same time, it should offer sufficient contrast of soft parts, so soft tissues and fat (e.g.: the infrapatellar fat pad) can be differentiated.

Ossification and closure of growth plates

Calcification of bone structures begins during gestation. At birth, only the diaphyses of long bones and the cranial bones are calcified, whereas the epiphyses are still cartilaginous, thus having the density of soft tissue, and cannot be distinguished from the soft tissues surrounding the bone. Subsequently, progressive calcification of the ossification centres located in the epiphyses, the apophyses and smaller-sized bones occurs. Table 3.1 shows the ages of onset and fusion of the different ossification centres in dogs and cats.

The metaphysis, located between the epiphysis and the diaphysis of long bones (fig. 3.1), can present slightly irregular margins in growing animals, especially in large breeds. It should not be mistaken for a periosteal reaction or for pathological osteolysis.

It is important not to mistake growth plates for fracture lines in young animals. In case of doubt, radiographic atlases can be consulted, although the best reference of normality is obtained by radiographing the contralateral limb of the same animal (provided the disease is not bilateral). In adult animals, the closed growth line can appear as a sclerotic band that binds the epiphysis with the metaphysis.

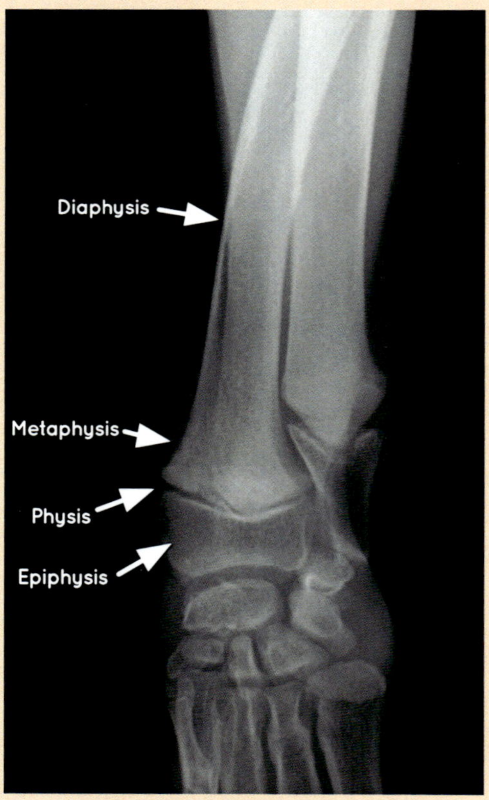

FIGURE 3.1. Dorsopalmar radiograph of the carpus of a healthy 10-week-old dog. The growth line (physis) appears as a soft tissue density band that separates the epiphysis from the metaphysis. The latter can present slightly irregular edges during growth, especially in large breed dogs. The metaphysis is joined to the bone diaphysis.

Osteolysis and osteogenesis

Bone lesions basically present in two forms: with bone destruction (osteolysis) and with new bone production (osteogenesis). The terms osteolysis and osteogenesis should not be mistaken for osteopaenia and sclerosis, although they are related. In osteopaenia, general reduction in radiopacity of a bone is observed, and the term sclerosis is used to describe increased bone radiopacity.

Several patterns in osteolysis and osteogenesis are described, and correct identification of the pattern leads to a more precise radiological diagnosis.

Patterns of osteolysis (fig. 3.2)

Geographical pattern

One or more areas of osteolysis appear, generally more than 1 cm in diameter and with well-defined edges, with a narrow zone of transition between the lesion and normal bone. Geographical lesions may or not have a sclerotic margin and are usually found in the bone marrow. The adjacent cortical zone can appear interrupted, thinned or displaced (expansile lesion). This pattern usually appears in benign or low-grade malignant lesions.

Moth-eaten pattern

Multiple osteolytic areas appear in different sizes, usually 3-10 mm in diameter, and may coalesce in the central area to form a bigger lesion. Margins are not well-defined and show a relatively wide area of transition to normal bone. They can be localised both in the bone marrow and cortex. The affected cortical zone usually appears irregularly eroded. This pattern usually appears in more aggressive processes, such as malignant tumours, osteomyelitis and multiple myeloma.

Permeative pattern

Many small-sized osteolysis zones appear, 1-2 mm, with pinpoint shapes. The margins of the lesion are ill-defined and show a relatively wide area of transition

TABLE 3.1 Ages of onset and fusion of the different ossification centres in the dog and the cat (taken from F.J. Barr, 2006; R. Dennis et al., 2001; J.P. Morgan, 1981; R.N. Smith, 1968, 1969 and G. Summer-Smith, 1966).

	Dog		Cat	
	Ossification centre appearance	Fusion	Ossification centre appearance	Fusion
Supraglenoid tubercle	6-9 weeks	3-7 months	7-9 weeks	4 Months
Humerus-proximal	1-2 weeks	10-13 months	1-2 weeks	18-24 months
Humerus- distal and medial parts of the condyle	2-4 weeks	6-9 weeks	2-5 weeks	3.5 months
Humerus- medial epicondyle	-	6 months	6-8 weeks	4 months
Humerus- condyle to remainder of the bone	-	5-8 months	-	4-4.5 months
Radius-proximal	3-5 weeks	5-11 months	3-4 weeks	5-7 months
Radius-distal	2-4 weeks	6-12 months	2-4 weeks	14-22 months
Ulna-olecranon	7-9 weeks	5-10 months	4-5 weeks	9-12 months
Ulna-anconeal process	-	3-5 months	-	-
Ulna-distal	7-9 weeks	6-12 months	3-4 weeks	14-24 months
Carpal bones	2-6 weeks	-	3-8 weeks	-
Metacarpals/metatarsals-proximal (finger 1)	3-5 weeks	6 months	-	-
Metacarpals/metatarsals-distal (fingers 2-5)	3-4 weeks	5-7 months	3-4 weeks	7-10 months
First phalanx-proximal	4-6 weeks	4-6 months	3-4 weeks	4-5 months
Second phalanx-proximal	5-7 weeks	4-6 months	3-4 weeks	4-5 months
Femur-greater trochanter	4-10 weeks	6-10 months	5-6 weeks	7-9 months
Femur-lesser trochanter	3-4 weeks	8-13 months	-	-
Femur-proximal	2-3 weeks	6-11 months	2 weeks	7-10 months
Femur-distal	3-4 weeks	6-11 months	1-2 weeks	13-19 months
Patella	8-9 weeks	-	8-9 weeks	-
Tibia-tibial tuberosity	7-9 weeks	6-8 months (to the epiphysis)	6-7 weeks	9-10 months (to the epiphysis)
Tibia-proximal	2-5 weeks	6-12 months	2-3 weeks	12-19 months
Tibia-distal	3 weeks	5-11 months	2-3 weeks	10-12 months
Tibia- medial malleolus	12 week	5 months	-	
Fibula-proximal	9-10 weeks	6-12 months	6-7 weeks	13-18 months
Fibula-distal	2-6 weeks	6-11 months	3-4 weeks	10-14 months
Calcaneus and astragalus	Birth- 1 week	-	Birth- 1 week	-
Other tarsal bones	2-6 weeks	-	2-7 weeks	-

to normal bone. The cortical zone usually appears irregularly eroded. It is characteristic of more aggressive bone lesions, such as highly malignant tumours or severe osteomyelitis.

Mixed pattern

A combination of the above-mentioned patterns can be found in a lesion, usually indicating evolution to the most aggressive type. This can be observed when a benign process becomes more active, becomes fractured or when it progresses to malignancy.

Osteopaenia

It is defined as a general reduction in bone radiopacity. It is usually accompanied by thinning of the cortices and apparent sclerosis of the subchondral bone. The most frequent causes of osteopaenia are:

- **Osteoporosis:** decreased bone calcification with reduced bone mass. A frequent cause for osteoporosis is secondary hyperparathyroidism of nutritional or renal origin. It can also appear after immobilisation of a limb (disuse osteoporosis) or as a sequela of distal fractures (post-traumatic osteoporosis).
- **Osteomalacia:** decreased bone calcification maintaining bone mass. It is caused by vitamin D deficiency and it is rare in small animals.

Patterns of osteogenesis (fig. 3.3)

A common characteristic of many skeletal lesions is new bone formation. This happens as a direct or indirect result of a lesion, infection, tumour or other local or systemic diseases. Most of the new bone is formed in the periosteum (periosteal reaction), although it can also be formed in the endosteum or bone trabeculae. It therefore corresponds to the bone response after an abnormal stimulus that can be short, repeated or maintained over time.

Several classifications of periosteal reactions have been made. The classification below has been sorted from moderate to high aggressiveness.

Solid periosteal reaction

Cortical thickening occurs, and may have smooth (chronic mild trauma, subperiosteal haematoma, panosteitis) or rough margins (trauma, inflammation of tissue adjacent to the bone).

Lamellated periosteal reaction

It is also known as "onion skin". New bone forms in layers due to repeated periosteum elevation periods. This reaction type is observed in many pathological processes, from focal trauma to bone infections and tumours.

Palisading periosteal reaction

It presents as a series of small bone columns perpendicular to the cortex. This type of reaction is usually observed in bacterial osteomyelitis and hypertrophic pulmonary osteoarthropathy.

Brush border periosteal reaction

Thin and short bone spicules are formed very close together and perpendicular to the cortex, occupying a wide cortical area. It can appear due to inflammation of tissue adjacent to the bone, in acute osteomyelitis or in early stages of bone neoplasms.

Spiculated periosteal reaction

Bone spicules are formed roughly set apart and perpendicular to the cortex. It is considered suggestive of malignancy.

Sunburst periosteal reaction

Bone spicules that irradiate from the lesion in various directions are formed. It is suggestive of lesion expansion through the cortex into adjacent soft tissue.

Amorphous periosteal reaction

Different sized, shaped and oriented new bone deposits appear in the soft tissues surrounding the damaged area of the bone. It is considered highly suggestive of malignancy.

Aggressive bone lesions versus non-aggressive

In order to classify a bone lesion as aggressive or non-aggressive several factors should be considered:

- Degree of lesion margin definition.

- Width of the zone of transition between damaged and healthy bone
- Pattern of osteolysis.
- Pattern of osteogenesis.
- Cortex involvement.
- Occurrence of sclerotic margins.
- Progress of the lesion over time.

Findings suggestive of aggressive and non-aggressive lesion are summarised in Table 3.2. When a lesion presents a combination of signs of both columns of the table, those which are more suggestive of aggressiveness should be considered.

Intra-articular bodies, osteophytes and enthesophytes

Intra-articular bodies are intra-articular bone fragments, or small fragments that are separated from the normal bone components of the joint.

Osteophytes are defined as small new bone formations, which develop at the joint margin (periarticular osteophytes) or adjacent to the joint margin (extra-articular osteophytes). Periarticular osteophytes are the most characteristic finding in degenerative joint disease (osteoarthritis).

Enthesophytes are distinguished from osteophytes only by their location, being formed at the origin or in-

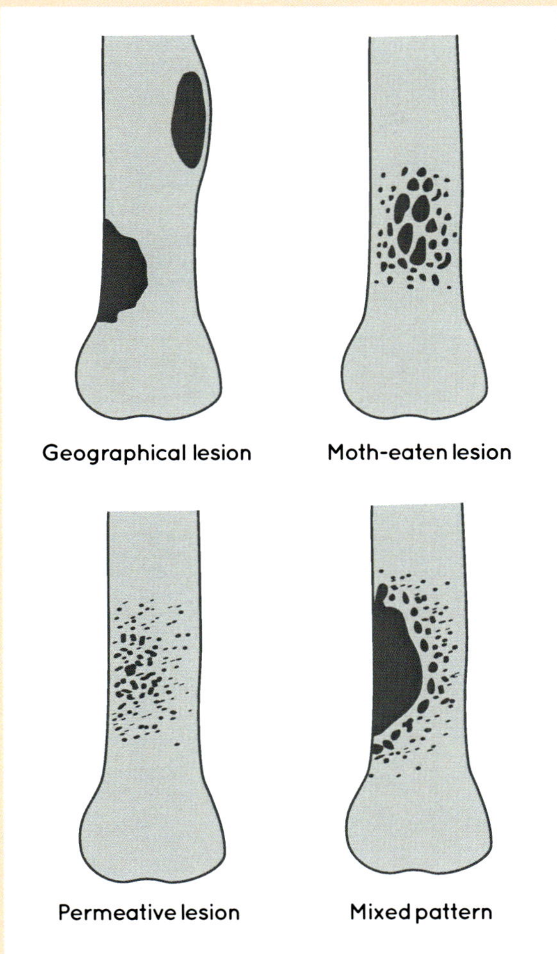

FIGURE 3.2. Diagram of the different radiological osteolysis patterns.

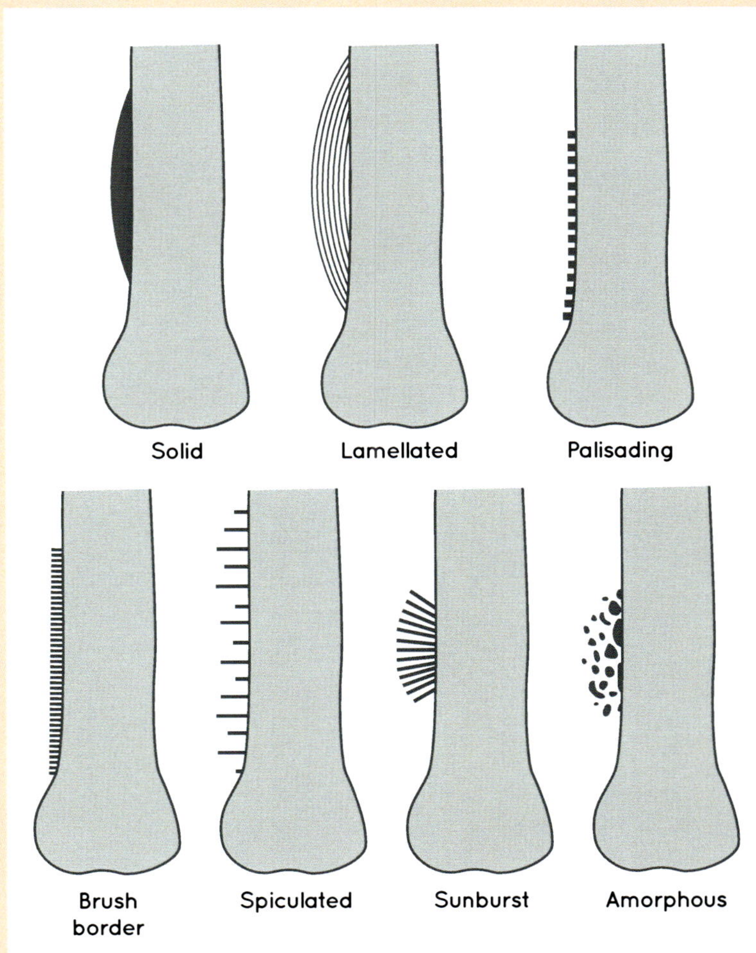

FIGURE 3.3. Diagram of the different periosteal reaction types.

TABLE 3.2 Radiological findings suggestive of aggressive bone lesions versus non-aggressive. When a lesion shows a combination of signs of both table columns, those which are more suggestive of aggressiveness should be considered.

NON-AGGRESSIVE BONE LESION Lesions due to trauma, degenerative, bone cysts, benign neoplasms.	AGGRESSIVE BONE LESION Malignancies, severe osteomyelitis
Well-defined edges.	Poorly-defined edges
Narrow zone of transition.	Wide zone of transition.
With or without geographical osteolysis.	Moth-eaten or permeative osteolysis.
The cortex can appear displaced or thinner, but does not usually present discontinuation.	Cortex discontinuation.
Solid or laminated periosteal reaction	Palisading, spiculated, sunburst or amorphous periosteal reaction.
With and without sclerotic margins.	Without sclerotic margins.
Slow progress or no changes.	Rapid progress.

sertion of a ligament or tendon. On radiographs, they are often indistinguishable from osteophytes.

Soft tissues

Soft tissues can show alterations associated to the presence of lesions in the appendicular skeleton. They often appear thicker due to inflammation or because of the presence of masses, although a reduction in size by muscular atrophy can also be appreciated.

Presence of gas in soft tissues (subcutaneous emphysema) is usually due to air penetration from the outside, in case of penetrating wounds or after surgery in the area, although it can also be caused by anaerobic infections.

Radiopaque foreign bodies or calcification zones in soft tissue can also be identified on radiographs. The latter can be mistaken for small bone fragments or overgrowths when localised next to the bone.

Other imaging techniques

In recent years, the use of ultrasonography has spread as a supplementary diagnostic technique to radiography for the evaluation of the musculoskeletal system. It is usually used to examine soft tissues and is of special interest in the study of muscular and tendon lesions. The associated joints and ligaments can also be examined, although very high resolution transducers and wide experience are required to correctly interpret the images for small animals.

Computed tomography offers excellent images of bone structures. It is specially indicated to evaluate less-evident bone lesions or those difficult to detect by radiography, or to examine anatomically complex joints such as the carpus or tarsus. It is also indicated for the preoperative assessment of bone deformations and complex fractures because three-dimensional image reconstruction at different angles enables the surgeon to know the exact location and morphology of the deformed bone or fragments in order to decide the most appropriate surgical approach.

In human medicine, magnetic resonance is the imaging technique of choice for the diagnosis of diseases of joints and soft tissues of the limbs. It is, however, limited for assessing bone structures, especially in those lesions that can mostly affect the bone cortex, given that it produces no signal. Despite this, it is most useful to evaluate bone tumours, osteomyelitis, haematomas and processes which cause bone necrosis. Due to the smaller size of the joints, its use in small animals is limited by the patient size and the resolution offered by the equipment.

Congenital, hereditary and developmental abnormalities

Chondrodysplasia

The term chondrodysplasia is applied to a wide group of diseases, all of them due to abnormal cartilage growth. It can affect long bone epiphyses, vertebral body epiphyses, long bone epiphyses and metaphyses, or a combination of the above.

One or several of the following radiological signs can be observed:

- Slower growth of long bones, which may appear shorter and thicker than normal.
- The physes can appear wider.
- Retained growth cartilage can be observed in the metaphyseal region.
- Calcification of the epiphyseal ossification centres can be delayed.
- Punctated or distorted epiphyses may be observed.
- Vertebral epiphyses can be partially or irregularly ossified.

Chondrodysplasia is classified based on the bone region that is mostly affected, as described below.

Epiphyseal chondrodysplasia

In dogs, it has been described in Beagles and Poodles. It is characterised by a delay in the calcification of the epiphyseal ossification centres. The epiphyses can have a punctate appearance and although ossification may be completed, they are often deformed, thus causing early onset of osteoarthritis. It has also been described in some cat breeds.

Physeal chondrodysplasia

It has been described for the Pointer breed and causes a disproportionate dwarfism. Marked widening of the physis is radiologically observed, especially in the radius, ulna and tibia. Long bones are shortened and curved. It is accompanied by articular cartilage erosion, thus causing early onset of osteoarthritis. The same process occurs in the Alaskan Malamute, although without articular cartilage erosion. It has also been described in cats.

Metaphyseal chondrodysplasia

It has been described in the Pyrenean Mountain Dogs. It basically affects long bone metaphyses and vertebrae. All long bone metaphyses appear wider, especially in the radius, ulna, tibia, metacarpals and metatarsals. Vertebral body epiphyses are irregularly or incompletely ossified. In the Labrador Retriever and the Samoyed, a form of oculoskeletal dysplasia has been described. It causes shortening and deformation of the limbs, associated with ocular defects.

Retained core of growth cartilage

In growing large and giant breed dogs, a retained core of growth cartilage can be observed, generally affecting the distal physis of the ulna, although it has also been described at other sites, such as the distal physis of the radius or the femur. It appears as a radiolucent triangular area that spreads from the physis to the metaphysis, with a sclerotic margin (fig. 3.4). It may cause limb deformity.

Retained core of growth cartilage can be observed associated with other pathological alterations of the physis, but in those cases the lesion usually has non sclerotic, ill-defined margins.

Polymelia

It indicates a higher number of limbs or parts of a limb than normal. Supernumerary fingers (polydactyly) are most frequent, especially observed in cats and other dog breeds such as the Pyrenean Mountain Dogs. Supernumerary fingers often start at the medial part of the limb and can include full or partial metacarpals or metatarsals and a variable number of phalanges. This abnormality is not usually clinically significant.

Ectrodactyly

The distal part of the limb appears split, with split phalanges, metacarpals, and carpal bones and associated abnormally to the radius and ulna (fig. 3.5). Aplasia, hypoplasia or fusion of distal bones in the limbs can occur. It is a rare alteration in cats and dogs, and considered hereditary in the latter.

Normal radiographic anatomy of the **appendicular skeleton**

http://goo.gl/z9vxXT

Hemimelia

Absence or hypoplasia of one of the bones forming a pair (most frequently affecting the ulna-radius, but also can affect the tibia-fibula).

Osteochondrosis and osteochondritis dissecans

Osteochondrosis is defined as a failure of endochondral ossification, resulting in thickening of the cartilage. The thickest areas do not receive enough quantity of nutrients, which results in necrosis and fissure formation in the affected area. When a chondral flap or an osteochondral fragment is separated from the adjacent subchondral bone, the process is called osteochondritis dissecans. The cartilage flap or even the osteochondral fragment cannot be radiologically identified in many patients, thus generally receiving the name osteochondrosis.

This developmental disease appears in young dogs of large and rapid growth breeds. Clinical signs usually appear between 6-9 months of age. It is usually bilateral, even though the animal may only present with lameness in one limb. It usually appears at specific anatomical locations and affects weight-bearing joint surfaces:

- Caudal or caudolateral aspect of the humeral head (fig. 3.6).
- Distal and medial aspect of the humeral condyle (fig. 3.7).

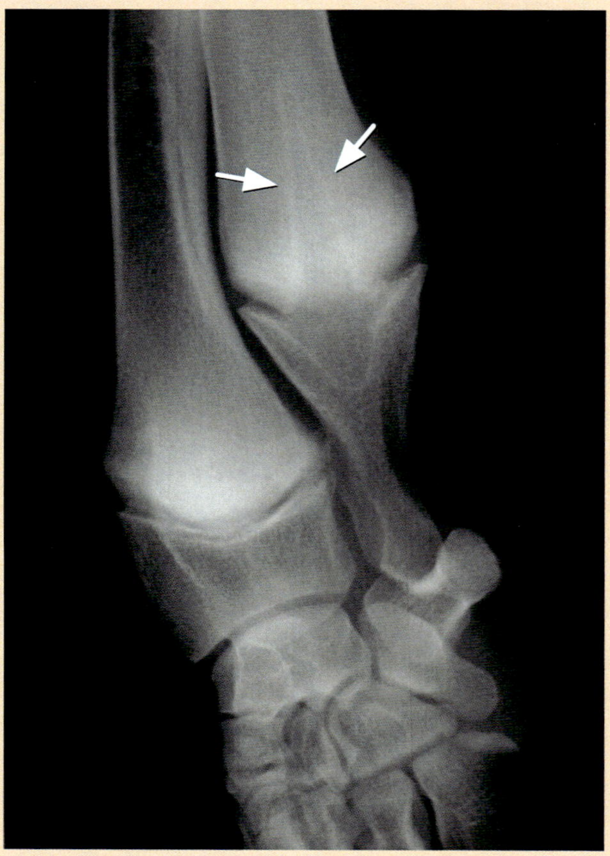

FIGURE 3.4. Enlarged image in mediolateral projection of the radius and distal ulna of a dog with retained core of growth cartilage of the ulna that appears as a radiolucent triangular area spreading from the physis to the metaphysis, with a thin sclerotic margin (arrows).

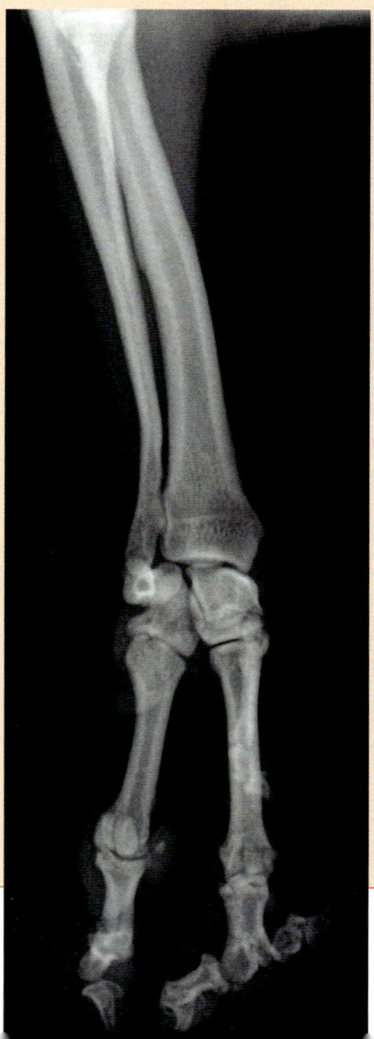

FIGURE 3.5. Dorsopalmar radiograph of the carpus, metacarpals and phalanges in a dog with ectrodactyly. The distal part of the limb appears split, with split phalanges, metacarpals, and carpal bones. In this case aplasia of some carpal bones is observed, as well as of metacarpals and phalanges in two fingers. Finger 2 shows duplicity of the medial and distal phalanges.

- Distal aspect of the lateral femoral condyle and less frequently, in the same area of the medial condyle.
- Medial or lateral trochlear edge of astragalus.

Flattening or concavity of the affected subchondral bone surface is radiologically observed, as well as sclerosis of the subchondral bone surrounding it. The cartilage flap is usually not observed, unless it is calcified. If osteochondral fragments are identified inside the joint, the clinical signs are usually more evident. Sacral osteochondrosis, which affects its craniodorsal edge, has also been described. It basically affects the German Shepherd and, less frequently, the Boxer and Rottweiler. Irregularity of the dorsal edge of the cranial vertebral endplate of the sacrum is observed. As in other sites, the osteochondral fragment is occasionally identified; in this example, on the vertebral canal floor.

Elbow dysplasia

Elbow dysplasia is a non-specific term that refers to a triad of developmental lesions which include:

- Osteochondrosis of the humerus.
- Ununited anconeal process of the ulna.
- Fragmentation of the medial coronoid process of the ulna.

One, two or all three lesions can be observed in one animal, and most frequently there is affectation of both limbs.

The anconeal process should fuse with the ulna at 5 months of age. Lack of fusion at this age is considered pathological. It affects large dog breeds, especially the German Shepherd. To adequately observe the lesion, the elbow radiograph should be taken in lateral projection, forcing flexion of the joint (fig. 3.8).

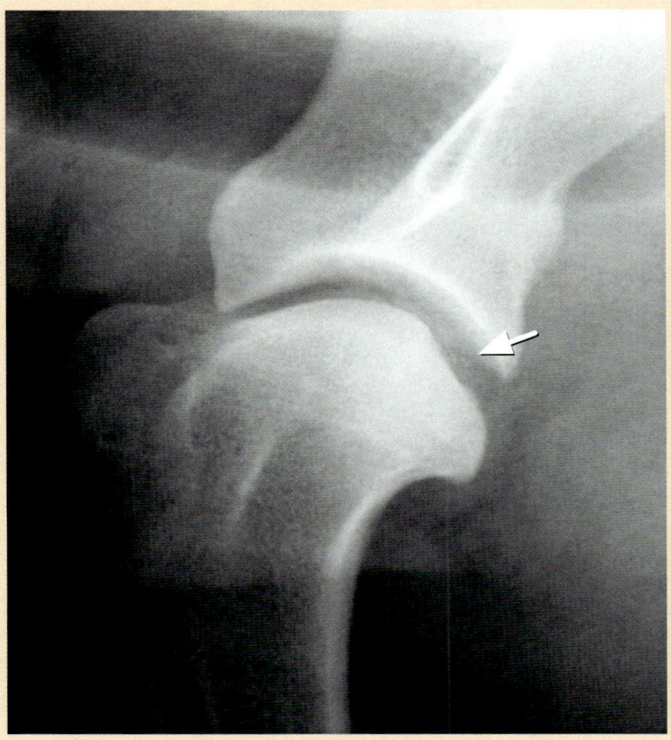

FIGURE 3.6. Mediolateral radiograph of the scapulohumeral joint of a dog with osteochondritis dissecans of the humeral head. A slight concavity in the margin of the humeral head and small osteochondral fragments are observed (pointed by the arrow).

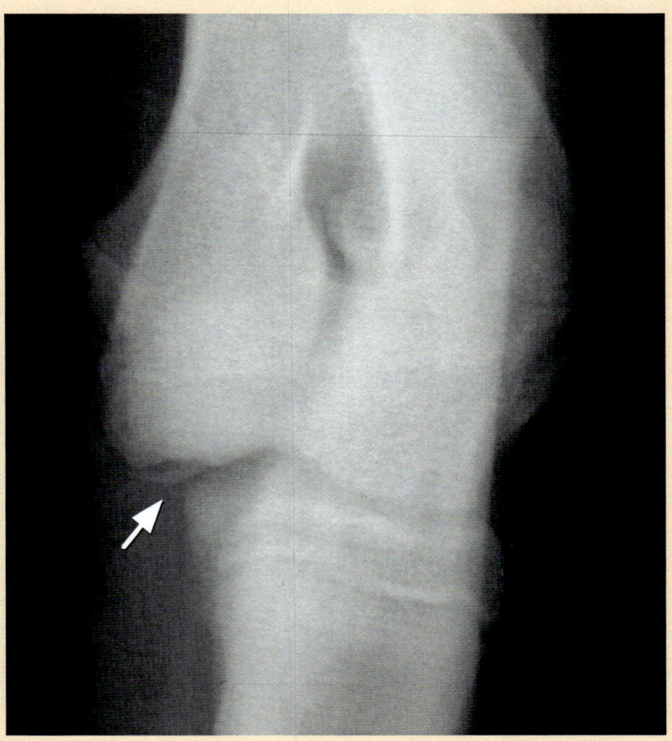

FIGURE 3.7. Craniocaudal oblique radiograph of the elbow of a dog with osteochondritis dissecans in the humeral medial condyle. A concavity in the distal and medial margins of the humeral condyle is observed and beside it, a small osteochondral fragment (pointed by the arrow).

Fragmentation of the medial coronoid process of the ulna affects large or medium breed dogs, more males than females, and clinical signs usually appear between 4-6 months of age. In many cases, the fragment is not identified on the radiograph due to superimposition with the radius, because it is partially adhered to the ulna or when it is basically made of cartilage. Thus, the radiological diagnosis is very frequently based on the observation of degenerative signs secondary to the primary lesion.

The radiographic signs that indicate fragmentation of the medial coronoid process of the ulna are:

- Visualisation of the bone fragment at the area where the medial coronoid process is located (rare) (fig. 3.9).
- Loss of definition or irregularity of the cranial edge of the medial coronoid process in mediolateral projection.
- Rounding of the medial edge of the medial coronoid process visible in craniocaudal projection.

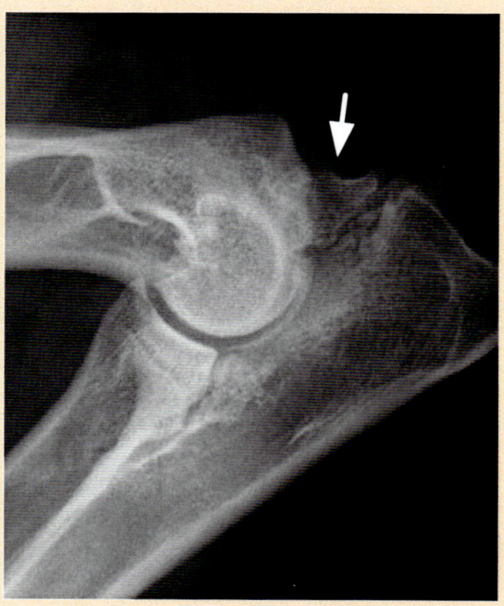

FIGURE 3.8. Mediolateral radiograph with hyperflexion of the elbow of a dog with ununited anconeal process of the ulna (arrow). The hyperflexion makes it easier to identify the lesion.

- Incongruence or subluxation of the elbow joint. Computed tomography is much more precise than radiography to evaluate joint incongruency (nonuniform contact of joint surfaces).
- Degenerative secondary signs: osteophyte formation at the proximal edge of the anconeal process, distal humerus, proximal radius, trochlear notch, and in the medial coronoid process itself; also, trochlear plate sclerosis.

Computed tomography is an excellent diagnostic alternative to identify this anomaly (fig. 3.10).

Hip dysplasia

The term hip dysplasia refers to an abnormal development of coxofemoral joints. It is a hereditary disease that can appear in any dog breed, but especially in large breeds, although also in medium and small breeds, as well as in cats. It is usually bilateral although it can also be unilateral (in approximately 11% of cases). At birth, the coxofemoral joint is normal but, due to the increase in joint laxity experienced by these animals, they develop a greater or lesser degree of subluxation/luxation and signs of degenerative joint disease (coxarthrosis).

The standard projection that is normally used when assessing hip dysplasia is ventrodorsal. In order to avoid diagnostic errors, a correct positioning is essential (fig. 3.11):

- Symmetric pelvis (it can be checked by comparing the two obturator foramina, which should be of the same size in the image, and the width of the wings of the ilium, which should also be the same).
- The femurs should appear in parallel.
- The patellas should appear aligned with the trochlear groove (to achieve this, internal rotation of the knees should be forced).
- The full pelvis and both knees should appear on the radiograph.

This projection is used to assess dysplasia when issuing official certificates, usually from 1 year of age.

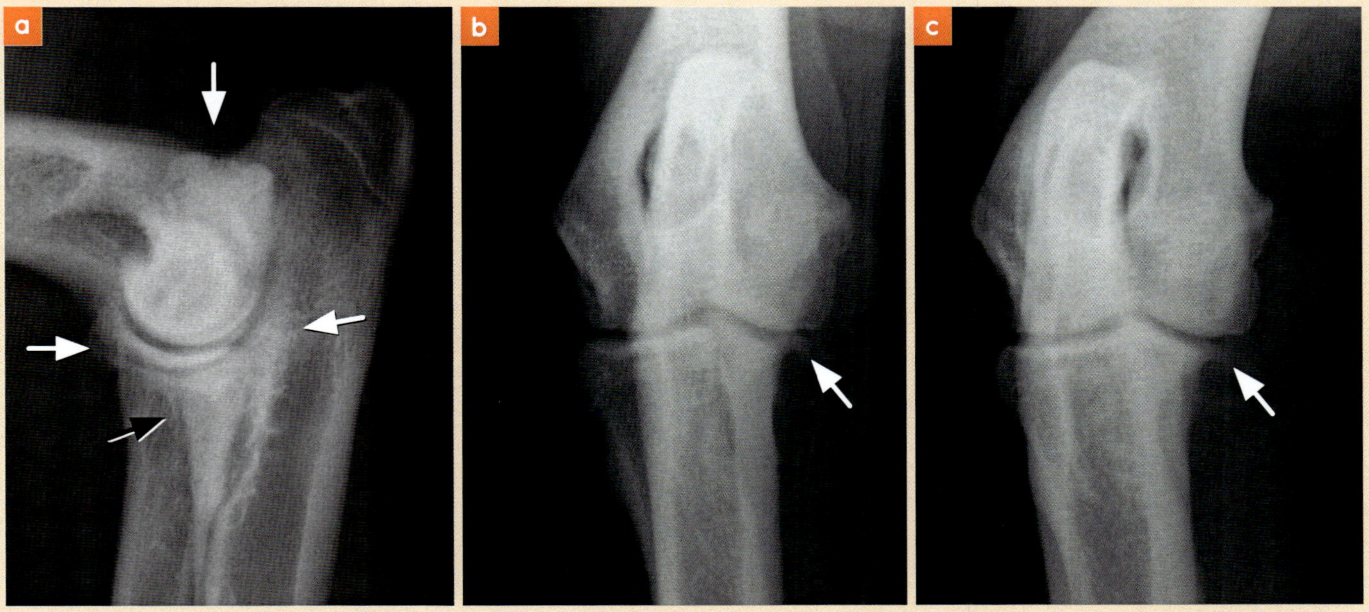

FIGURE 3.9. Mediolateral (a), craniocaudal (b) and oblique caniolateral-caudomedial radiographs of a dog with fragmentation of the medial coronoid process of the ulna. The fragment cannot be identified in the image (a), but the flattening of the cranial margin of the medial coronoid process of the ulna (black arrow) and secondary degenerative signs (white arrows) with osteophyte formation in the distal margin of the caudal humerus and cranial margin of the proximal radius can be identified, as well as sclerosis in the trochlear notch. The small fragment is observed in the image (b), and it is more evident in (c) due to the obliquity of the radiograph.

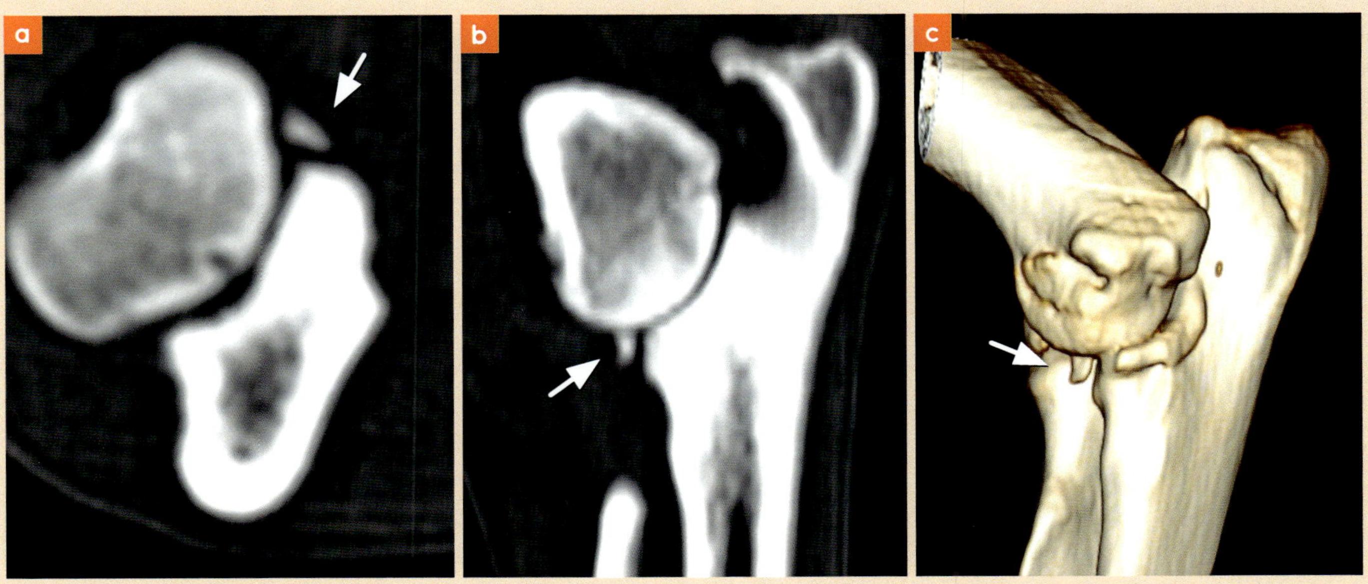

FIGURE 3.10. Computed tomography images in transverse plane (a), sagittal reconstruction (b) and volumetric reconstruction (c) of the elbow of a dog with fragmentation of the medial coronoid process of the ulna. In the three images the arrows are pointing at the fragment. The fragment is easily identified in the image (a) because there is no structural superimposition in these types of images. By means of post-processing computer programmes, multiplanar reconstructions can be performed (in any plane of space), as well as volumetric reconstructions (three-dimensional) that may more or less contribute to the diagnosis.

Radiographic signs for dysplasia include:

- Femoral head subluxation or luxation: usually the acetabular coverage of the femoral head is at least 50 %. When there is coxofemoral subluxation, widening of the medial joint space will be observed (fig. 3.12). The degree of luxation is also measured by the Norberg angle, that requires specific templates or angle-measuring devices. In digital radiography, the angle can be measured using specific post-processing tools (fig. 3.13).
- Signs of joint degeneration (fig. 3.14):
  - Acetabular remodelling (usually flattening), with rounding of the cranial acetabular edge.
  - Femoral head and neck remodelling.
  - Periarticular osteophyte formation on the edges of the femoral head and the acetabulum.
  - A sclerotic line appearing on the femoral neck called Morgan's line. It is due to osteophyte formation at the caudal aspect of the femoral neck and is considered an early sign of coxoarthrosis.
  - Subchondral sclerosis of the acetabular edge.

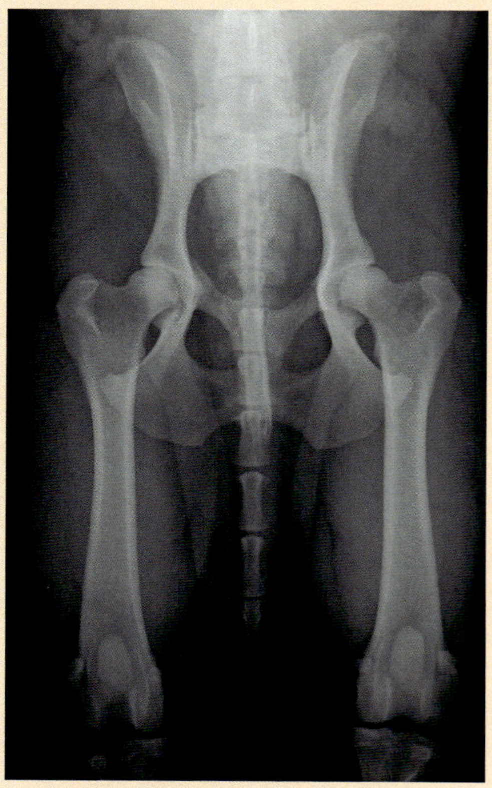

FIGURE 3.11. Ventrodorsal radiograph of a healthy dog's hip. To correctly assess coxofemoral joints, the pelvis should appear symmetric, the femurs in parallel and the patellas aligned with the trochlear channel.

Dysplasia is less prevalent in cats than in dogs. In the cat, most degenerative changes appear at the craniodorsal edge of the acetabulum, whereas remodelling of the femoral head and neck is less frequent.

The Norberg angle is measured at the intersection of two lines: one drawn between the centres of both femoral heads, and another one starting at the centre of each femoral head and moving tangentially to the craniolateral acetabular edge. The Norberg angle measures 105° or more in most healthy dogs, and at least 95° in healthy cats. Inferior measurements are suggestive of dysplasia. The smaller the angle value is, the higher the subluxation degree, and therefore the severity of the dysplasia. Nevertheless, it is important to remark that there are many factors influencing the correct measurement of this angle, such as the positioning of the femurs and pelvis and changes in the acetabular edge.

Femoral inclination and anteversion angles can also be measured as assessment criteria of the degree of dysplasia. The cervicofemoral inclination angle should measure between 130° and 145° under normal conditions, although when the positioning of the animal is not perfect, it is easy to obtain wrong measurements. To measure the anteversion angle, the patient should be placed in such manner that the X-ray beam penetrates in parallel to the longitudinal axis of the femur; its normal value is between 12° and 45°.

The PennHIP method is a way to assess the degree of laxity of the coxofemoral joint at an earlier stage, from 16 weeks of age. Three radiographic projections are used: the standard ventrodorsal with the femurs pulled into extension; a ventrodorsal projection with compression of both coxofemoral joints; and a ventrodorsal with distraction of both joints. A specific device is used to cause the distraction. The distraction index is calculated by dividing the distance from the femoral head centre to the centre of the acetabulum, between the radius of the femoral head. The value of this index can vary from 0 to 1. A value of 0 indicates perfect joint congruity and a

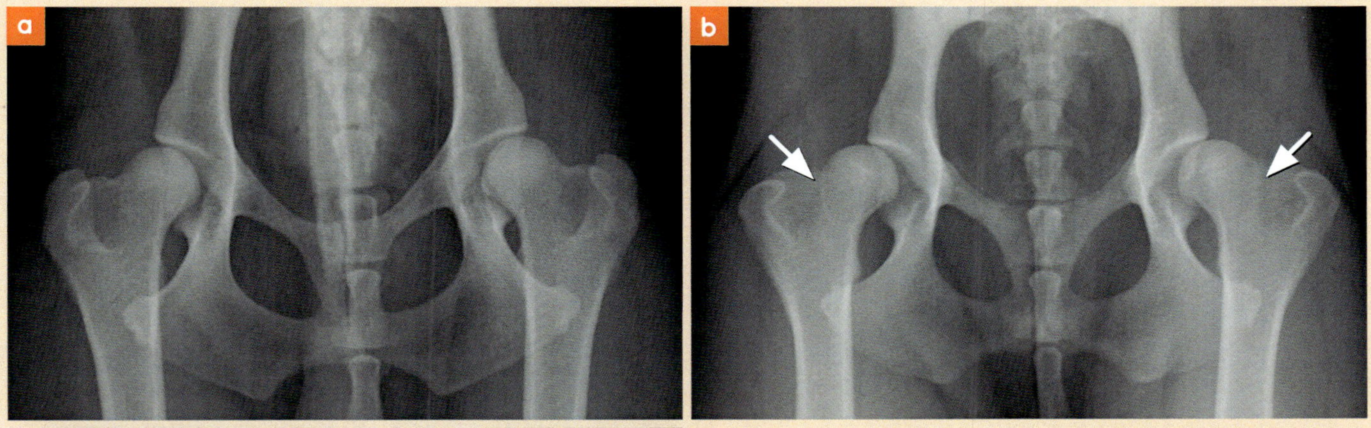

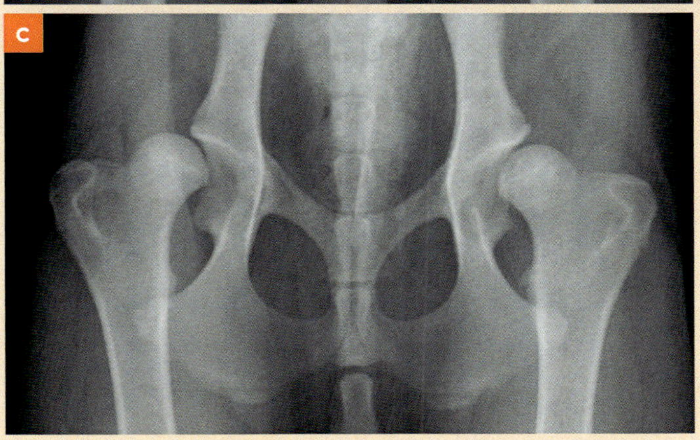

FIGURE 3.12. Enlarged images in ventrodorsal projection of the hip of three dogs with several degrees of coxofemoral subluxation suggestive of mild (a), moderate (b) and serious (c) dysplasia. A sclerotic line in both femoral necks is observed in image (b). This line is called Morgan's line and is suggestive of joint degeneration (arrows).

Normal radiographic anatomy of the **hip**

http://goo.gl/uiEtpX

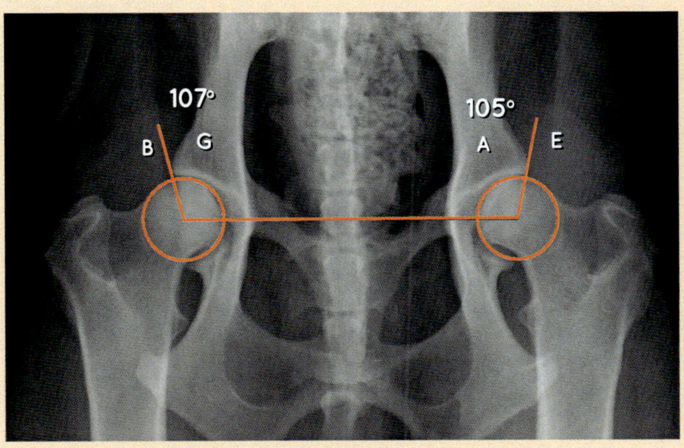

FIGURE 3.13. Enlarged image in ventrodorsal projection of the hip of a healthy dog, on which the Norberg angle has been measured using digital image post-processing tools. The value of this angle is 105° or higher in healthy animals.

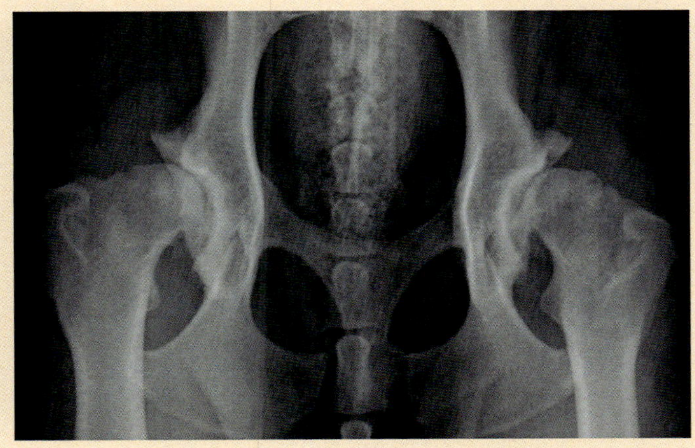

FIGURE 3.14. Enlarged image in ventrodorsal projection of the hip of a dog with severe coxoarthrosis caused by dysplasia. Marked remodelling of the acetabula, and femoral heads and necks is observed, with periarticular osteophyte formation at the edges of the femoral and acetabular heads, as well as subchondral sclerosis of the acetabular edge.

value of 1 indicates complete luxation. This method was developed by researchers from the University of Pennsylvania, where an international database is elaborated and there are specific courses to obtain official certification as a PennHIP certified technician.

Hypertrophic osteodystrophy

Also called metaphyseal osteopathy or metaphyseal osteodystrophy. It affects young dogs between 2 and 7 months of age, generally large and giant breeds. It is uncertain how this disease is originated, but in some cases it has been related to distemper and nutritional alterations (an excessive administration of vitamin complexes is thought to cause onset, but this is not clear). Great Danes and Weimaraners could be somewhat predisposed. Clinically, the animal can develop fever and the metaphysis area of long bones appears swollen, warm and painful. It is generally self-limiting and is usually resolved in a few weeks, although most severe cases can cause premature or abnormal closure of growth lines as a sequela.

Radiological signs (fig. 3.15):

- Lesions are usually bilateral and symmetrical.
- A radiolucent band usually appears at the metaphysis, parallel to the epiphyseal line. This sign is more evident in the distal metaphysis of the radius, ulna and tibia, although it may affect the metaphyses of all long bones.
- A sclerotic band usually appears at the metaphysis, parallel to the radiolucent band.
- Inflammation of the soft tissues adjacent to the affected metaphysis.
- In advanced stages, calcified areas are formed around the metaphysis, apparently separated from the bone cortex by a radiolucent band. These areas can extend to the diaphysis.
- Remodelling of the affected areas takes place over time. Sometimes, the growth plate is prematurely or abnormally closed, thus causing deformation of the affected bone(s).

Panosteitis

This disease causes inflammation of the diaphyses of long bones in youngs large breed dogs. It affects more males than females, and German Shepherds could be more predisposed. It typically appears in animals between 5 and 18 months of age, but it has also been detected in dogs up to 7 years. It is clinically characterised by episodes of acute lameness, that may affect one or several limbs and it does not always appear simultaneously in all affected limbs (alternating lameness). During the examination, pain is observed at deep palpation of the affected limbs.

With regard to the radiographic signs (fig. 3.16):

- They may appear in one or several bones.
- Areas of focal increased density (sclerosis) are observed in long bone marrow, usually in the femur, humerus, radius, ulna and tibia.
- An irregular thickening of the cortical endosteum can be observed.
- A solid and smooth periosteal reaction can be appreciated.
- With time, resolution of bone marrow sclerotic lesions can make the bone trabecular pattern seem to be more marked than usual. Cortical thickness may persist.

Femoral head avascular necrosis

It is also called Legg–Calvé–Perthes disease or femoral head aseptic necrosis. It is a developmental disease that appears in young dogs between 4 and 11 months of age, of small or miniature breeds. Normally, the process is unilateral (fig. 3.17) and less frequently bilateral (fig. 3.18). It results from a deficit in vascular supply to the femoral head epiphysis that produces subchondral bone necrosis. In early stages of the disease, small radiolucent areas are observed with an irregular morphology at the femoral head, which then evolves to deformation and flattening of the femoral head and neck, that may cause coxofemoral subluxation.

Incomplete ossification of the humeral condyle

It is a hereditary disease mainly affecting dogs from Spaniel breeds, although it has also been described in dogs from medium and large breeds. The two ossification centres that appear at the humeral condyle fuse at approximately 84 days from birth. Once skeletal maturation is complete, those animals with incomplete ossification will maintain a thin fissure between

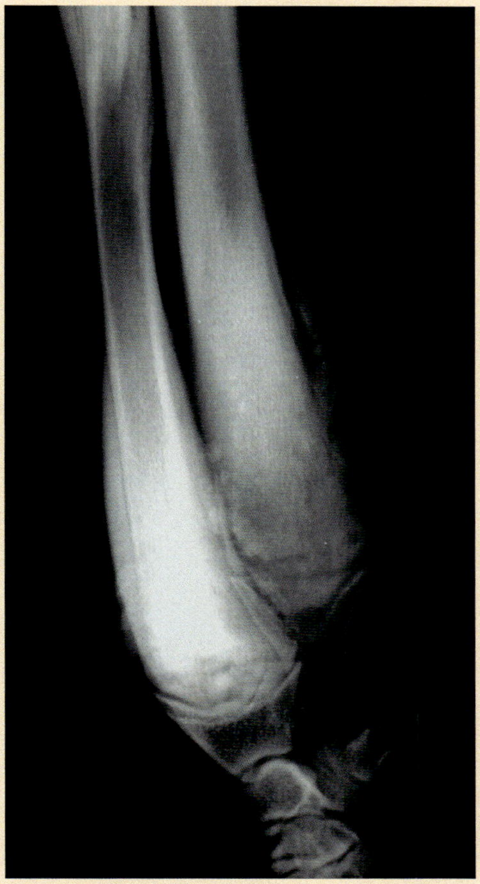

FIGURE 3.15. Mediolateral radiograph of radius and ulna of a dog with hypertrophic osteodystrophy. A radiolucent band in the metaphysis parallel to the epiphyseal line is observed, as well as solid periosteal reaction and calcified areas surrounding the metaphysis and part of the diaphysis, apparently separated from the bone cortex.

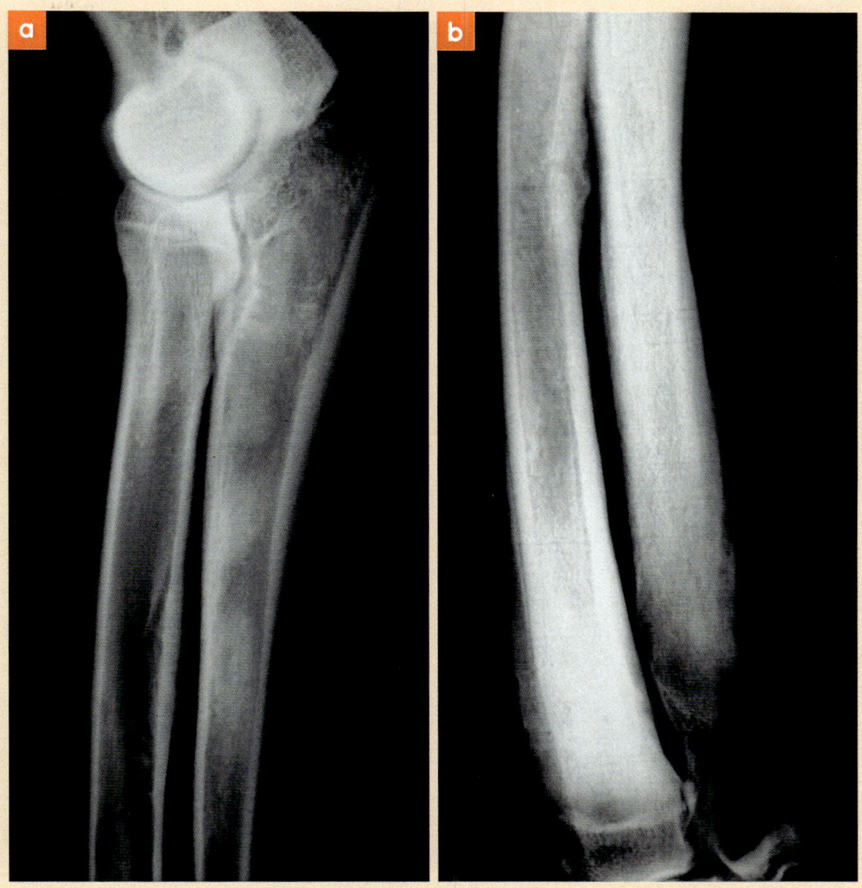

FIGURE 3.16. Enlarged image of the radius and ulna in mediolateral projection of 2 dogs with panosteitis. Focal sclerotic areas in the ulnar diaphysis are observed in image (a). In image (b) increased bone marrow density is more diffuse and affects the radius and the ulna, that also present endosteal and periosteal growth of solid type.

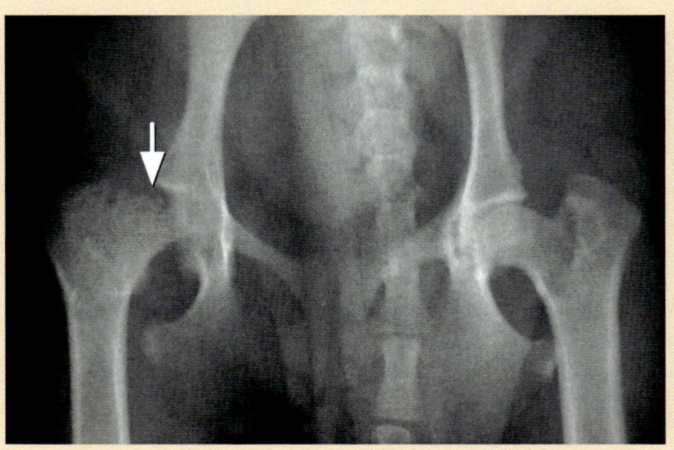

FIGURE 3.17. Enlarged image of the hip on a ventrodorsal radiograph of a dog with unilateral right avascular necrosis in the femoral head (Legg-Calvé-Perthes disease). The appearance of necrotic areas in the femoral head causes osteolysis, which induces femoral head and neck deformities over time (arrow).

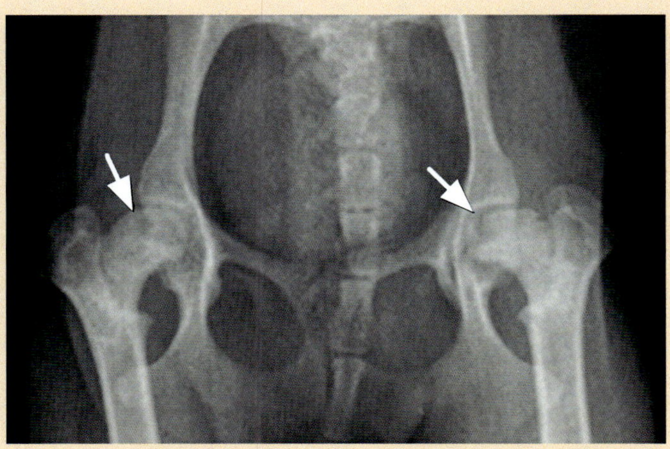

FIGURE 3.18. Enlarged image in ventrodorsal projection of the hip of a dog with bilateral avascular necrosis in the femoral head (Legg-Calvé-Perthes disease). Both femoral heads have small osteolytic areas (arrows) and appear slightly deformed. Even when it is bilateral, radiological changes do not appear at the same time in both femurs in many cases.

both halves of the condyle, thus predisposing them to pathological fractures at that site.

Fractures

Fractures are classified as:

- Closed (intact skin) or open (skin defect in the area) (fig. 3.19).
- Simple (single fracture line), comminuted (several fracture lines interconnect at one point or plane, thus dividing the bone in three or more fragments) or multiple (several fracture lines that do not interconnect, in the same or different bones).
- Transverse, oblique, spiral or irregular, depending on the fracture line direction.
- Complete (affects the whole bone diameter) or incomplete (e.g. greenstick fracture).
- Articular or nonarticular fracture, if it affects the joint or not.
- Avulsion fracture: it separates the insertion site of a muscle (fig. 3.20), ligament or tendon.
- Stress or fatigue fracture (caused by repeated mild trauma).
- Compression or impacted fractures: the end of one of the fragments jams into the other (fig. 3.21); shortening of the bone can be observed and it is more frequent in vertebrae.

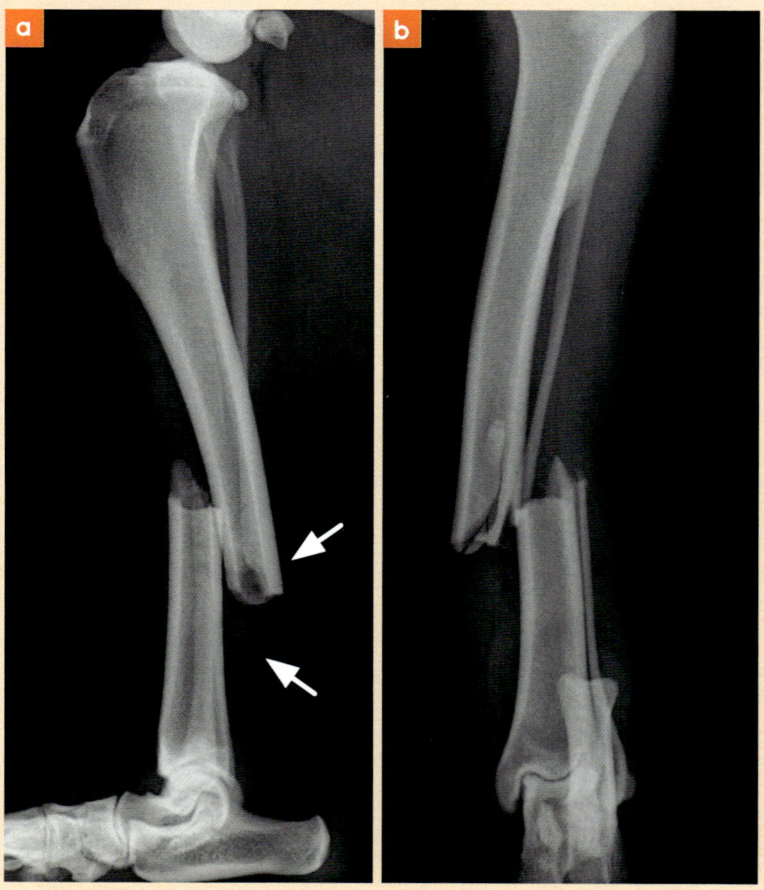

FIGURE 3.19. Mediolateral (a) and craniocaudal (b) radiographs of the tibia and fibula of a dog with an open fracture in both bones. The presence of small areas with gas density in surrounding soft tissues (arrows) is a radiological sign indicative of an open fracture.

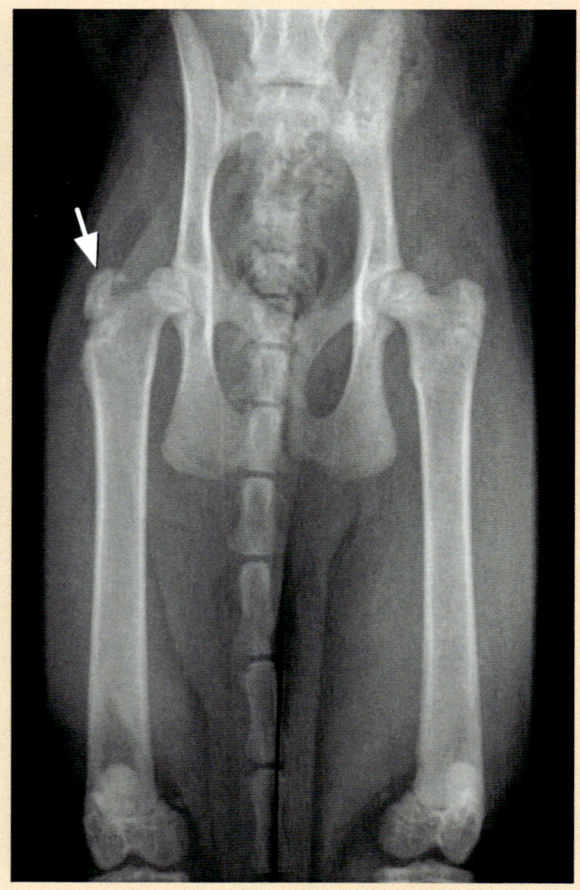

FIGURE 3.20. Ventrodorsal radiograph of the hip of a cat with an avulsion fracture in the greater trochanter of the right femur (arrow), in which the gluteus medius and profundus are inserted.

- Salter-Harris fractures (see box and fig. 3.22 y 3.23): they affect the physis.
- Pathological fractures: they are caused by another disease (processes that cause osteopaenia, tumours, bone cysts, osteomyelitis).

Immediately after surgical resolution of the fracture, a radiograph will allow the assessment of: the degree of fracture reduction (contact between the fragments); the alignment of the fragments; and the correct placement of the osteosynthesis material. In further radiological checks, the following will be examined: bone callus evolution; possible displacement of the fragments or the osteosynthesis material; rupture of the osteosynthesis

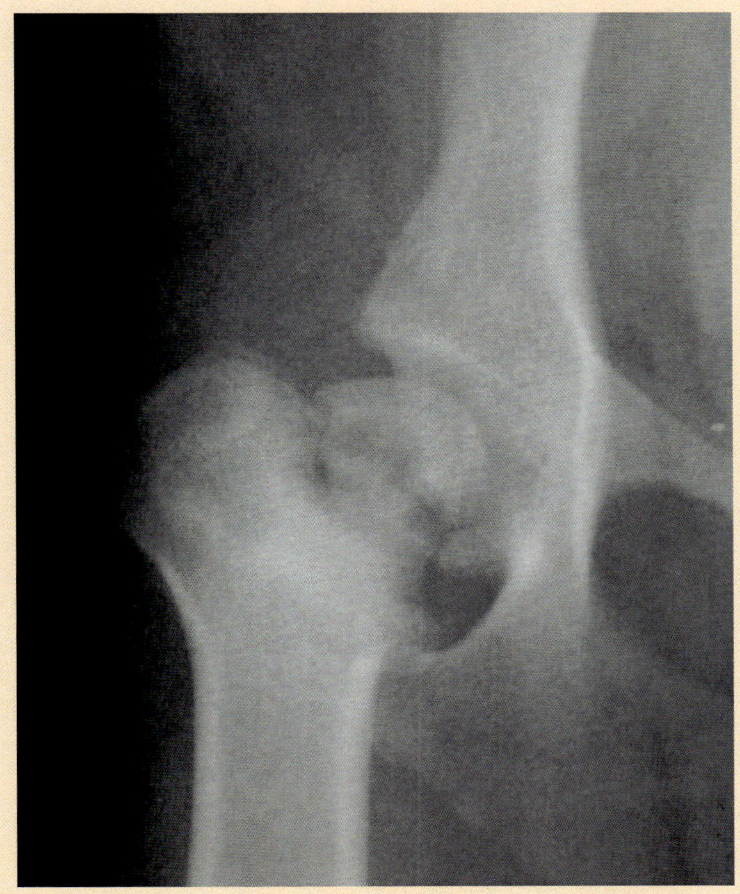

FIGURE 3.21. Enlarged image in ventrodorsal projection of the right coxofemoral joint of a dog with an impacted femoral neck fracture. Femoral neck shortening is caused by the fracture.

SALTER-HARRIS FRACTURES

Fractures that affect the physis are classified in 6 types (Salter-Harris classification) (fig. 3. 22):

- **Type I:** the fracture occurs along the physis.
- **Type II:** the fracture line crosses the physis and also divides part of the metaphysis.
- **Type III:** the fracture line crosses the physis and also divides part of the epiphysis.
- **Type IV:** the fracture line crosses the physis and also divides part of the metaphysis and of the epiphysis (fig. 3.23).
- **Type V:** impacted or compressed fracture hat occurs at the physis level. It may completely or partially affect the physis. This is the type of fracture that may cause premature closure of the distal growth plate in the ulna.
- **Type VI** (rare): it is a consequence of trauma that only affects part of the physis thus causing its partial closure (asymmetric). This type has been added later to the classification and some authors think it should not be included.

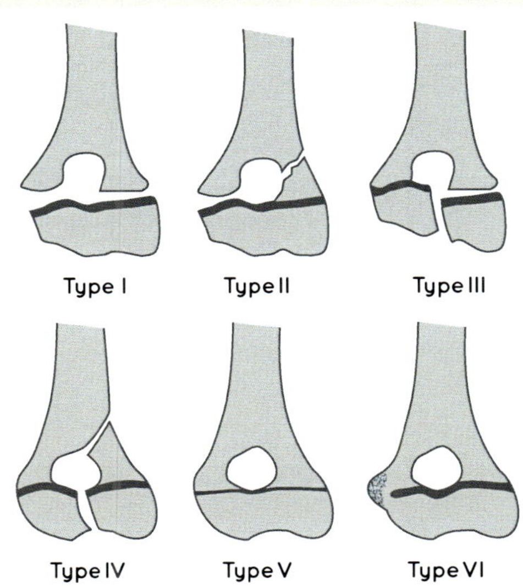

FIGURE 3.22. Diagram of the classification of Salter type fractures.

material (fig. 3.24); and abnormalities in the adjacent soft tissues. The occurrence of radiolucent bands surrounding the osteosynthesis material indicates mobility of the material or infection (fig. 3.25). Nevertheless, an artefact with the same appearance (radiolucent lines surrounding metallic implants) has been described in digital radiography, due to overuse of the edge-enhancement tool. This has already been corrected in many modern equipment.

Progression in a fracture healing depends on several factors:

- Type of bone.
- Type of fracture.
- Age of the patient.
- Treatment method.
- Other systemic diseases.
- Vascular supply.

Table 3.3 shows the average healing time for a fracture in a dog depending on the age and type of treatment method used (Brinker, 1978; Butterworth, 2006).

Post-traumatic osteoporosis is a common sequela of many long bone distal fractures and can be especially acute in young animals. It is often wrongly called **disuse osteoporosis**. Post-traumatic osteoporosis develops distal to the fracture (fig. 3.26), whereas disuse osteoporosis (caused by limb immobilisation) affects the whole limb. Once the fracture has formed a solid callus and the bone is again rigid, bone density returns quickly to normal in both types of osteoporosis.

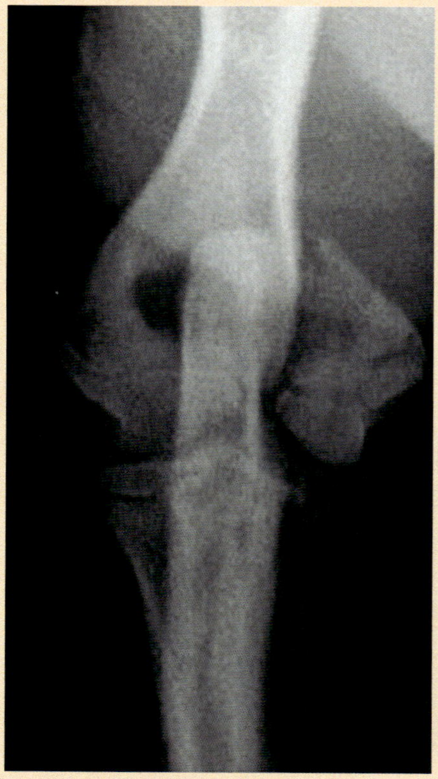

FIGURE 3.23. Craniocaudal radiograph of the elbow of a 10-week-old dog with a type IV Salter fracture (the fracture line crosses the distal physis of the humerus splitting part of the epiphysis and part of the metaphysis).

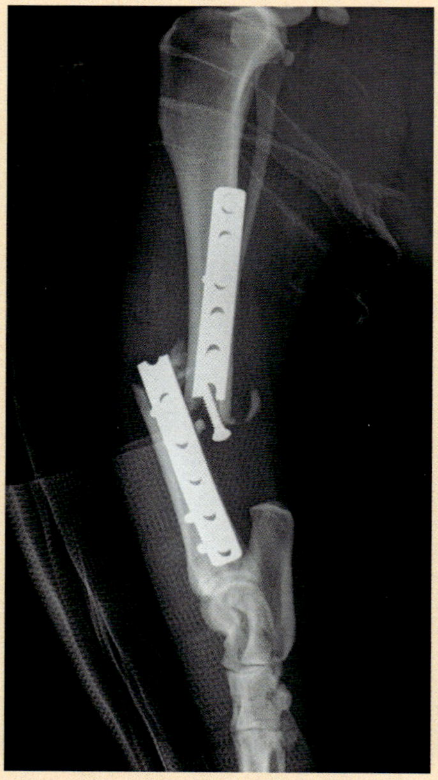

FIGURE 3.24. Mediolateral radiograph of the tibia and fibula of a dog with a broken osteosynthesis plate, which was applied as treatment for a fracture of both bones. The central screw looks displaced and multiple small fragments can be identified surrounding the fracture focus. The shadow of the dressing can be observed in the image.

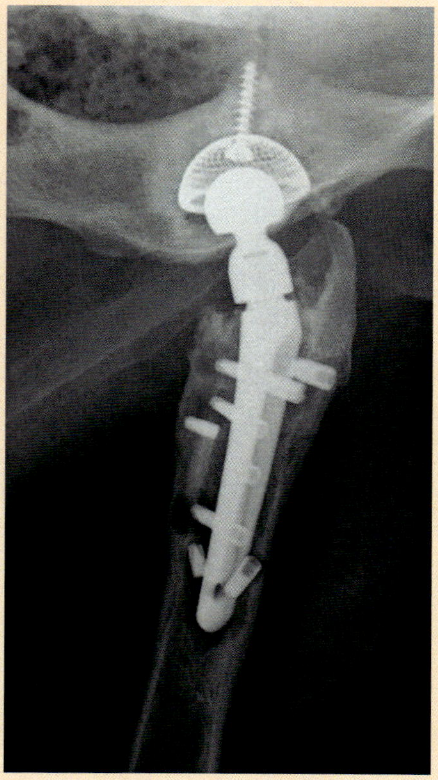

FIGURE 3.25. Enlarged image in mediolateral projection of the femur of a dog that shows some degree of mobility of a hip prosthesis. Radiolucent bands surrounding the rod can be seen, as well as rupture of several screws.

Normal radiographic anatomy of the **tibia and fibula**

http://goo.gl/v8eu8k

TABLE 3.3 Average healing time for a fracture in a dog depending on the age and treatment method used (W.O. Brinker, 1978; S.J. Butterworth, 2006).

Age	Resolution time according to treatment	
	Dressing External fixators Intramedullary needles	Osteosynthesis plate
< 3 months	2-3 weeks	1 month
3-5 months	4-6 weeks	2-3 months
6-12 months	5-8 weeks	3-5 months
> 12 months	7-12 weeks	5-12 months

The main complications from fractures are:

- **Delayed union:** callus formation is slower than normal.
- **Non-union:** callus is not formed; it can be atrophic (end of fragments are pointed) (fig. 3.27) or hypertrophic (bone forms around the ends of the fragments, but they do not bind; the shape of the ends looks like an "elephant's foot" (fig. 3.28).
- **Defective consolidation:** fragments are bound, but not correctly aligned (fig. 3.29).
- **Exuberant callus:** splinters of bone incorporate to the callus, due to mobility of the fracture focus or to infection.

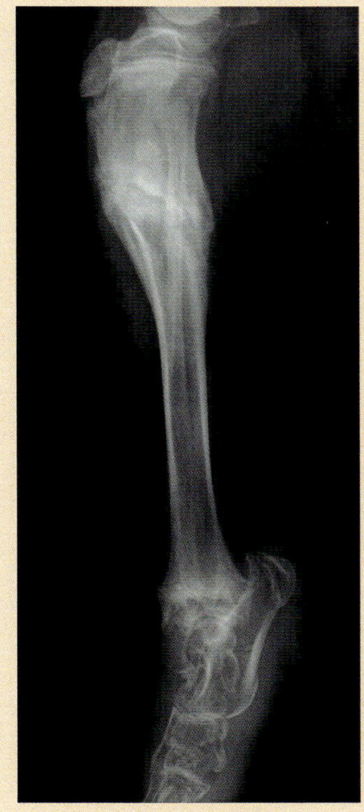

FIGURE 3.26. Mediolateral radiograph of the tibia and fibula of a dog with a consolidated fracture in both bones as well as post-traumatic osteoporosis. The osteoporosis develops distal to the fracture (in this case, more marked in the tarsus and metatarsals), unlike desuse osteoporosis that affects the whole limb.

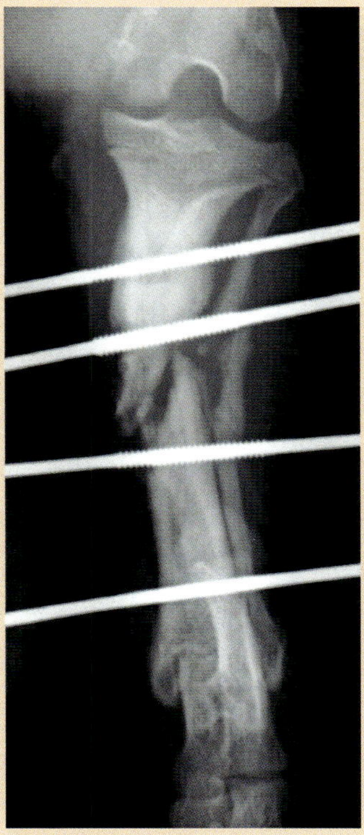

FIGURE 3.27. Craniocaudal radiograph of the tibia and fibula of a dog with atrophic nonunion of a tibial fracture. The fragment ends appear pointed. The external fixators and a double fibula fracture can be observed in the image.

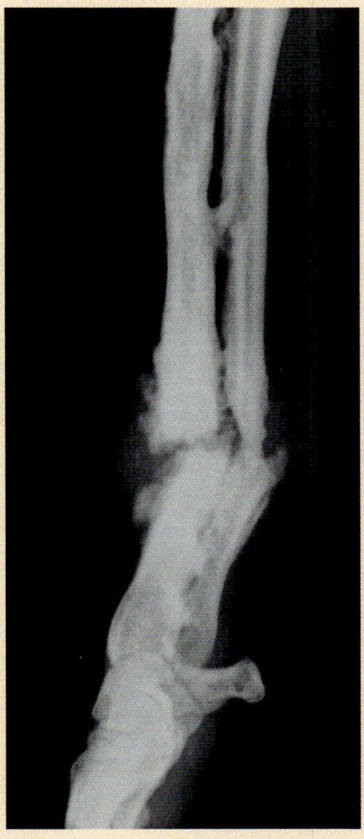

FIGURE 3.28. Mediolateral radiograph of the radius and the ulna of a dog with hypertrophic nonunion of the radial fracture. The fragment ends appear separated, sclerotic and new bone is forming around them. Nonunion of an ulnar fracture is also observed, with the proximal fragment looking atrophic and the distal, hypertrophic.

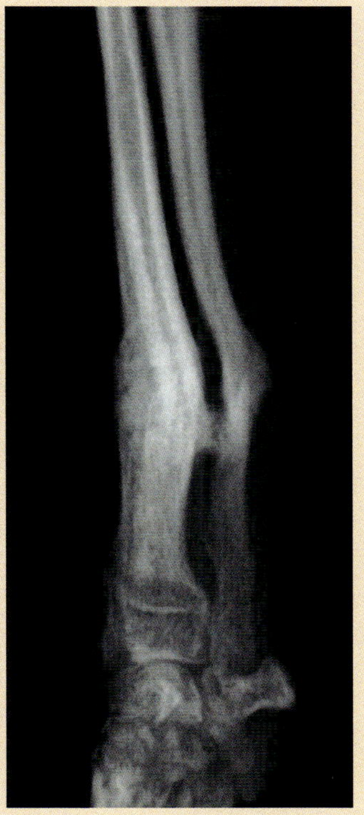

FIGURE 3.29. Mediolateral radiograph of the radius and the ulna of a dog with defective consolidation of a fracture in both bones.

Normal radiographic anatomy of the **radius and ulna**

http://goo.gl/clzWz2

- **Osteomyelitis:** infection will be suspected when osteolysis is observed surrounding the material, together with an atypical periosteal reaction and marked soft-tissue tumescence, that may look like emphysema (focal gas accumulations) in some cases.
- **Neoplastic development:** may appear after several years, especially if the osteosynthesis material was not removed or the fracture resolution was very complicated. Its cause is unknown but it could be related to chronic inflammation.

Deformities due to growth plate alteration

Growth plate lesions cause slowed-down or arrested growth, and its consequences can be:

- Shortening of the affected bone(s).
- Angulation of the affected bone(s).
- Subluxation of adjacent joints.

The degree of bone shortening depends on the specific contribution that the damaged plate has in global bone growth and on the stage of growth when the lesion is produced.

Angulation or curvature of the affected bone takes place when the lesion affects more than one area in the plate, or when the affected bone is part of a pair (e.g. radius-ulna).

The most significant deformities occur by lesion of the proximal or distal growth plate of the radius and of the distal growth plates of the ulna, femur or tibia.

Due to its conical shape, the distal growth plate of the ulna is especially prone to lesions. Sometimes, premature growth line closure can be observed with no previous evident trauma. When distal growth of the ulna is slowed-down or arrested and the radius continues growing at a normal pace, cranial and medial curvature of the radius occurs, as well as valgus (lateral) deviation of the hand, elbow subluxation and proximal migration of the ulna styloid process (fig. 3.30). This deformity is called radius curvus.

When the lesion affects the distal radial growth plate, the radius is shortened with respect to the ulna, that keeps growing at a normal pace. The radial head separates from the humeral condyle, widening the joint space (fig. 3.31). Medial widening of the distal radial epiphysis occurs, which usually causes valgus deviation of the hand, although it is sometimes in the opposite direction (in varus, to the medial area).

Proximal growth plate lesions of the radius are much less frequent and cause similar radiographic signs to those of the distal plate, but the distal radius remains normal and there is no hand deviation.

Bone tumours and osteomyelitis

Bone tumours

Benign bone tumours are rare, and include: osteomas, generally appearing as radiodense masses of amorphous bone; chondromas, with less radiopacity than osteomas; and osteochondromas, appearing as single cartilaginous exostoses.

Malignant bone tumours (osteosarcoma, fibrosarcoma, haemangiosarcoma, chondrosarcoma) appear as aggressive bone lesions, usually single, mainly located at the following metaphyses: proximal of the humerus, distal of the radius, distal of the femur and proximal or distal of the tibia (fig. 3.32). Chondrosarcomas usually affect the ribs, pelvis, or skull.

Primary bone tumours can appear as lesions with various degrees of osteolysis and osteoproliferation. The zone of transition between the lesion and normal bone is usually wide and poorly defined, and the periosteal reaction of spiculated, sunburst or amorphous type. For years, tumours were thought to have a characteristic periosteal reaction that was called Codman triangle (fig. 3.33), and corresponds to a small triangular bone area located at the edge of the lesion. Today, it is known that it is formed when the periosteum gets broken and lifted “for any reason” and, although it is generally considered suggestive of

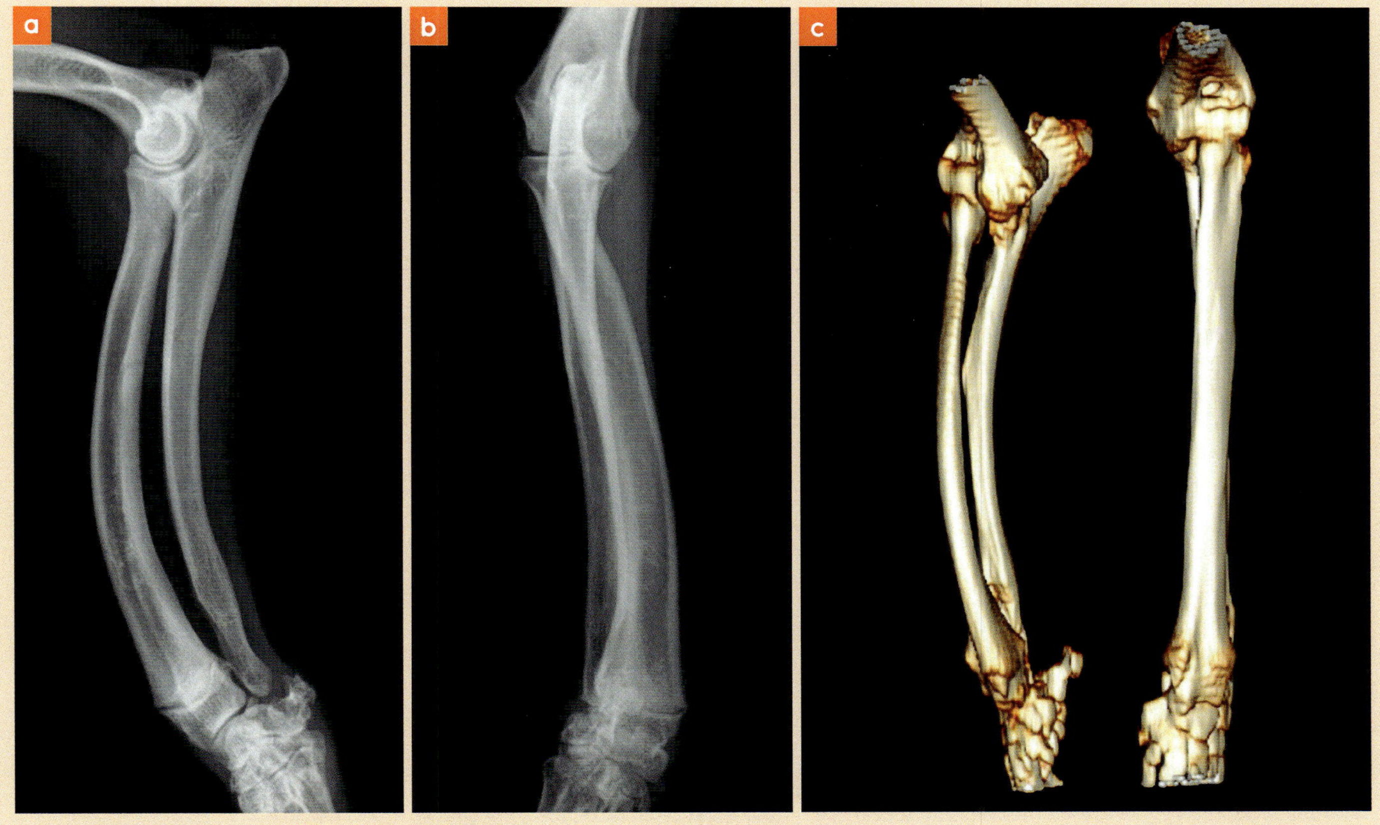

▲ FIGURE 3.30. Radiographic images in mediolateral (a) and craniocaudal (b) projection of the radius and ulna of an 8-month old dog with radius curvus. Computed tomography image of the same patient (c). As previous trauma has caused premature closure of the distal growth line of ulna, the radius is curved cranially and medially. This causes elbow subluxation and valgus deviation of the hand. Accessory carpal bone deformity can be also observed, as well as a fragment caudal distal to the distal epiphysis of the radius. Both findings are related to the prior trauma. The image (c) shows computed tomographic-based volumetric reconstruction of both limbs, where the damaged limb can be compared in detail to the normal limb. The degree of deformity can therefore be easily assessed, as well as the degree of angulation of the affected limb. This is of special interest when planning surgical treatment.

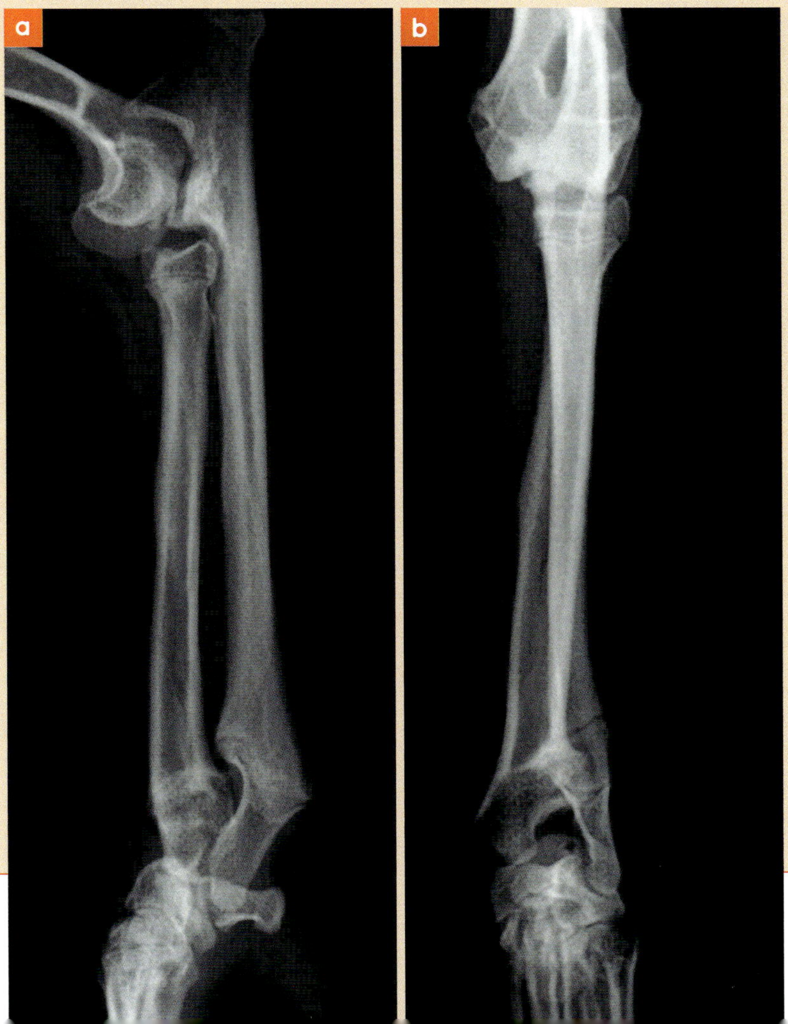

◀ FIGURE 3.31. Mediolateral (a) and craniocaudal (b) radiographs of the ulna of a dog with a short radius. The radius is shortened by premature closure of the distal radial growth line, with the proximal epiphysis migrating distally, which causes elbow joint incongruity. The distal part of the ulna and the radius seems deformed.

malignancies, it can also be associated to subperiosteal haematoma and inflammatory processes.

Primary tumours do not normally "cross" the joint and extend to adjacent bone. They can be the cause for secondary pathological fractures. As lung metastases are frequent, it is advised to always perform a radiological thoracic study when these types of bone lesions are observed.

Bone metastases often appear as multiple aggressive lesions, generally more osteolytic than primary tumours (fig. 3.34).

Multiple myeloma results from neoplastic proliferation of bone marrow plasma cells. It produces multiple focal lesions that affect long bones, vertebrae and ribs at the same time.

Malignant soft-tissue tumours adjacent to the bone may secondarily affect nearby bone structures. In these cases, the typical radiological finding is marked tumefaction of soft tissues together with osteolytic, rather than osteoproliferative changes in the adjacent bone (it may affect several bones depending on the primary tumour extension). Subungual squamous cell carcinoma is a typical example of a malignant tumour of soft tissues usually affecting adjacent bones (fig. 3.35), which appears more frequently in large breed dogs with black coat.

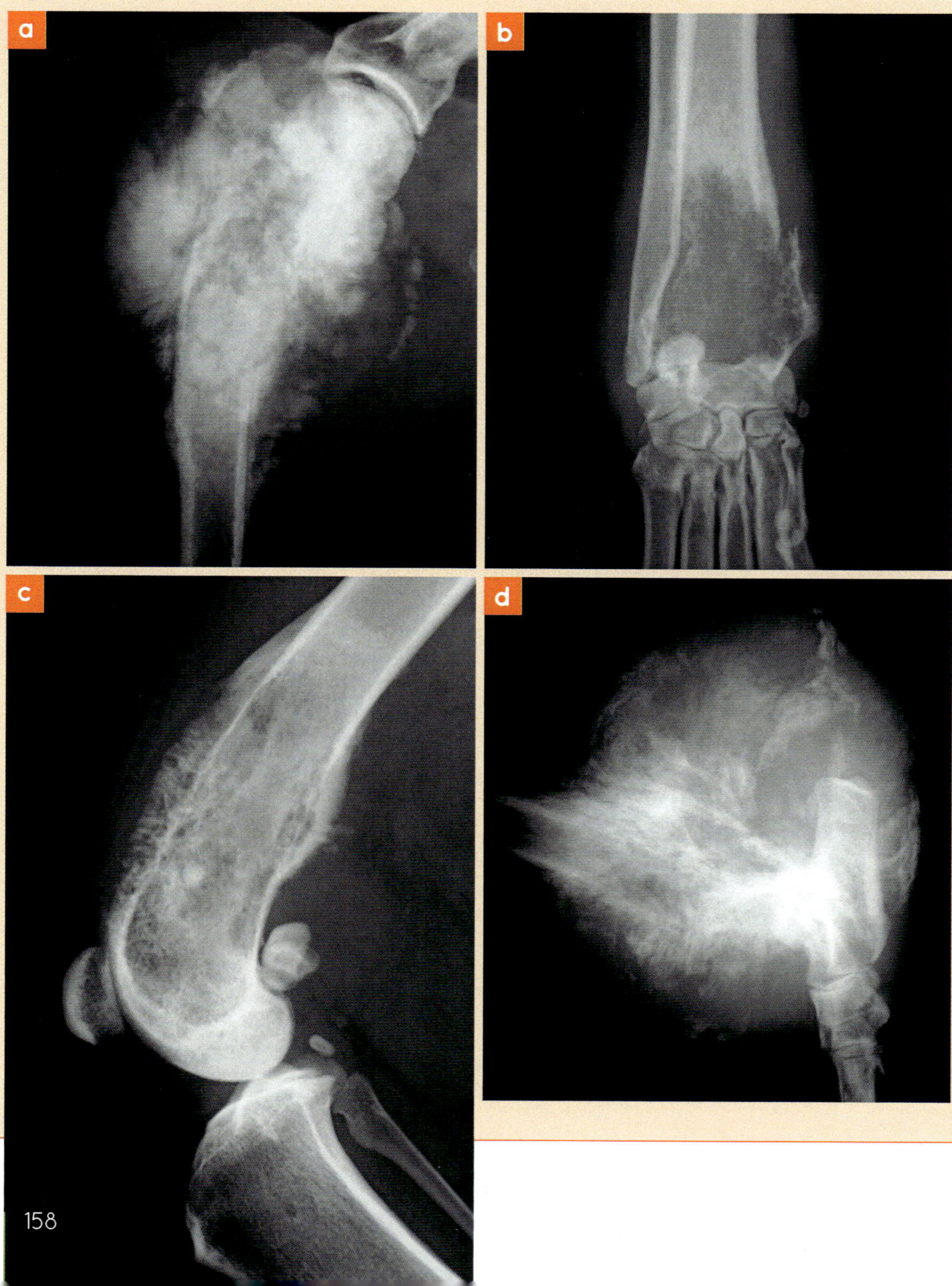

FIGURE 3.32. Images of the most common sites for bone neoplasms: proximal humerus (a), distal radius (b), distal femur (c) and proximal or distal tibia (d). The lesion in image (a) is mostly osteoproliferative with amorphous periosteal reaction, which is highly suggestive of malignancy. The lesion in image (b) is mostly osteolytic with mixed geographical pattern at its central area and infiltrating at its peripheral area. The cortex is interrupted at its medial margin. Image (c) shows a moth-eaten osteolytic pattern and solid periosteal reaction at the caudal and cranioproximal aspects of the lesion. Palisading periosteal reaction can be observed at the medial and distal cranial edge of the lesion. The marked mixed periosteal reaction (sunburst and amorphous) in image (d) makes it somewhat difficult to identify the pathological fracture in the patient's affected area.

Osteomyelitis

It is usually a sequela of surgical fracture repair (fig. 3.36), although it can also appear in open fractures. Sometimes the infection is produced haematogenously.

In the acute phase, aggressive periosteal reaction is observed, with some degree of cortical and trabecular osteolysis and inflammation of the adjacent soft tissues. In chronic phases, bone proliferation surrounding the lesion occurs, an irregular periosteal reaction is maintained and a well-defined central osteolytic area may remain (sequestrum).

In practice, it is not possible to safely differentiate osteomyelitis from a bone neoplasm only by radiological imaging. A biopsy is always required to confirm diagnosis.

Nutritional and metabolic alterations

Balanced bone production and resorption is maintained in healthy adults. Numerous factors play a role to control this equilibrium, mainly the level of some hormones such as the parathyroid hormone and calcitonin (both are produced in the parathyroid gland), growth hormone, glucocorticoids and vitamin A, among others.

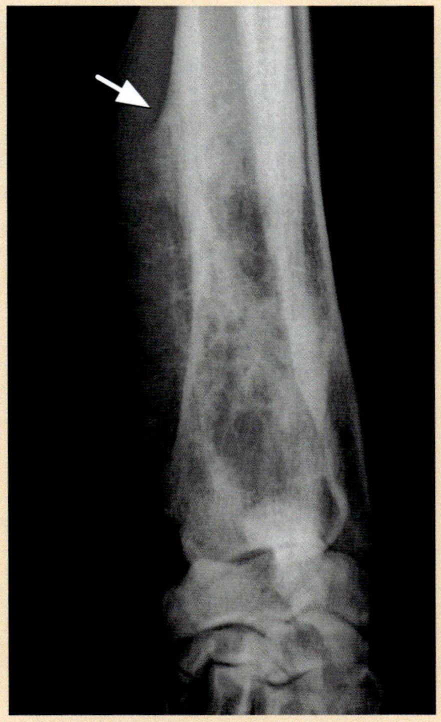

FIGURE 3.33. Enlarged image in craniocaudal projection of the radius and ulna of a dog with a bone neoplasm (osteosarcoma). The osteolysis pattern is moth-eaten, the zone of transition between the damaged and the normal bones is relatively wide, the periosteal reaction is spiculated, and a triangular bone overgrowth that corresponds to the so-called Codman triangle (arrow) can be identified at its medial and proximal edge.

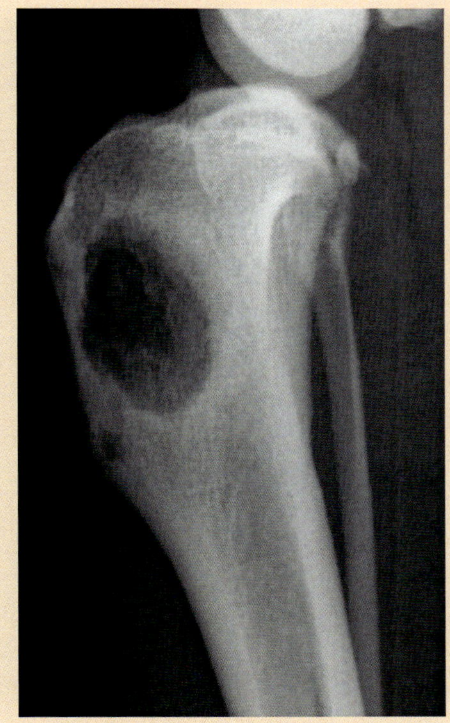

FIGURE 3.34. Enlarged image in mediolateral projection of the tibia of a dog with bone metastases in the tibial proximal metaphysis. Two osteolytic lesions are observed, one that is larger and the smaller one situated craniodistal from the first.

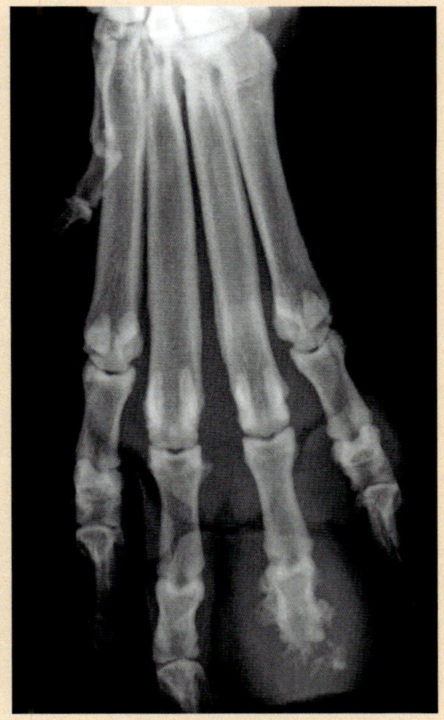

FIGURE 3.35. Dorsopalmar radiograph of the metacarpals and phalanges of a dog with a soft-tissue tumour that is secondarily affecting adjacent bones. The soft-tissue tumour is a squamous cell carcinoma that has destroyed the third phalanx of the fourth finger almost completely. It is also causing palisading periosteal reaction in the second phalanx of the same finger, thus indicating it is also affected.

Bone is a living tissue that can reflect metabolic alterations and nutritional imbalances, that sometimes lead to increased bone production, although they more frequently cause increased resorption with subsequent bone density loss. Density changes in bone can be detected by conventional radiography but not at an early stage. In order to be evident on a radiograph, 30-50 % of bone calcium should be lost to reduce its opacity. Bone densitometry, a more sensitive and precise technique, is used in human medicine to evaluate changes in bone density.

Secondary nutritional hyperparathyroidism

It is also called nutritional osteodystrophy. It usually affects growing animals, especially cats, that feed on a low-calcium diet, or with an inappropriate calcium/phosphorus ratio (e.g. when they feed exclusively on meat, with a high phosphorus and low calcium content). Hypocalcaemia stimulates parathyroid hormone production. Radiological signs are (fig. 3.37):

- Decreased bone radiopacity.
- Thinning of long bone cortex.
- A double cortical line caused by resorption of intracortical bone may be observed (rare).
- Secondary pathological fractures may be observed.
- Deformed bone limbs due to old pathologic fractures may be observed.
- Pelvic and vertebral deformity can appear.
- Fast calcification of bone structures after introducing a balanced diet.

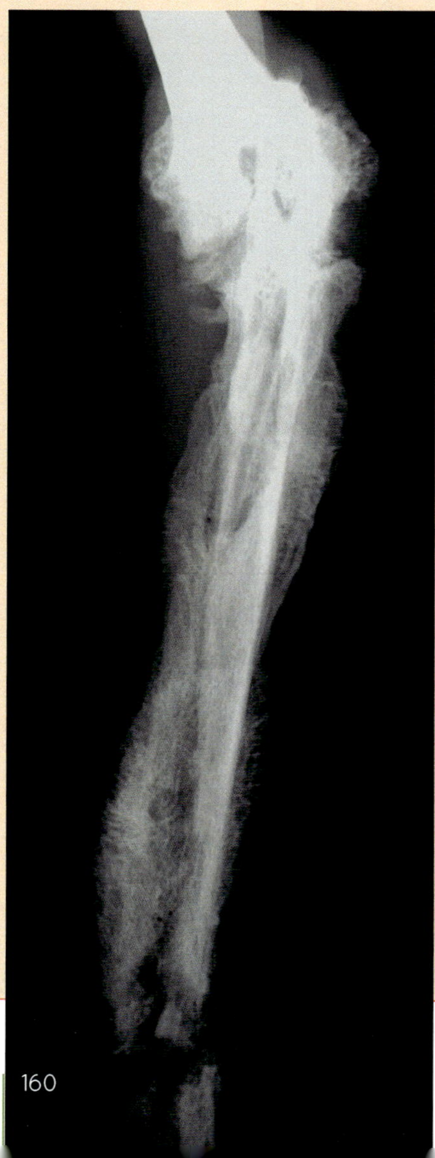

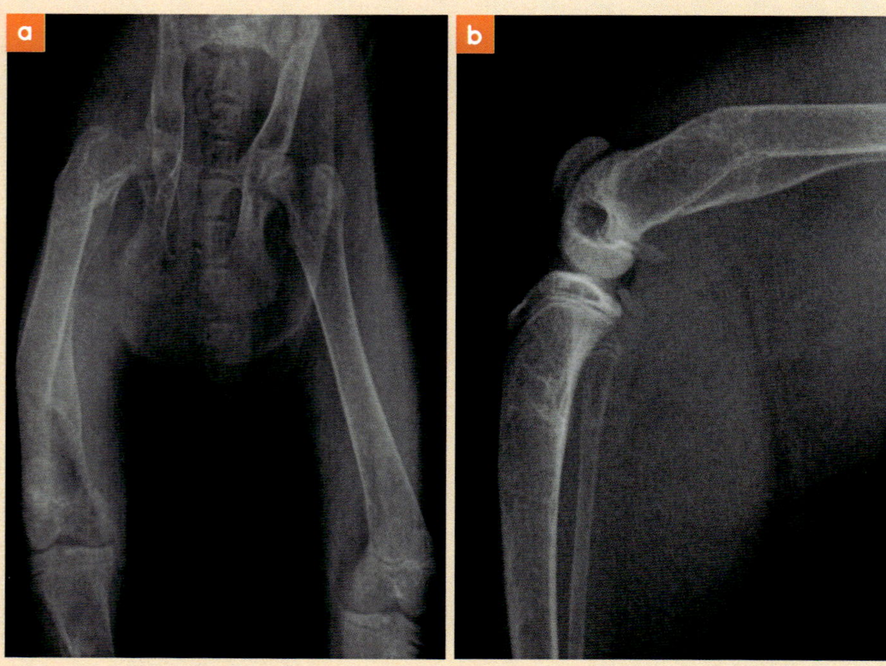

FIGURE 3.37. Ventrodorsal radiograph of the hip (a) and mediolateral radiograph of the knee (b) of a young cat with secondary nutritional hyperparathyroidism. Osteopaenia causes decreased bone radiopacity and thinning of the cortex. The right femur appears deformed by two old pathological fractures (due to osteopaenia) in the proximal third and the distal third of the diaphysis. In these cases, pelvic and vertebral deformity can be frequently observed.

FIGURE 3.36. Craniocaudal radiograph of the radius and ulna of a dog with osteomyelitis that appeared after surgical fracture repair. The radiograph was taken after removing the osteosynthesis material and the fracture remains visible at the distal third of the diaphyses of both bones. Palisading periosteal reaction is observed.

Secondary renal hyperparathyroidism

It appears in animals with chronic renal failure. Reduced glomerular filtration rate causes phosphorous retention, thus reducing blood calcium levels. This stimulates parathyroid hormone production. It usually appears in older dogs, but it can also be detected in young patients with renal dysplasia. The radiographic findings in long bones are similar to those described in secondary nutritional hyperparathyroidism, but the most significant bone changes usually affect the skull (see chapter 5).

Hypophyseal dwarfism

It mostly affects the German Shepherd and it is caused by abnormal growth hormone production (sometimes also with hypothyroidism). Unlike other metabolic or hereditary diseases also causing dwarfism, it causes proportional dwarfism. Radiological signs are:

- Delayed calcification of the epiphyseal ossification centres.
- Delayed closure of growth lines.
- Incomplete epiphysis ossification when the skeletal maturation of the animal concludes.

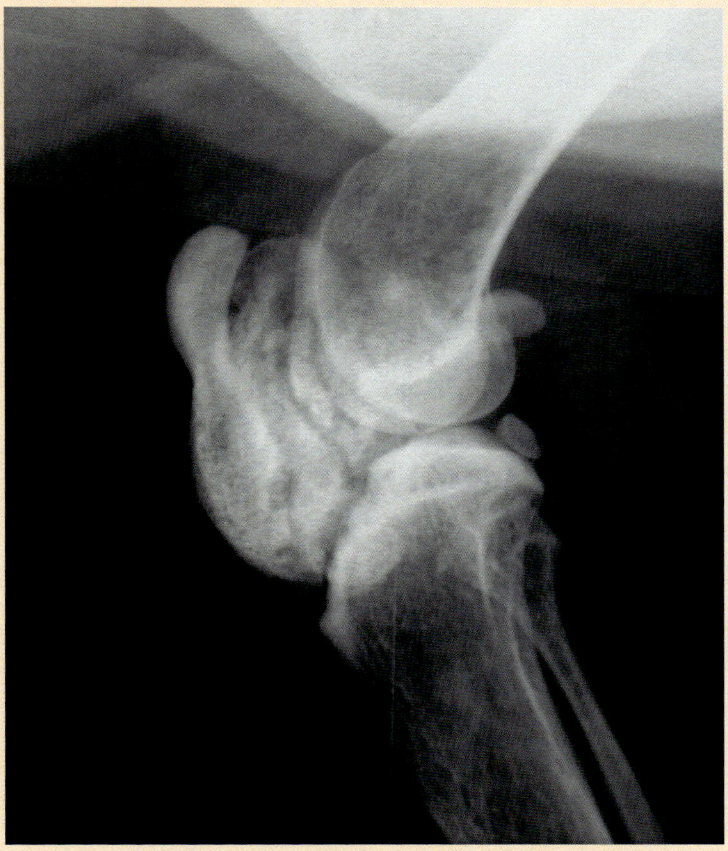

FIGURE 3.38. Mediolateral radiograph of the knee of a cat with hypervitaminosis A. The cat has a localised osteoproliferative lesion on the cranial aspect of the joint. In these cases, similar lesions can be observed in long bone metaphyses and vertebrae.

Normal radiographic anatomy of the **knee**

http://goo.gl/KmOI4v

Hypervitaminosis A

This disease affects cats that ingest excessive amount of vitamin A (usually in liver-based diets). Clinically these animals have spine stiffness, lameness and pain when the neck is being handled. In young animals, delayed development may occur. Radiological signs are:

- Irregular bone growths in long bone metaphyses and around the joints (fig. 3.38).
- Exostosis in vertebrae, usually cervical and thoracic, sometimes causing the spinous processes to fuse.

It is important not to mistake the radiographic image for a neoplasm.

Joint disease

Joints are the regions of the locomotor system where movement takes place. Apart from this dynamic function, they are responsible for the skeleton functioning as an elastic set, and therefore, better prepared to bear pressure and stretching than a rigid block. The bones that integrate joints should keep interrelated in order to fulfil these functions.

Luxations and subluxations

Luxations are the complete loss of the normal congruity between the joint surfaces of two bones (fig. 3.39). When there is still a certain amount of apposition between them, the term subluxation is used (fig. 3.40). Luxations and subluxations are relatively easy to diagnose radiologically, although they are sometimes not evident on one of the orthogonal views. They may be caused by trauma, although they can also have a congenital origin or appear secondarily to developmental abnormalities. The most frequent congenital luxations are those affecting the elbow (fig. 3.41) and the shoulder, although they can affect other joints. They cause marked remodelling of the articular surfaces by degeneration.

Patellar subluxation or luxation can have a traumatic or congenital origin. Congenital subluxation/luxation is more common in small breeds, in which it appears medially and is accompanied by femoral and tibial deformity (they adopt the shape of a 5) (fig. 3.42). In large and giant breeds, congenital patellar luxation or luxation associated with development abnormalities is usually lateral (fig. 3.43).

Degenerative joint disease

The most frequent joint disease is degenerative joint disease, also called **osteoarthritis** or **arthritis**. It can be primary (idiopathic) or secondary to other developmental or acquired diseases. It is radiologically characterised by: synovial fluid leakage (in joints where it can be detected, for example in the knee by partial obliteration of the infrapatellar fat pad); initial widening and further narrowing of the joint space; subchondral bone sclerosis; and periarticular osteophyte formation (fig. 3.44).

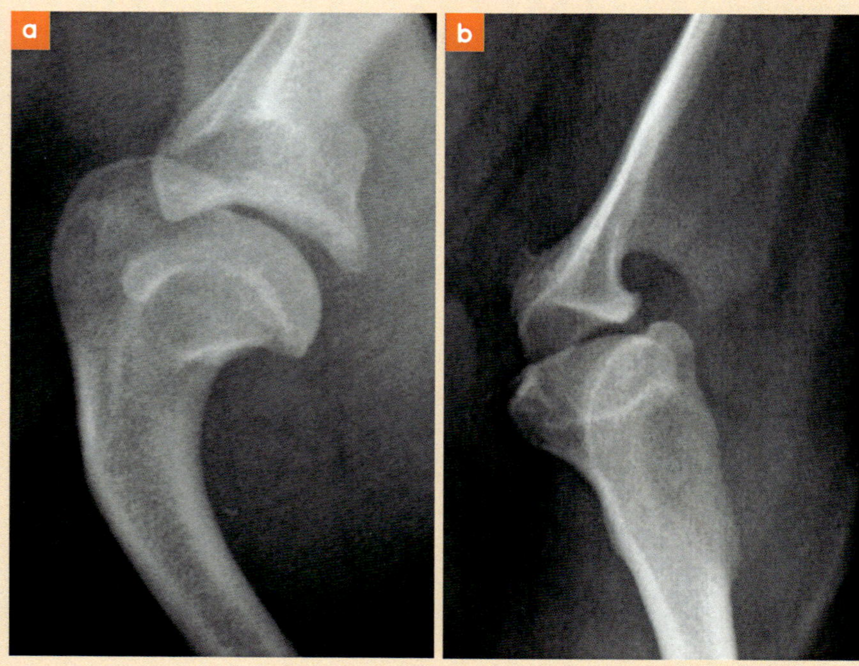

FIGURE 3.40. Mediolateral (a) and craniocaudal (b) radiographs of the elbow of a dog with scapulohumeral subluxation.

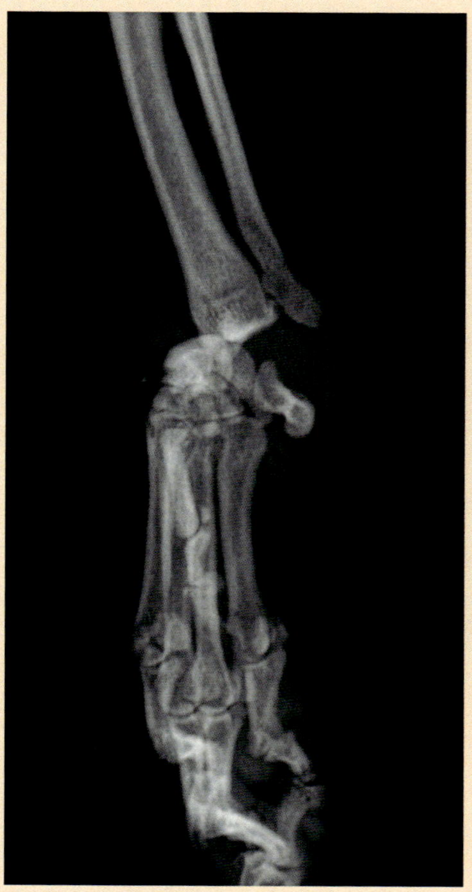

FIGURE 3.39. Mediolateral radiograph of the carpus of a dog with antebrachiocarpal joint luxation.

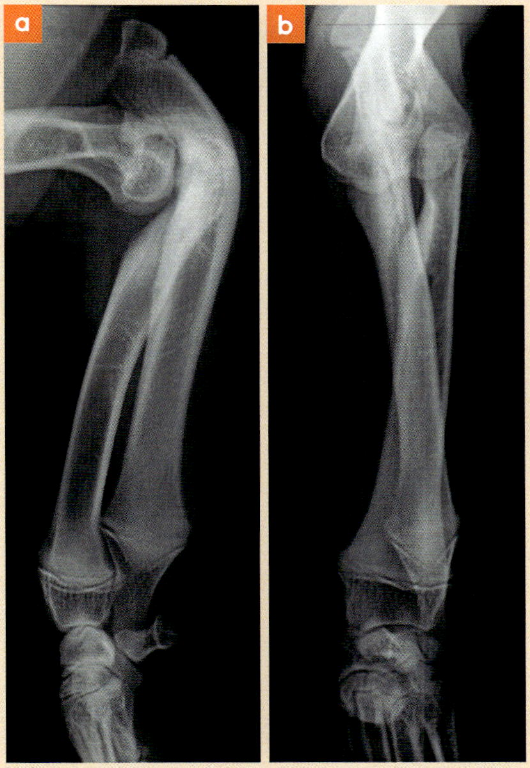

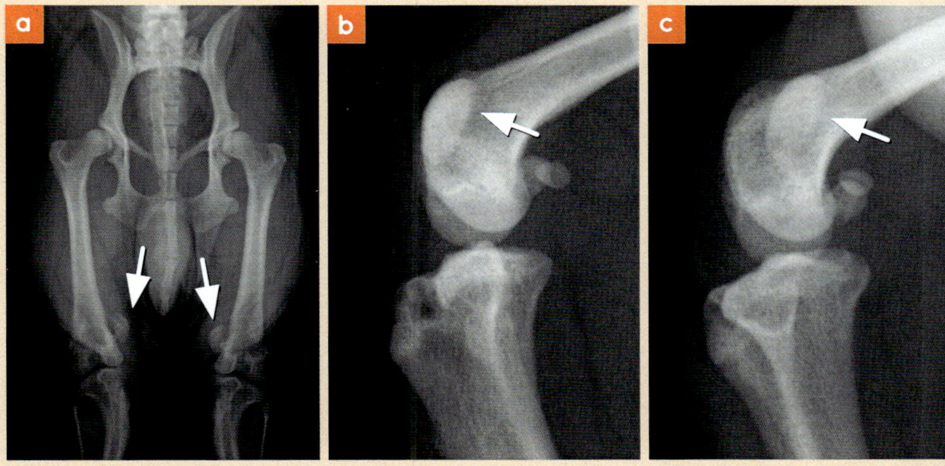

FIGURE 3.42. Ventrodorsal radiograph of the hip (a) and mediolateral radiograph of the left (b) and right knees (c) of a dog with bilateral medial patellar luxation (arrows). In image (a), the tibia looks curved medially. In images (b) and (c) the patella looks superimposed on the distal femur.

◀ FIGURE 3.41. Mediolateral (a) and craniocaudal (b) radiographs of the radius and ulna of a dog with congenital luxation of the elbow. The proximal part of radius and ulna is very deformed and normal alignment between the humerus and the radial head is lost.

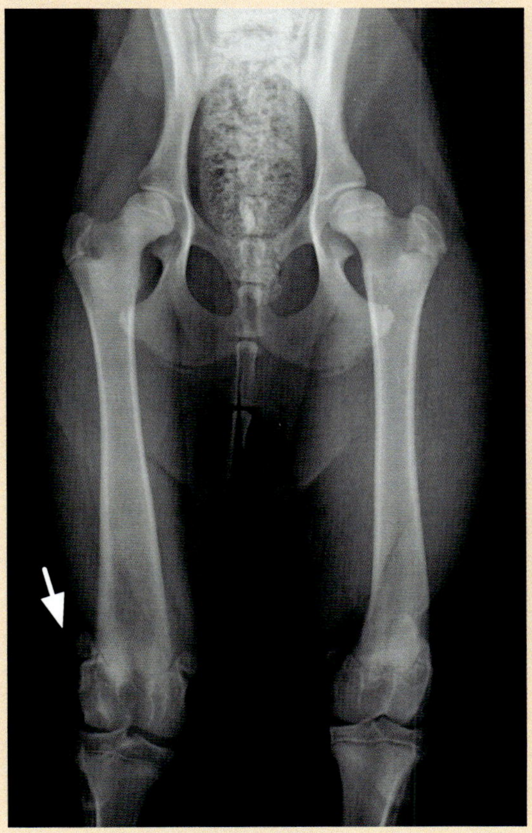

FIGURE 3.43. Ventrodorsal radiograph of the hip of a dog with lateral right patellar luxation.

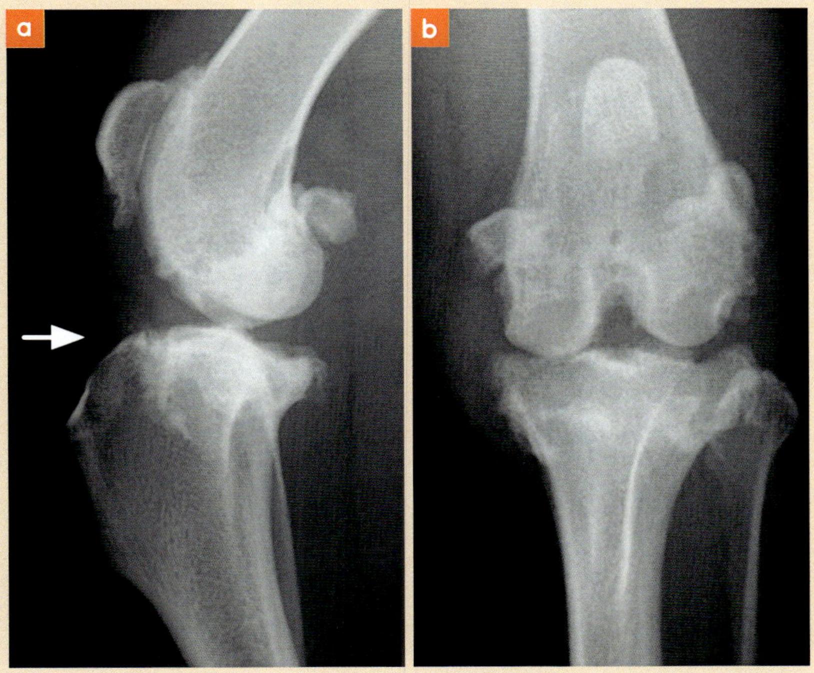

FIGURE 3.44. Mediolateral (a) and craniocaudal (b) radiographs of the knee of a dog with severe degenerative joint disease. Osteophytes and enthesophytes appear at the femoral trochlea, along the distal and proximal patellar margins, on the sesamoid bones in the gastrocnemius and popliteus muscles, on the tibial plate, and on the lateral edges of the lateral condyles and medial edges of the medial femoral and tibial condyles. The presence of synovial fluid leakage can be assessed on the mediolateral radiograph based on the degree of obliteration (narrowing) of the infrapatellar fat pad. In this case, it appears much reduced (arrow), which is indicative of a moderate to severe synovial fluid leakage.

Normal radiographic anatomy of the **carpus**

http://goo.gl/QOYeGC

Infection

Septic arthritis may appear as a consequence of penetrating wounds affecting the joint, although they are also spread haematogenously. In the latter, one or several joints may be affected. Although the image could be mistaken for severe arthritis, the associated soft-tissue inflammation is normally higher. Subchondral bone defects may appear and periarticular osteophytes usually have a more aggressive appearance (fig. 3.45). Secondarily, infection can spread to the bone.

Immune-mediated polyarthropathy

The term refers to the set of joint diseases with an immune-mediated origin. They are classified as erosive and non-erosive. It typically affects multiple joints, thus the term polyarthropathy. When inflammation of multiple joints is observed, haematogenous septic arthritis or immune-mediated polyarthropathy must be considered in the differential diagnosis.

Inflammation of soft tissues and synovial fluid leakage (when it is detectable in the joints) are usually observed on radiographs in **non-erosive immune-mediated polyarthropathy**, with no apparent bone abnormalities (fig. 3.46).

Erosive immune-mediated polyarthropathy is less frequent. In addition to the changes described in

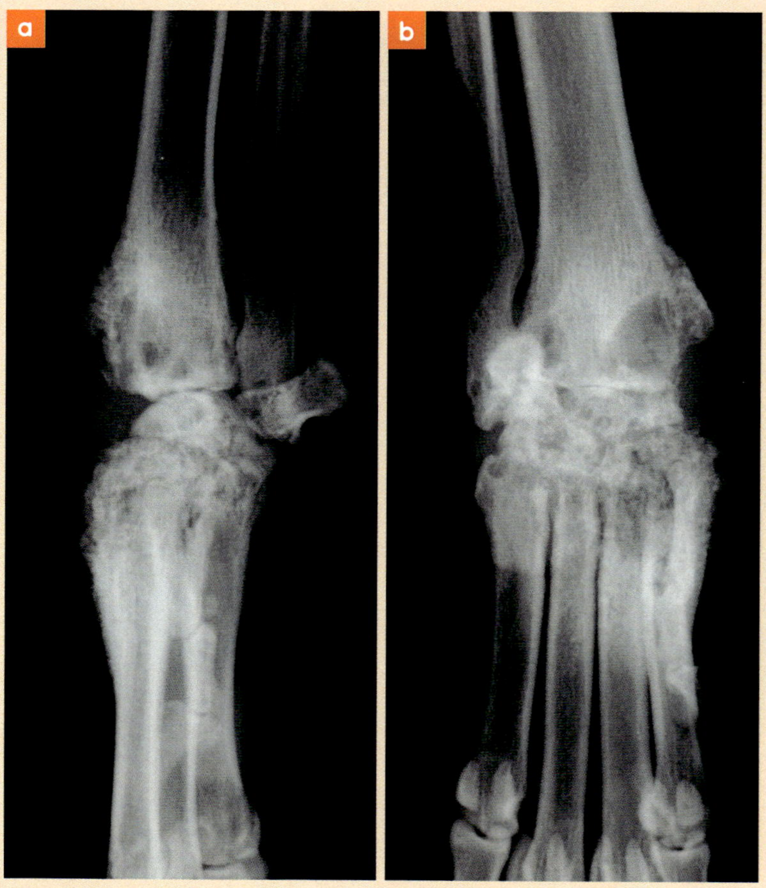

FIGURE 3.45. Mediolateral (a) and dorsopalmar (b) radiographs of the carpus of a dog with septic arthritis. Numerous osteolytic areas appear on the joint surfaces of every bone forming the joint. Periarticular osteophytes look more aggressive than those caused by degenerative joint disease.

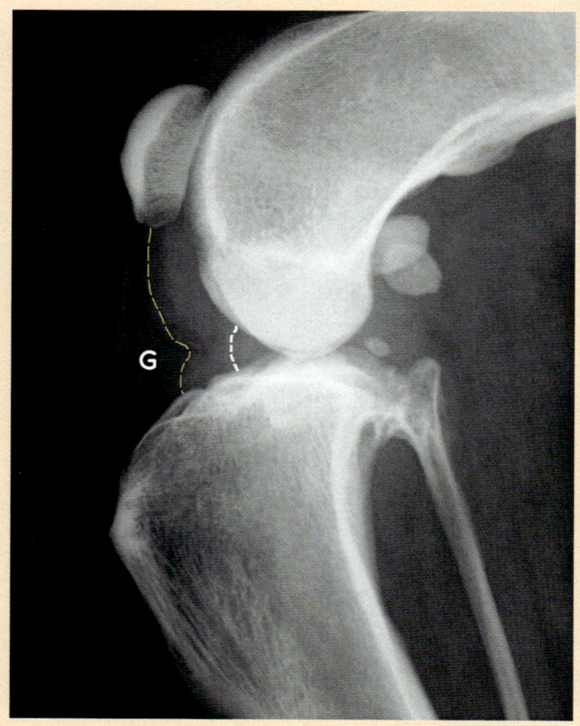

FIGURE 3.46. Mediolateral radiographs of the knee of a dog with non-erosive immune-mediated polyarthropathy. Signs of moderate synovial fluid leakage are observed, not accompanied by evident alteration in the bones that make up the joint. In the knee, synovial fluid leakage is assessed based on the degree of obliteration of the infrapatellar fat pad (G). The white dotted line shows the normal limit of synovial fluid and the yellow dotted line shows this patient's limit, which is easy to identify by the contrast between the fluid (soft tissue opacity) and the infrapatellar fat pad (fat opacity).

the non-erosive form, joint edge erosion is observed (fig. 3.47) and in many cases, aggressive periosteal reaction. The most common type of erosive polyarthropathy in the dog is rheumatoid arthritis. However, it is rare in dogs and cats. It usually affects the distal joints of small and miniature breed dogs. In cats, the most striking radiographic finding is periosteal reaction and it has only been described in young male cats.

Joint tumours

Joint neoplasms are not frequent. They usually cause marked soft tissue inflammation, widening of the medial joint by soft tissue proliferation and marked erosion of the joint margins and subchondral bone, with well-defined osteolysis areas (fig. 3.48).

Other appendicular skeleton abnormalities

Pulmonary hypertrophic osteopathy

It is also called Marie's disease, hypertrophic osteopathy or pulmonary hypertrophic osteoarthropathy. This disease is usually associated with the presence of lesions in the thorax (generally masses), although it has also been described linked to abdominal diseases. It is clinically characterised by affecting older dogs, that present with hot and painful inflammation of the distal limb area, as well as lameness. The first affected bones are the phalanges. If the primary cause is resolved, it is a reversible process.

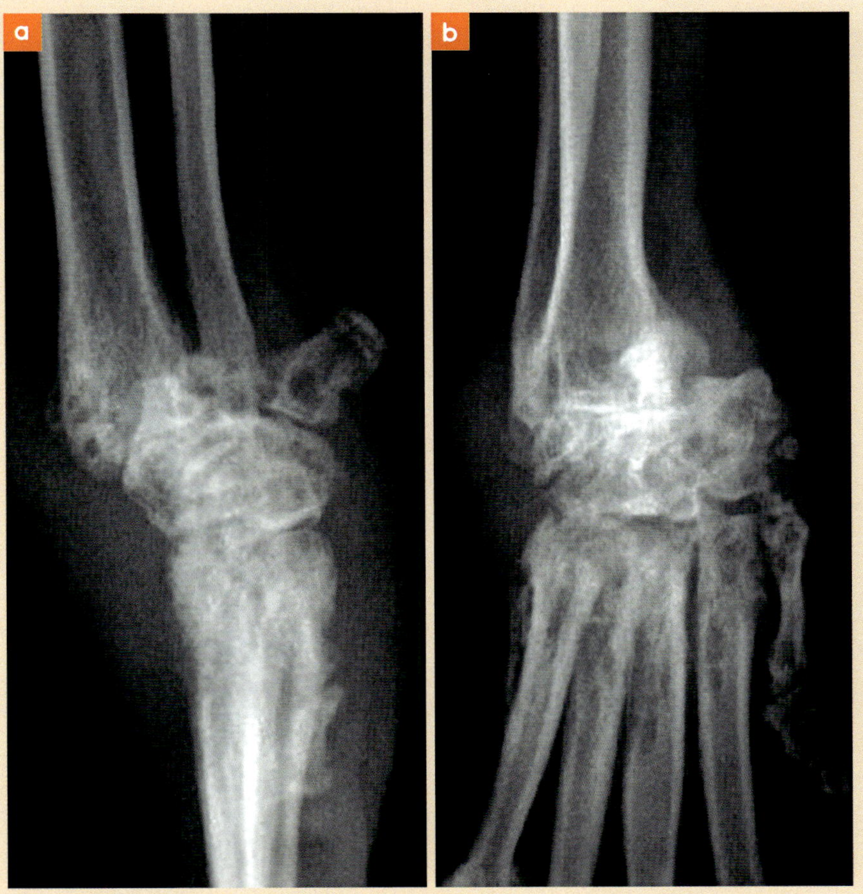

FIGURE 3.47. Mediolateral (a) and dorsopalmar (b) radiographs of the carpus of a dog with erosive immune-mediated polyarthropathy. Marked tumescence of the soft tissues surrounding the joint is observed, as well as osteolytic lesions (erosive) in the joint surfaces of all bones that make up the joint, extending even to the metacarpal diaphysis.

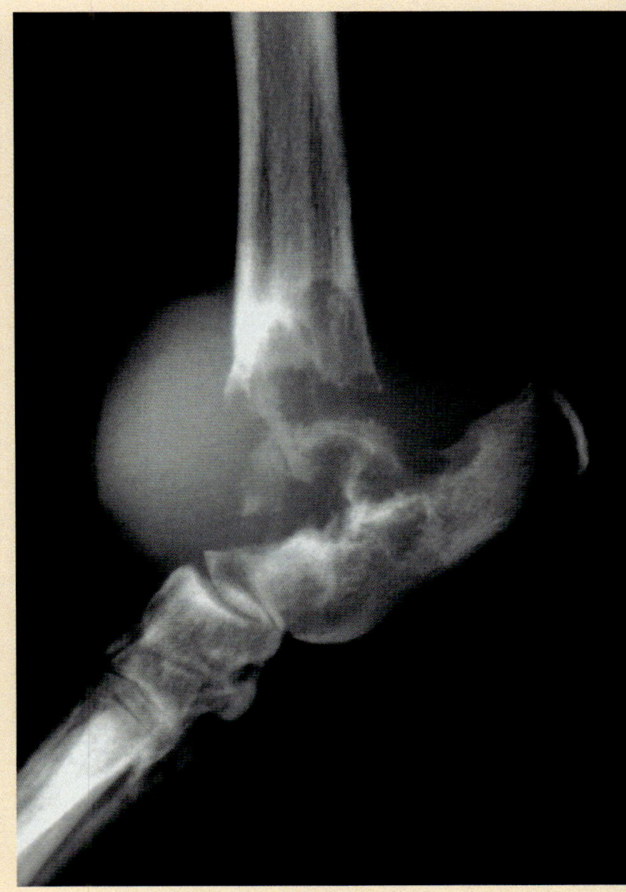

FIGURE 3.48. Mediolateral radiograph of the tarsus of a dog with a joint neoplasm. Marked soft tissue tumescence is observed, as well as great destruction (osteolysis) of the joint edges.

Normal radiographic anatomy of the **metacarpals and phalanges**

http://goo.gl/15uLT9

Self-assessment cases

http://goo.gl/1tpZJd

Radiographic signs are (fig. 3.49):

- Palisading periosteal reaction.
- Initial lesions tend to be distal and may affect the four limbs.
- Lesions may be bilaterally symmetrical.
- Marked soft-tissue inflammation.

To evaluate the presence of possible lesions in both anatomical regions, thoracic and abdominal radiographs should always be taken.

Circumscribed calcinosis

It presents as ectopic calcification foci in soft tissues, generally periarticularly located (fig. 3.50). It usually affects young large breed dogs, especially the German Shepherd.

Multiple cartilaginous exostoses

It is an benign osteoproliferative disease that appears in growing dogs. Exostoses in long bone metaphyses, vertebrae and ribs are evident on radiographs. It usually does not have clinical significance, unless the lesions cause excessive compression of certain anatomical structures such as the spinal cord, but this is rare. Lesions cease to grow when skeletal maturation of the animal concludes. Exceptionally, cases of affected adults and continued growth of the lesions after skeletal maturation have been described.

A similar disorder has been described in cats, although it may be of viral origin. Lesions appear in adult cats and they grow progressively. They are similar to those caused by hypervitaminosis A.

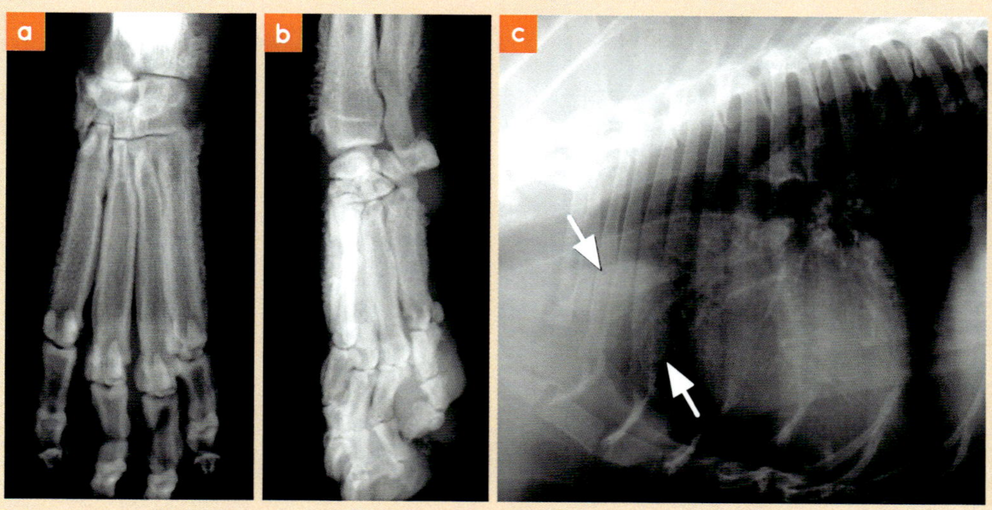

FIGURE 3.49. Dorsopalmar (a) and mediolateral (b) radiographs of the carpus, metacarpals and phalanges, as well as lateral thoracic radiograph (c) of a dog with pulmonary hypertrophic osteopathy (Marie's disease) and a pulmonary neoplasm. Palisading periosteal reaction is observed in the long bones (radius, ulna, metacarpals and phalanges). Pulmonary hypertrophic osteopathy is usually associated with mass-type thoracic and abdominal lesions, in this case a pulmonary mass.

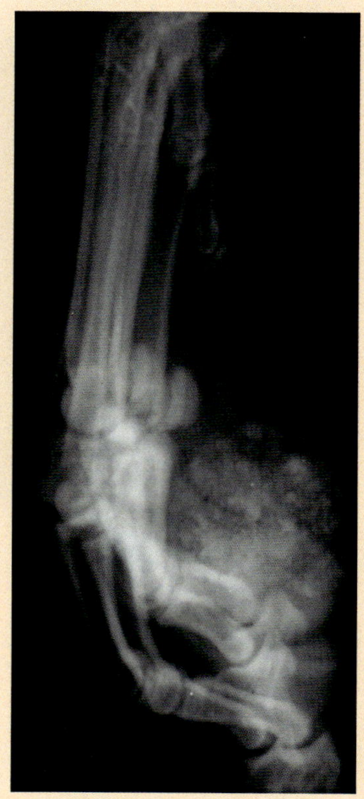

FIGURE 3.50. Mediolateral radiograph of the metacarpals and phalanges of a dog with circumscribed calcinosis. A lesion formed by calcification foci is observed in the palmar area of the hand. It is a benign lesion that is usually periarticularly located and it is more frequent in young dogs, especially in German Shepherds.

Spine

4

Principles of interpretation

Both dogs and cats have 7 cervical vertebrae, 13 thoracic vertebrae, 7 lumbar vertebrae, 3 sacral vertebrae and a variable number of coccygeal vertebrae. Each anatomical region of the spine has different characteristics, and it is necessary to know them in order to interpret radiographs correctly. These are described in the following boxes.

Good-quality images are essential to carry out a thorough assessment of the spine. That is why it is recommended to take radiographs under sedation, using appropriate positioning accessories (radiolucent blocks, tape and sand bags).

In lateral projection, the longitudinal axis of the spine has to be parallel to the cassette, which is achieved by

Thoracic spine

- T11 is the anticlinal vertebra (its spinous process is vertical instead of being directed caudally or cranially).
- T10-T11 is the anticlinal intervertebral space, which is the narrowest intervertebral space.
- The heads of the ribs appear cranial to their corresponding vertebrae.

Cervical spine

- C1 has a large transverse process (wings of the atlas).
- C2 is the largest vertebra and has a process in the cranioventral area of its body, called the odontoid process, or dens.
- The C2-C3 and C7-T1 intervertebral disc spaces are usually narrower than the rest.
- C6 has a large, characteristic ventral lamina.
- The spinous process of C2 must be adjacent to or superimposed on the arch of C1.

Lumbar spine

- The cat's lumbar vertebrae are longer than those of the dog.
- The ventral border of L3 and L4 can appear slightly blurry in dogs, especially in large breeds, which is due to the crura of the diaphragm being superimposed (this image should not be confused with that of a lesion).

Sacrum and coccygeal vertebrae

- The three vertebrae that form the sacrum are usually fused.
- Coccygeal vertebrae have haemal processes, which should not be confused with spondylosis deformans.

Normal radiographic anatomy of the **cervical spine**

http://goo.gl/ys5mNu

placing a radiolucent block under the cervical area and another one under the lumbar area (fig. 4.1). To ensure that the sagittal plane of the vertebrae is parallel to the cassette, it is necessary to place blocks in order to slightly elevate the position of the limbs. If the spine is twisted when taking a lateral radiograph, the transverse processes of each vertebra will be separated in the image (fig. 4.2).

Lateral rotation of the spine should be avoided when taking a radiograph in ventrodorsal projection. If the position of the patient is correct, the spinous processes will be aligned and centred with the vertebral bodies in the image (fig. 4.3).

A complete study of the spine should include two cervical radiographs (one centred on C3-C4 and another one on C6-C7), a thoracic radiograph (centred on T6-T7) and a thoracolumbar radiograph (centred on T13-L1). Usually, the previous clinical assessment of the patient allows the location of the region or regions of the spine that may be injured, which narrows the radiographic study down to the affected area.

Spinal radiographs taken in forced flexion or extension may be useful for the diagnosis of certain diseases, such as atlantoaxial, cervical or lumbosacral instability. However, they should always be taken after standard radiographs in a neutral position. If these radiographs show an abnormal position of the vertebrae, radiographs in forced positions will not be recommended, since they can cause serious compressive lesions of the spinal cord. We should also always handle the patient very carefully when a fracture of luxation of the spine is suspected, since we could worsen the clinical picture.

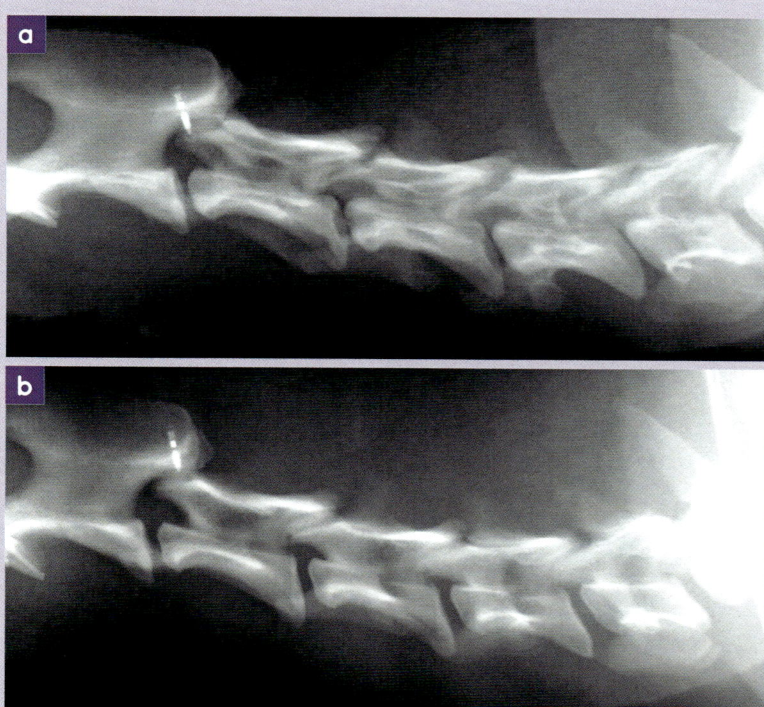

FIGURE 4.1. Poorly positioned lateral radiograph of the cervical spine of a dog (a) and lateral radiograph of the same region with correct positioning (b), after placing a radiolucent block under the neck so the longitudinal axis is parallel to the cassette. In the first radiograph, it is not possible to assess the intervertebral disc spaces in an appropriate way, since the X-ray beam penetrates obliquely through them.

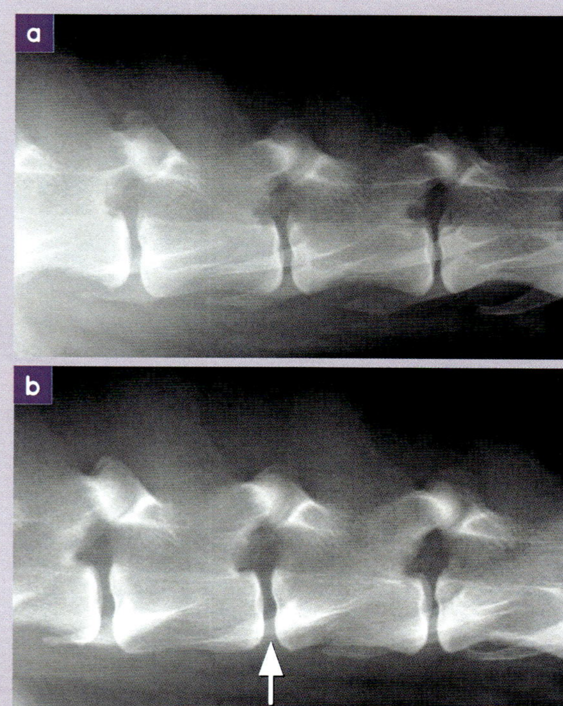

FIGURE 4.2. Enlarged images of the lumbar region of a dog, obtained in lateral projection, before (a) and after (b) placing a positioning block that slightly elevates the position of the limbs, so the sagittal plane of the vertebrae is parallel to the cassette. The perfect superimposition of the transverse processes of each vertebra (arrow) indicates that the radiograph was taken correctly.

Myelography

Myelography is the contrast technique most frequently used to assess the spine (fig. 4.4). It is based on the introduction of a contrast medium in the subarachnoid space. As it involves certain risks, it should be carried out only when considered absolutely necessary, generally when the choice of surgical treatment depends on the results of this test. Magnetic resonance imaging is an excellent alternative.

Myelograms must be performed under general anaesthesia. Before administering the contrast medium, it is necessary take plain radiographs with correct positioning. The contrast media of choice are low-osmolarity, nonionic iodinated contrast agents, such as iohexol or iopamidol, since they are less neurotoxic and remain longer in diagnostic concentrations in the subarachnoid space than other water-soluble agents. They are used at concentrations from 200 to 350 mg I/ml (the higher the concentration of iodine, the better defined the contrast columns will be in the images) and at doses of 0.3 ml/kg or 50 mg I/kg. The administered volume depends on the size of the animal and on the region that is going to be examined:

- **Small dogs and cats** (1-5 kg): 1.5-2 ml.
- **Medium-size dogs** (5-15 kg): 1.5-3 ml.
- **Large dogs** (15-35 kg): 3-5 ml.
- **Giant breed dogs** (+ 35 kg): 8-9 ml maximum.

The contrast medium may be introduced in the cisterna magna or in the lumbar area. Spinal needles are used for this purpose (25-mm needles for cats and

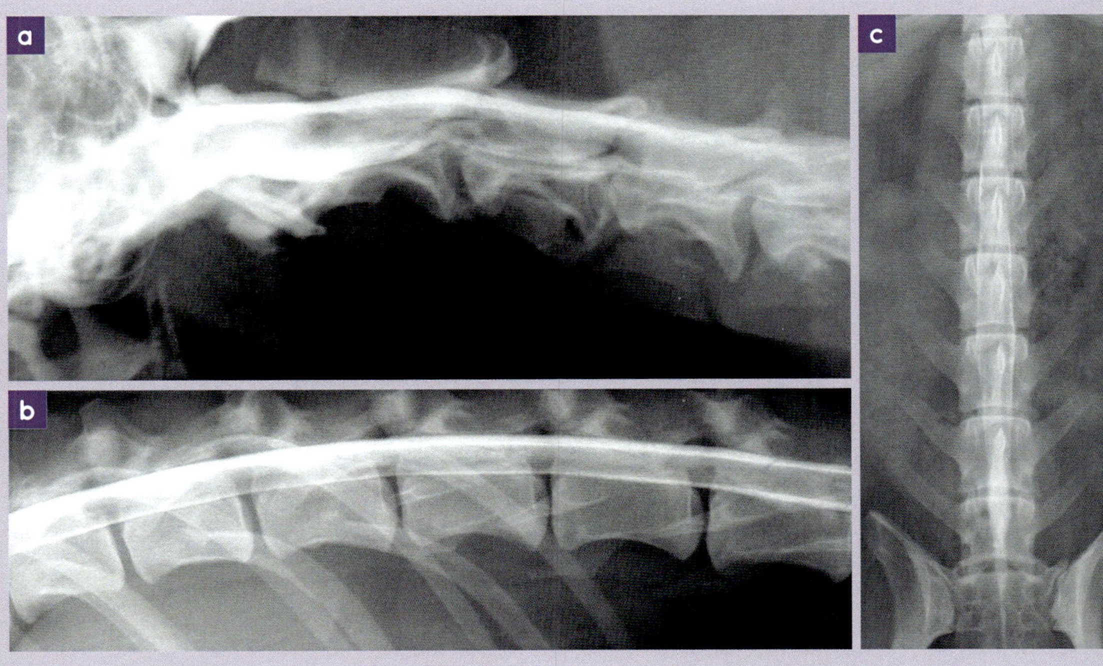

FIGURE 4.4. Usual myelographic pattern of the cervical region in lateral projection (a), thoracolumbar region in lateral projection (b) and lumbar region in ventrodorsal projection (c).

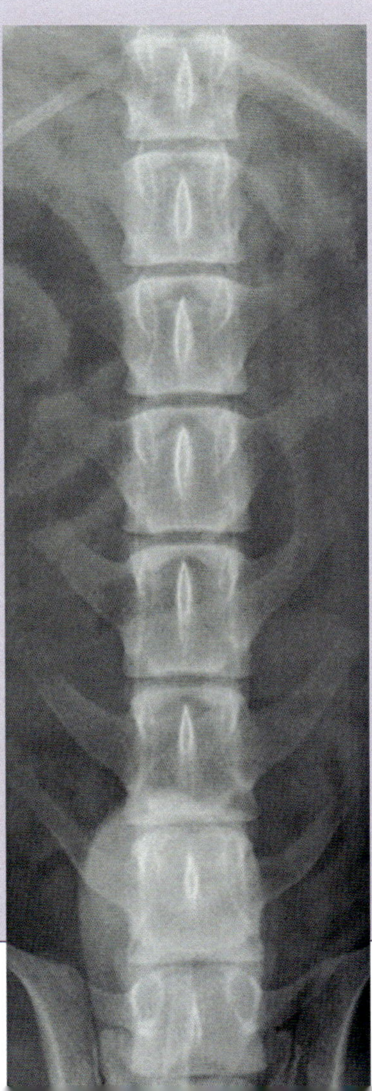

FIGURE 4.3. Ventrodorsal radiograph of the lumbar spine in a dog. The centred position of the spinous processes with respect to the vertebral bodies indicates that the radiograph was taken correctly.

small dogs, 40-mm needles for medium-size dogs and 75-90-mm needles for large dogs) and maximum asepsis should be maintained when performing the injection.

In order to perform a cisternal injection (cisternal myelography), the patient should be placed in lateral recumbency and its head bent at a 90-degree angle with respect to the neck. It is important to make sure this movement does not cause the obstruction of the airways. If the table can be inclined, it should be tilted 15 degrees upwards approximately. Alternatively, radiolucent positioning blocks may be used to elevate the patient's head and neck. The technique is described in the box below.

It is recommended to allow an amount of cerebrospinal fluid similar to the volume of contrast medium that is going to be injected to flow out and analyse a sample. The injection of the contrast medium is performed slowly, in 2 to 3 minutes approximately. If the head has not previously been elevated, it is indispensable to do it at that moment, to ensure that the contrast material flows caudally and does not leak into the cerebral ventricles. If resistance is felt when administering the contrast medium, the injection should be stopped and the needle withdrawn.

If there is a compression site, the contrast column may fail to pass beyond the lesion, in which case it is not possible to determine the real extension of the area of compression.

In lumbar myelography, the contrast medium is injected in the subarachnoid space in the lumbar area. It is more difficult to perform and more traumatic, since the needle is inserted into the spinal cord. Two advantages of this technique are that the lumbar and thoracic areas are properly filled and that, in many cases, the contrast material can reach sites located cranial to an area of compression. The technique is described in the box below.

The injection of a contrast medium in the spinal cord may be lethal (severe paresis or paralysis in lumbar injections cranial to L4-L5, or death of the animal in cisternal injections). If the contrast medium is injected in the epidural space, the contrast columns will be very irregular and difficult to analyse.

Although it would be recommended to inject the contrast agent as close as possible to the area where

Puncture technique for cisternal myelography

In order to carry out the puncture, the depression between the external occipital protuberance and the dorsal lamina of the atlas should be palpated. The needle is inserted in the median line of this depression, at a slight angle in cranial direction and slowly moving forward. The bevel should be directed caudally. It is possible to feel some degree of resistance when going through the nuchal ligament. If the needle is positioned correctly, cerebrospinal fluid (CSF) will flow out. If blood flows out together with CSF, it is usual to carry on with the procedure. However, if only blood flows out, the needle must be removed and the injection should be attempted again with a new needle. In case of piercing through the bone, the needle should be redirected.

Puncture technique for lumbar myelography

In order to carry out a lumbar myelogram, the animal is placed in sternal recumbency, with the spine arched. This is achieved by extending the hind limbs forward. The spinal needle is inserted in the L5-L6 disc space in dogs and in the L6-L7 disc space in cats. The needle is moved forward, going through the spinal cord, until reaching the floor of the canal. The bevel of the needle should be directed cranially. When reaching the floor of the canal, the needle is removed slightly and the introducer needle is withdrawn. If CSF flows out, this indicates that the needle has correctly been placed. If no CSF flows out, the position of the needle may be checked by taking a radiograph or by means of fluoroscopy. An additional check can be made by introducing a small amount of contrast and examining its position in a radiographic image.

Attempting to enter in the dorsal subarachnoid space without going through the spinal cord is possible, by frequently removing the introducer needle to check if CSF flows out, but this is not easy.

the lesion is suspected to be located, the simplest and safest technique is cisternal myelography, which helps to determine the area of most lesions.

The subarachnoid space is larger in the cisterna magna. The spinal cord has a larger diameter in the cervical-thoracic region and in the central area of the lumbar region. The ventral column often appears slightly elevated at the intervertebral disc spaces, which should not be confused with spinal cord compression.

It should be borne in mind that the contrast medium is progressively absorbed, and will therefore no longer be evident in the image after approximately 50 minutes.

An **extradural lesion** causes the contrast column to be elevated or displaced at the site of compression. This is accompanied by a narrowing of the opposite column (fig. 4.5). This type of lesions includes herniated discs, thickening of the dorsal longitudinal ligament, thickening of the ligamentum flavum, haematomas, epidural fat deposits, deformations of the vertebral body, luxations, vertebral subluxations and fractures, cervical or lumboscral spondylopathy and abscesses, granulomas and extradural tumours.

An **intradural-extramedullary lesion** causes focal enlargement of the subarachnoid space (fig. 4.6). This type of lesions includes intradural tumours (e.g. neurofibroma, meningioma), as well as haemorrhages, oedema or intradural granulomas.

An **intramedullary lesion** causes divergence of the contrast columns at the site of the lesion (fig. 4.7).

Normal radiographic anatomy of the **thoracic spine**

http://goo.gl/JVcZYS

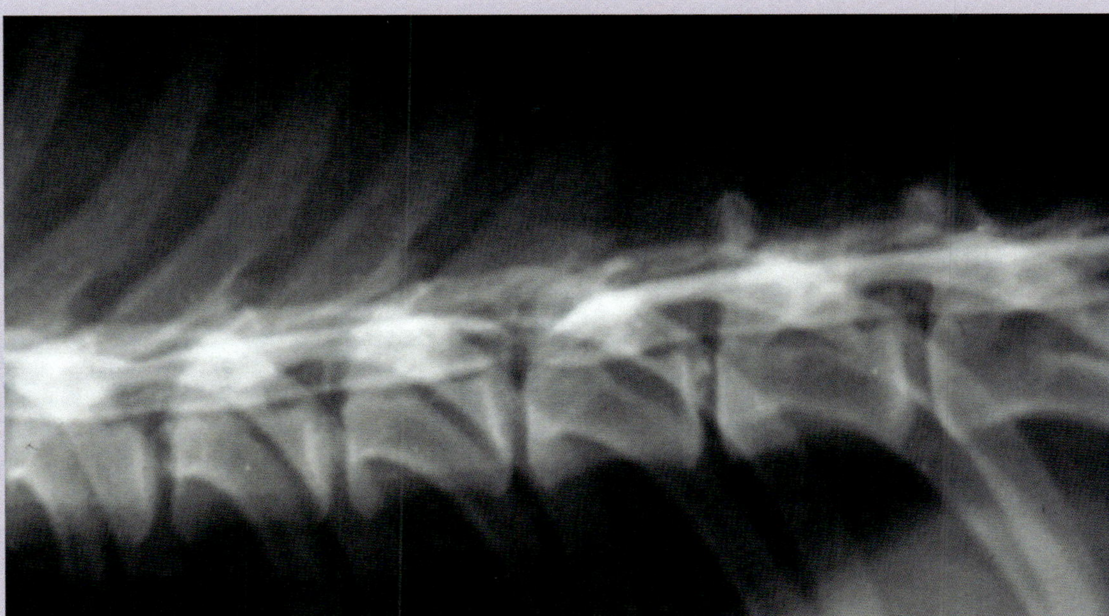

FIGURE 4.5. Myelographic pattern of an extradural lesion.

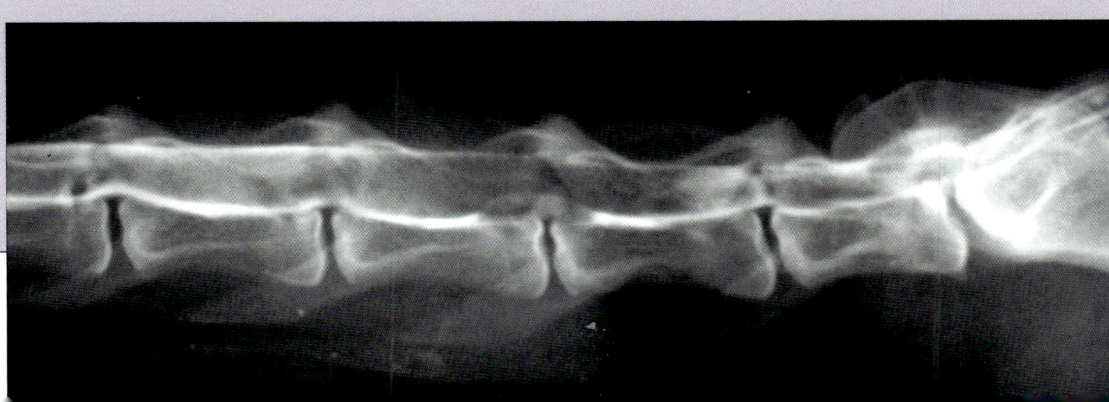

FIGURE 4.6. Myelographic pattern of an intradural-extramedullary lesion. The contrast medium surrounds the lesion located in the subarachnoid space.

There may be an interruption of the contrast column at the site of the lesion, cranial to the lesion in a cisternal myelogram, or caudal to the lesion in a lumbar myelogram. This type of lesions includes intramedullary tumours (e.g. ependymoma, astrocytoma), intramedullary haemorrhage or oedema, hydromyelia, syringomyelia and granulomatous meningoencepahlitis.

Other contrast techniques may be used to examine the spine instead of myelography, but their application is much more limited. Epidurography involves introducing the contrast medium (intentionally, not by mistake) in the epidural space, generally at the sacrococcygeal junction. It has been recommended for the detection of lesions in the cauda equina. The interpretation of the results of this technique is often difficult. Discography involves introducing a contrast medium in the intervertebral disc space, but is hardly used in cats and dogs.

Computed tomography offers excellent images of the bones that form the spine, but it is not as good as magnetic resonance imaging for the definition of its soft tissues.

Congenital disorders

Hemivertebra

It is due to an incomplete development of the vertebral body. It may affect one or several vertebrae. Hemivertebrae may have a butterfly shape on ventrodorsal radiographs (fig. 4.8) or a "wedge" shape on lateral or ventrodorsal radiographs (fig. 4.9). Compensatory morphological changes in the adjacent vertebrae can usually be observed.

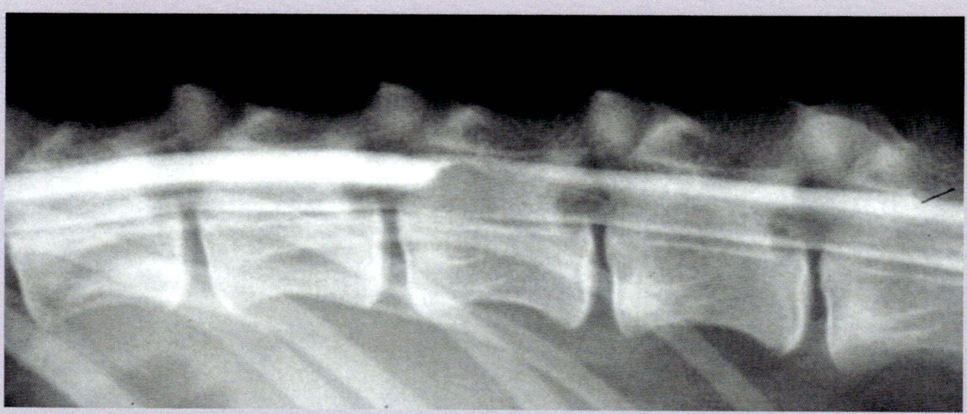

FIGURE 4.7. Myelographic pattern of an intramedullary lesion. The width of the contrast columns decreases around the spinal cord lesion. An enlargement of the dorsal contrast column, cranial to the site of the lesion, can be observed.

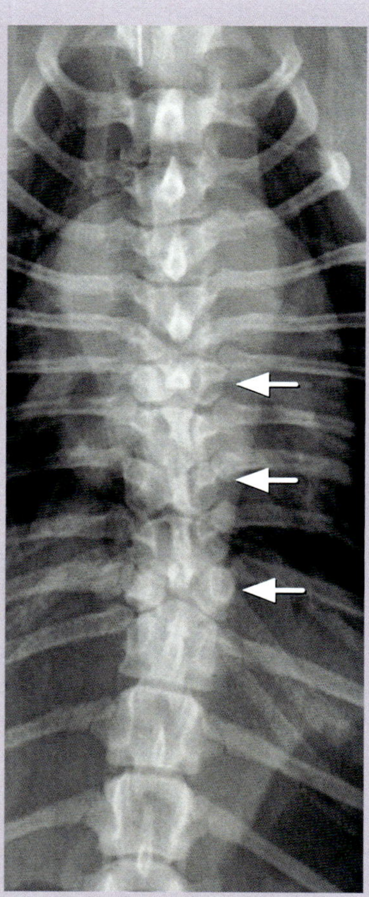

FIGURE 4.8. Ventrodorsal radiograph of the thoracic spine of a Bulldog with several "butterfly" vertebrae (arrows).

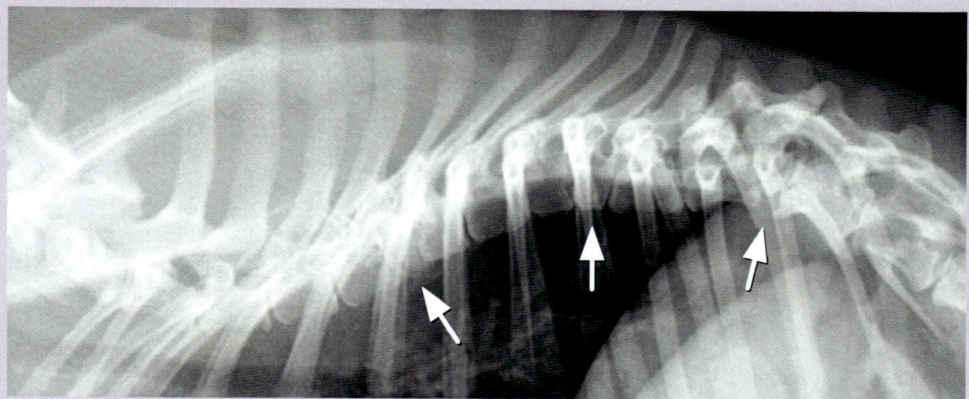

FIGURE 4.9. Lateral radiograph of the thoracic spine of a dog with several "wedge" vertebrae (arrows).

Normal radiographic anatomy of the **lumbosacral spine**

http://goo.gl/dV0lox

Hemivertebrae generally appear in the thoracic spine and are usually associated with kyphosis (dorsal displacement of the spine). They occasionally become clinically significant when they cause spinal cord compression, which can be assessed by means of myelography or advanced techniques (magnetic resonance imaging –fig. 4.10.– or computed tomographic myelography).

Block vertebra

Two or more adjacent vertebral bodies appear partially or totally fused, with no intervertebral disc (fig. 4.11). This generally has no clinical significance.

Transitional vertebra

This occurs when the vertebrae of the atlantoaxial, cervical-thoracic, thoracolumbar, lumbosacral or sacroccygeal junction have morphological characteristics of the vertebrae of both regions (they totally or partially have the shape of the previous or next vertebra):

- Lumbarisation: the S1 vertebra appears separated from the rest of the sacrum, and may have one or two transverse processes, similar to those of the lumbar vertebrae.
- Sacralisation: the transverse process of L7 is fused with the wing of the sacrum and may articulate with the ilium. This alteration may cause lumbosacral instability and degeneration of the intervertebral disc

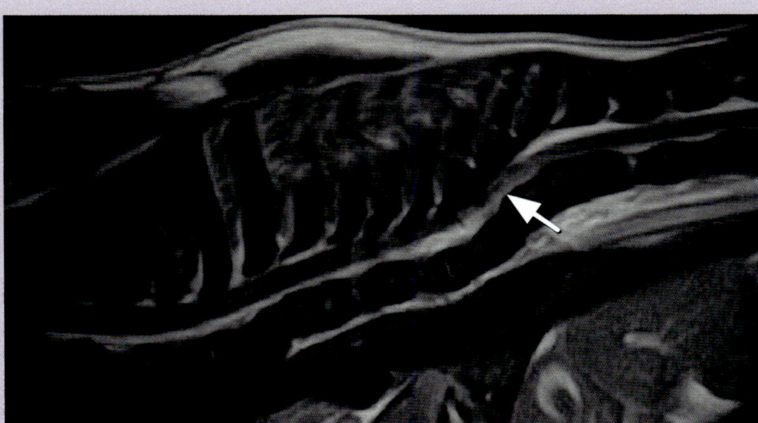

FIGURE 4.10. Magnetic resonance image of the thoracolumbar spine of a dog with multiple vertebral deformations causing angulation of the spinal canal and spinal cord compression (arrow).

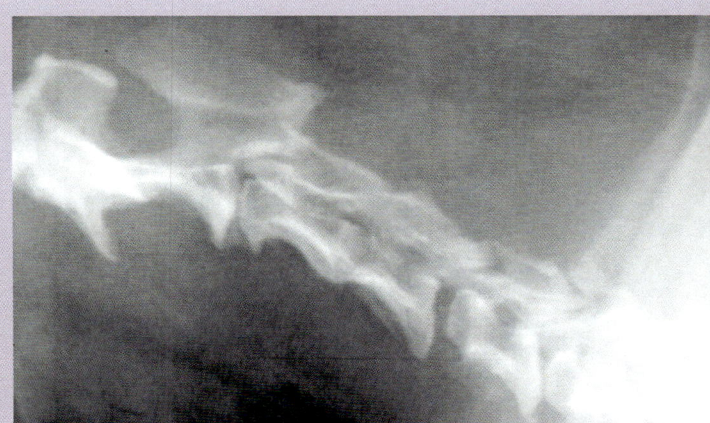

FIGURE 4.11. Lateral radiograph of the cervical spine of a dog whose C3 and C4 are fused (block vertebra).

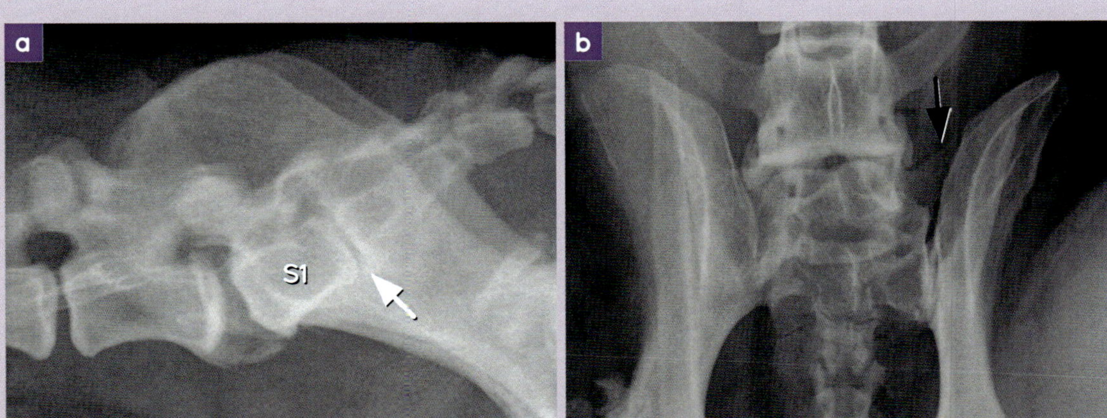

FIGURE 4.12. Lateral (a) and ventrodorsal (b) views of the lumbosacral area of the spine of a dog with lumbarisation of the sacrum. On the lateral view, a radiolucent line (white arrow) can be seen, which separates the S1 vertebra from the rest of the sacrum. On the ventrodorsal view, a transverse process (black arrow) can be identified on S1. Spondylosis at L7-S1 can be observed on both radiographs.

Normal radiographic anatomy of the **cervical spine**

http://goo.gl/ys5mNu

(fig. 4.13), leading to cauda equina syndrome. It may also make the correct positioning of the animal more difficult when taking a ventrodorsal radiograph of the hip.

- Partial or complete fusion of S3 with Cc1.
- A T13 transitional vertebra may have a transverse process instead of the rib (fig. 4.14). Vestigial ribs may be observed, and appear as structures with mineral density in soft tissues. This variation is relatively frequent. Therefore, when planning a spine surgery, it is recommended to always take radiographs in the two projections, since an image in lateral projection could lead to an error when locating the exact vertebra or intervertebral disc space.
- A transitional L1 vertebra may have a rib instead of a transverse process.
- A transitional C7 vertebra may have a rib instead of a transverse process.
- Occipitalisation of the atlas.

Morphological changes may be unilateral or bilateral and, except for those affecting the lumbosacral junction, they do not usually have any clinical significance.

Spina bifida

It is a very uncommon anomaly. It is due to a failure in the closure of the neural arch and may affect one or more vertebrae. It can be associated with a protrusion of the meninges through the defect. It is best viewed on ventrodorsal radiographs. If there is a failure in the fusion of the spinous processes, the image will show a double spinous process in the affected vertebrae. In mild cases, the patient may not display any clinical signs.

Instability syndromes

They are associated with congenital anomalies that may worsen with growth, or with acquired lesions secondary to instability. They affect three anatomical regions: atlantoaxial, cervical and lumbosacral.

Atlantoaxial instability

Atlantoaxial instability or subluxation usually appears as a congenital anomaly in small and miniature breeds, such as Yorkshire Terriers, Chihuahuas, Pomeranians or Poodles. It may be due to agenesis or hypoplasia of the odontoid process, to a lack of fusion of this process with the axis, or to a stretching or rupture of the ligament holding it.

It can also appear in other breeds, and is generally associated with an injury that has caused a fracture of the process or a lesion of the ligament.

On lateral radiographs, an increase in the distance between the dorsal arch of the atlas and the spinous process of the axis can be observed, accompanied by an angulation of the floor of the spinal canal at the atlantoaxial junction (fig. 4.15). Slightly bending the animal's neck can help identify these findings, although there is a risk of worsening the patient's clinical picture.

Cervical instability

It is also called Wobbler disease, cervical spondylopathy, caudal cervical spondylomyelopathy or cervical vertebral malformation. It affects large or giant breeds, especially Great Danes and Dobermans, and has also been described in Basset Hounds. The affected animals present with progressive discoordination of the hind limbs and, on occasions, of the forelimbs. The symptoms usually appear between 3 to 10 months of age, although they may also appear at a later age, especially in the Doberman breed.

Various vertebral disorders associated with this syndrome have been described. The vertebrae that seem to be most frequently affected are C5, C6 and C7, although it may also appear in the C2, C3 and C4 vertebrae.

The radiographic signs that may be observed are:

- Alteration in the shape of the affected vertebra or vertebrae.
- Narrowing of the cranial part of the affected vertebra or vertebrae, which gives the spinal canal the aspect of a "funnel" or triangle.
- The cranial articular processes may appear deformed or be absent.
- If there is subluxation (fig 4.16), lateral images obtained with the neck flexed will show the cranial end of

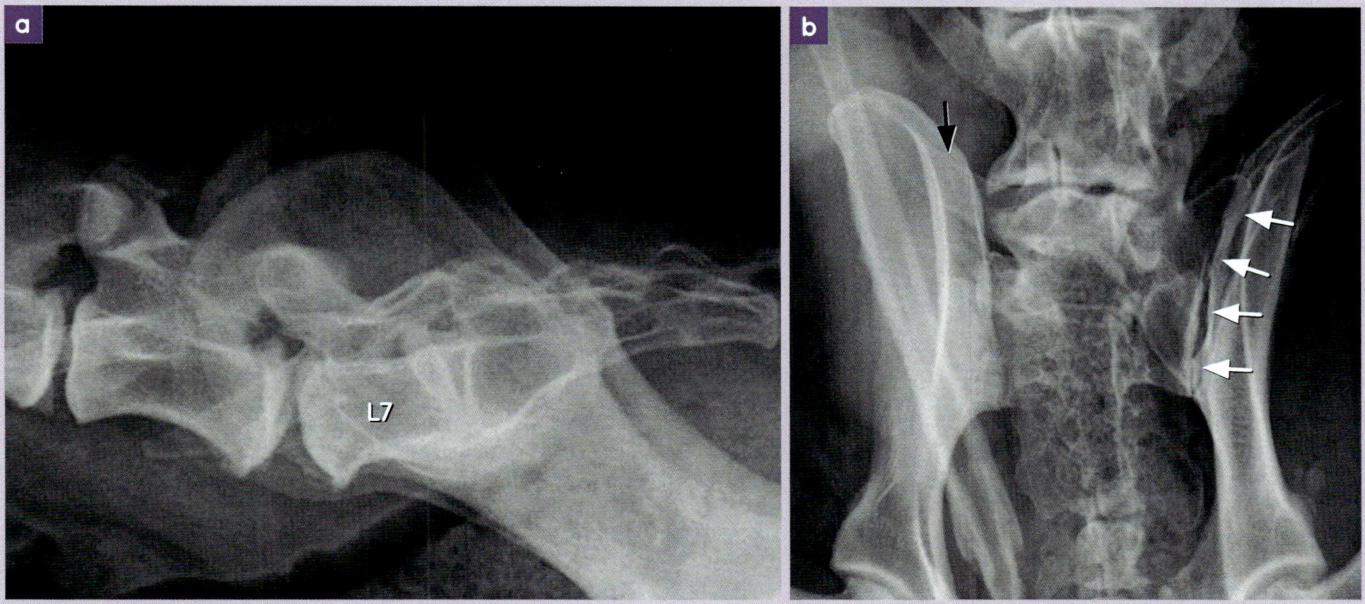

FIGURE 4.13. Lateral (a) and ventrodorsal (b) radiographs of the lumbosacral area of the spine of a dog with sacralisation of L7. On the lateral radiograph, L7 appears shortened. On the ventrodorsal radiograph, a fusion of the left margin of L7 with the sacrum may be observed (white arrows), while in the right side L7 has a transverse process.

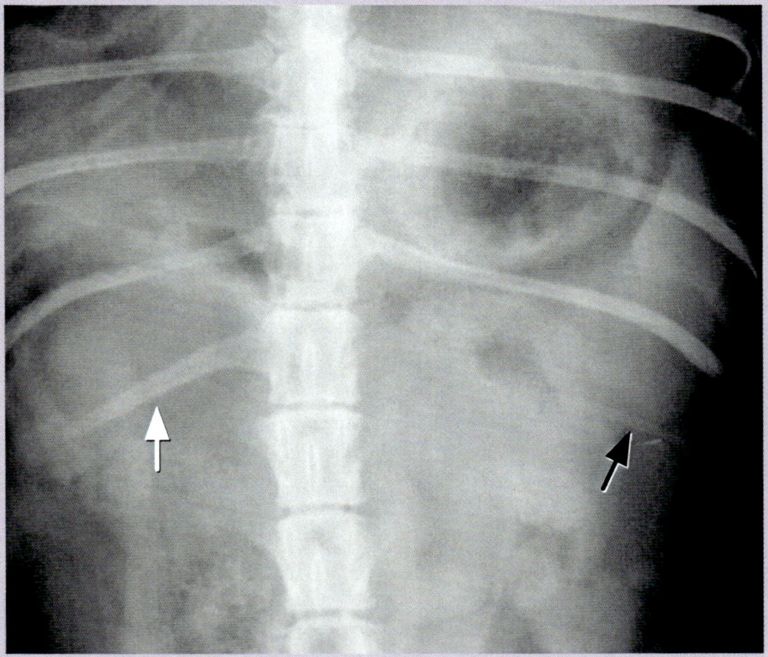

FIGURE 4.14. Ventrodorsal radiograph of the thoracolumbar spine of a dog with transitional T13. This vertebra has an extended right transverse process (white arrow), and a vestigial rib in the left cranial abdomen can be observed (black arrow).

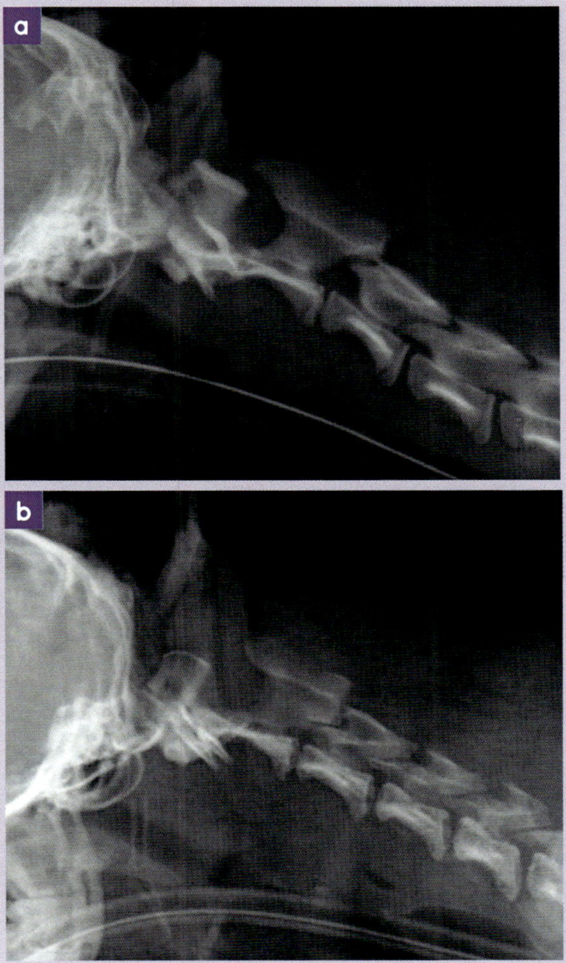

FIGURE 4.15. Enlarged image of the cervical spine on a lateral radiograph of a Yorkshire Terrier with no vertebral anomalies (a) and of a dog of the same breed with atlantoaxial subluxation (b).

Normal radiographic anatomy of the **lumbosacral spine**

http://goo.gl/dV0lox

Normal radiographic anatomy of the **coccygeal spine**

http://goo.gl/zrhALG

the affected vertebra protruding dorsally towards the spinal canal. It should be taken into account that, when the neck is flexed, the cranial end of the vertebrae is always raised to some degree, which should not be confused with a pathological subluxation.

- The intervertebral disc space cranial to the affected vertebra may be enlarged and the affected discs may be calcified.
- There may be new bone formation and sclerosis of the end-plates of the vertebral bodies.
- The myelogram may show spinal cord compression. This should not be confused with the normal image obtained with the neck flexed, in which a certain degree of elevation of the contrast column is observed in the areas located on the intervertebral disc spaces.
- Ventral compression indicates a prolapsed disc or hypertrophy of the dorsal longitudinal ligament, while dorsal compression indicates hypertrophy of the ligamentum flavum.

On occasions, taking radiographs in flexion, extension or with cervical traction can show subluxations that were not detected in a neutral position. These lesions are termed dynamic lesions. In the case of adynamic lesions, there are no differences with the image obtained in neutral position. The movements of the neck should be carried out carefully so as not to worsen the clinical status of the animal.

Lumbosacral instability

It is also called lumbosacral stenosis, lumbosacral malformation or cauda equina syndrome. It is characterised by the presence of a narrowing of the spinal canal or of the intervertebral foramina, which causes a compression of the nerves that form the cauda equina. It may be congenital or acquired in origin, and generally affects large breed dogs, especially German Shepherds. It may also appear in cats.

The most frequently observed radiographic findings associated with this anomaly are of the degenerative type: spondylosis deformans and sclerosis of the caudal end of L7 and of the cranial end of the sacrum (fig. 4.17). It is sometimes possible to observe a reduction of the L7-S1 intervertebral disc space, a reduction of the dorsoventral diameter of the spinal canal at the level of L7 or of the sacrum and/or a central displacement of the sacrum with respect to the position of L7 (fig. 4.18). This latter finding may be constant or inconstant, and may appear alone, or become more noticeable when a radiograph is taken in hyperflexion or hyperextension.

There is no direct correlation between the clinical signs and the radiological findings. In fact, some patients with symptoms show a normal image of the lumbosacral junction on plain radiographs while many patients with radiographic evidence of L7-S1 spondylosis do not present with any clinical signs. Myelography or epidurography may help in the diagnosis, although magnetic resonance imaging is the most appropriate technique for the assessment of this disease (fig. 4.19).

Degenerative intervertebral disc disease

Each disc is formed by an annulus fibrosus (fibrous ring) and a nucleus pulposus. This latter is composed of a homogeneous gelatinous material. The annulus fibrosus is much thicker in its ventral part than in its dorsal part (this is why ventral protrusions are rare, and would not affect the spinal cord in any case). Discs are covered dorsally by the longitudinal ligament, which runs through the floor of the spinal canal. This ligament is reinforced by other ligaments in the area between T1 and T10, so herniated discs in this area are rare.

The most appropriate projection to examine intervertebral disc spaces (IVDS) is the lateral one.

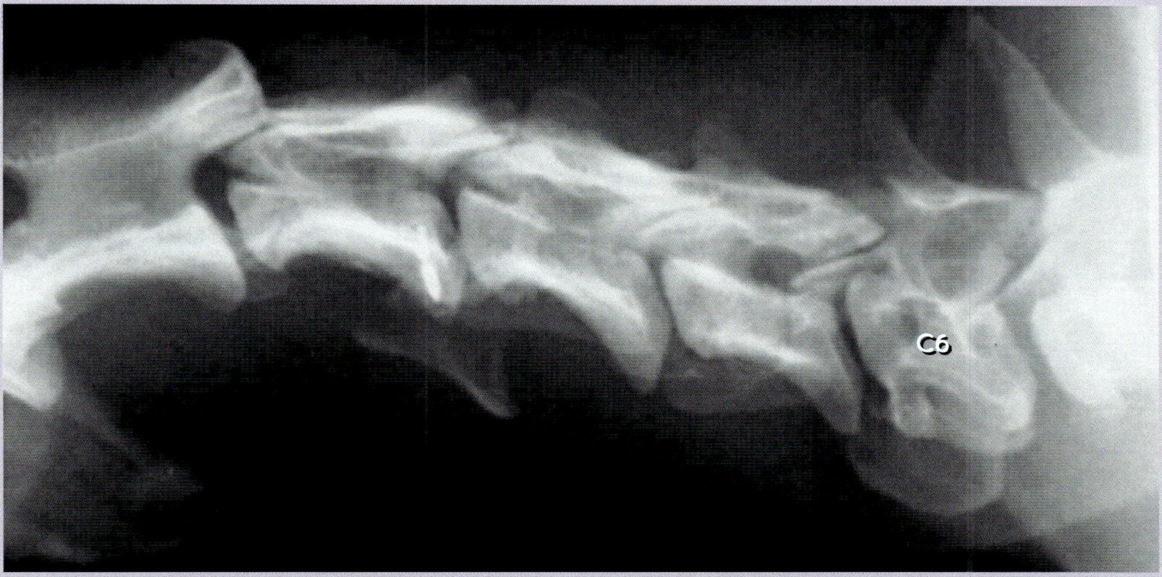

FIGURE 4.16. Lateral radiograph of the cervical spine of a Great Dane with Wobbler disease. The C6 vertebra is subluxated, which causes a marked narrowing of the spinal canal in this area.

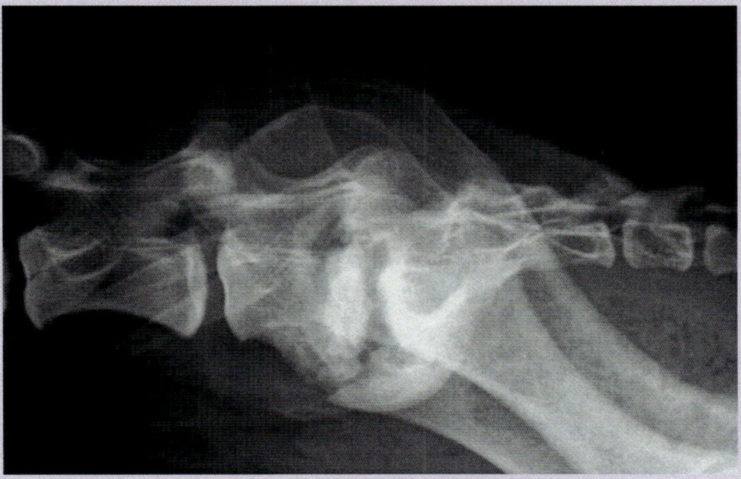

FIGURE 4.17. Lateral radiograph of the lumbosacral area of the spine of a dog with spondylosis deformans at L7-S1 and sclerosis of the caudal end of L7 and of the cranial end of the sacrum. These findings of a degenerative nature indicate lumbosacral instability.

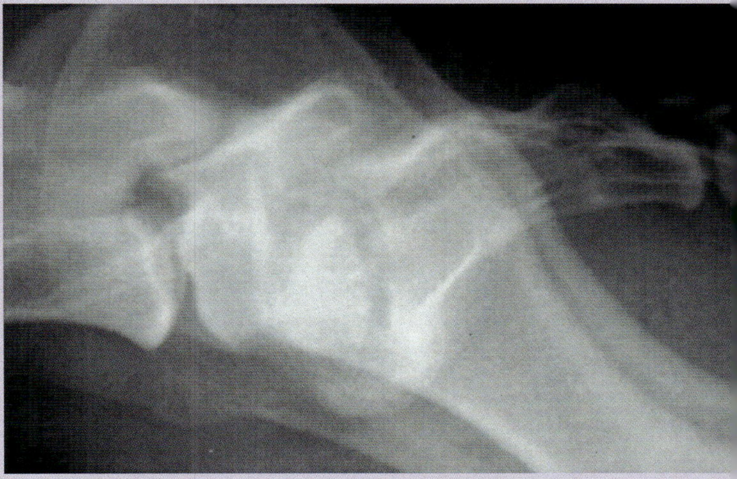

FIGURE 4.18. Lateral radiograph of the lumbosacral area of the spine of a dog with ventral displacement of the sacrum with respect to L7, reduction of the L7-S1 intervertebral disc space and spondylosis deformans at L7-S1. These findings indicate lumbosacral instability.

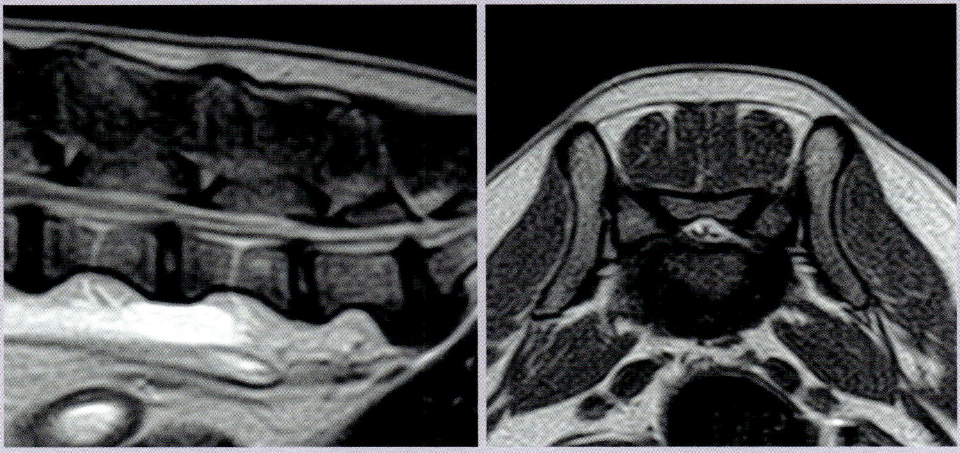

FIGURE 4.19. Magnetic resonance images in sagittal and transverse plane of the L7-S1 disc in a dog with lumbosacral instability. The images show degenerative changes and protrusion of the disc, which causes a compression of the cauda equina.

Radiolucent positioning blocks should be placed under the cervical and lumbar spine, in order to try to make the spine parallel (not curved) to the cassette. The obliquity of the peripheral X-rays of the beam makes it necessary to centre the radiograph appropriately on the IVDS where a lesion is suspected (fig. 4.20). On each radiograph, it is only possible to assess the centred IVDS and the spaces immediately cranial and caudal to it. If the area that we are going to examine is wider, several radiographs should be taken, centring the images on different sites.

The IVDS at the cervicothoracic junction and at the lumbosacral junction are slightly narrower than the others. The IVDS located between T10 and T11 may also be slightly narrower in normal conditions. If no radiolucent positioning blocks are placed under the cervical or lumbar spine, the width of the IVDS may appear falsely reduced, due to the curvature of the spine.

Disc degeneration is a phenomenon related with age. Problems occur when the degeneration process is faster than usual. Two types of degeneration are distinguished:

- **Hansen type I:** it is generally observed in chondrodystrophic breeds, in which a degeneration of the nucleus pulposus at early ages is frequently observed (many animals have calcified discs, with no clinical significance). With time, the annulus fibrosus also degenerates, which can cause its rupture and subsequent bulging out of the nucleus pulposus into the spinal canal, which is called extrusion of the disc material.
- **Hansen type II:** more common in non-chondrodystrophic breeds, in which degenerative changes occur more slowly, and rarely cause calcification. A protrusion of the disc (with no rupture of the annulus fibrosus) usually occurs. The disc moves to a greater or lesser extent towards the spinal canal and may cause different degrees of spinal cord compression.

In cases of type I extrusion, clinical signs appear in an acute manner, with pain, neurological deficiency and paralysis. In cases of type II protrusion, the clinical picture is less dramatic, and progressive ataxia and neurological deficiency are usually observed.

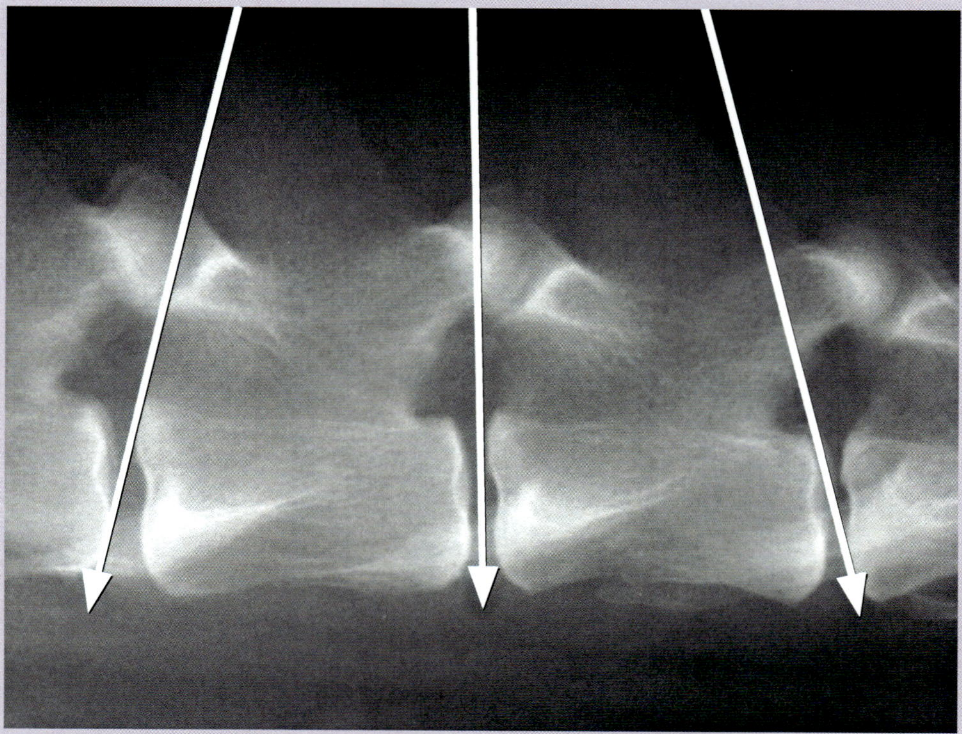

FIGURE 4.20. Representation of the direction of entry of the X-ray beam through the intervertebral spaces. Since the X-ray beam is divergent, only the central rays of the beam are aligned with the intervertebral disc space on the radiograph. The farther the spaces are from the centre of the beam, the more oblique the direction of entry of the X-rays in the other intervertebral disc spaces will be.

The radiological signs that may appear in degenerative intervertebral disc disease are:

- Disc calcification (more frequent in chondrodystrophic breeds). This finding alone is not diagnostic of disc prolapse, but does indicate its degeneration (fig. 4.21).
- Narrowing of the affected IVDS (fig. 4.22).
- Observation of calcified disc material in the spinal canal (fig 4.23). It is also sometimes possible to identify non-calcified disc material when this is located in the area of the intervertebral foramen.
- Appearance of a pattern of ventral or ventrolateral extradural lesion on the myelogram.

The radiological signs should always correlate with the clinical symptoms, although the finding of spinal cord compression on the myelogram is always significant. An acute protrusion of the disc may be accompanied by a normal image in plain radiographs. Old lesions may not have any clinical significance, and may be accompanied by sclerosis of the end-plates of the adjacent vertebral bodies and spondylosis deformans (fig. 4.24).

Other disorders of the spine

Scoliosis, kyphosis and lordosis

Scoliosis is defined as an abnormal curvature of the spine in lateral direction, and is therefore best visualised on ventrodorsal radiographs (fig. 4.25). Kyphosis is defined as an anbormal curvature of the spine in dorsal direction (fig. 4.26), while lordosis occurs in ventral direction (fig. 4.27). These are therefore best observed on lateral radiographs.

These disorders may be congenital, idiopathic or may appear associated with other diseases affecting the spine. They do not usually have clinical significance.

Spondylosis deformans

It is a degenerative alteration, characterised by the development of bony growths in the ventral area of the cranial and/or caudal end-plates of the vertebral bodies (fig. 4.28). These formations tend to increase in size and even to fuse with the adjacent vertebrae, thus forming true bone bridges (fig. 4.29). They may also grow

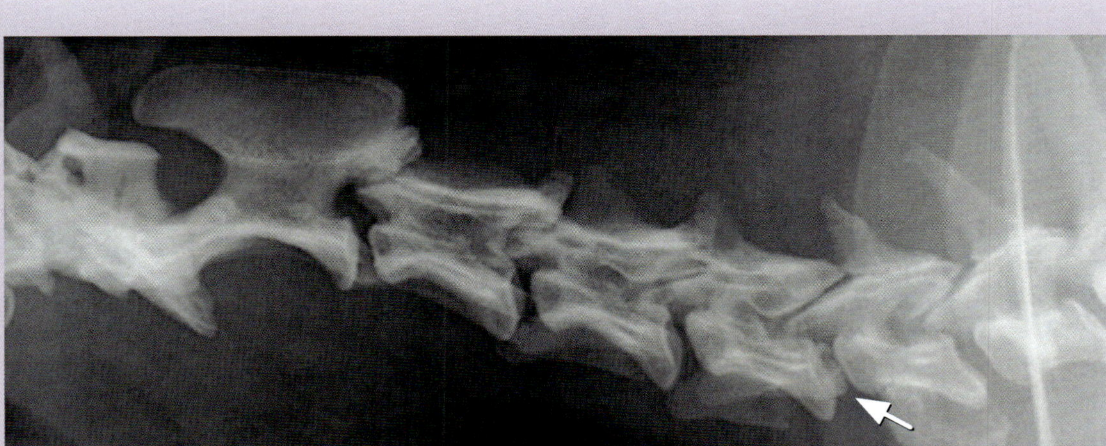

FIGURE 4.21. Lateral radiograph of the cervical spine of a dog with calcification of the C5-C6 intervertebral disc (arrow). Calcification is a finding that indicates disc degeneration.

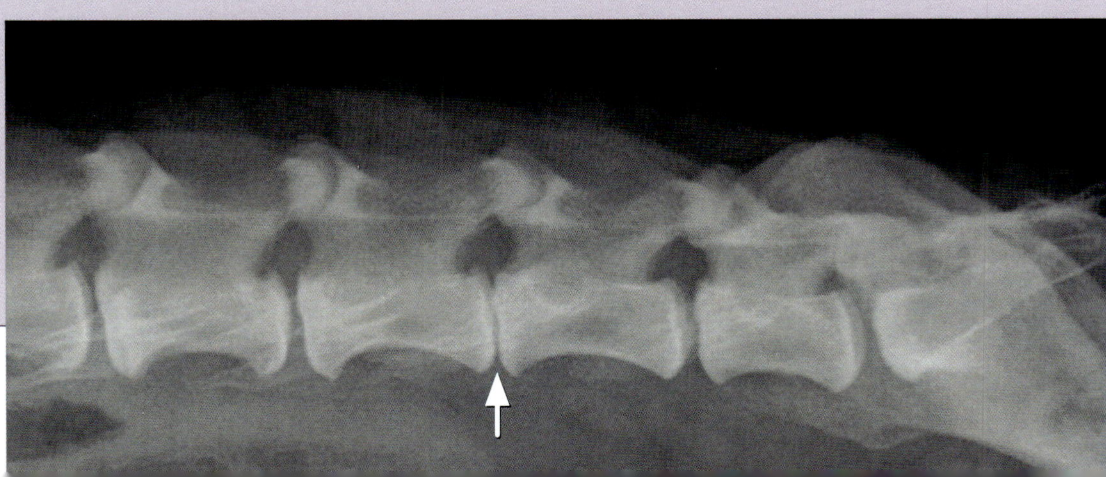

FIGURE 4.22. Lateral radiograph of the lumbar spine of a dog with a narrowing of the L5-L6 intervertebral disc space (arrow), which indicates disc disease.

on the lateral aspect of the end-plates of the vertebrae, but this is less frequent (fig. 4.30).

There are usually no clinical signs, although the lateral overgrowths may exceptionally compress the nerve roots at their exit through the intervertebral foramen.

It may affect wide segments of the spine, especially in Boxers. Large overgrowths may be observed in this breed, even at very early ages (fig. 4.31).

Dural ossification

It is characterised by the formation of bony plaques in the dura mater, which may be visible or not on a plain radiograph. When they are observed, they appear as thin lines of mineral density running parallel to the floor of the spinal canal (fig. 4.32). They usually have no clinical significance.

Spondyloarthrosis (degenerative joint disease)

It occurs in the intervertebral joints. A deformation of the joint facets due to the formation of osteophytes is generally observed (fig. 4.33). It is observed more frequently in the lumbar region and occasionally, in the cervical region.

Inflammation and infection

The inflammation of the vertebrae is called spondylitis, and may be accompanied or not by an infection. It usually causes new bone formation in the ventral area of the body of the affected vertebra or vertebrae (fig. 4.34). It is important to remember that the ventral margin of L3 and L4 may appear poorly defined due to the crura of the diaphragm being superimposed. This should not be confused with spondylitis.

Vertebral infection is termed osteomyelitis or spondylopyosis. It is characterised by the appearance of an aggressive lesion, which may affect one or several vertebrae, with an osteolytic and osteoproliferative component (fig. 4.35). The infection may extend to the spinal canal, causing meningitis and myelitis. In many cases, it is related to the penetration of foreign bodies (e.g. grass awns), although it may also be associated with penetrating wounds or infections through the haematogenous route.

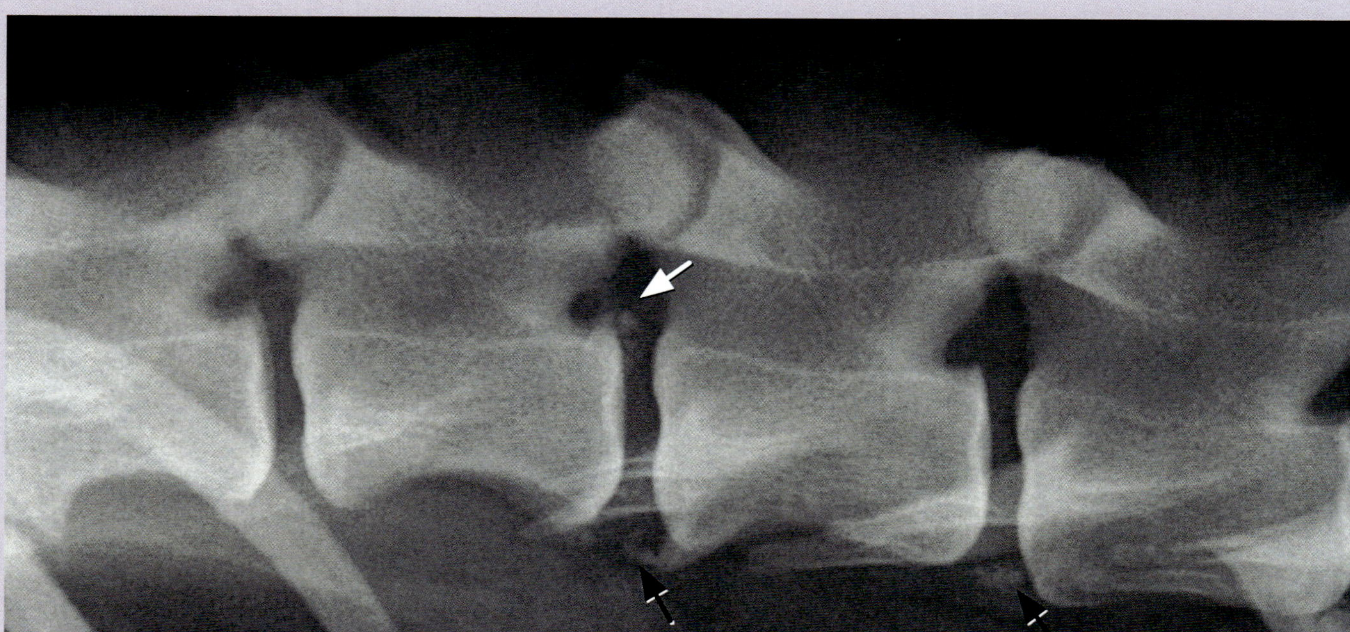

FIGURE 4.23. Enlarged image of the lumbar spine of a dog in lateral projection, in which calcified disc material is observed, immediately dorsal to the L2-L3 intervertebral disc space (white arrow), as well as in the ventral areas of the L2-L3 and L3-L4 disc spaces (black arrows).

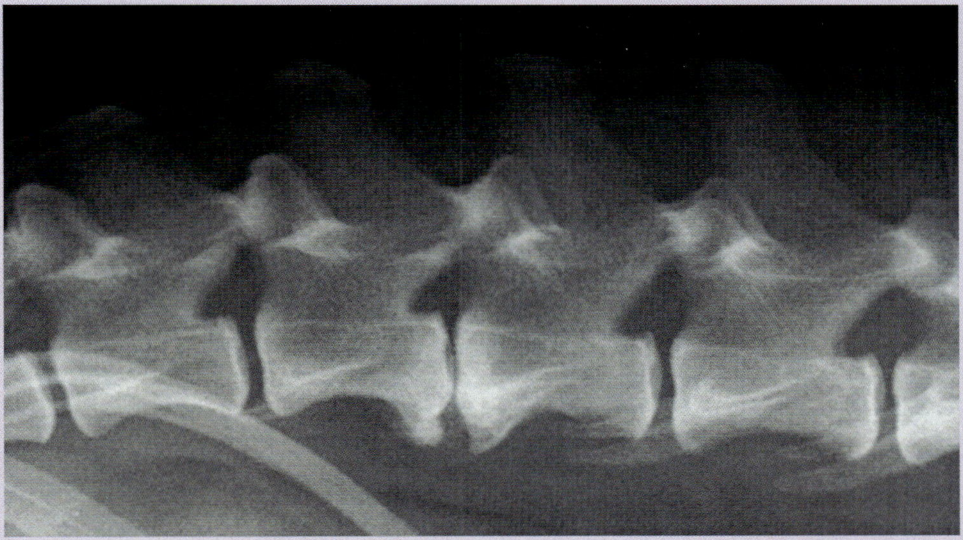

FIGURE 4.24. Enlarged image of the lumbar spine on a lateral radiograph of a dog with a narrowing of the L2-L3 intervertebral disc space, sclerosis of the caudal margin of L2 and cranial margin of L3 and spondylosis deformans at L2-L3. The sclerosis and spondylosis suggest a possible old disc lesion.

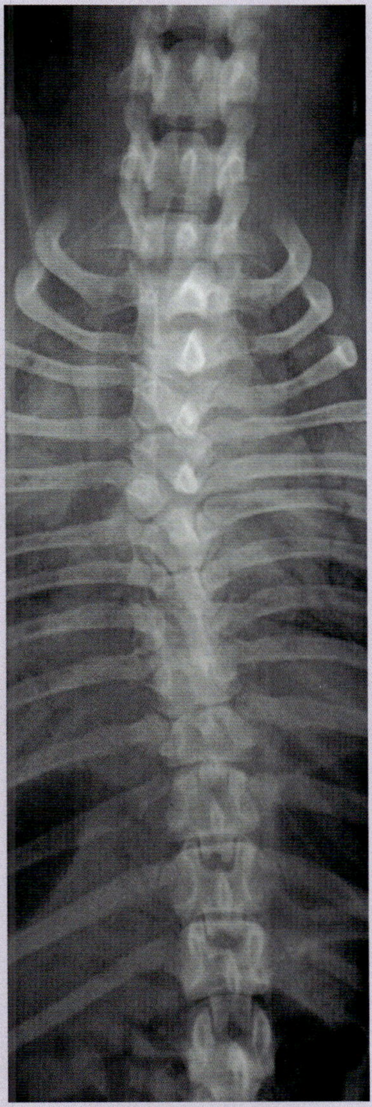

FIGURE 4.25. Ventrodorsal radiograph of the thoracic spine of a dog with scoliosis (displacement of the spine in lateral direction). Scoliosis commonly appears associated with multiple vertebral deformations.

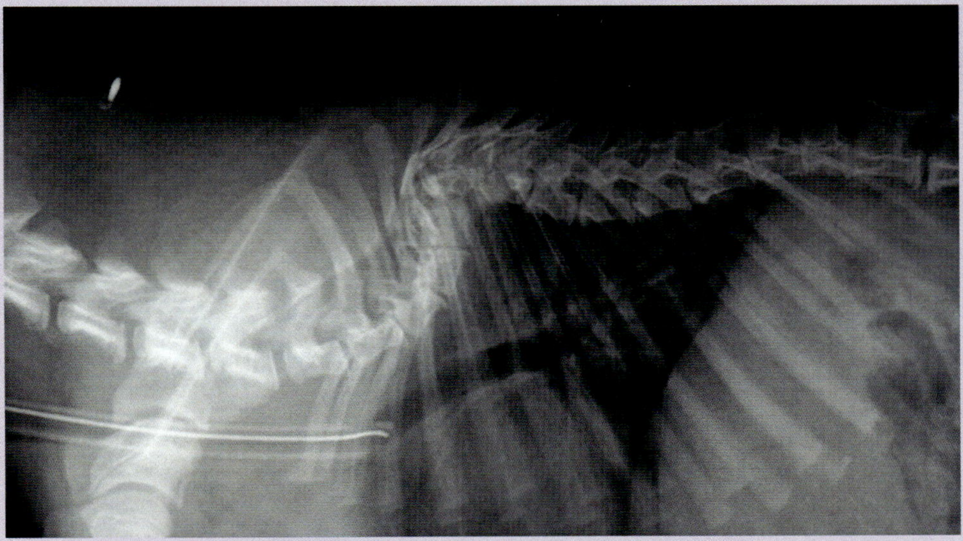

FIGURE 4.26. Lateral radiograph of the thoracic spine of a dog with kyphosis (displacement of the spine in dorsal direction). Kyphosis commonly appears associated with multiple vertebral deformations.

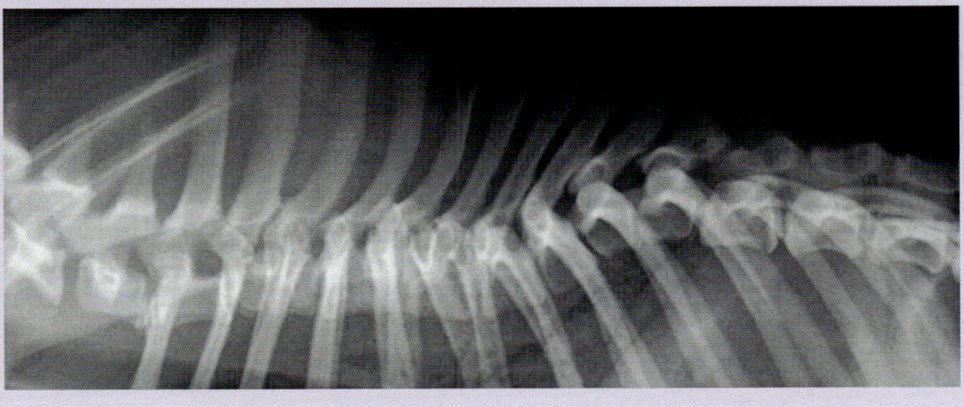

FIGURE 4.27. Lateral radiograph of the thoracic spine in a dog with lordosis (displacement of the spine in ventral direction). Lordosis commonly appears associated with multiple vertebral deformations.

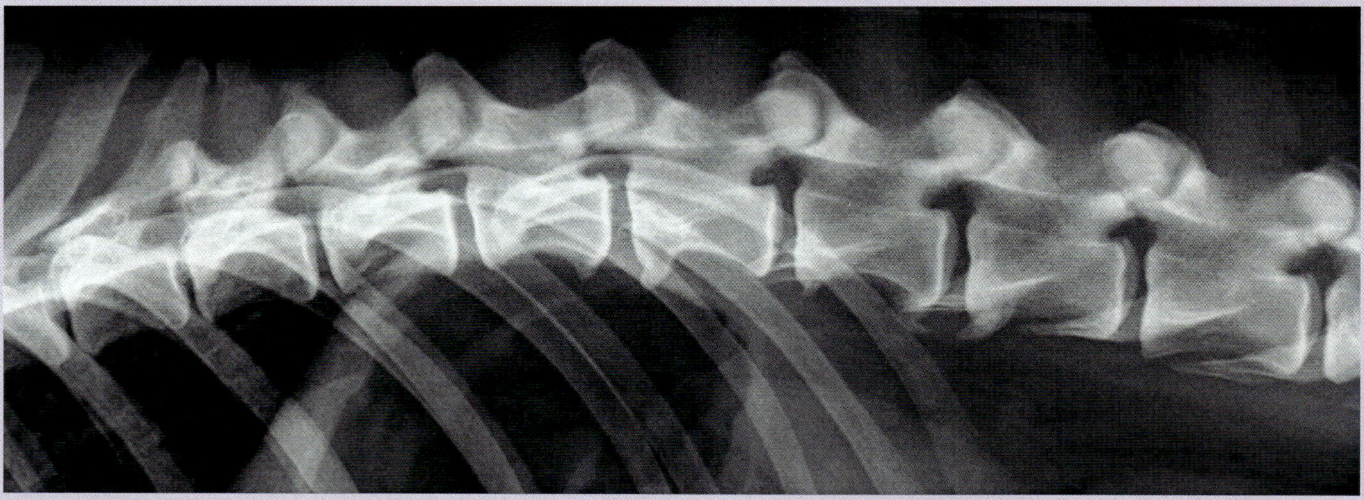

FIGURE 4.28. Lateral radiograph of the thoracolumbar spine of a dog with mild spondylosis deformans at T13-L1, L1-L2 and L2-L3.

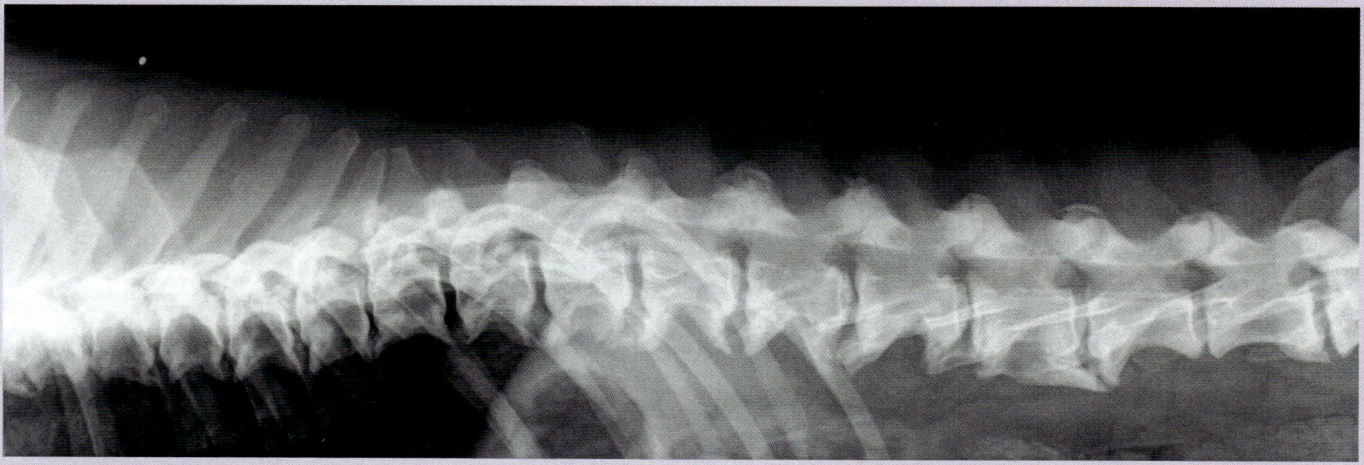

FIGURE 4.29. Lateral radiograph of the thoracolumbar spine of a dog with marked spondylosis deformans affecting all the thoracic and lumbar vertebrae.

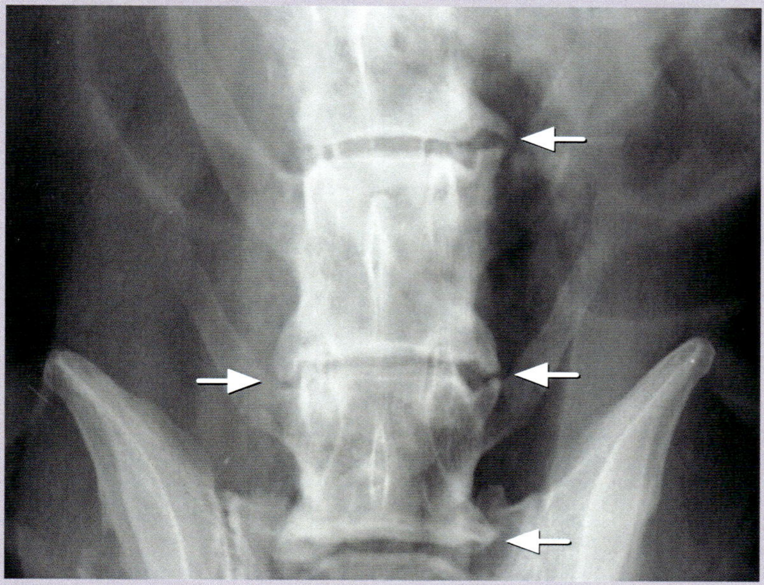

Normal radiographic anatomy of the **thoracolumbar spine**

http://goo.gl/uRwvcn

Normal radiographic anatomy of the **lumbar spine**

http://goo.gl/fONLCq

FIGURE 4.30. Enlarged image of the lumbar spine on a ventrodorsal radiograph of a dog with lateral spondylosis deformans at L5-L6, L6-L7 and L7-S1 (arrows).

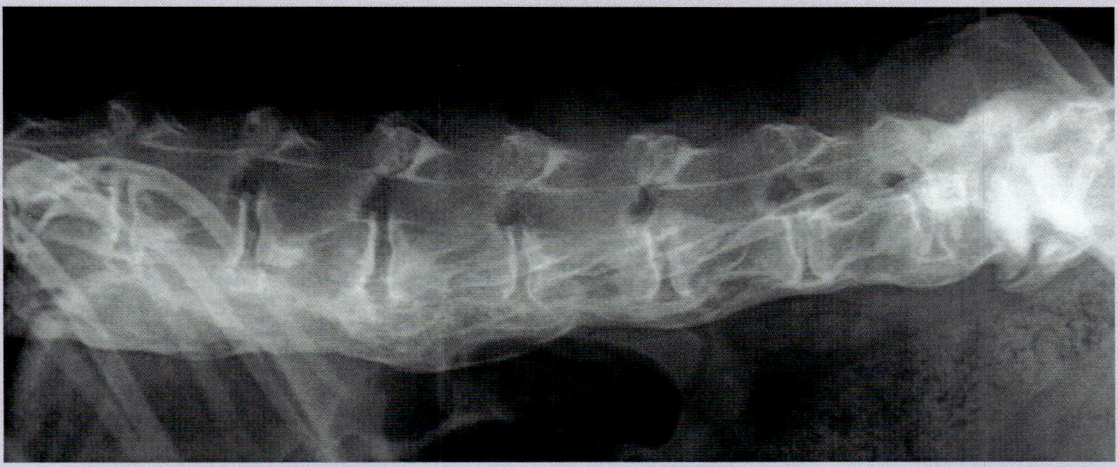

FIGURE 4.31. Lateral radiograph of the lumbar spine of a Boxer with marked spondylosis deformans affecting all the lumbar vertebrae.

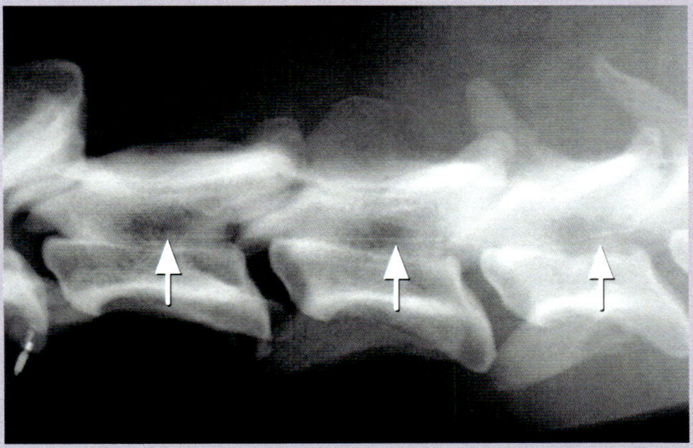

FIGURE 4.32. Enlarged image of the cervical spine on a lateral radiograph of a dog with dural ossification (arrows).

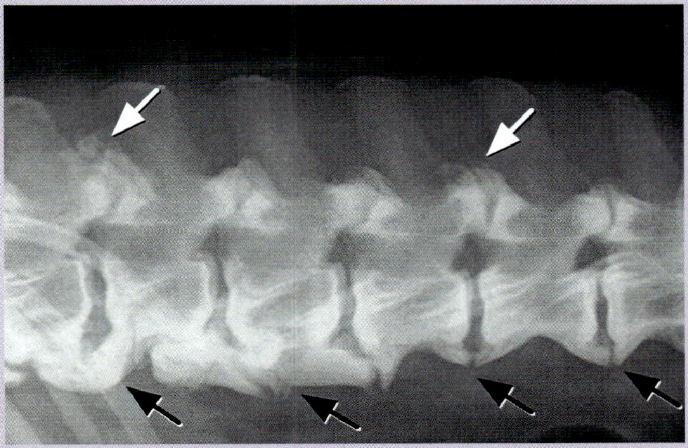

FIGURE 4.33. Enlarged image of the lumbar spine on a lateral radiograph of a dog with spondyloarthrosis. The joint facets appear deformed, with large osteophytes at L2-L3 and L5-L6 (white arrows). The vertebral bodies show spondylosis deformans (black arrows).

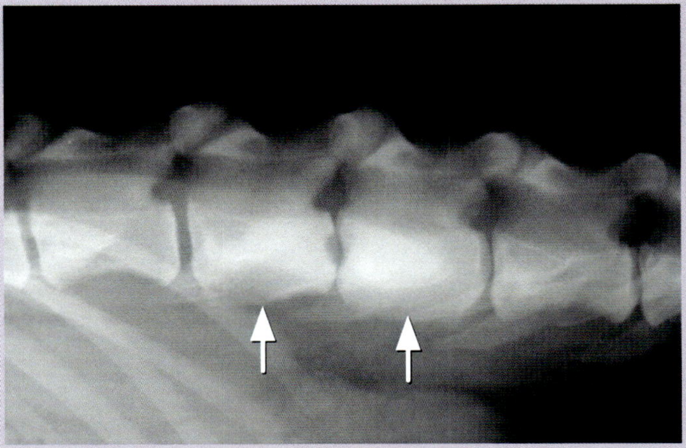

FIGURE 4.34. Enlarged image of the lumbar spine on a lateral radiograph of a dog with spondylitis at L2 and L3. The regular overgrowth of the ventral margin of both vertebrae (arrows) indicates inflammation of the vertebral bodies. In addition, the L2-L3 intervertebral disc space appears reduced and with initial signs of osteolysis of the caudal margin of L2 and cranial margin of L3, which suggests a disc infection at initial stage.

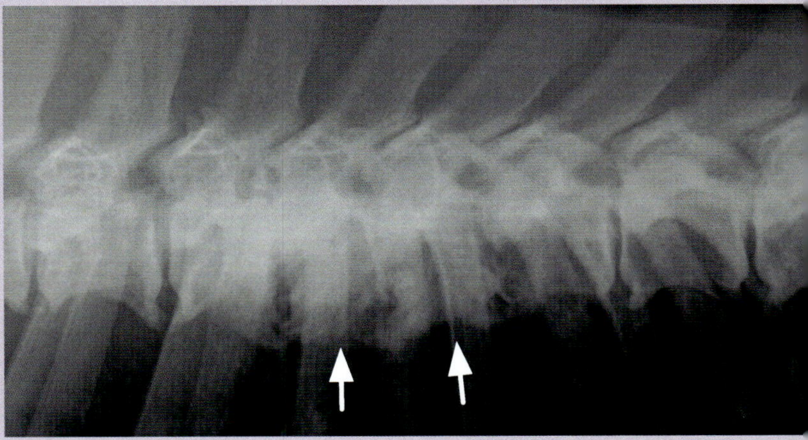

FIGURE 4.35. Enlarged image of the thoracic spine of a dog with spondylopyosis (vertebral osteomyelitis). The irregular overgrowth of the ventral margin of the affected vertebrae (arrows) indicates vertebral infection.

Normal radiographic anatomy of the **lumbosacral spine**

http://goo.gl/dV0lox

The term discospondylitis is used when an infectious process affects the intervertebral disc and the end-plate of the adjacent vertebral bodies. The infection may extend to the meninges and spinal cord. The radiograhic image varies according to the moment at which the diagnosis is carried out (fig. 4.36):

- At initial stages, it is possible to observe osteolysis and irregularity of the end-plates of the vertebral bodies adjacent to the affected disc or discs, which cause a narrowing of the intervertebral disc space (fig. 4.37).
- New bone formations on the ventral and lateral aspect of the affected vertebrae, which is similar spondylosis deformans, but if they are secondary to discospondylitis, they are usually more extended and have a more aggressive aspect.
- Over time, bone is produced in the areas where it had been destroyed, resulting in a narrowing of the intervertebral disc space. Fusion of the vertebral bodies may even take place (fig. 4.38). Sclerosis of the end-plates of the affected vertebral bodies is observed and the ventral new bone acquires a more regular and well-defined image (similar to that of spondylosis).

Fractures and luxations

They are generally caused by trauma, although they may also be secondary to other lesions (pathological fractures). The ease with which a vertebral fracture is identified on radiographs depends on the degree of displacement of the fragments (fig. 4.39). In cases of fractures by compression, the image shows an apparent loss of vertebral body height. Radiographs must be obtained in two projections (lateral and ventrodorsal), handling the patient with maximum care to avoid worsening potential spinal cord damage. It should be borne in mind that, during the recovery period, the bone callus may cause a spinal cord compression.

Fractures of spinous or transverse processes are not usually clinically significant (fig. 4.40).

Complete luxations are easily identifiable on plain radiographs. The ease with which a vertebral subluxation is identified depends on the degree of displacement of the affected vertebrae (fig. 4.41). In normal conditions, the body of L4 may have a position that is slightly ventral to that of L3, which should not be confused with pathological subluxation.

Both in spinal fractures and luxations, a vertebral displacement of more than 2/3 of the diameter of the spinal canal is considered a sign indicating severed spinal cord (fig 4.42).

Tumours

Tumours in vertebrae are quite rare. The tumours that usually affect vertebrae are osteosarcomas, chondrosarcomas and mestastases of primary tumours of a different origin. Neoplasms located in the vertebrae are usually more osteolytic than osteoproliferative (fig. 4.43). Associated pathological fractures may occur.

The spine is a site of predilection for myelomas, which have a radiographic pattern that is characterised by the appearance of numerous small, round osteolytic areas in the long bones and spine. Bone lymphoma may also present a multifocal pattern, with lesions that are predominantly osteolytic.

Metastases usually appear as aggressive bone lesions located in the spine and other bones. The bone metastases of some pelvic tumours, especially prostate carcinoma, have a peculiar image, since they affect the surrounding bones (last lumbar vertebrae, sacrum and pelvis), causing lesions that are fundamentally proliferative (fig 4.44). These lesions are sometimes detected before the primary tumour.

Hypervitaminosis A

It usually affects cats from 2 to 4 years old that ingest excessive amounts of liver. It is much less frequent in dogs. The excess of vitamin A causes the growth of subperiosteal bone. In young animals, an asymmetric longitudinal growth of the long bones occurs. In adults, bone exostoses develop essentially in the cervical and thoracic spine, ribs and around the limb joints, and can lead to ankylosis of these joints and of the vertebrae.

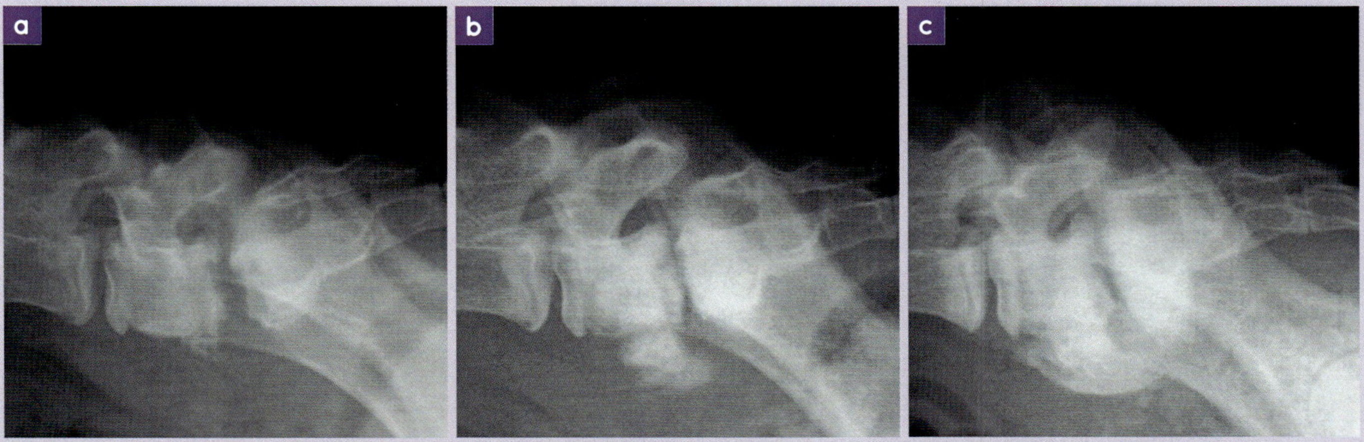

FIGURE 4.36. Images of the lumbosacral area of the spine on a lateral radiograph of a young dog with discospondylitis at an initial (a), intermediate (b) and advanced or chronic (c) stage.

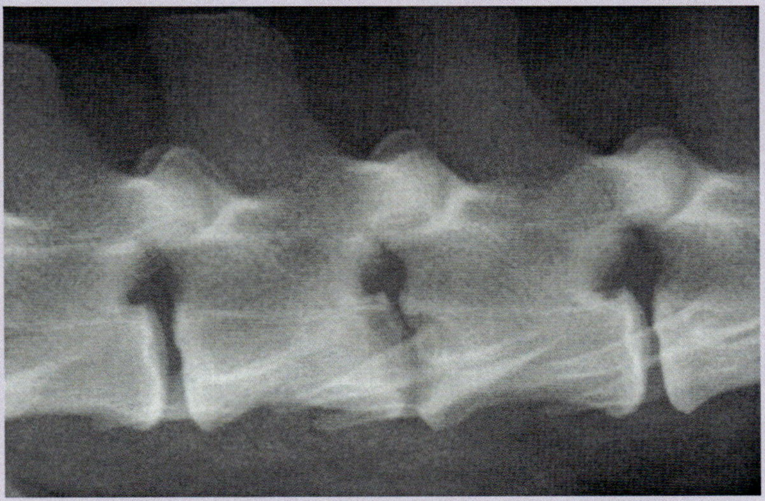

◀ FIGURE 4.37. Enlarged image of the lumbar spine on a lateral radiograph of a dog with discospondylitis at L2-L3 at an initial stage.

▼ FIGURE 4.38. Enlarged lateral cisternal myelogram showing the thoracic spine of a dog with discospondylitis at an advanced or chronic stage. The affected vertebrae appear fused, with ventral overgrowths with regular margins. The lesions cause an interruption of the contrast columns (arrow) located cranial to the lesion.

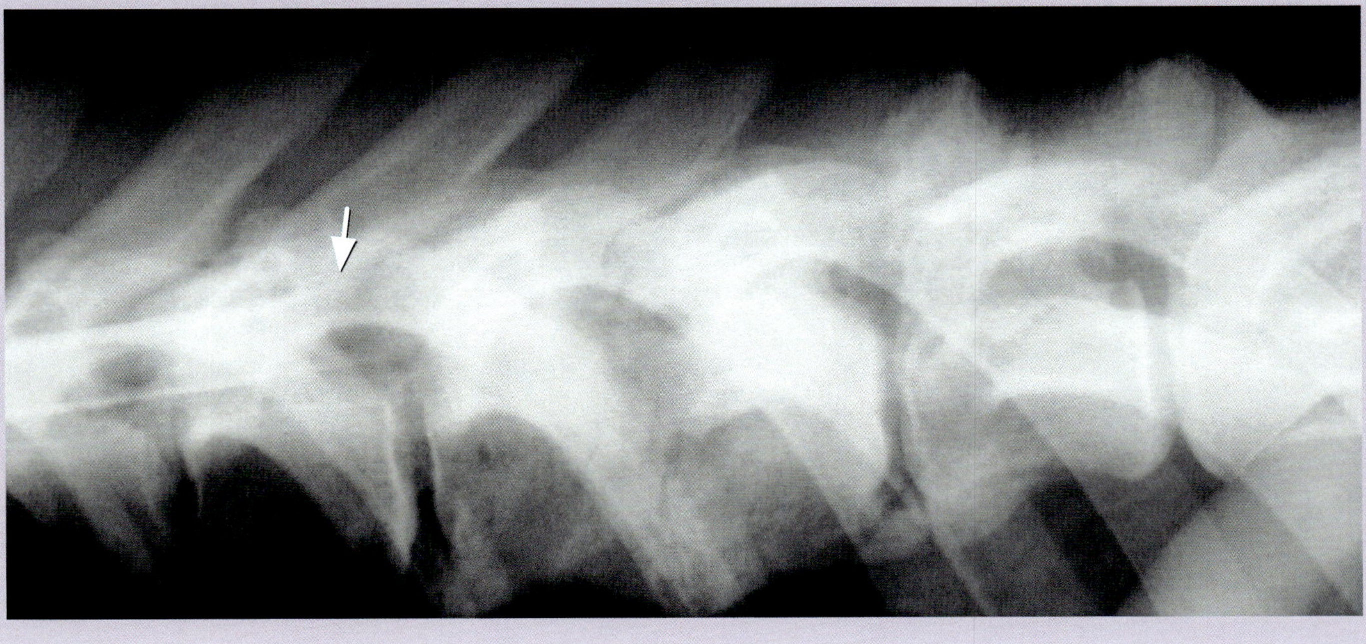

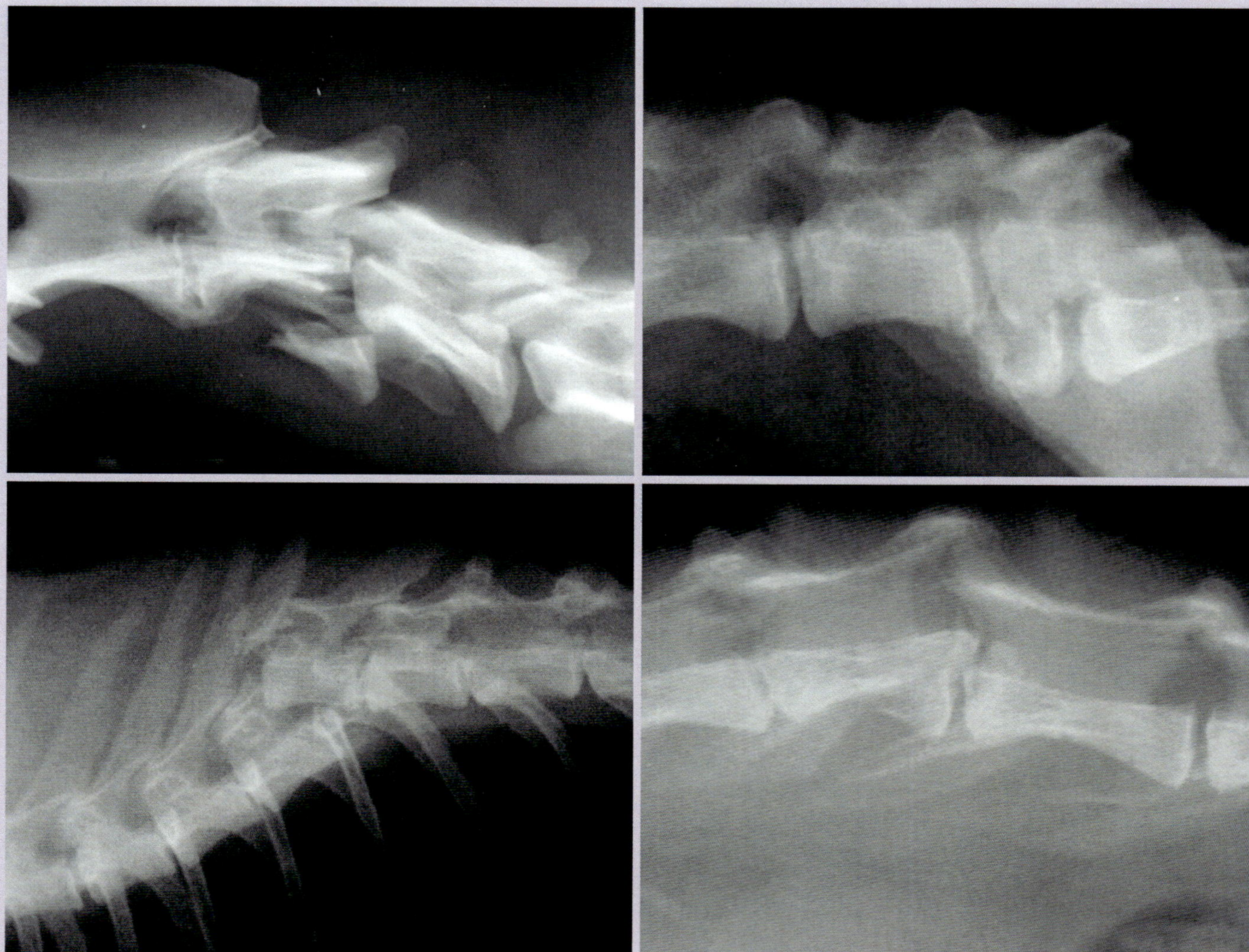

FIGURE 4.39. Images of various vertebral fractures.

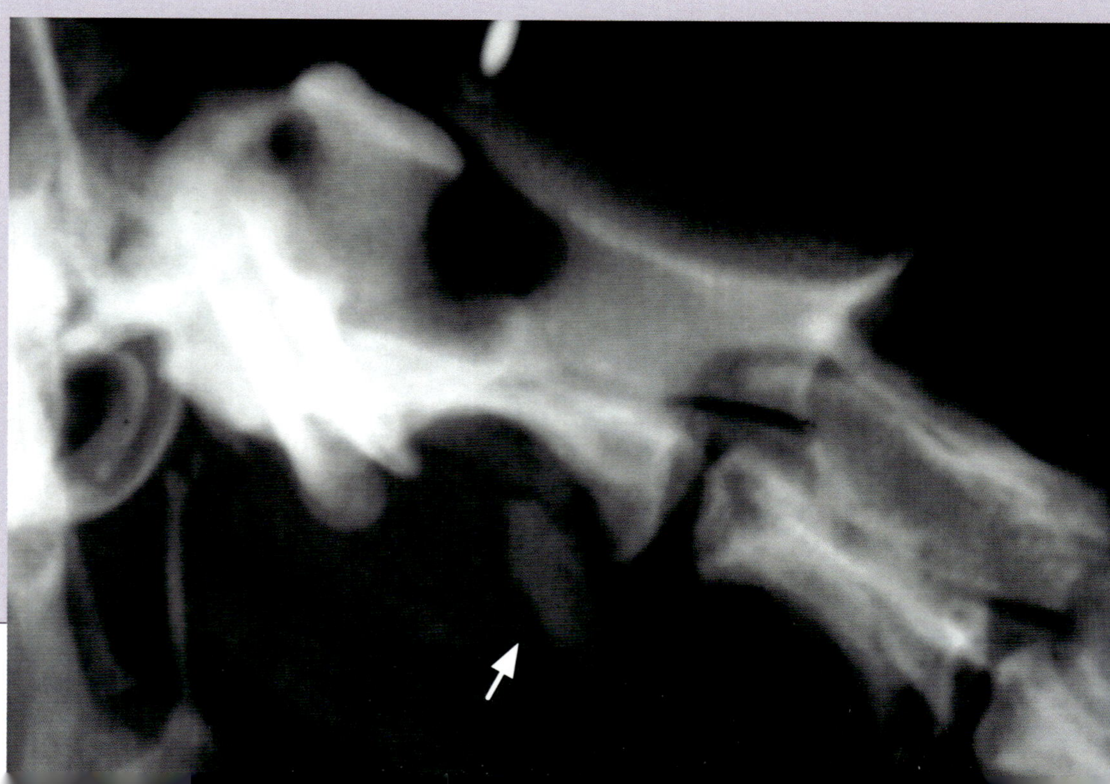

FIGURE 4.40. Enlarged image of the cervical spine on a lateral radiograph of a dog with a fracture of the transverse process of the axis (arrow).

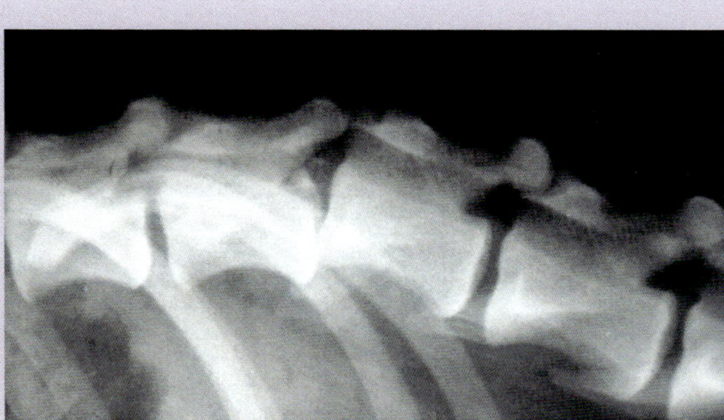

FIGURE 4.41. Enlarged image of the lumbar spine on a lateral radiograph of a dog with L1-L2 subluxation.

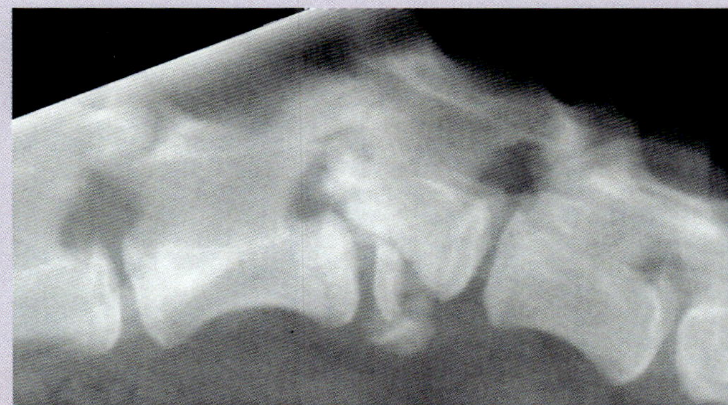

FIGURE 4.42. Enlarged image of the lumbar spine on a lateral radiograph of a dog with a comminuted fracture of L6. The displacement of L6 exceeds 2/3 of the diameter of the spinal canal, which indicates a severed spinal cord.

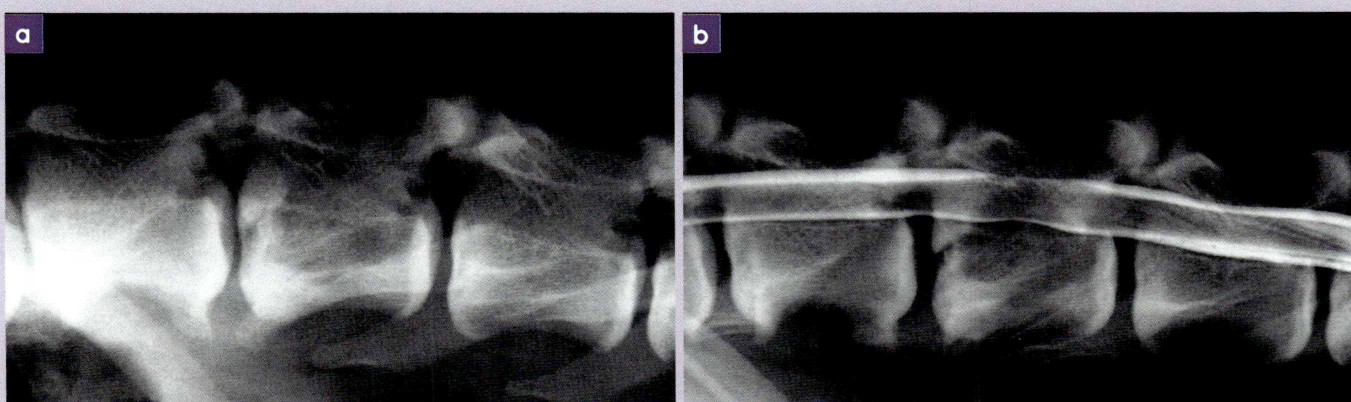

FIGURE 4.43. Enlarged image of the lumbar spine on a lateral radiograph of a dog with osteorsarcoma of L2. The tumour appears as an osteolytic geographic lesion on the plain radiograph (a). On the myelogram (b), it has an extradural pattern.

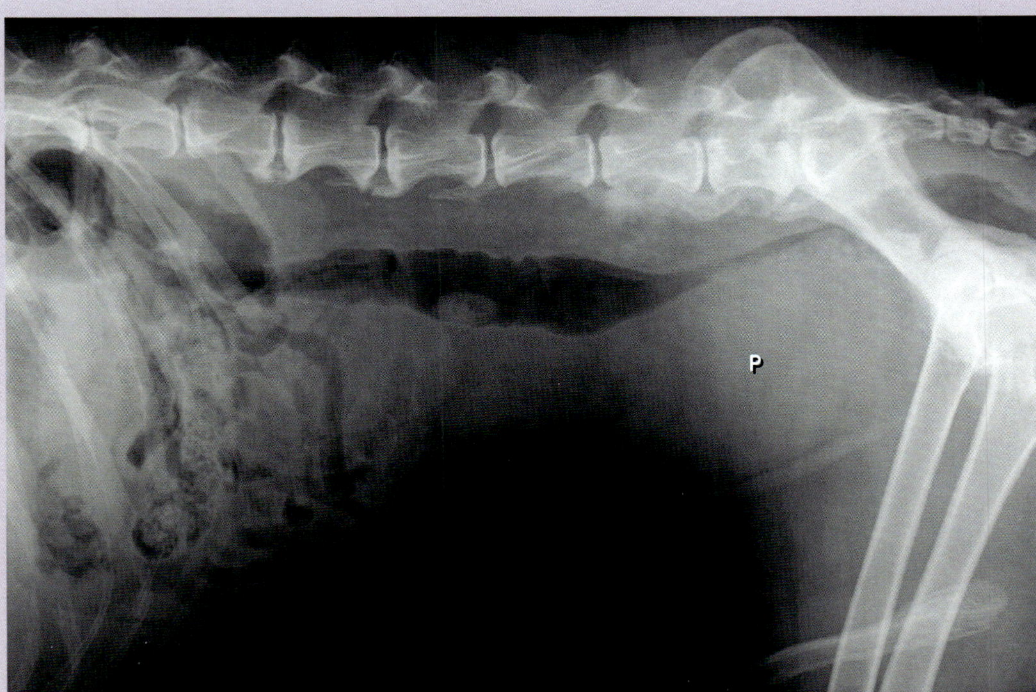

FIGURE 4.44. Lateral radiograph of the abdomen of a dog with prostate carcinoma (P). The L6 vertebra shows irregular overgrowth of its ventral margin, which corresponds to metastases of the prostatic tumour. Spondylosis at L6-L7 and L7-S1 is also observed.

Self-assessment
cases

http://goo.gl/qvfCZ9

Mucopolysaccharidosis can cause similar lesions in the vertebrae. It is due to an alteration in the catabolism of mucopolysaccharides associated with the malfunctioning of an enzyme. It has been described in Siamese cats and Teckel dogs.

Multiple cartilaginous exostoses

It is an uncommon anomaly, which is characterised by osteoproliferative benign lesions in the metaphyses of the long bones, ribs and vertebrae of young dogs (fig. 4.45). The growth of the lesions generally stops when skeletal maturity is reached. It is not usually clinically significant, unless the lesions invade the spinal canal or the intervertebral foramina, causing compression of the spinal cord or nerve roots. Exceptionally, a late evolution to osteosarcoma or chondrosarcoma has been described.

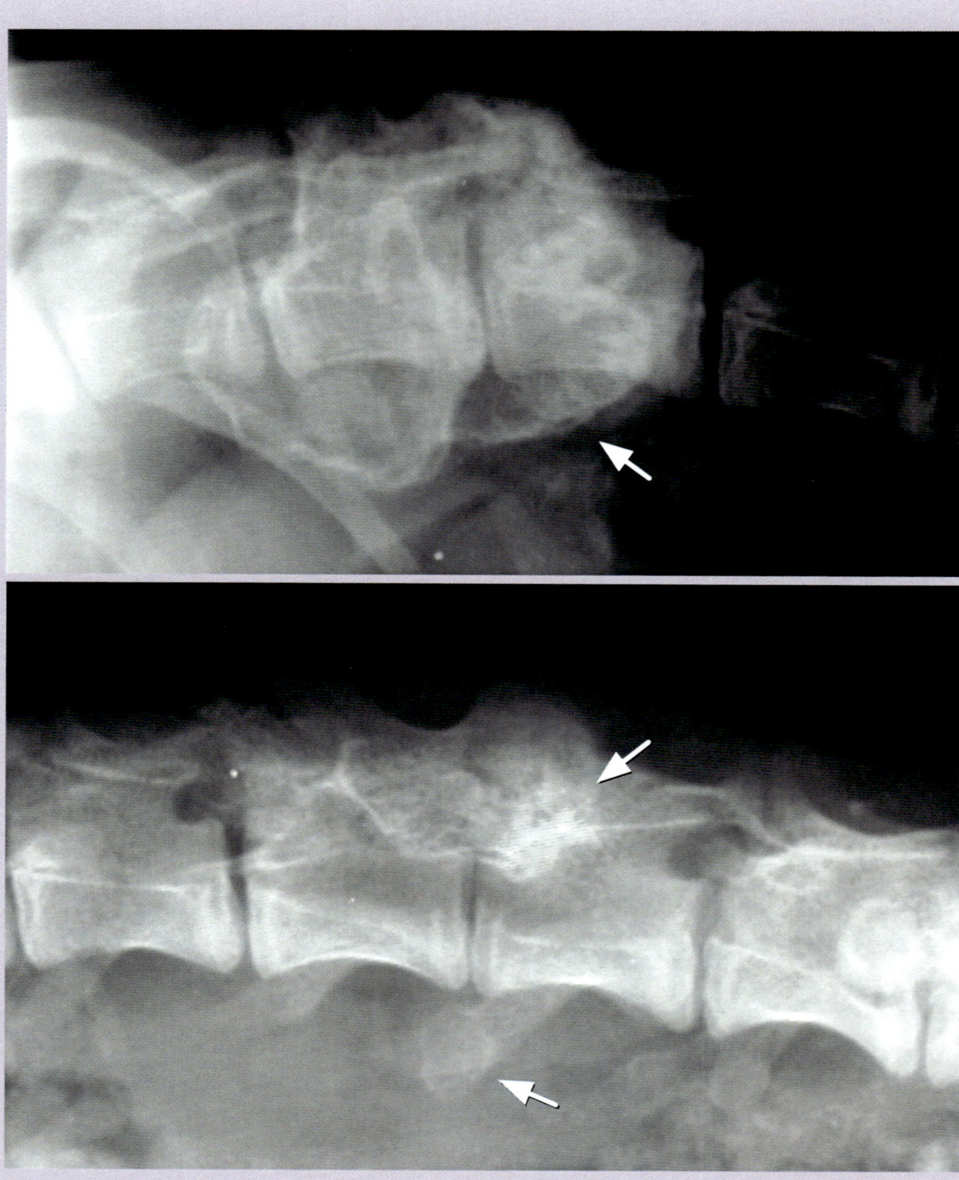

FIGURE 4.45. Enlarged images of the lumbar spine on lateral radiographs of a young dog with multiple cartilaginous exostoses, which appear as benign osteoproliferative lesions in the vertebrae (arrows).

Head

5

Principles of interpretation

The head is an extremely complex anatomical region, formed by approximately 50 bones, numerous teeth and various soft tissues. In addition, its morphological characteristics considerably vary depending on the species, and in the canine species, depending on the breed. Three basic conformations of the skull have been described:

- **Dolichocephalic:** nasal area longer than the cranial cavity.
- **Mesaticephalic:** the nasal area has approximately the same length as the cranial cavity.
- **Brachycephalic:** nasal area shorter than the cranial cavity.

In order to correctly interpret radiographs of the head, it is essential for the animal to be correctly positioned, since the radiological interpretation will often be based on the symmetrical image of the skull. Performing the radiological study under sedation or anaesthesia is recommended to obtain good-quality images. If an endotracheal tube is used, it will sometimes be necessary to remove it at the moment of taking the radiograph, so that it is not superimposed with the anatomical structures that are going to be assessed in the image. In some cases, it will also be necessary to change the position of the tongue, especially when taking a ventrodorsal open-mouth radiograph.

As it is an extremely complex anatomical region, comparing the images obtained with those that are included in atlases of normal radiographic anatomy is very useful. When the lesions affect only one side of the head, the contralateral half may also be used as reference for normality.

A wide variety of projections may be used to assess the different clinically important regions of the head. The choice of projections will be made according to the region that is to be examined.

- Cranial vault: lateral and ventrodorsal projections.
- Nasal cavity and frontal sinuses: lateral, ventrodorsal open-mouth or dorsoventral intraoral (occlusal) and rostrocaudal tangential (also termed "skyline") projections.
- Mandible, maxilla and temporomandibular joint: lateral, dorsoventral, dorsoventral intraoral (to assess maxilla), ventrodorsal intraoral (to assess mandible), lateral oblique and rostrocaudal open-mouth (for temporomandibular joints) projections.
- Teeth: lateral oblique and intraoral (dorsoventral, ventrodorsal and lateral) projections.
- Auditory system: dorsoventral, lateral oblique and rostrocaudal open-mouth projections.
- It will sometimes be useful to take radiographs centred on the lesion, which will provide complementary information to that provided by standard projections.

Radiographs provide valuable information of the bone structure of the head, but are usually not very useful to assess soft tissues in this anatomical region. Ultrasonography may help to characterise lesions located in superficial soft tissues and is of great interest for the study of the eyeball and retrobulbar space. However, the diagnostic imaging techniques that offer the most complete diagnostic information about this anatomical region are computed tomography and magnetic resonance imaging. Both provide

Normal radiographic anatomy of the head **lateral view**

http://goo.gl/JE5G8d

Normal radiographic anatomy of the head **dorsoventral view**

http://goo.gl/iqa8CR

tomographic images of the patient (with no superimposition of structures) with excellent detail of intra- and extracranial anatomical structures. In general, magnetic resonances imaging is more appropriate to assess soft tissues, while computed tomography offers more detailed images of bone structures.

Cranial vault

Congenital hydrocephalus

It is more frequent in miniature breeds such as the Chihuahua, Pomeranian, Yorkshire Terrier, etc. It may be asymptomatic or manifested by various neurological disorders. The radiological signs that may be associated with this disease are excessive enlargement of the cranial vault, thinning of the bones that form it, persistence of the fontanelles in the adult animal and relatively homogeneous appearance of the intracranial content (due to the loss of the normal sulci of the brain) (fig. 5.1a and b).

An ultrasound examination may be very useful to assess the degree of dilatation of the ventricular system when the fontanelle is large enough to allow good contact of the transducer and good penetration of the ultrasound beam (fig. 5.1c).

Occipital dysplasia

As with hydrocephalus, this congenital alteration also mainly affects miniature breeds and can have little clinical significance. Rostrodorsal-caudoventral radiographs are particularly useful for its radiological assessment. The main radiological sign is the abnormal dorsal enlargement of the foramen magnum, which acquires a "lock" shape (fig. 5.2). This anomaly is sometimes associated with atlantoaxial subluxation.

Fractures

Fractures located in the cranial vault are generally difficult to visualise on radiographs, since the displacement of the fragments is usually minimal (fig. 5.3). The areas of greater inflammation of the soft tissues are a useful guide and the patient should be positioned so that these areas are centred on the radiograph (fig. 5.4).

Computed tomography is an excellent option to assess patients in which a skull fracture is suspected, since in addition to providing detailed information about bone structures, it will also allow the evaluation of possible associated intracranial lesions.

Tumours

Osteosarcomas are the bone tumours that most frequently appear in this area of the skull. As in other anatomical regions, these tumours usually appear on radiographs as aggressive lesions with an osteoproliferative and osteolytic component, and with marked swelling of the adjacent soft tissues (fig. 5.5).

Osteomas and osteochondromas are occasionally identified in this region. Osteomas tend to be more sclerotic and delimited than osteosarcomas, and sometimes have a "cauliflower" shape (fig. 5.6).

As in other anatomical regions, aggressive soft-tissue neoplasms (e.g. squamous cell carcinomas, melanomas, fibrosarcomas, etc.) may also affect the bones of the skull in a secondary manner (fig. 5.7).

Nasal cavity and sinuses

In radiographic images obtained in dorsoventral or ventrodorsal projection, the nasal cavity appears divided into two halves by the nasal septum, formed by the vomer bone and nasal cartilage. The nasal conchae appear as thin lines of mineral density in the rostral part of the cavity (dorsal and ventral nasal conchae) and as thicker swirls of mineral density in the caudal area of the cavity (ethmoid labyrinth or ethmoid conchae).

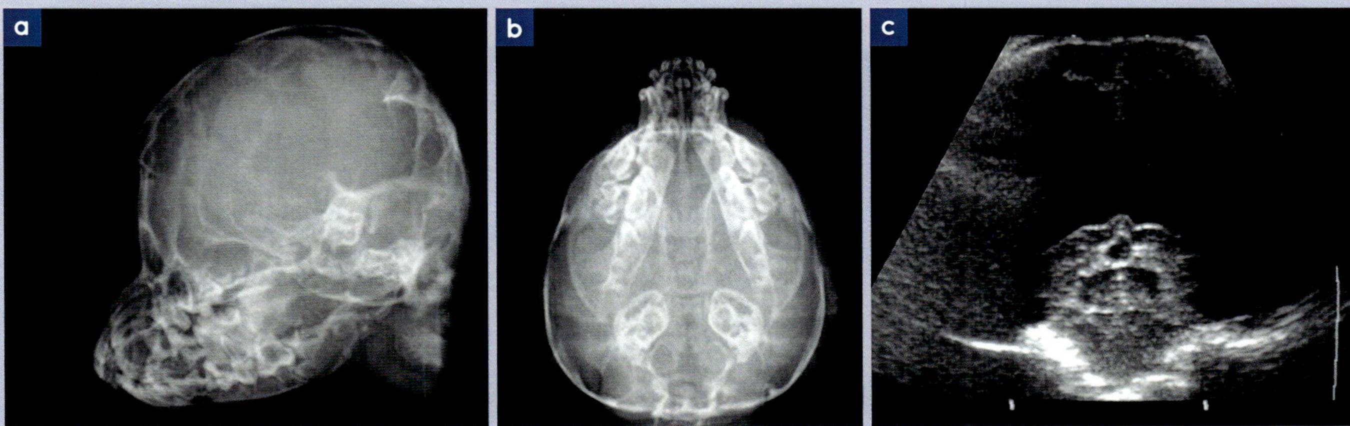

FIGURE 5.1. Lateral (a) and dorsoventral (b) radiographs of the head of a dog with congenital hydrocephalus. The radiographs show enlargement of the cranial vault and thinning of the bones. The ultrasound scan (c) shows marked dilatation of the lateral ventricles.

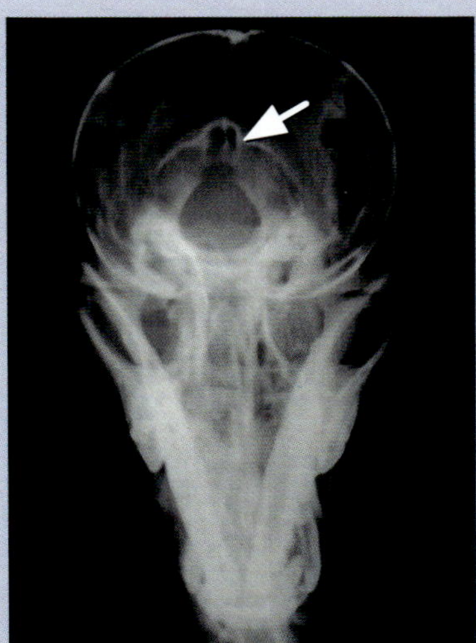

FIGURE 5.2. Rostrodorsal-caudoventral view of the head of a dog with occipital dysplasia. The foramen magnum has an abnormal dorsal extension (arrow).

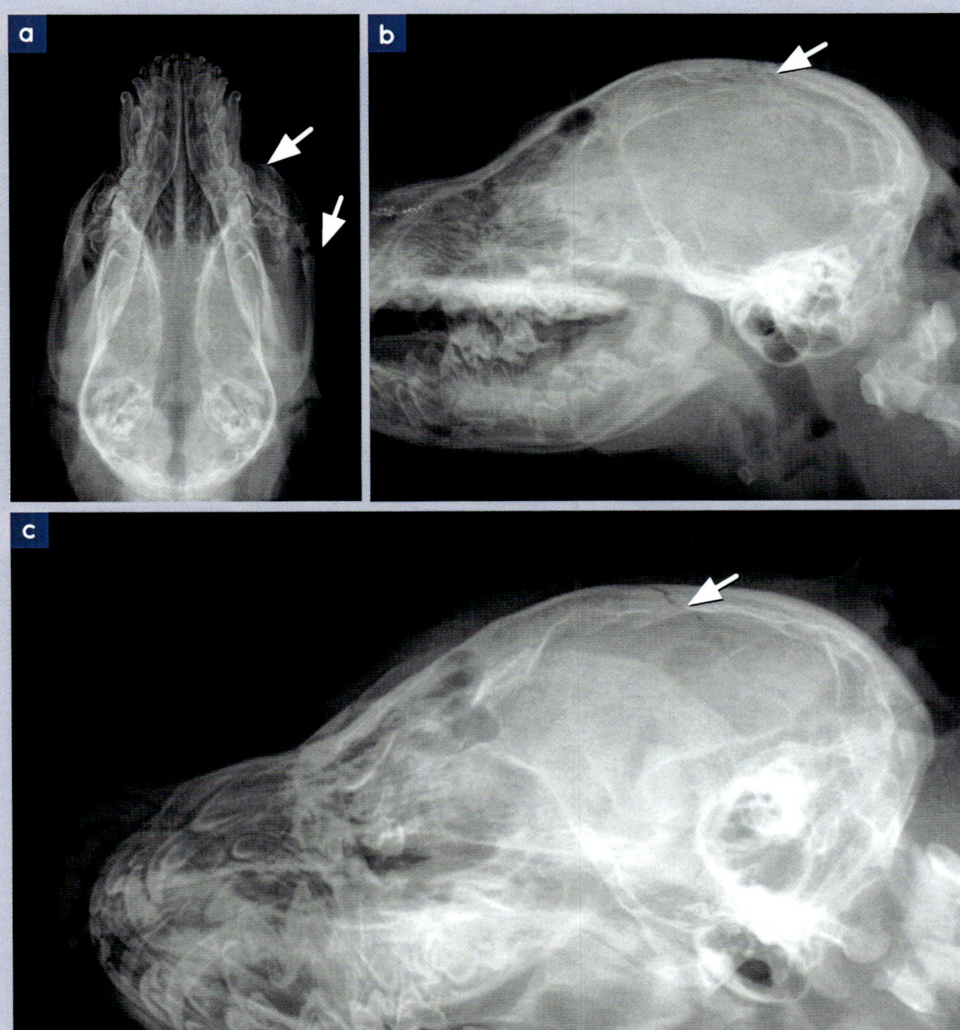

FIGURE 5.3. Dorsoventral (a), lateral (b) and lateral oblique (c) radiographs of the head of a young dog with multiple fractures of the skull. The arrows indicate several lines of fracture located in the left maxillary and zygomatic bones, as well as in the medial area of the cranial vault. This latter is better visualised on the lateral oblique radiograph (c) and should not be confused with a normal suture line.

Normal radiographic anatomy of the head
rostrodorsal-caudoventral view

http://goo.gl/shdAWX

Normal radiographic anatomy of the head
lateral oblique view
(tympanic bulla)

http://goo.gl/alQAHX

Foreign bodies

Mineral or metallic density foreign bodies located in the nasal cavity are usually easy to identify on radiographs. However, those with a radiographic density similar to that of soft tissues and fluids (radiolucent foreign bodies), such as grass awns, sticks, small plastic objects, etc., usually cannot be visualised in the image, although the signs of associated focal rhinitis they cause are often identified.

Fractures

Fractures affecting the nasal bone (fig 5.8) or the frontal sinuses (fig. 5.9) may be difficult to diagnose. There is usually depression of the bone fragments, which is accompanied by inflammation of the adjacent soft tissues and, in many cases, subcutaneous emphysema as air escapes to the adjacent tissues.

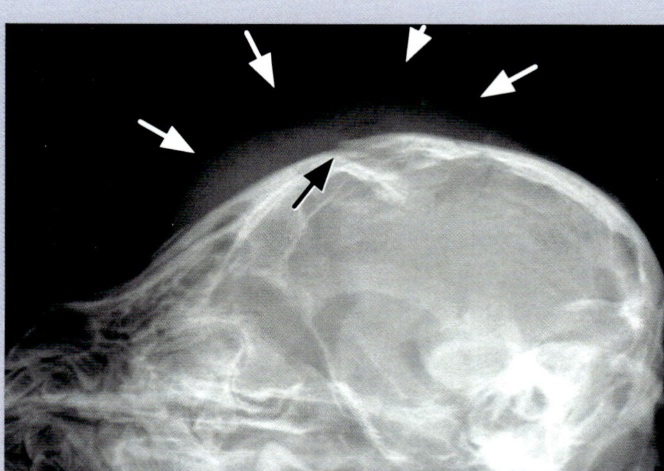

FIGURE 5.4. Enlarged image of the cranial vault of a young dog in lateral oblique projection. The radiograph was centred on the area of inflammation of the soft tissues (white arrows), which allowed the identification of a cranial fracture (black arrow), which was not visible on the standard lateral radiograph.

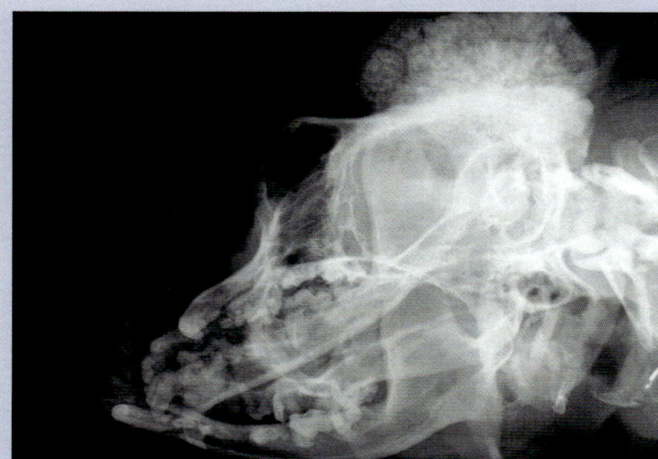

FIGURE 5.5. Lateral oblique radiograph of the head of a dog with a markedly osteoproliferative bone lesion located in the cranial vault. The radiograph was centred on the lesion to improve its visualisation. Histological diagnosis: osteosarcoma.

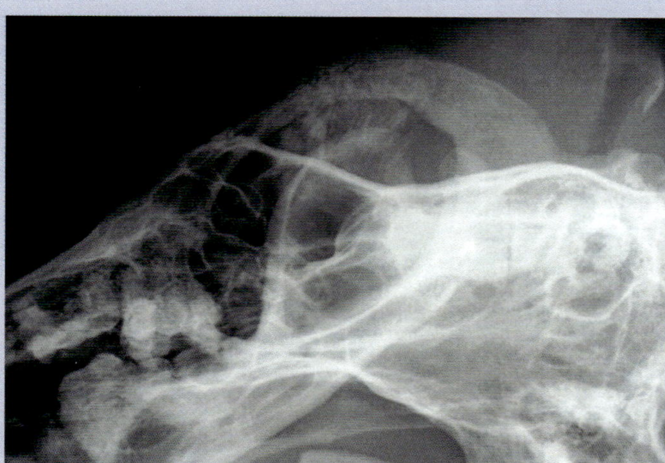

FIGURE 5.6. Enlarged image in lateral oblique projection of the region of the zygomatic bone of a dog with an osteoproliferative lesion in the central area of the zygomatic arch. The radiograph was centred on the lesion to improve its visualisation. Histological diagnosis: osteoma.

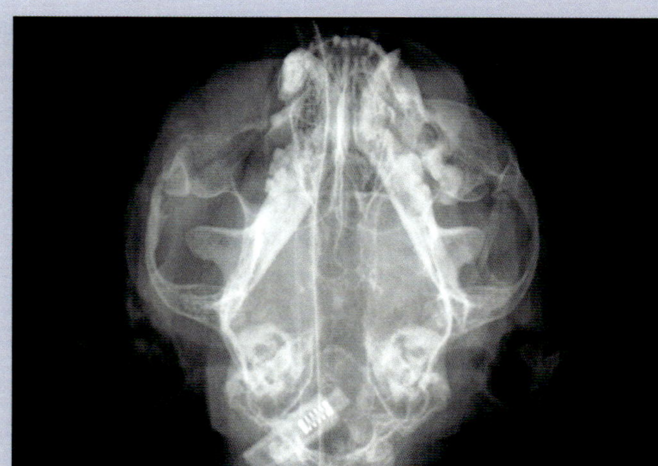

FIGURE 5.7. Dorsoventral radiograph of the head of a cat with a soft-tissue neoplasm (squamous cell carcinoma) that affects the adjacent bone and partially destroys the rostral part of the right zygomatic arch and the lateral area of the maxilla of the same side.

Rhinitis

Rhinitis secondary to bacterial infections and lymphoplasmatic rhinitis usually lead to increased radiographic density of the nasal cavity, accompanied or not by increased density of the frontal sinuses, although the nasal conchae are usually still well-differentiated in the image (fig. 5.10). In acute processes, there may not be any evident alterations of the cavity in the radiographic image.

Hyperplastic chronic rhinitis may cause, together with an increase in the radiopacity of the cavity, a loss of differentiation of the nasal conchae due to a thickening of the mucosa and the presence of exudate between them (fig. 5.11).

Normal radiographic anatomy of the head **ventrodorsal open-mouth view**

http://goo.gl/cPJEs6

It is more difficult to assess the image of the nasal conchae in cats, since under normal conditions they have a more irregular pattern than in dogs. It is important to bear this aspect in mind when assessing

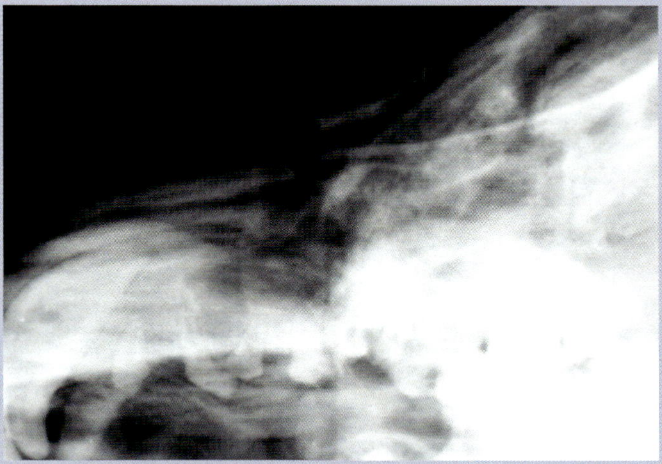

FIGURE 5.8. Enlarged image of the nasal region on a lateral oblique radiograph of a dog with a fracture of the nasal bone. The radiograph was centred on the lesion to improve its visualisation.

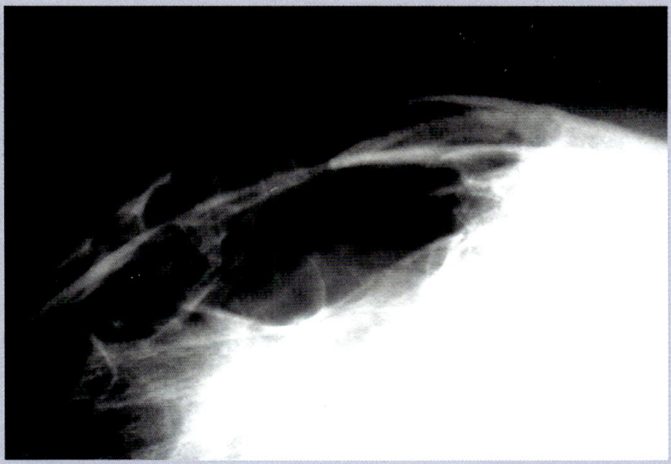

FIGURE 5.9. Enlarged image of the frontal region on a lateral oblique radiograph of a dog with a fracture of the frontal bone. The radiograph was centred on the lesion to improve its visualisation.

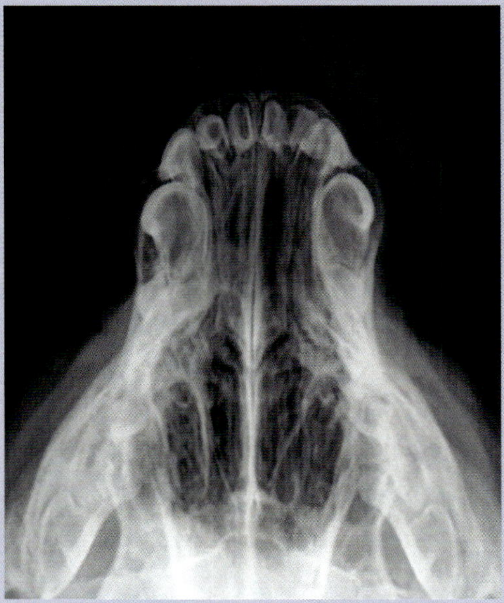

◀ **FIGURE 5.10.** Enlarged image of the nasal cavity on a ventrodorsal open-mouth radiograph of a young dog with bacterial rhinitis. An increase in the radiopacity of the right nasal cavity may be observed.

FIGURE 5.11. Enlarged image of the nasal cavity on a ventrodorsal open-mouth radiograph of a dog with chronic hyperplastic rhinitis. An increase in the radiopacity of the left nasal cavity is observed, especially in the middle third, where the nasal conchae are difficult to differentiate (this is attributed to the thickening of the mucosa and the presence of exudate between them). ▶

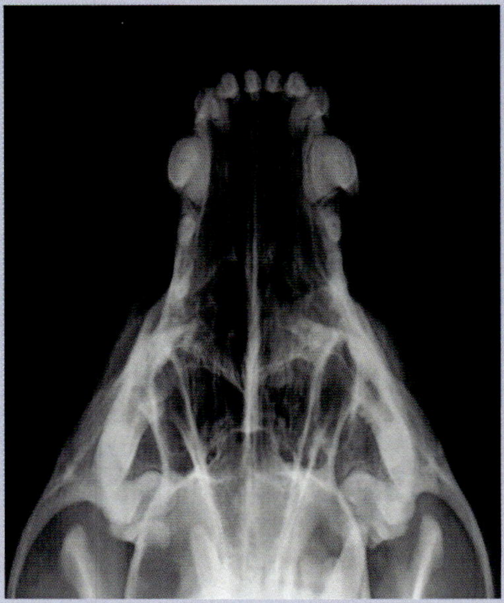

a possible case of feline chronic rhinitis, since it may cause a disorganisation or destruction of the conchae (fig. 5.12).

Fungal rhinitis, especially that caused by *Aspergillus*, is destructive. Radiographically, it is usually possible to observe a mixed pattern with a combination of areas of increased density and osteolytic areas, which cause a loss of differentiation of the nasal conchae as a result of their destruction (fig. 5.13). At advanced stages, displacement or erosion of the vomer bone may be observed, although it is not very frequent. The density of the frontal sinuses may also be increased, with or without a thickening of the bone wall.

Tumours

In small animals, approximately two thirds of nasal tumours are carcinomas and the other third are sarcomas. Nasal lymphoma, which is more common in cats, has also been described.

The radiographic image of nasal tumours may vary depending on the type of tumour and how long it has been present. The least aggressive tumours, as well as those detected at initial or early stages, have a similar radiographic image to that of rhinitis, characterised by a localised or diffuse increase in the density of the nasal cavity (fig. 5.14), which may or not affect the frontal sinuses. These findings usually appear in a unilateral manner in the case of neoplasms. The most aggressive tumours, or those detected at later stages of the disease, usually have a fairly destructive aspect, with loss of the characteristic pattern of the nasal conchae, displacement and/or destruction of the nasal septum and vomer bone, and invasion of other adjacent bones (fig. 5.15). The image may be similar to that caused by aggressive rhinitis, generally of fungal origin, so a differential diagnosis usually cannot be made based only on the radiological findings.

Nasal tumours sometimes extend to superficial planes and lead to the formation of an external soft-tissue mass, causing facial deformities (fig. 5.16). This is more typical in cases of tumours than in cases of rhinitis. Nasal neoplasms may also invade the cribriform plate and penetrate into the cranial cavity. They may thus affect the brain. Although extension of the tumour to the frontal sinus is also possible, the

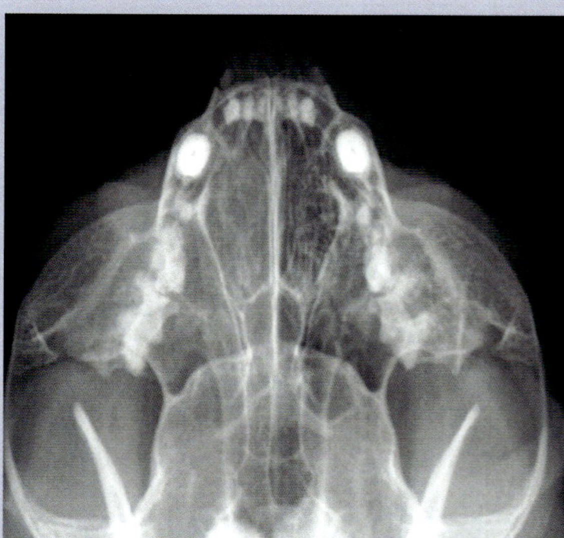

FIGURE 5.12. Enlarged image of the nasal cavity on a ventrodorsal open-mouth radiograph of a cat with chronic rhinitis. It is possible to observe an increase in the radiopacity of the right nasal cavity with a loss of differentiation of the nasal conchae.

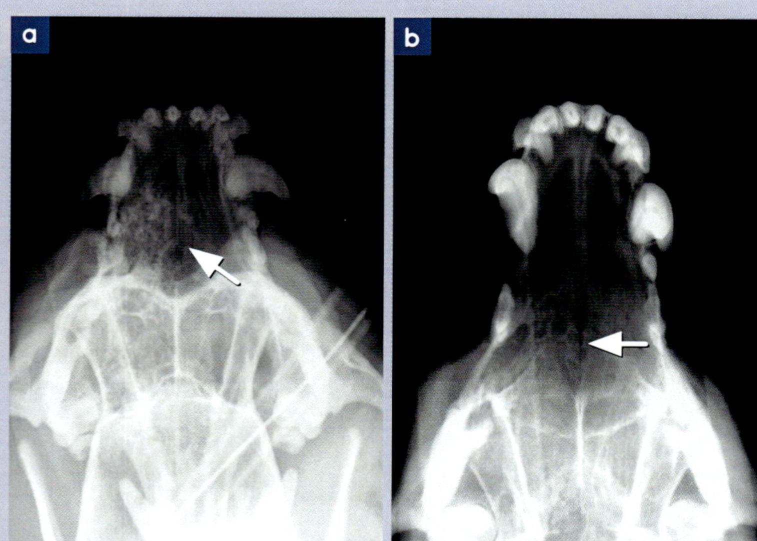

FIGURE 5.13. Enlarged images of the nasal cavity on ventrodorsal open-mouth radiographs of two dogs with fungal rhinitis caused by *Aspergillus*. In radiograph (a), it is possible to observe a mixed osteoproliferative and osteolytic lesion in the middle and caudal third of the right nasal cavity, increased radiopacity in the left nasal cavity and partial destruction of the vomer bone (arrow). Radiograph (b) shows multiple osteolytic areas in the middle third of the right nasal cavity (arrow), an increase in the radiopacity of both nasal cavities and disappearance of a great part of the vomer bone.

increase in density that is often observed in the ipsilateral sinus is usually due to the development of obstructive sinusitis, more than to a neoplastic invasion of the sinus (fig 5.17).

Normal radiographic anatomy of the head
rostrocaudal tangential view

http://goo.gl/LOV8jQ

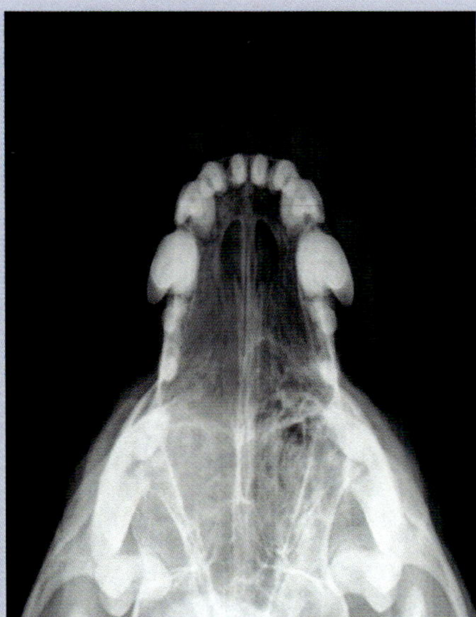

FIGURE 5.14. Enlarged image of the nasal cavity on a ventrodorsal open-mouth radiograph of a dog with a nasal neoplasm. An increase in the radiopacity of both nasal cavities may be observed, with marked loss of differentiation of the nasal conchae on the right. Histological diagnosis: adenocarcinoma.

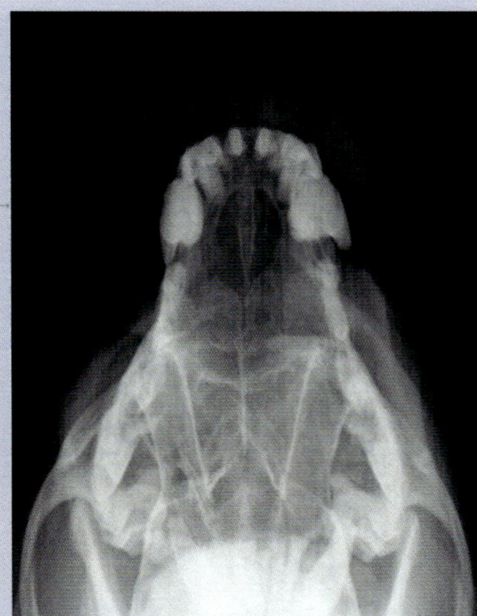

FIGURE 5.15. Enlarged image of the nasal cavity on a ventrodorsal open-mouth radiograph of a dog with a nasal neoplasm. It is possible to observe an increase in the radiopacity of both nasal cavities, with partial destruction of the vomer bone and loss of the normal pattern of the nasal conchae. Histological diagnosis: adenocarcinoma.

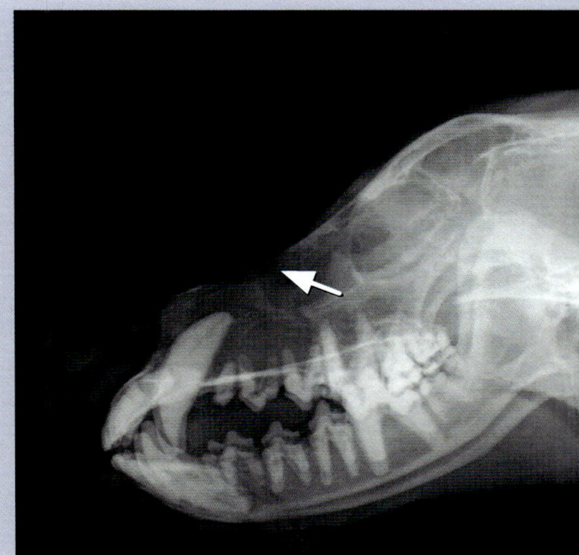

FIGURE 5.16. Lateral radiograph of the head of a dog with a nasal neoplasm. Partial destruction of the nasal bone (arrow) and inflammation of the adjacent soft tissues may be observed.

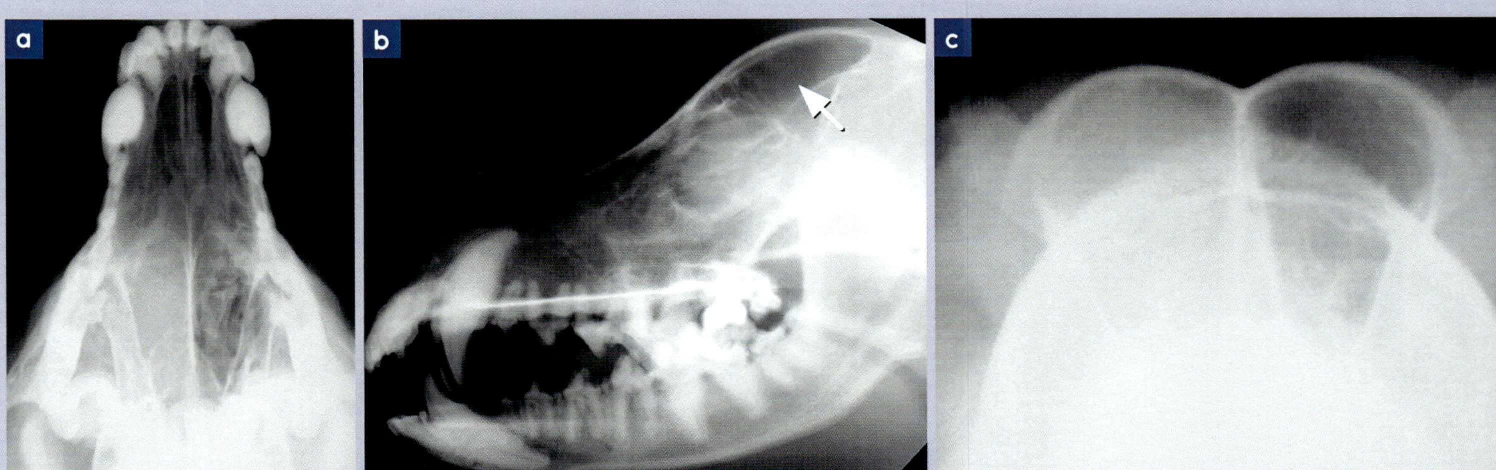

FIGURE 5.17. Enlarged image of the nasal cavity on a ventrodorsal open-mouth radiograph (a), lateral radiograph of the head (b) and rostrocaudal tangential radiograph of the frontal sinuses (c) of a dog with a nasal neoplasm. The ventrodorsal open-mouth radiograph shows an increase in radiopacity in the middle and caudal third of the right nasal cavity, with absence of the normal pattern of the conchae in both areas. The lateral radiograph shows an increase in radiopacity in the frontal sinuses (arrow), although it is not possible to determine whether it is uni- or bilateral on this view. The rostrocaudal tangential radiograph allows us to determine that the increase in radiopacity only affects the right frontal sinus. This can be attributed to obstructive sinusitis secondary to the presence of the mass in the ipsilateral nasal cavity, or to a neoplastic invasion of the sinus.

Normal radiographic anatomy of the head **lateral oblique view (mandible)**

http://goo.gl/alQAHX

Normal radiographic anatomy of the head **dorsoventral occlusal view**

http://goo.gl/iqa8CR

Nasal lymphoma in cats may cause an increase in the radiographic density of the nasal cavity, accompanied or not by bone destruction (fig. 5.18).

Computed tomography and magnetic resonance imaging are both appropriate for the assessment of nasal tumours. Computed tomography is indicated to analyse the involvement of the bone structures with greater precision, while magnetic resonance imaging is appropriate if the animal has neurological signs that make us suspect a secondary extension of the tumour to the brain through the cribrifom plate.

The frontal bone is a common location for osteosarcomas. Adenocarcinomas and squamous cell carcinomas may also appear in this location and affect the sinuses in a secondary manner (fig. 5.19).

Mandible, maxilla and temporomandibular joint

Fractures

Fractures of the mandible may appear in the symphysis (especially in cats) (fig. 5.20) or in the body of the mandible (fig. 5.21). They are identified with greater or lesser difficulty depending on the degree of displacement of the fragments. The lateral oblique and ventrodorsal intraoral projections are the most appropriate to examine these fractures. In order to assess fractures of the maxilla, the ventrodorsal open-mouth or dorsoventral intraoral projections are used (fig. 5.22).

The fractures that affect the components of the temporomandibular joint are usually difficult to diagnose. Computed tomography offers an excellent alternative for the diagnosis of this type of lesion.

Luxation

In order to assess a possible luxation or subluxation of the temporomandibular joint, it is recommended to take dorsoventral and lateral radiographs, as well as right and left lateral oblique radiographs with elevation of the rostral part of the head (they improve the visualisation of the temporomandibular joint, which is located closer to the cassette) (fig. 5.23). It will often be useful to compare both the lateral and lateral oblique radiographs with the mouth open and with the mouth closed.

The luxation of the temporomandibular joint is more frequent in cats than in dogs. It usually appears as a sequela of trauma, may be uni- or bilateral and is often associated with a fracture of the mandible. Clinically, the affected animals cannot close their mouth completely, have poor dental occlusion with lateral displacement of the mandible and suffer from excessive salivation. This problem may be difficult to identify on radiographs. The condyloid process of the mandible usually appears displaced in rostral and dorsal direction (fig. 5.24). Associated fractures of the condyloid process of the mandible or of the mandibular fossa of the temporal bone may also be observed.

Temporomandibular subluxations are difficult to identify on radiographs (fig. 5.25). However, computed tomography is an excellent alternative to diagnose this type of lesion.

Temporomandibular dysplasia

This uncommon congenital alteration has been described on a more frequent basis in the Basset Hound, followed by the Irish Setter. It is usually unilateral. The mandibular fossa of the temporal bone of the affected animals is usually flattened, the retroarticular process may sometimes be absent and subluxation may be present when open-mouth and closed-mouth radiographs are compared.

Degenerative joint disease

The signs of degenerative disease of the temporomandibular joint include narrowing and irregularity of the articular space and formation of periarticular osteophytes. It may appear as a sequela of dysplasia, trauma or otitis media.

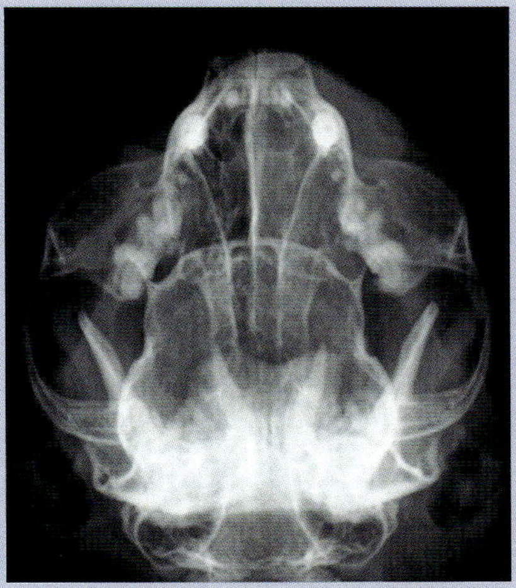

FIGURE 5.18. Ventrodorsal open-mouth radiograph of the head of a cat with a nasal neoplasm. An increase in the radiopacity of the left nasal cavity, with displacement of the rostral third of the vomer bone to the right, may be observed. Histological diagnosis: nasal lymphoma.

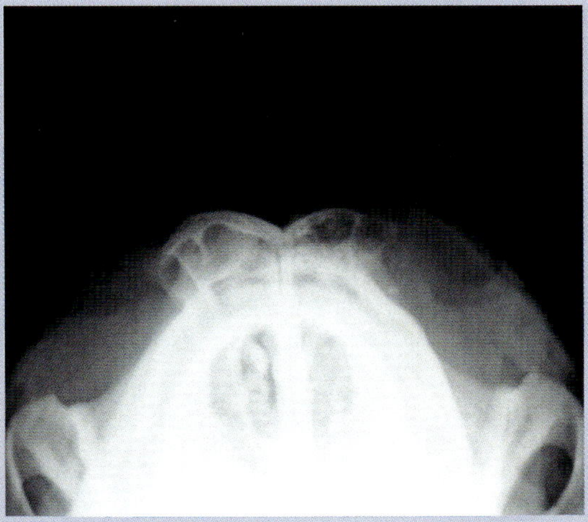

FIGURE 5.19. Rostrocaudal tangential radiograph of the frontal sinuses in a dog with a soft-tissue neoplasm in the left frontal area. Marked swelling of the soft tissues and partial destruction of the left frontal sinus may be seen. Histological diagnosis: carcinoma.

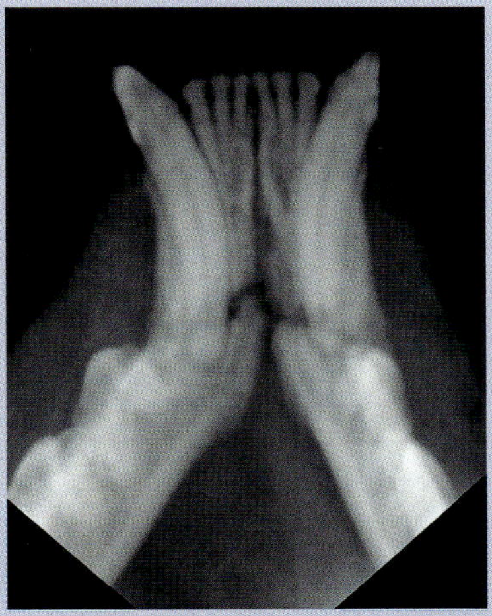

FIGURE 5.20. Ventrodorsal intraoral radiograph of the mandible of a cat with a fracture of the symphysis and rostral area of the left and right mandibles.

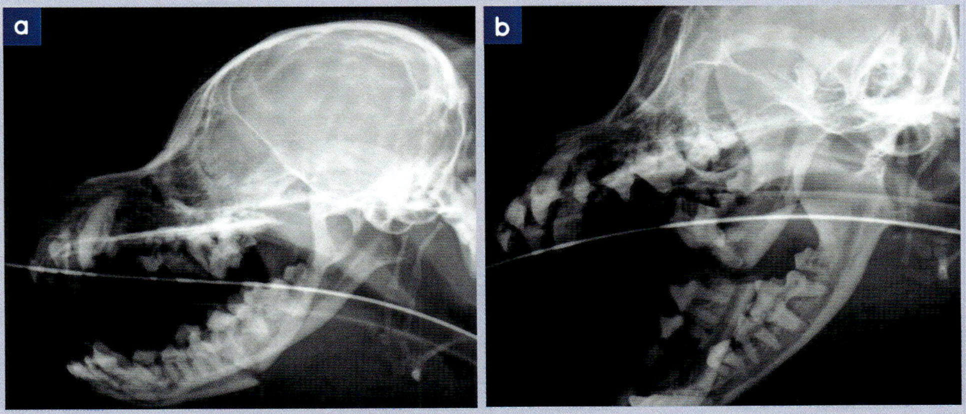

◀ **FIGURE 5.21.** Lateral (a) and lateral oblique (b) radiographs of the head of a dog with an oblique fracture of the body of the right mandible. The fracture is better visualised on the oblique radiograph.

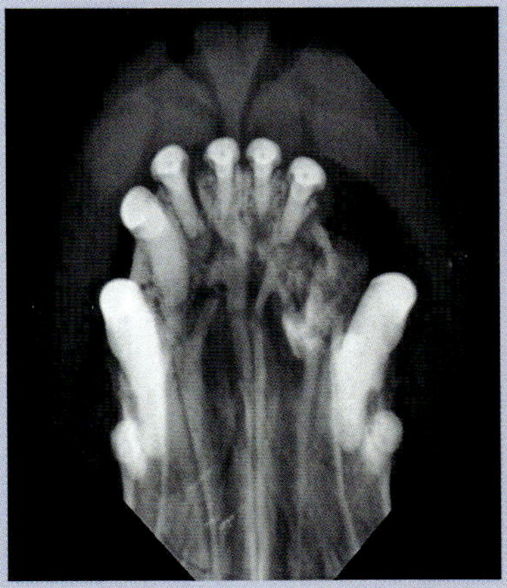

FIGURE 5.22. Dorsoventral intraoral radiograph of the maxilla of a dog with a comminuted fracture of the rostral area of the maxilla. Several lines of fracture may be observed and the upper left third incisor is missing.

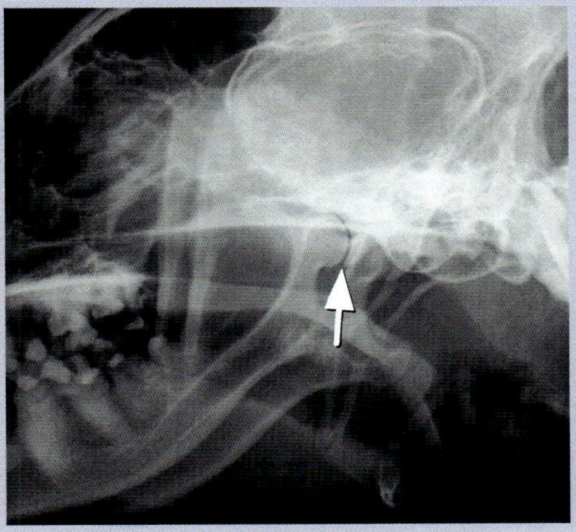

FIGURE 5.23. Lateral oblique radiograph with elevation of the rostral part of the head of a healthy dog. This radiograph offers a good image of the temporomandibular joint that is closest to the cassette (arrow).

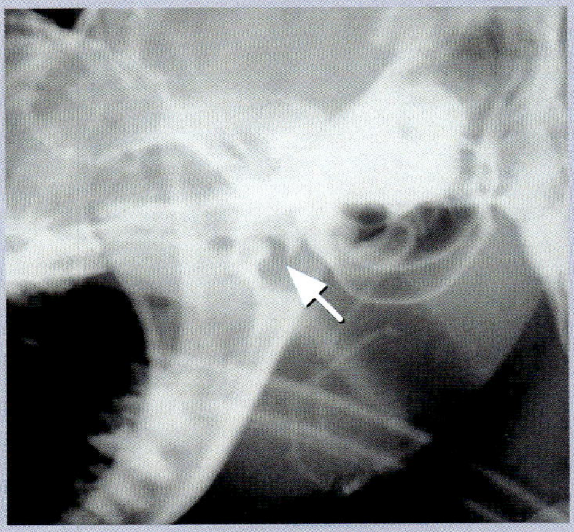

FIGURE 5.24. Lateral oblique radiograph with elevation of the rostral part of the head of a cat with luxation of the temporomandibular joint (arrow).

Normal radiographic anatomy of the head **lateral oblique view (temporomandibular joint)**

http://goo.gl/alQAHX

Tumours

The most frequent malignant oral tumours are squamous cell carcinomas, fibrosarcomas and malignant melanomas. They appear on radiographs as soft-tissue density masses, which generally infiltrate the adjacent bone, thus leading to the appearance of an aggressive bone lesion (fig. 5.26). Some teeth may be lost or displaced (fig. 5.27). When these radiological findings are observed, other diseases such as primary bone neoplasm and osteomyelitis, should be considered in the differential diagnosis.

Craniomandibular osteopathy

It is also known as "lion's jaw". This disease appears in young dogs, of 3 to 18 months of age, especially in the West Highland White Terrier, although it has also been described in the Boston Terrier, Cairn Terrier, Scottish Terrier and, exceptionally, in the Labrador Retriever and Doberman Pinscher. Clinically, it is possible to observe inflammation of the mandible, difficulty to pick up food, pain when opening the mouth or when chewing, and fever. On radiographs, a marked osteoproliferative reaction is observed in the affected areas, which may be the right and left mandibles (fig. 5.28.), the tympanic bullae and the petrous part of the temporal bone (fig. 5.29). The temporomandibular joint, and therefore its mobility, may also be affected. The changes may be uni- or bilateral. The dorsal area of the cranial vault may also appear enlarged, although its aspect is usually not as irregular as in other regions (fig. 5.30). Bone proliferation usually stops when the skeleton stops growing and a restructuring of these lesions sometimes occurs.

Secondary renal hyperparathyroidism

It is also called renal osteodystrophy or "rubber jaw". The reduction in the degree of glomerular filtration causes retention of phosphorus, which reduces calcium levels in blood. This stimulates the production of parathyroid hormone. This disease seems to affect the mandible and maxilla. It usually appears in older dogs, but can also be detected in young patients with congenital renal dysplasia. Clinically, it may be characterised by the appearance of dental disease, excessive salivation, loss of teeth or

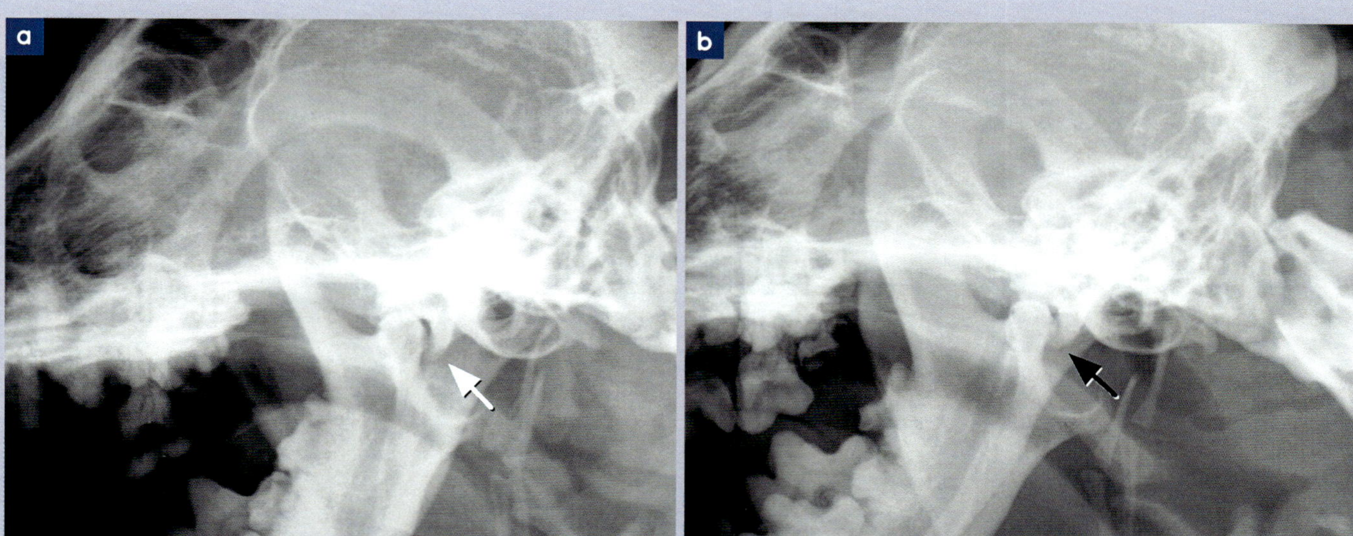

FIGURE 5.25. Right (a) and left (b) lateral oblique radiographs with elevation of the rostral part of the head of a dog with temporomandibular subluxation. The right temporomandibular joint (white arrow) is better visualised on the right lateral oblique radiograph, and the left joint (black arrow) is better visualised on the left lateral oblique radiograph.

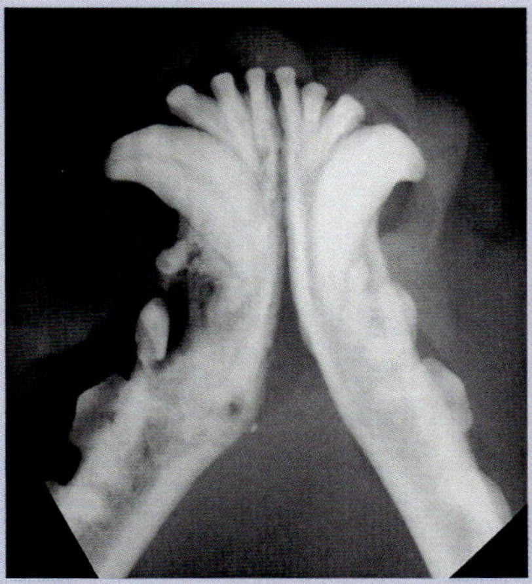

FIGURE 5.26. Ventrodorsal intraoral radiograph of the mandible of a dog with an oral soft-tissue neoplasm. Osteolysis is observed in the rostral end of the right mandible, with displacement of the lower right first and second premolars, which is indicative of secondary bone involvement. Histological diagnosis: melanoma.

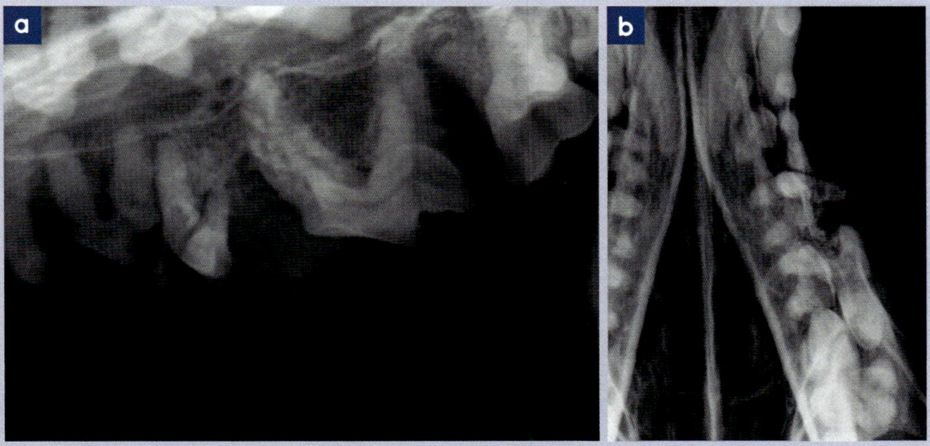

FIGURE 5.27. Enlarged images of the left maxillary area on left lateral oblique (a) and ventrodorsal (b) radiographs of the head of a dog with an oral soft-tissue neoplasm. It is possible to observe a mass of soft tissue located between the upper left third and fourth premolars, which causes the rostral displacement of the third premolar and the loss of the normal bone structure in the area adjacent to the lesion. This is compatible with secondary bone involvement. Histological diagnosis: fibrosarcoma.

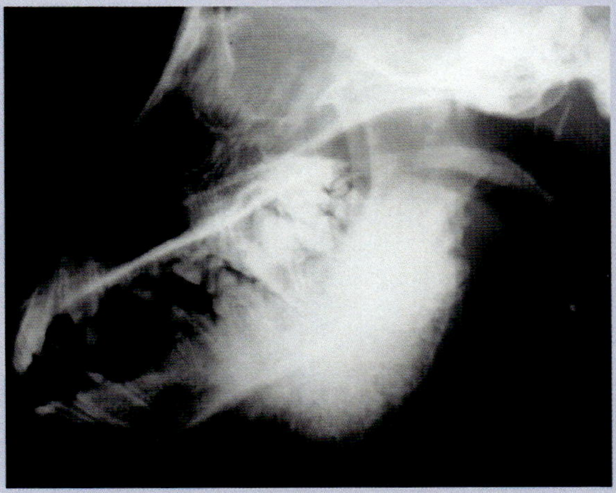

FIGURE 5.28. Enlarged image of the mandibular region on a lateral radiograph of the head of a dog with craniomandibular osteopathy that affects the two mandibles.

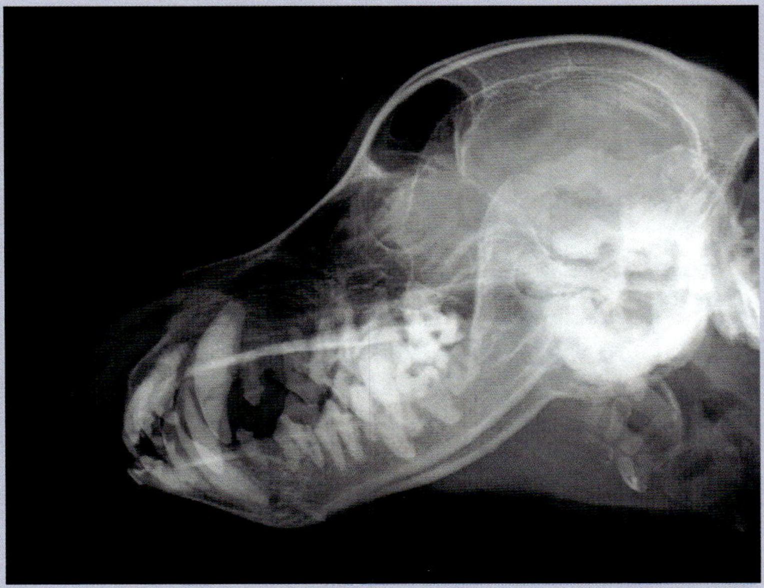

▲ FIGURE 5.29. Lateral radiograph of the head of a dog with craniomandibular osteopathy that affects the tympanic bullae and the petrous region of the temporal bone.

Normal radiographic anatomy of the head
lateral view
http://goo.gl/JE5G8d

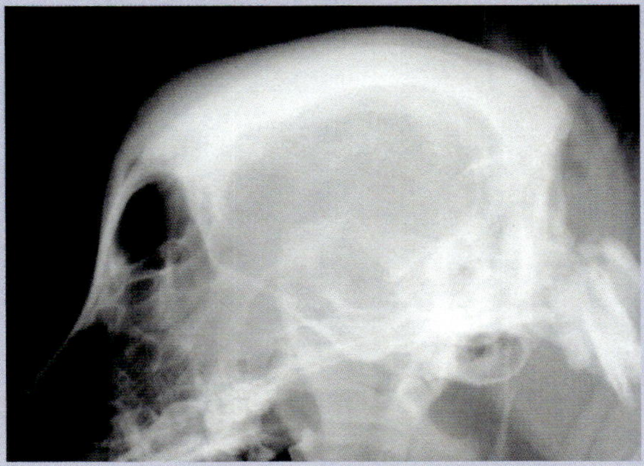

◀ FIGURE 5.30. Enlarged image of the cranial vault on a lateral radiograph of a dog with craniomandibular osteopathy.

Normal radiographic anatomy of the head **dorsoventral view**

http://goo.gl/iqa8CR

respiratory problems due to maxillary collapse. The radiographic signs include demineralisation of the mandible and/or maxilla, loss of the lamina dura and formation of radiolucent halos around the dental roots. At advanced stages, the mineral density of teeth markedly contrasts with the demineralised surrounding bone (fig. 5.31). In chronic processes, there may be demineralisation of the long bones of the limbs.

Teeth

A tooth is formed by a root (part embedded in the bone) and crown (part located in the mouth cavity). The bone that is located between the teeth is called alveolar crest. The dentin, enamel and cement are radiopaque. The pulp cavity and periodontal membrane have soft-tissue density (fig. 5.32). The pulp cavity decreases in size with age. The periodontal membrane appears surrounded by a thin layer of mineral density, which corresponds to the lamina dura.

Although many dental disorders can be identified by using conventional cassette-film systems, in some cases it will be useful to take intraoral radiographs with dental film.

The dental formulas of the dog and cat are shown in table 5.1.

Table 5.1. Dental formulas of the dog and cat.

Species	Deciduous teeth	Permanent teeth
Cat	2 x (I 3/3 C 1/1 PM 3/2) = 26	2 x (I 3/3 C 1/1 PM 3/2 M 1/1) = 30
Dog	2 x (I 3/3 C 1/1 PM 2/2 M 1/1) = 28	2 x (I 3/3 C 1/1 PM 4/4 M 2/3) = 42

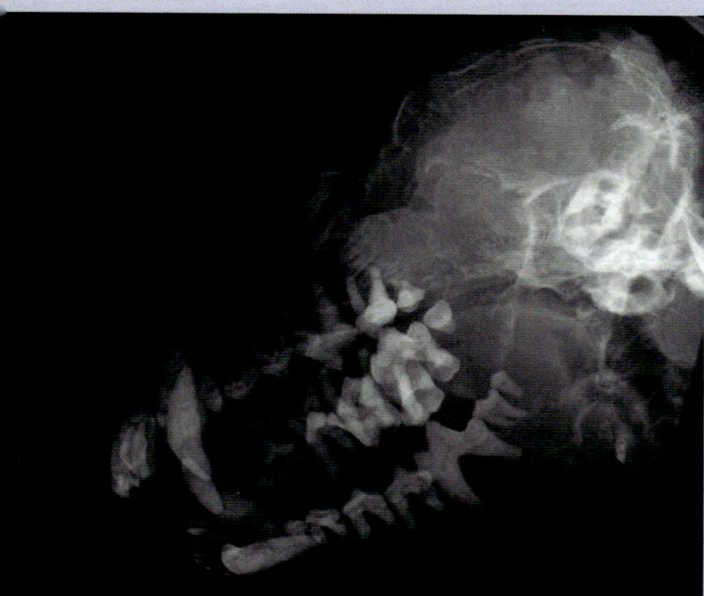

FIGURE 5.31. Lateral oblique radiograph of the head of a dog with secondary renal hyperparathyroidism ("rubber jaw"). Marked demineralisation of the mandible, maxilla, zygomatic arches and cranial vault may be observed. The frontal bone appears depressed. The density of the teeth contrasts to a large extent with that of the demineralised bone.

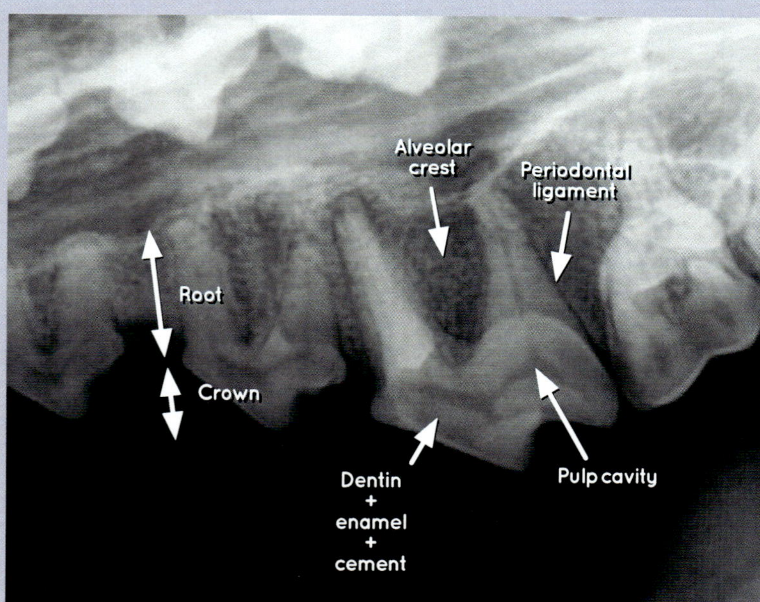

FIGURE 5.32. Enlarged image of the maxillary region of a healthy dog in oblique lateral projection. Parts of the teeth.

Normal radiographic anatomy of the head **ventrodorsal open-mouth view**

http://goo.gl/cPJEs6

Caries

They appear as a radiolucent effect in the crown of the affected tooth. In dogs, they are most often observed on the upper first molar.

Periodontal disease

Periodontal disease is common in adult animals. It is characterised on radiographs by a widening of the periodontal space, loss of lamina dura and lysis of the trabecular bone located around the tooth (fig. 5.33).

Periapical abscess

Periapical abscesses may appear associated with periodontal disease, caries or fractures of dental roots. They give rise to the formation of a radiolucent halo around the root of the affected tooth, caused by the destruction of the alveolar bone. Resorption of the dental root, which appears thinner and with an irregular outline, may also be observed (fig. 5.34). In dogs, infections of the fourth maxillary premolar may lead to the formation of a fistulous tract that usually opens to the exterior under the eye.

Auditory system

In order to assess the auditory system, it is recommended to take a ventrodorsal radiograph, which allows the examination of the ear canals, a rostrocaudal open-mouth radiograph, in which the two tympanic bullae may be observed, and right and left oblique lateral radiographs, which improve the visualisation of the bulla closest to the chassis.

In cats, an additional projection has been described, the rostroventral-caudodorsal oblique projection with a 10-degree angle, which offers a good image of both bullae in this species (fig. 5.35).

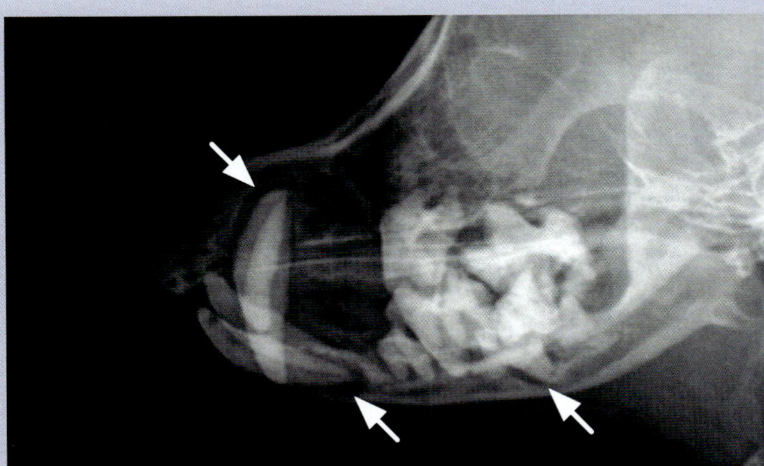

FIGURE 5.33. Enlarged image of the maxillary and mandibular region on a lateral radiograph of the head of a dog with periodotontal disease. Radiolucent halos around several dental roots (arrows) and the absence of numerous teeth may be observed.

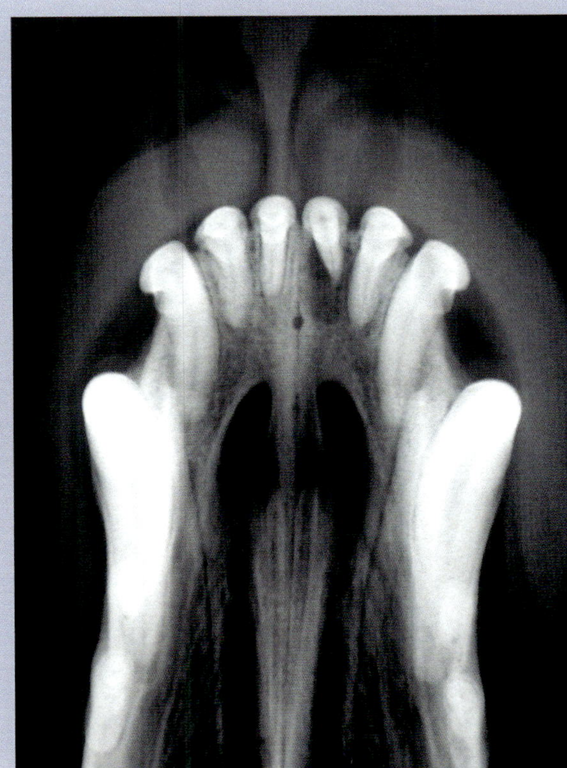

FIGURE 5.34. Enlarged image of the maxillary region on a ventrodorsal open-mouth radiograph of the head of a dog with a periapical abscess. A radiolucent area around the root of the upper left first incisor is observed, with partial resorption of this dental root.

The ear canals appear as gas density tracts lateral to the tympanic bullae on ventrodorsal radiographs. On lateral oblique and rostrocaudal open-mouth radiographs, the tympanic bulla appears as an approximately round structure containing air, limited by a thin wall of mineral density (fig. 5.36). The image is slightly different in cats, since they have a bone division that creates two compartments, one internal and the other external (fig. 5.37).

Otitis externa

Otitis externa is diagnosed clinically and in many cases does not cause any evident alteration of the radiographic image of the ear canals. Obstruction of the affected canal or canals is sometimes observed and it is common to find calcification of the walls in chronic processes (fig. 5.38).

Otitis media

It is usually secondary to chronic otitis externa. The left and right lateral oblique views, as well as the rostrocaudal open-mouth view, are the most appropriate to assess this alteration. The radiological signs indicative of otitis media are thickening and/or irregularity of the bone wall of the tympanic bulla, as well as increased radiographic density in its interior (fig. 5.39). The process may be uni- or bilateral (fig. 5.40). If the osteoproliferative reaction is very marked, it may eventually affect the temporal bone and temporomandibular joint. A normal radiographic image of the bullae does not rule out otitis media. Both computed tomography and magnetic resonance imaging are excellent techniques for the evaluation of this disease.

Tumours

The most frequent tumours of the ear canal are squamous cell carcinomas and adenocarcinomas of the mucous glands. They appear as soft-tissue masses that may cause obstruction of the ear canal and secondary involvement of the bulla and adjacent bone structures (fig. 5.41).

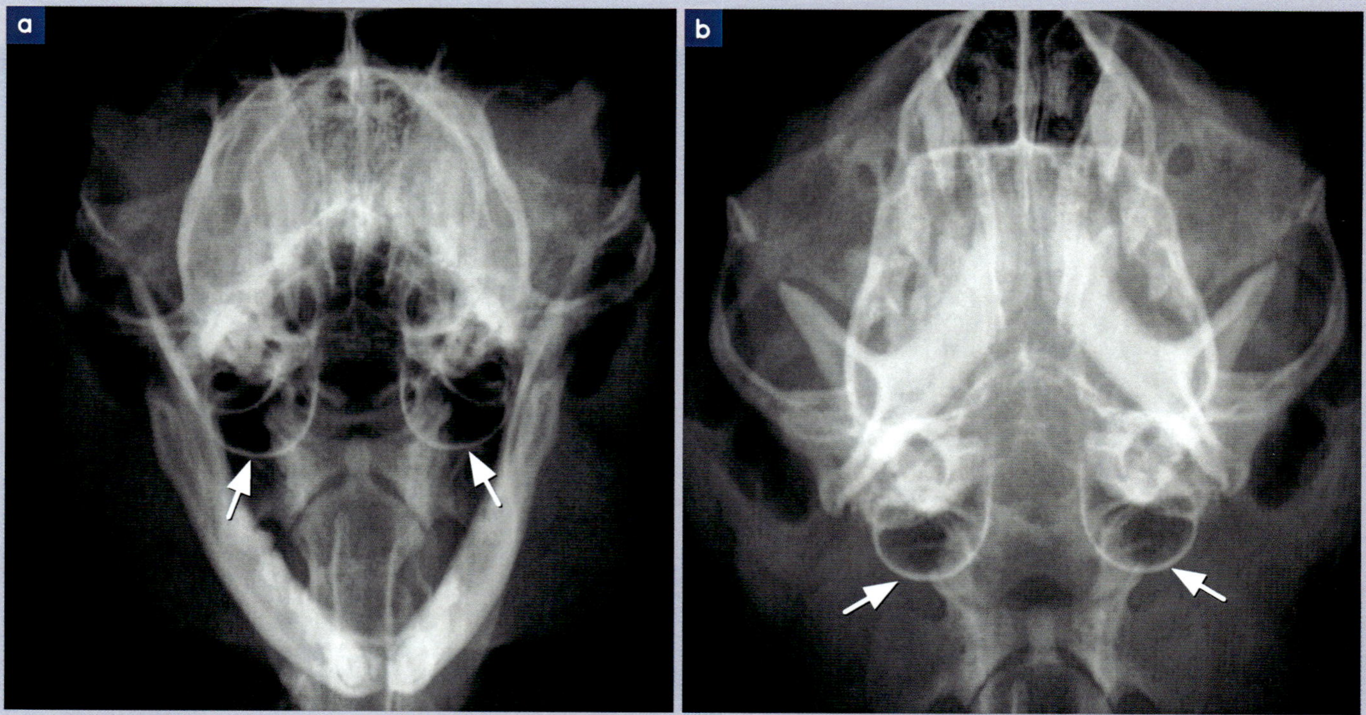

FIGURE 5.35. Rostrocaudal open-mouth (a) and rostroventral-dorsoventral oblique (b) radiographs of the head of a healthy cat. Both views are appropriate for the assessment of the tympanic bullae (arrows) in cats.

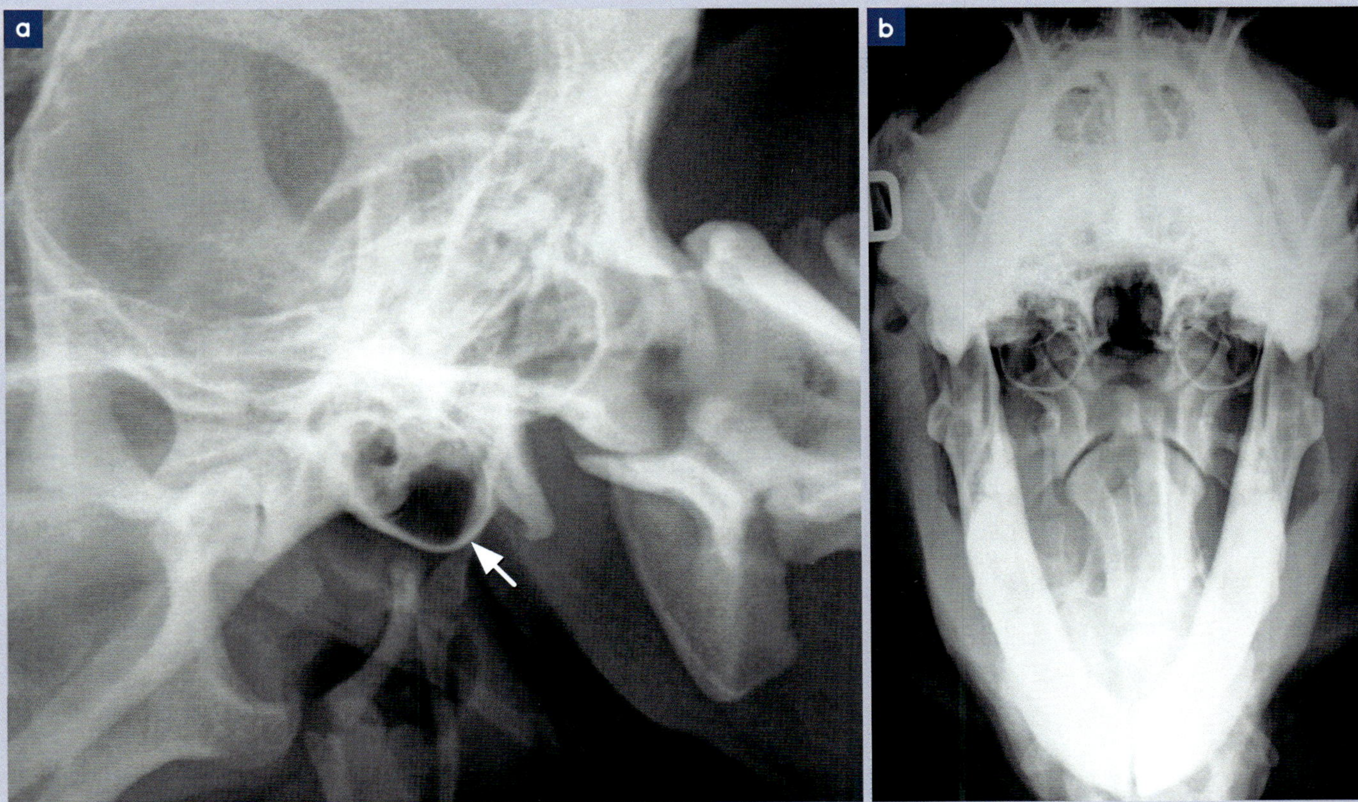

FIGURE 5.36. Enlarged image of the left tympanic bullae (arrow) on lateral oblique (a) and rostrocaudal open-mouth (b) radiographs of the head of a healthy dog.

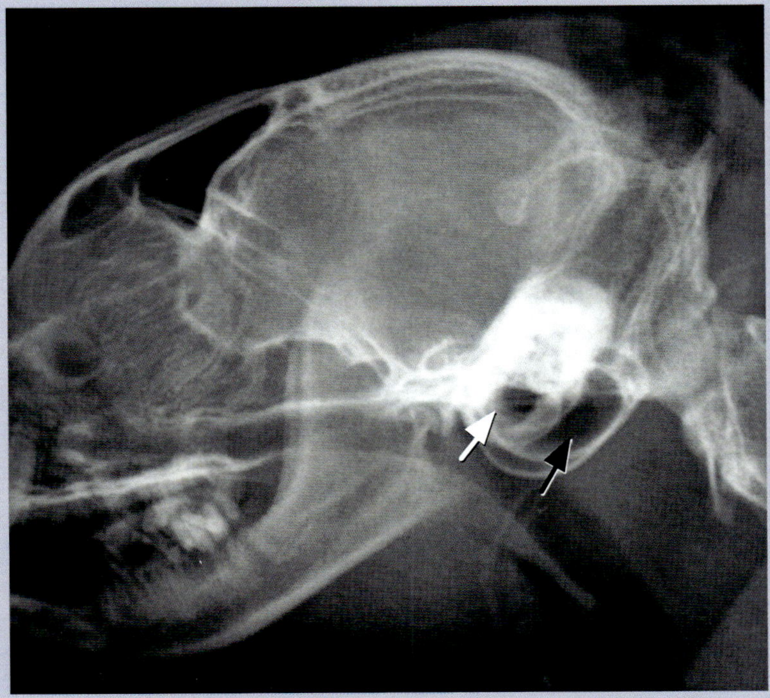

FIGURE 5.37. Lateral radiograph of the head of a healthy cat. In cats, the tympanic bullae have a bone division that separates an internal compartment (white arrow) from an external compartment (black arrow).

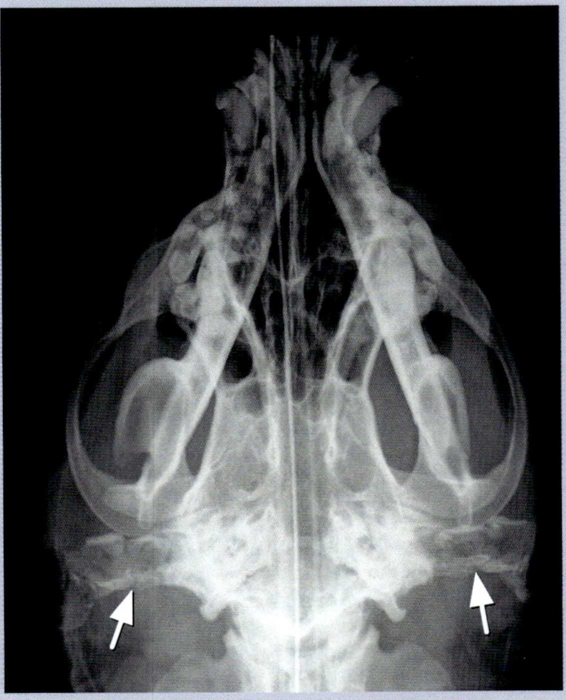

FIGURE 5.38. Dorsoventral radiograph of the head of a dog with otitis externa. Calcification of the ear canals is observed (arrows).

Normal radiographic anatomy of the head **rostrocaudal open-mouth view**

http://goo.gl/LOV8jQ

Self-assessment cases

http://goo.gl/bxl8Ap

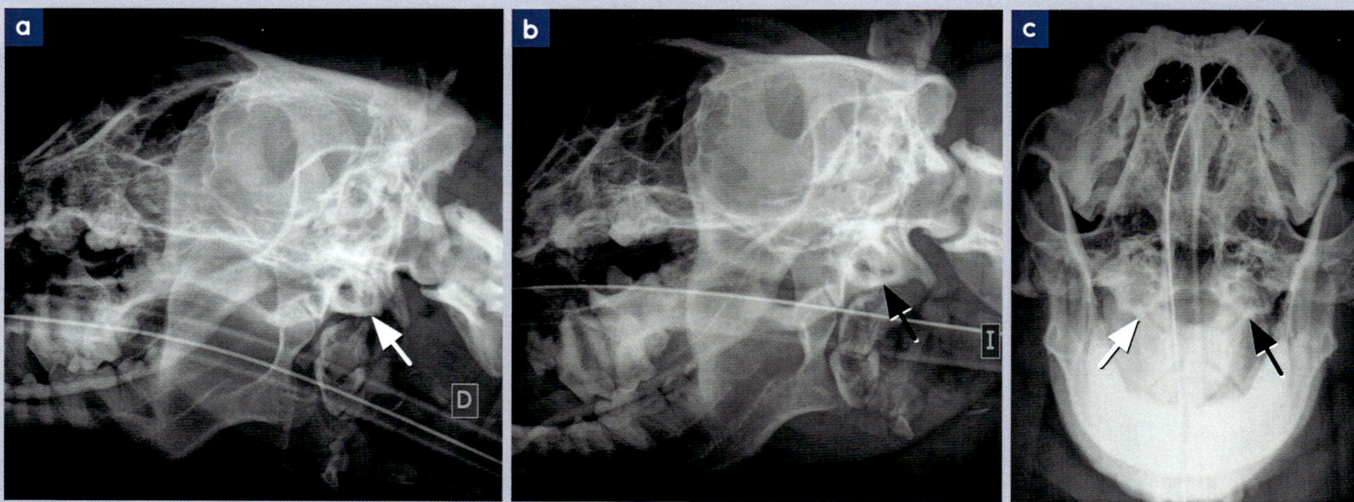

FIGURE 5.39. Enlarged images of the tympanic bullae on right (a) and left (b) lateral oblique radiographs and on a rostrocaudal open-mouth radiograph of the head of a dog with bilateral otitis media. Both the right tympanic bulla (white arrows) and the left tympanic bulla (black arrows) have a thickened wall and increased radiographic density in their interior. Both ear canals are calcified.

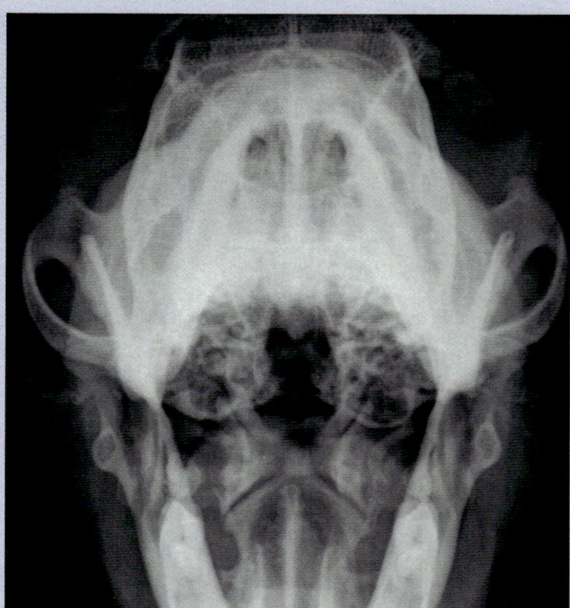

FIGURE 5.40. Enlarged image of the tympanic bullae on a rostrocaudal open-mouth radiograph of the head of a dog with right unilateral otitis media. Thickening and irregularity of the wall of the right tympanic bulla may be observed.

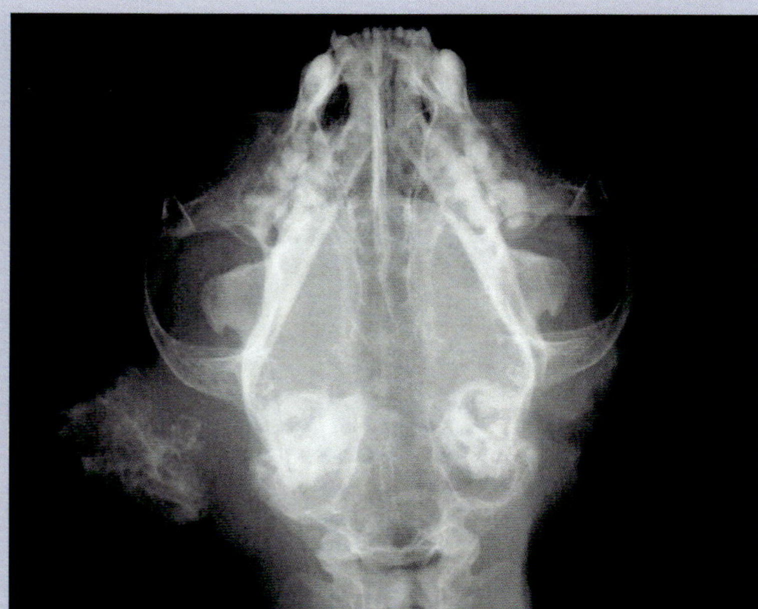

FIGURE 5.41. Dorsoventral radiograph of the head of a cat with a tumour of the ear canal. A partially calcified soft-tissue mass may be observed in the area of the right ear canal. Diagnosis: adenocarcinoma of the mucous glands.

Most common diagnostic errors 6

The main disadvantages of radiography against other diagnostic imaging techniques are the limited differences of opacity in the image (gas, fat, soft tissues and fluids, mineral and metal) and the superimposition of structures, which often causes a loss of diagnostic information as well as optical effects that may lead to errors in the diagnosis. Diagnostic errors are also frequently caused by apparently anomalous images due to a poor position of the patient when the radiograph was taken, the use of incorrect exposure values, an inappropriate administration of the contrast agent, and by a poor knowledge of the normal anatomical variations of certain structures.

This chapter reviews the most common diagnostic errors divided by anatomical regions and includes a specific reference to those that are typical of digital radiography in the last section. Many of them have already been mentioned in the corresponding chapters of this book.

Note: the text includes references to the figures in this chapter as well as to other figures that have already appeared in previous chapters.

Abdomen

Lack of abdominal fat, wet hair

Very thin (fig. 6.11) or young animals have very little intraabdominal fat, which makes the identification of abdominal structures more difficult. This image may be mistaken for that caused by ascites, peritonitis or peritoneal carcinomatosis. The image produced by overlying wet hair, for example when a radiograph is taken after an abdominal ultrasound in which gel was applied to enhance the transmission of ultrasonic waves, should not be confused with that of these diseases either.

Underexposure and overexposure

A greatly underexposed abdominal radiograph (taken with very low exposure values) may also give a false appearance of increased and more homogeneous radiopacity than normal, which should not be confused with peritoneal disease. On the other hand, on a highly overexposed abdominal radiograph (taken with very high exposure values), the decrease in radiopacity caused by the technical error may be confused with that caused by a pneumoperitoneum.

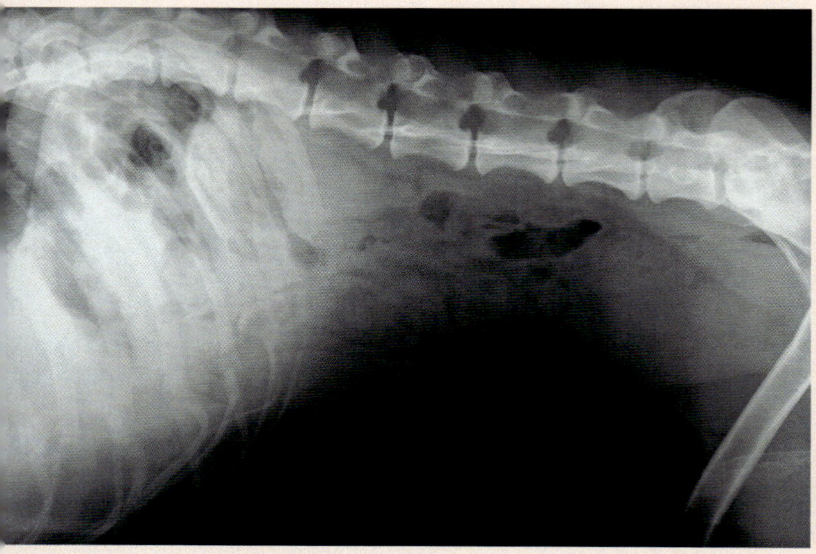

FIGURE 6.1. Lateral radiograph of the abdomen of a very thin, healthy dog. The abdominal organs appear poorly differentiated due to the lack of intraabdominal fat. This could be confused with ascites, peritonitis or peritoneal carcinomatosis. In case of doubt, an ultrasound scan will allow us to establish a precise diagnosis.

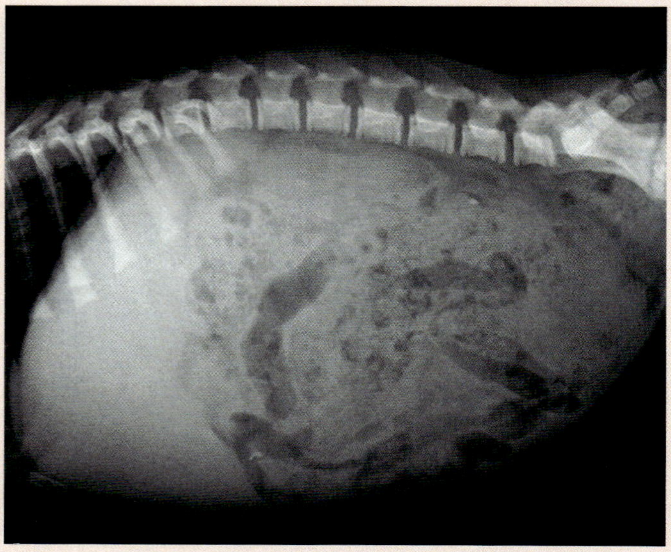

FIGURE 6.2. Lateral radiograph of the abdomen of a healthy young dog. The abdominal organs appear poorly differentiated due to the lack of intraabdominal fat, which is normal in young animals. We should not confuse this image with that caused by ascites, peritonitis or peritoneal carcinomatosis. In case of doubt, an ultrasound scan will allow us to establish a precise diagnosis.

Caudal hepatic border depending on thoracic conformation

The caudal hepatic border is usually seen at the level of or slightly beyond the costal arch on lateral radiographs. In order not to give an incorrect diagnosis of increase or reduction in the size of the liver, it must be borne in mind that, in breeds with a deep and narrow thorax, the whole shadow of the liver may be located in the thoracic cage (false appearance of decrease in size) while, on the other hand, the caudal hepatic border extends beyond the limit of the costal arch to a greater extent in breeds with a wide and shallow thorax (false appearance of increase in size).

Physiological organomegaly in young animals

It should be remembered that young animals display a certain degree of organomegaly in comparison with adult animals. This should be taken into account in the first months of life so as not to make an incorrect diagnose of increase in the size of the abdominal organs.

False impression of splenomegaly

It is also important to highlight that splenomegaly is assessed in function of the thickness of the shadow of the spleen, since its length depends on the position of the tail of the spleen when taking the radiograph. A long shadow with no increase in its thickness does not indicate splenomegaly (fig. 1.32).

Gestation before foetal mineralisation

Before day 45 of pregnancy in the dog and between days 36 and 45 in the cat, the pregnant uterus appears increased in size, but the mineralised foetal structures cannot be differentiated in it (fig. 1.76). We may therefore mistake pregnancy for pathological dilatation of the uterus. Performing an abdominal ultrasound scan will allow us to establish a differential diagnosis.

Superimposition of the prepuce and os penis

The shadow of the prepuce on a ventrodorsal radiograph may be mistaken for the shadow of the bladder or for a mass. Especially on rotated radiographs, the shadows of the prepuce and os penis may create optical effects of superimposition on the hip that may be confused with lesions of the latter.

"Pseudomasses"

Some normal abdominal images may produce a pseudomass effect. Thus, a very distended bladder filled with fluids may be mistaken for masses originated by pathological causes in other organs (fig. 1.57). The fat that accumulates in the falciform ligament of obese cats creates a shadow ventral to the liver that reminds of a mass, although its density, which is lower than that of soft tissues, facilitates its identification as fat (fig. 1.9). The superimposition of the two kidneys on lateral radiographs creates an optical effect since their radiographic densities add up, which may be confused with the presence of a third structure in the area. Another example of pseudomass is the markedly round image that the normal pyloric antrum may have on right lateral radiographs. This is a classical example of a possible diagnostic pitfall, as it may be confused with a mass or with a round foreign body (fig. 6.3).

False thickening of the gastric or intestinal wall

Although this has already been mentioned in the corresponding section, it is important to highlight that one of the most important errors that may be made when assessing an abdominal radiograph is to diagnose a thickening of the gastric (fig. 1.96) or intestinal (fig. 1.113) wall. In the image, it is impossible to distinguish a wall that is really thickened from a normal wall with fluid or mucus adjacent to it, which gives a false impression of increase in thickness. The thickness of the walls of the stomach and intestine must be assessed by ultrasonography.

Increase in the amount of gastric and intestinal fluid/gas

A predominance of fluid (fig. 6.4) or gas (fig. 6.5) content in the small intestine is considered to be indicative of enteritis, but it is important to highlight that these findings alone do not mean there is a disease process. In a similar way, a very dilated stomach filled with gas in a nervous animal may be exclusively due to aerophagia and may not have any pathological significance.

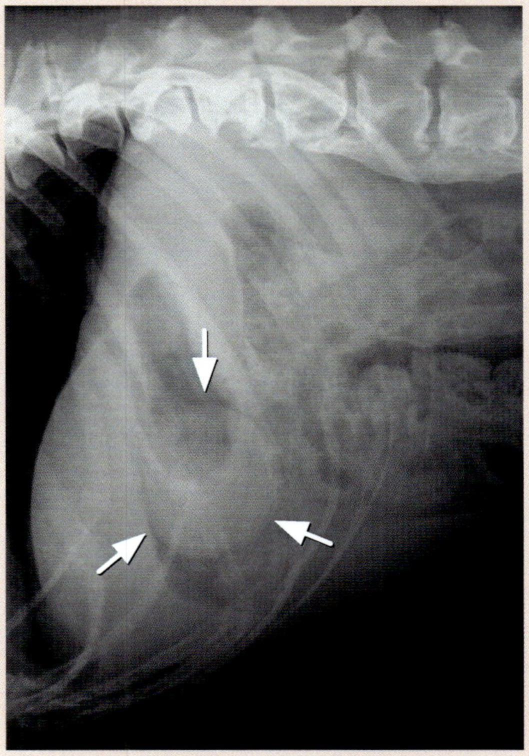

FIGURE 6.3. Enlarged image of the abdomen on a lateral radiograph of a healthy dog. The pyloric antrum (arrows) has a round aspect due to the normal accumulation of fluid/mucus on this view. This image may be confused with a round foreign body or with a mass.

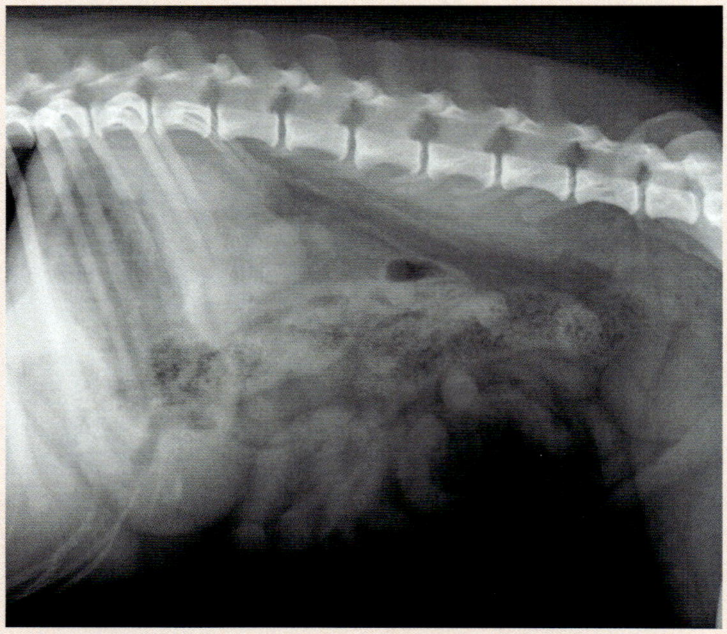

FIGURE 6.4. Lateral radiograph of the abdomen of a healthy dog. In the image, it is possible to observe a marked predominance of fluid content (fluid/mucus) in the small intestine, which is not accompanied by alterations of its diameter. This finding alone does not have any pathological significance, although it sometimes appears associated with processes of enteritis. However, it would be a serious error to establish a diagnosis of enteritis based only on this radiological sign.

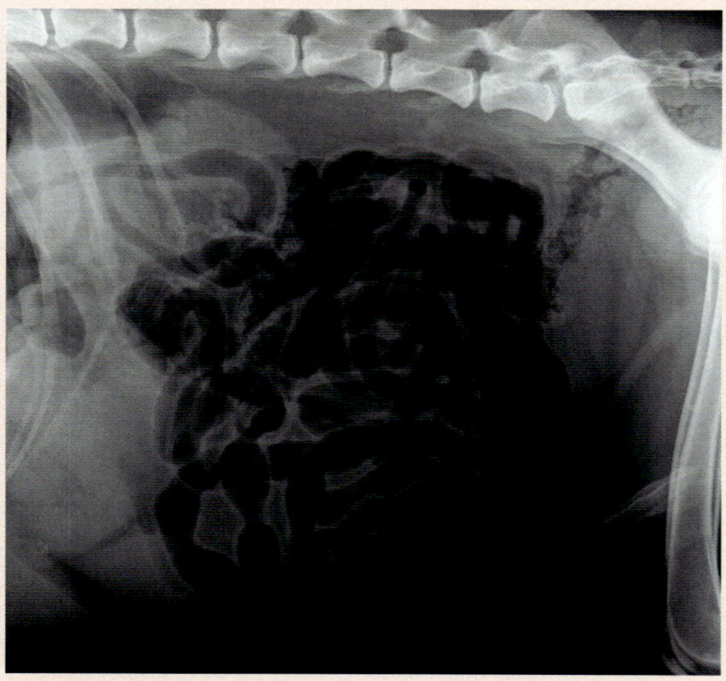

FIGURE 6.5. Lateral radiograph of the abdomen of a healthy dog. In the image, it is possible to observe a marked predominance of gas content in the small intestine, which is not accompanied by alterations of its diameter. This finding alone does not have any pathological significance, although it sometimes appears associated with processes of enteritis. As in the case of a predominance of fluid, it would be a serious error to diagnose enteritis based only on this radiological finding.

Anatomical variations of the gastrointestinal tract in cats

The accumulation of loops of the small intestine in the centre of the abdomen in obese cats is due to the tendency shown by these animals to accumulate fat in the peripheral areas of the abdomen (fig. 1.9), and this finding should therefore not be attributed to pathological causes.

The radiographs of some cats also show a band of fat density in the gastric wall, which is considered an incidental finding with no clinical significance.

Intestinal particularities in dogs

The caecum in dogs often appears dilated, with gas content and a C-shape in the right cranial area of the abdomen on ventrodorsal radiographs (fig. 1.130), and superimposed on the descending colon on lateral radiographs. It is important not to confuse it with a segment of abnormally dilated small intestine so as not to make an incorrect diagnosis of intestinal obstruction.

Some dogs have a longer colon than normal, which is called **redundant colon** and is considered a normal anatomical variation.

Peristaltic waves

A wavy appearance of the wall of the small or large intestine may sometimes be observed. This finding is indicative of an inflammatory or diffuse infiltrative process if it persists on various radiographs taken at different times, but when it is an isolated finding in a radiographic study, it is usually due to the appearance of a peristaltic wave when the radiograph was taken (fig.6.6).

Inappropriate doses of contrast agent

With regard to contrast techniques, the most frequent cause of diagnostic errors is the administration of an inappropriate dose of contrast medium. For instance, if positive-contrast gastrography is used to evaluate gastric emptying and a lower dose than recommended is administered, the rate of emptying will be slower, while if an excessive dose is administered it will be faster. The results of the test will therefore not be objective.

Patterns of contrast medium accumulation

When carrying out a barium study of the small intestine in small dogs, it is possible to observe out-pouchings in the contrast column as this goes through the duodenum. These are called **pseudoulcers** (fig. 6.7), and are due to the focal accumulation of the contrast medium in areas with lymphatic tissue. In approximately 30% of cats, it is also possible to observe a peculiar image of the duodenum when administering barium, which is referred to as the "string of pearls" sign (fig 6.8), and is due to strong segmental contractions of the duodenal wall with no pathological significance. This image is similar to the one that the presence of a linear foreign body may cause in any intestinal segment.

Presence of gas bubbles

When retrograde urethrography or positive-contrast cystography are used, it is easy to confuse the image created by the gas bubbles that were introduced when the patient was catheterised with real filling defects caused by calculi or clots (fig. 1.162). These gas bubbles usually have a round morphology, while calculi and clots usually have a more irregular shape and distribution.

Contrast diffusion

Finally, on retrograde urethrograms in males, it is possible to observe the passage of a small amount of contrast medium to the prostatic ducts. This finding does not have any pathological significance, unless it is accompanied by a focal accumulation of contrast material in cavities or cystic areas.

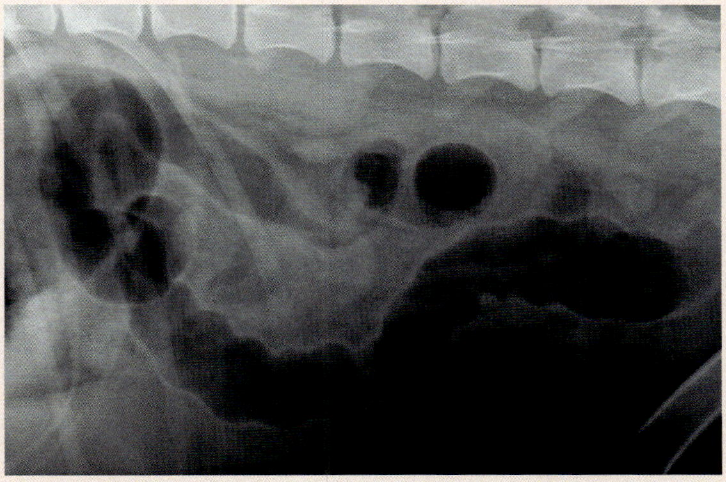

FIGURE 6.6. Enlarged image of the abdomen on a lateral radiograph of a healthy dog. The wavy appearance of the large intestinal wall may be due to an inflammatory process, but it may also be due to normal peristalsis. The persistence of this image on serial radiographs is considered indicative of a disease.

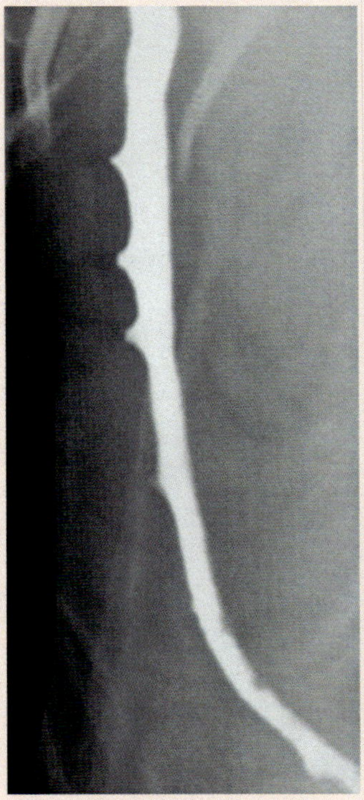

FIGURE 6.7. Enlarged image of the duodenum 20 minutes after administering barium by oral route to a healthy dog. The out-pouchings that appear on the lateral aspect of the contrast column are due to the presence of normal lymphatic tissue in the duodenal wall. This image may be confused with ulcers, which is why it is referred to as pseudoulcers.

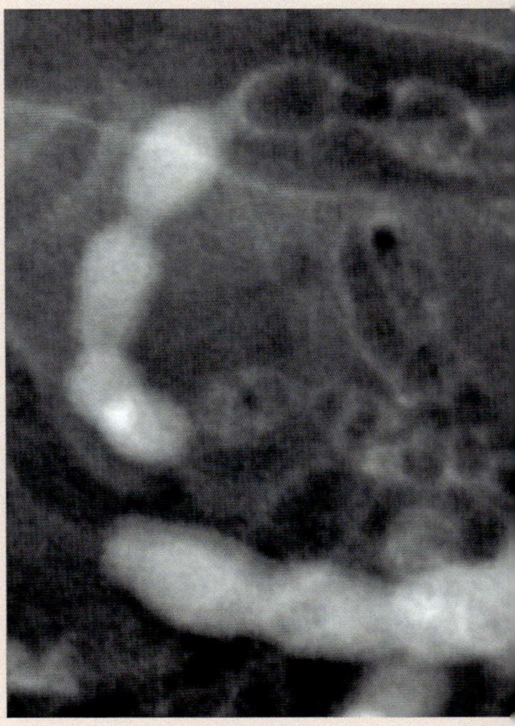

FIGURE 6.8. Enlarged image of the duodenum 30 minutes after administering barium by oral route to a healthy cat. The wavy appearance of the duodenal wall is due to normal peristaltic contractions and is termed "string of pearls" sign. It may be confused with the image of a linear foreign body.

Neck and thorax

Confusion of the hyoid apparatus with foreign bodies

When the presence of a foreign body in the neck is suspected, the bones that form the hyoid apparatus should not be confused with foreign bodies in the pharynx. If a real foreign body is detected on a lateral radiograph, its exact location should always be confirmed by taking a ventrodorsal radiograph.

Cricopharyngeal sphincter

When administering a contrast agent by oral route and evaluating its passage from the orophraynx to the oesophagus, it is important not to confuse the image of the cranial oesophageal sphincter (cricopharyngeal sphincter) with a filling defect or "mass effect" due to pathological causes.

Cutaneous nodules and nipples

Cutaneous nodules may have a similar image to nodular lesions in the lung. The same may sometimes occur when nipples are superimposed (fig. 6.9) on rotated radiographs. In case of doubt, the thoracic wall should be examined thoroughly and a small amount of barium should be applied on the cutaneous lesion or nipple to repeat the radiograph.

Calcification associated with age

Calcification of the costochondral junctions associated with age, which has no clinical significance, should not be confused with aggressive bone lesions (fig. 2.7). On ventrodorsal radiographs, these calcifications may create a false effect of calcified nodular lesions in the lung (fig. 6.10).

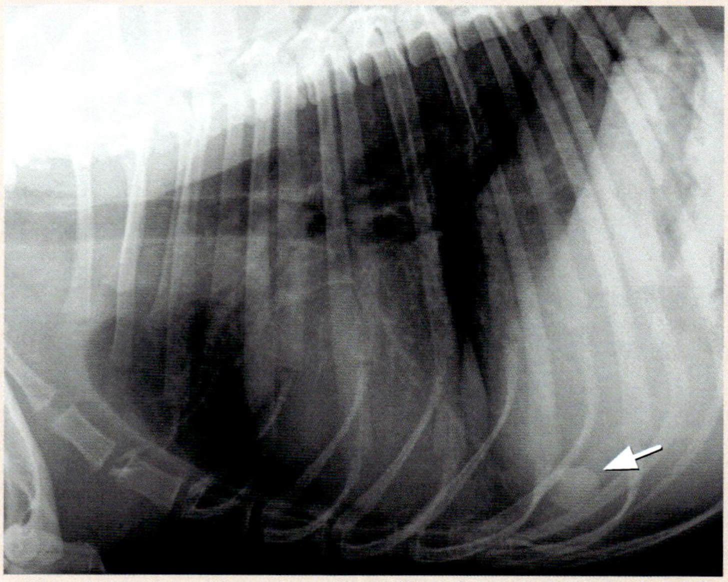

FIGURE 6.9. Lateral radiograph of the thorax of a healthy dog. The arrow indicates a hyperplastic nipple, which, due to the rotated position of the thorax, is superimposed on the ventral area of the shadow of the liver and may be mistaken for a calculus in the gallbladder or for a nodular lesion in the lung.

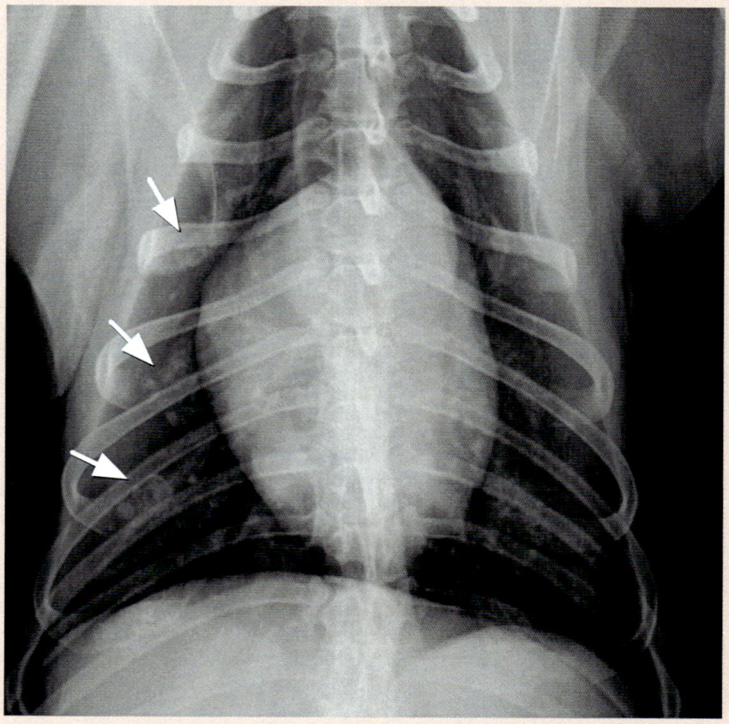

FIGURE 6.10. Ventrodorsal radiograph of the thorax of a healthy dog. The arrows show calcifications of the right costochondral junctions. These should not be confused with aggressive bone lesions or calcified nodular lesions in the lung.

Folds of skin

The folds of skin that form when the patient is placed on the cassette may create well-defined shadows of soft-tissue density surrounded by gas, which should not be confused with diseases (fig. 2.1c).

Rib curvature and costal cartilage calcification

Chondrodystrophic breeds sometimes show a peculiar curvature of the ribs and costal cartilages towards the inside of the cavity, in the area proximal to the costochondral junction. This creates shadows of soft-tissue density that may be similar to a pleural or pulmonary lesion.

Costal cartilages may appear partially calcified in cats, which may produce a false appearance of fractures.

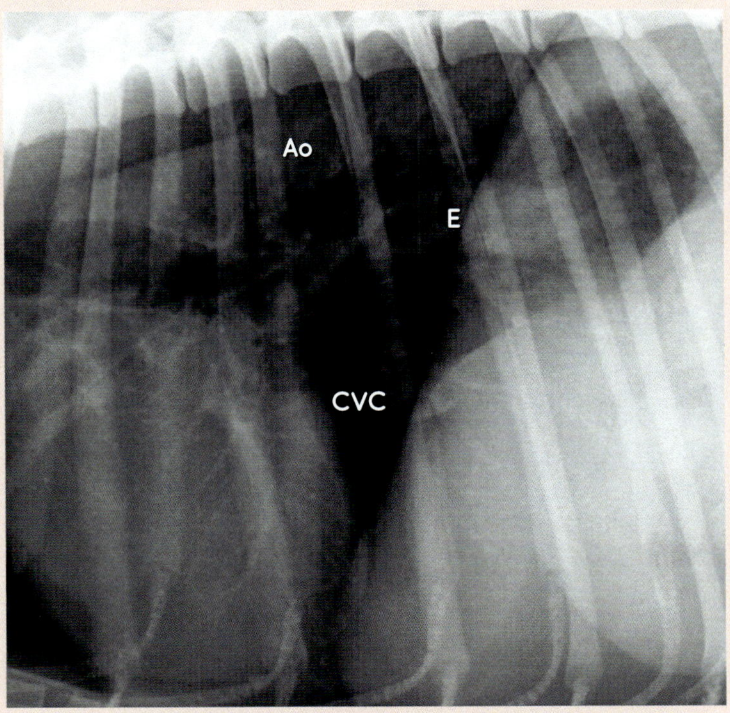

FIGURE 6.11. Left lateral radiograph of the thorax of a healthy dog. It is possible to observe a band of soft-tissue density in the caudodorsal area of the thorax, between the aorta (Ao) and the caudal vena cava (CVC). This shadow is due to the retention of fluid or mucus in the caudal area of the thoracic oesophagus (E), and is not considered pathological unless it persists on serial radiographs.

False alterations of the trachea

Minimal variations in the diameter of the trachea between inspiration and expiration are physiological. The rotation of the thorax at the moment when a lateral radiograph is taken may cause the oesophagus and/or muscles and the trachea to be superimposed, thus creating a false image of tracheal collapse. This type of image may also be caused by the so-called **redundant tracheal membrane**, by displacement of the dorsal wall of the trachea in ventral direction. This process has no clinical significance in the patient (fig. 2.15). The thoracic trachea may have a slightly wavy course if the radiograph is taken with the patient's head or neck in an incorrect position. In addition, a false dorsal displacement of the trachea may appear when the radiograph is taken with the median plane of the thoracic cavity inclined on the cassette (fig. 2.2) (this is corrected by placing a positioning block that elevates the sternum). In obese animals, it is possible to observe a right displacement of the trachea on ventrodorsal radiographs, caused by the excessive accumulation of fat in the mediastinum, not by pathological causes. In order not to make an incorrect diagnosis of tracheal hypoplasia, it is important to remember that the diameter of the trachea is proportionally smaller in brachycephalic breeds, especially in the Bulldog (fig. 2.19).

False alterations of the oesophagus

The presence of minimal accumulations of gas in the oesophageal lumen is not considered pathological (fig. 2.20), unless it persists over time. The accumulation of a small amount of fluid/mucus in the distal area of the thoracic oesophagus (fig. 6.11), just before going through the oesophageal hiatus of the diaphragm, is also considered physiological. This finding is more frequent on left lateral radiographs than on the right lateral ones. When barium is administered, the temporary retention of a small amount of contrast medium between the folds of the oesophageal wall is not considered significant, but if it persists over time it would be considered indicative of oesophagitis. We should also remember that the oesophagus may appear moderately dilated in anaesthetised animals (fig. 2.21), so as not to make an incorrect diagnosis of pathological dilatation in these cases.

Mediastinum in brachycephalic breeds and obese animals

In brachycephalic breeds, the shadow of the mediastinum is wider compared with other breeds. In obese animals the mediastinum may also appear enlarged, which could be similar to the image of a mediastinal mass or effusion, especially on ventrodorsal and dorsoventral radiographs. On lateral radiographs, fat may cause a more or less noticeable elevation of the cardiac silhouette (fig.2.44).

False impression of cardiomegaly

A false impression of cardiomegaly may be given by rotated radiographs (they show evident increased cardiosternal contact —fig. 2.2—) and expiratory radiographs (the small volume of the lung gives a false impression of increased cardiac size —fig. 6.12—). We should also remember that in old cats, the heart tends to be in greater contact with the sternum due to the progressive elongation of the aorta. This could be confused with an increase in the width of the cardiac silhouette (fig. 2.53). The cardiac silhouette should not be assessed on ventrodorsal and dorsoventral radiographs when the thorax is in rotated position, since it may result in incorrect diagnoses of increased right or left heart size, depending on the side to which the patient has been rotated (fig. 2.3). The accumulation of fat in the pericardial space that may appear in obese animals may also create a false image of increased cardiac size.

The organomegaly observed in young animals also affects the heart.

Thymus

The thymus is observed until approximately 6 months of age and should not be confused with pleural or pulmonary lesions (fig. 2.45).

Coronary vessels

A serious diagnostic error is to mistake pulmonary vessels for coronary vessels (fig. 6.13). These latter have the same radiopacity as the myocardium, so they cannot be differentiated on a radiograph with no contrast.

False pleural effusion

Various normal structures may be mistaken for a pleural effusion on a radiograph. In cats, it is normal to observe a minimal retraction of the dorsocaudal border of the caudal pulmonary lobes (fig. 2.4), while the same finding would be indicative of a mild pleural effusion in dogs. Thickening or calcification of the pleura with no pathological significance may also be confused with a mild pleural effusion.

False pulmonary alterations

The costal cartilages may have the appearance of interlobar fissures, although they can be differentiated since the cartilage is straighter and its junction with the rib can be identified.

Folds of skin may cause an artefact known as **pseudopneumothorax**, which is termed this way because it produces a marked difference of radiopacity between the areas lateral and medial to the fold of skin, resulting in a very dark lateral area (fig. 2.36). This may be mistaken for a pulmonary retraction due to the presence of gas in the pleural space.

The radiopacity of the lung may appear falsely increased in obese animals (because of the summation

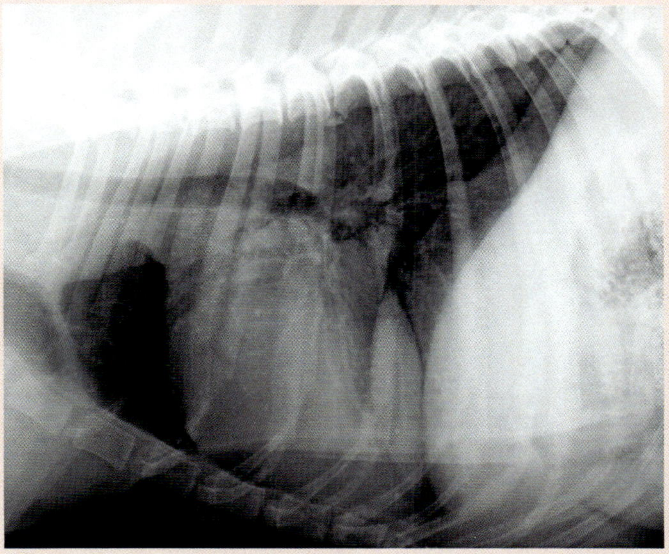

FIGURA 6.12. Lateral radiograph of the thorax of a healthy dog. The radiograph was taken in expiration, which causes a false appearance of cardiomegaly due to the smaller volume of the lung and superimposed shadow of the diaphragm and cardiac silhouette.

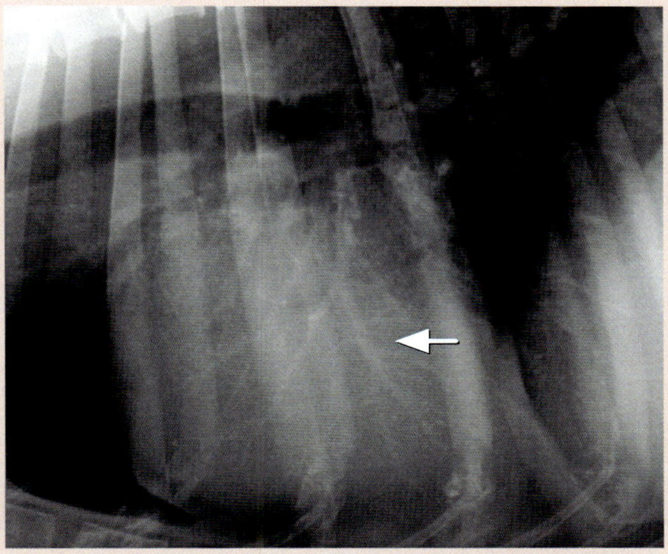

FIGURE 6.13. Enlarged image of a lateral radiograph of the thorax of a healthy dog. Mistaking the pulmonary vessels (arrow), which appear superimposed on the cardiac silhouette, for coronary vessels is a serious diagnostic error. Coronary vessels have the same radiopacity as the cardiac wall and therefore cannot be identified on a plain radiograph.

with the density of the subcutaneous fat and limitation of the degree of pulmonary expansion due to the presence of fat in the mediastinum) on underexposed or expiratory radiographs, which should not be confused with a real interstitial pattern due to pathological causes. If the radiograph is overexposed, a false reduction of pulmonary radiopacity is observed, which should not be confused with emphysema or pulmonary hypovascularisation.

The appearance of signs of atelectasis in the lower part of the lung is a usual finding in animals that have remained in lateral recumbency for a long period of time, especially if they have been anaesthetised. The alveolar pattern caused by atelectasis can be differentiated from that caused by oedema, pneumonia or haemorrhage, because a displacement of the mediastinal structures to the side where the atelectasic lung is located will appear on ventrodorsal and dorsoventral radiographs (fig. 2.97).

The superimposed pulmonary vessels and ribs may create shadows of greater radiopacity that are similar to nodular lesions in the lung. It is also possible to confuse the transversal shadows of those vessels that run parallel to the X-ray beam with nodules, in which case we should evaluate the adjacent vascular structures to determine whether the diameter of the shadows corresponds or not with that of the vessels in the area (fig. 6.14). Pleural and pulmonary calcifications (fig 2.39) are usually small and it is difficult to mistake them for pulmonary metastases, as these are very rarely calcified. The presence of calcified sludge in the gallbladder may be confused with areas of pleural or pulmonary calcification, or with pulmonary nodules (fig. 6.15). The location of the gallbladder on the two projections allows differentiation and in case of doubt, an abdominal ultrasound examination may be performed. The shadow of the gastric fundus on left lateral radiographs may also be mistaken for a lesion in the dorsocaudal area of the thorax (fig. 6.16).

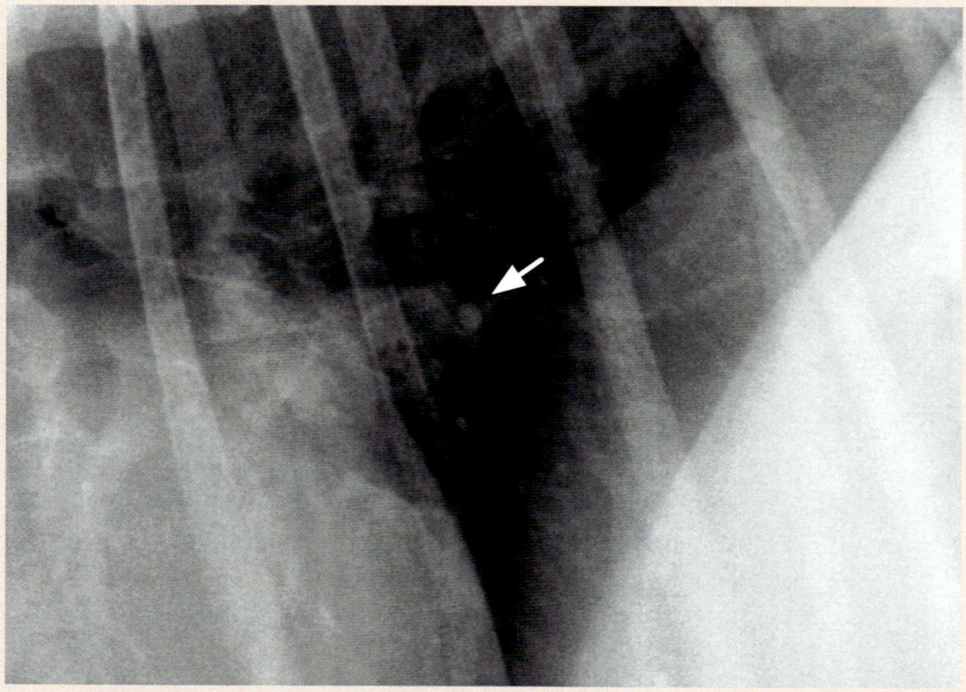

FIGURE 6.14. Enlarged image of a lateral radiograph of the thorax of a healthy dog. The arrow indicates the transverse image of a normal pulmonary vessel, which could be confused with a pulmonary nodular lesion. In order not to make an incorrect diagnosis, we must check whether other vessels in the area have a similar diameter. In case of doubt, a more precise diagnosis may be established with the help of computed tomography.

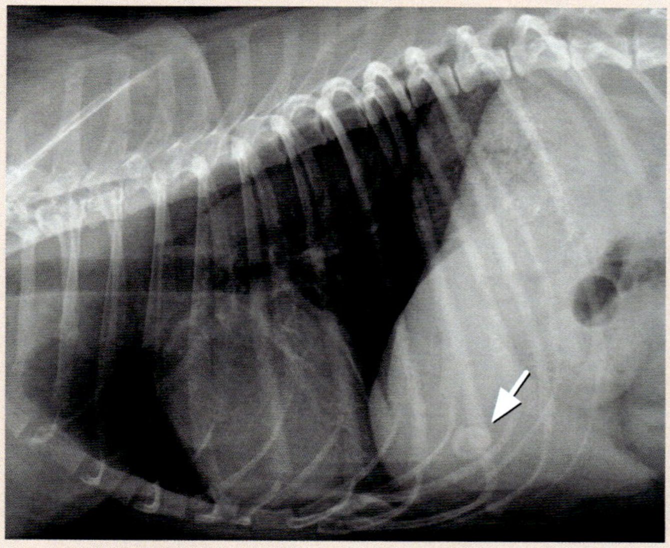

FIGURE 6.15. Lateral radiograph of the thorax of a healthy dog. The arrow shows a calculus/gallbladder sludge, which may be mistaken for a calcified nodular lesion in the lung.

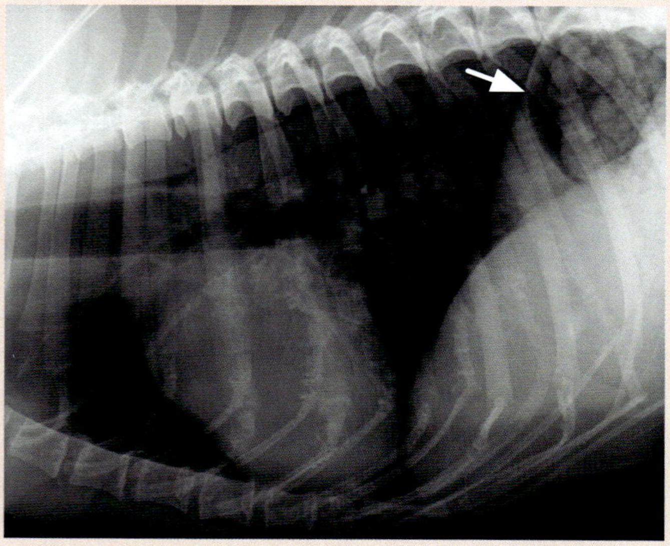

FIGURE 6.16. Left lateral radiograph of the thorax of a healthy dog. The arrow indicates the image of the normal gastric fundus (with gas and food content), which shows an apparently more cranial position on the left lateral view than on the right lateral view. This image may be mistaken for a pulmonary lesion.

Appendicular skeleton

Radiographic technique

An error that is often made when evaluating the appendicular skeleton is not to take two orthogonal projections, since some lesions are evident in only one of them (e.g. fractures with little displacement, joint subluxations) (fig. 6.17).

Overexposure of the radiograph may lead to an incorrect diagnosis of osteopaenia, as the bone appears less radiopaque in the image.

Age and breed

Growth lines in young animals should not be mistaken for fractures (fig. 6.18) and it is therefore recommended to use an atlas with radiographic images of animals throughout their development in case of doubt. It should be remembered that large-breed dogs may have slightly irregular metaphyseal margins, which may be confused with a periosteal reaction or with osteolysis. It is also important to be familiarised with the peculiar morphology of bones in chondrodystrophic breeds (e.g. Basset Hound).

Incorrect positioning of the patient

The most frequent cause of diagnostic errors in the assessment of the appendicular skeleton is the incorrect positioning of the patient when taking the radiograph. This is especially significant in the examination of some joints such as the coxofemoral joint, as its image is greatly altered by minimal rotations of the pelvis. When this joint is rotated to one side, it is

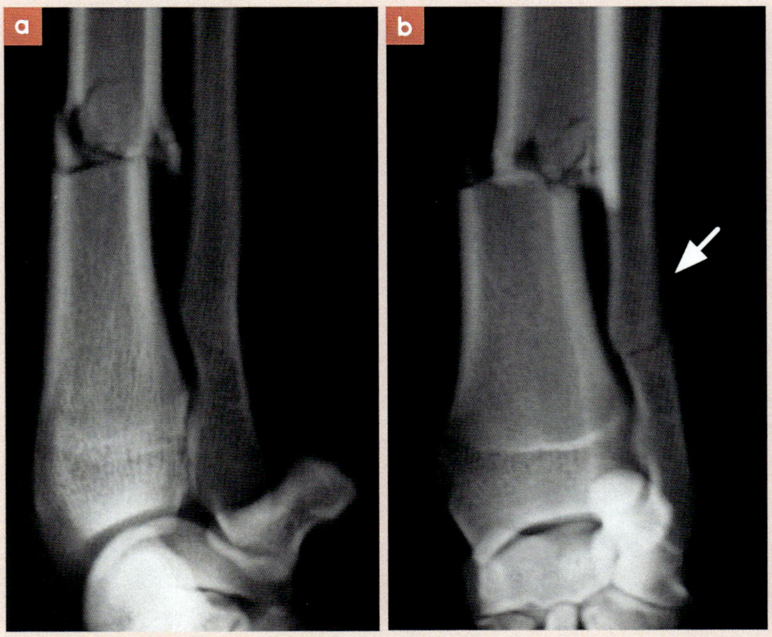

FIGURE 6.17. Enlarged images in mediolateral (a) and craniocaudal (b) projection of the radius and ulna of a dog with a fracture of both bones. The fracture of the ulna (arrow) is not visible on the mediolateral view and would therefore not be diagnosed if this radiograph alone were taken.

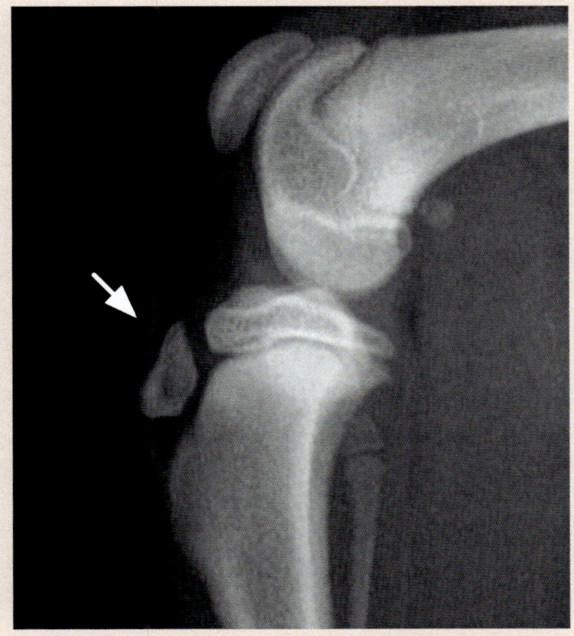

FIGURE 6.18. Mediolateral radiograph of the tibia of an 11-week-old, healthy dog. The growth plate of the tibial tuberosity (arrow) appears separated from the metaphysis until 6-8 months of age, which could be confused with an avulsion fracture of the tuberosity.

possible to see it in the image because the obturator foramen of the same side appears smaller and the shadow of the wing of the contralateral ilium appears narrower. In these conditions, reduced acetabular coverage (false increase of the joint space) on the side to which the pelvis is rotated, and greater acetabular coverage (false reduction of the joint space) in the contralateral joint will be observed (fig. 6.19). The position of the femurs will also affect the width of the joint space, which means that for a proper assessment of the joint, the femurs must remain parallel, with the patellas aligned with the trochlear groove.

The integrity of the sacroiliac joints is not assessed properly when the pelvis is rotated, since one of the joints will appear falsely enlarged, which could be confused with a luxation of subluxation.

Clavicle and sesamoid bones

Two important anatomical variations among those that may lead to diagnostic errors are vestigial clavicles (fig. 6.20) and some sesamoid bones that do not appear in a constant manner in dogs. Vestigial clavicles appear as small structures with mineral opacity medial to the head of the humerus. The sesamoid bone in the tendon of origin of the supinator muscle sometimes appears on radiographs of the elbow joint, craniolateral to the head of the radius. A sesamoid bone may also be observed in some cases on the lateral plantar aspect of the tarsometatarsal joint or in it. Sesamoid bones may also appear in the iliopubic ligament, and these are located cranial to the pubic eminence of the pelvis on lateral radiographs.

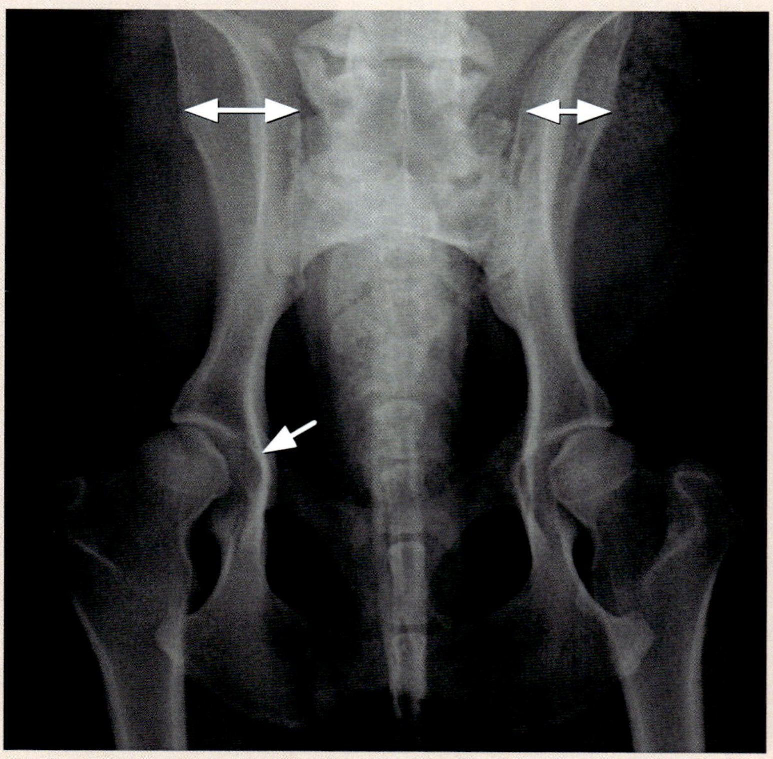

FIGURE 6.19. Ventrodorsal radiograph of the hip of a dog with a mild degree of hip luxation due to dysplasia. We can detect that the pelvis is rotated to the right side because the obturator foramen appears smaller and the shadow of the wing of the ilium is narrower. Due to this rotation, the right hip joint space (arrow) appears falsely increased, while in the left hip joint, the acetabular coverage is falsely increased.

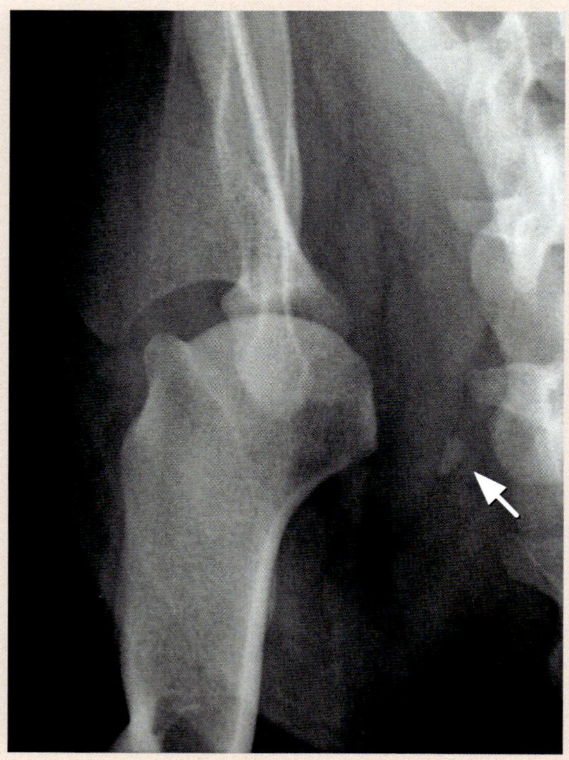

FIGURE 6.20. Caudocranial radiograph of the scapulohumeral joint of a healthy dog. The arrow shows the vestigial clavicle, which is sometimes observed in dogs. It is bilateral and should not be mistaken for a pathological calcification of the soft tissues of the area.

Spine

Incorrect positioning of the patient

The main source of diagnostic errors in the assessment of the spine is the incorrect positioning of the patient when taking a radiograph. If no radiolucent positioning blocks are used to elevate the cervical and lumbar spines, these remain curved towards the cassette/X-ray table, causing an evident narrowing of the intervertebral disc spaces (fig. 6.21). Even if the position of the spine is correct, only the intervertebral disc spaces that are most centred in the image should be evaluated, since the X-ray beam penetrates through them more obliquely as these spaces are farther away from its centre, thus creating a false narrowing in the image.

In order for the median plane of the spine to be parallel to the cassette, it is necessary to place radiolucent positioning blocks between the limbs or under them. If this is not done, the spine is rotated and the transverse processes of each side appear separated in the image. The most ventral ones may easily be confused with spondylosis deformans.

Overexposure and underexposure

Overexposure or underexposure of the radiograph may cause a false alteration of the radiopacity of the vertebrae, which we may be confused with osteopaenia o sclerosis.

Superimposed structures

The superimposition of the large bowel containing gas or faeces on the sacrum or pelvis may create an image similar to that of lines of fracture in these structures.

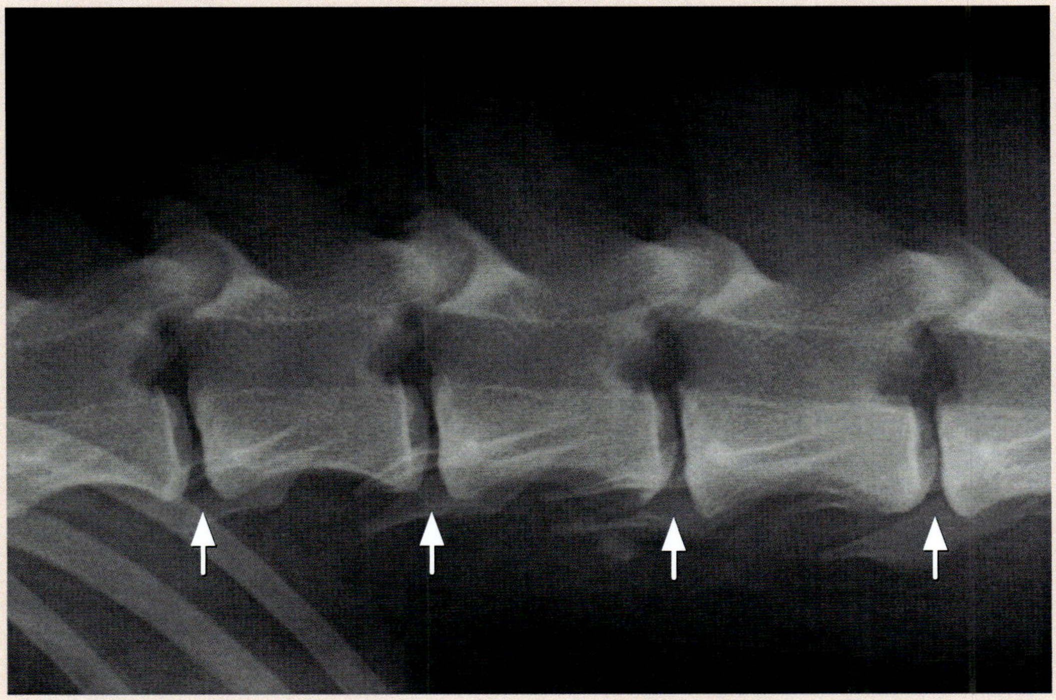

FIGURE 6.21. Enlarged image of the lumbar spine on a lateral radiograph of a healthy dog. When an area of the spine (cervical or lumbar) is curved towards the cassette/X-ray table, a false narrowing of the intervertebral disc spaces (arrows) will be observed on the radiograph. This defect is corrected by placing a radiolucent positioning block under the spine to ensure its axis is parallel to the cassette. In this image, the transverse processes of each vertebra appear at a different height, which indicates that the spine is rotated on its longitudinal axis (this can be corrected by placing a radiolucent positioning block between the limbs). The most ventral transverse processes may be confused with spondylosis deformans.

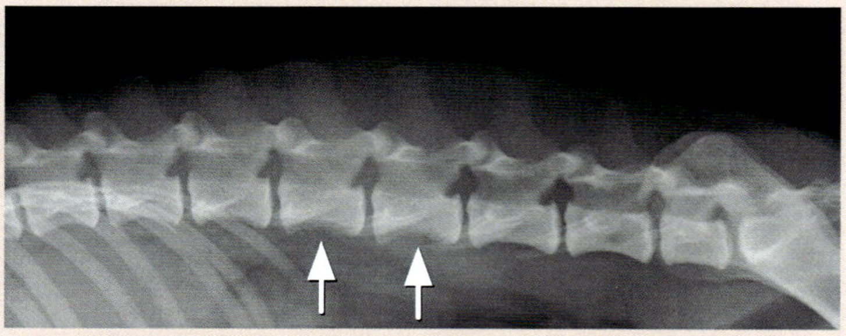

FIGURE 6.22. Lateral radiograph of the lumbar spine of a healthy dog. The ventral margin of the vertebral body of L3 and L4 (arrows) appears less defined due to the insertion of the crura of the diaphragm. This finding is more evident in large breed dogs.

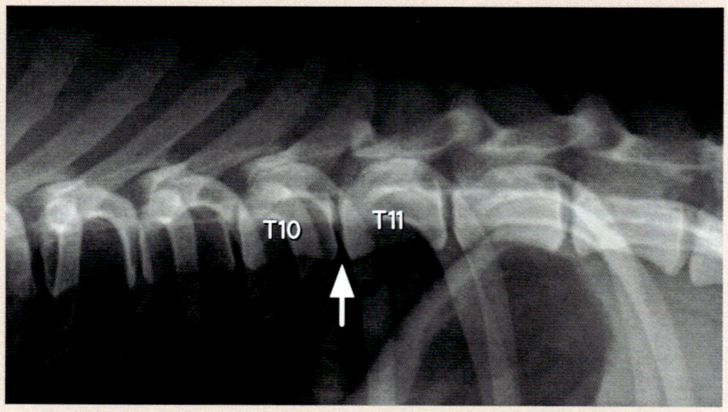

FIGURE 6.23. Enlarged image of the thoracic spine on a lateral radiograph of a healthy dog. A mild narrowing of the T10-T11 intervertebral disc space (arrow) can be seen when compared with the others. This is considered a normal anatomical variation.

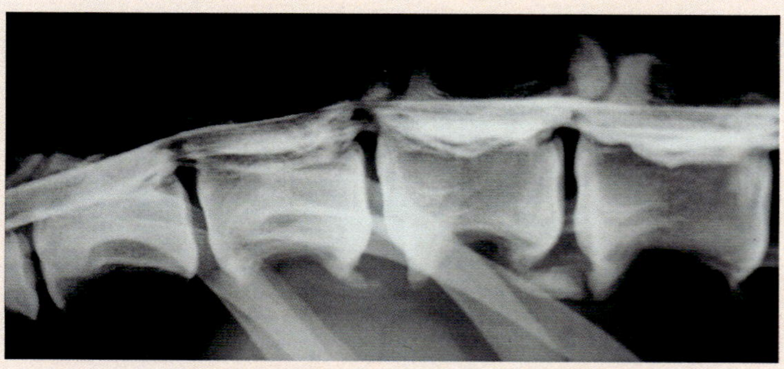

FIGURE 6.24. Enlarged image of the thoracolumbar area of the spine on a lateral radiograph of a dog that has received an injection of an iodinated contrast agent in the subarachnoid space for a myelogram, and in the extradural space by mistake, which creates irregularities in the margin of the contrast columns.

Normal anatomical variations

Some normal anatomical variations that may be mistaken for diseases are: the lack of definition of the ventral margin of the body of L3 and L4, due to the insertion of the crura of the diaphragm (fig 6.22) (more evident in large breed dogs); the narrowing of the T10-T11 intervertebral disc space, as it is an anticlinal space (fig 6.23); and the presence of haemal processes at the ends of the coccygeal vertebrae, which may be confused with spondylosis deformans.

Contrast medium in extradural space

If the contrast medium is introduced by mistake in the epidural space instead of in the subarachnoid space when performing a myelogram, the contrast columns will have a very irregular morphology (fig. 6.24) and making a precise diagnosis will thus be more difficult.

Head

Incorrect positioning of the patient

Most of the interpretation errors made when evaluating radiographs of a patient's head are due to a poor positioning of the patient. In this region, it is essential not to rotate the skull, especially on dorsoventral and ventrodorsal radiographs (fig. 6.25), since the symmetry or lack of symmetry of the structures is a key element on which the diagnosis of many diseases of this anatomical region is based.

On ventrodorsal open-mouth radiographs, the superimposition of the tongue should be avoided, since it may create a false image of mass in the nasal cavity (fig. 6.26).

Rostrocaudal tangential radiographs may provide images of a false increase in radiopacity of the frontal sinuses due to a poor positioning of the patient, or to the actual morphology of the sinuses and nasal bone depending on the breed (fig. 6.27).

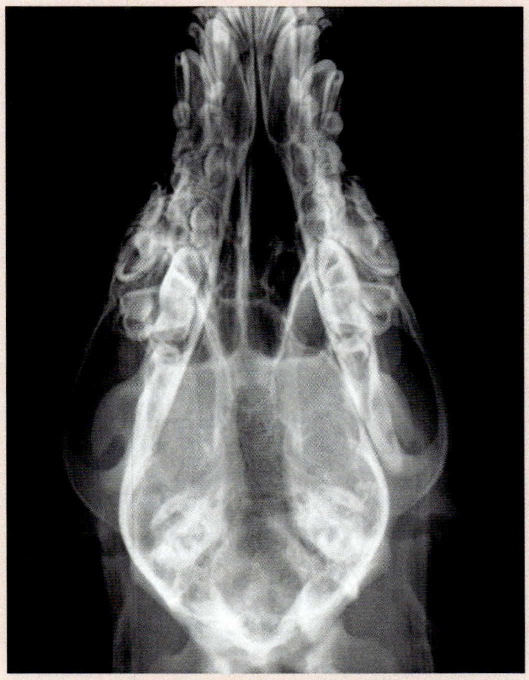

FIGURE 6.25. Dorsoventral radiograph of the head of a healthy young dog (superimposed deciduous and permanent teeth are observed). The rotation of the head increases the summation effect of the right mandible and nasal cavity of the same side, which hinders the correct assessment of this region of the skull.

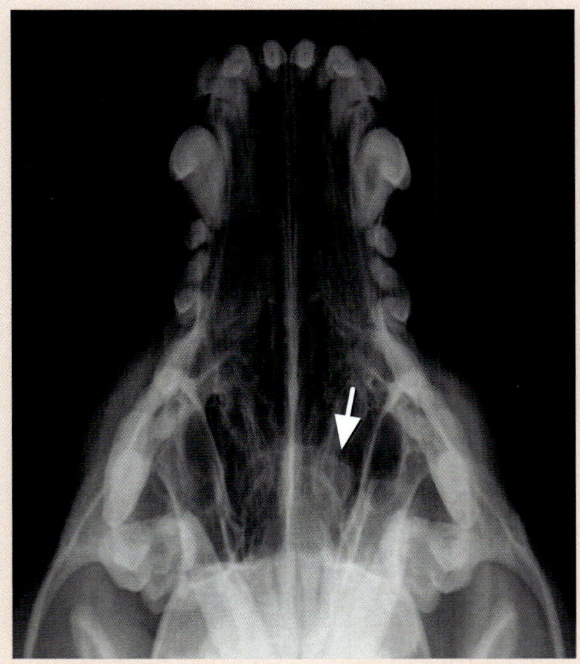

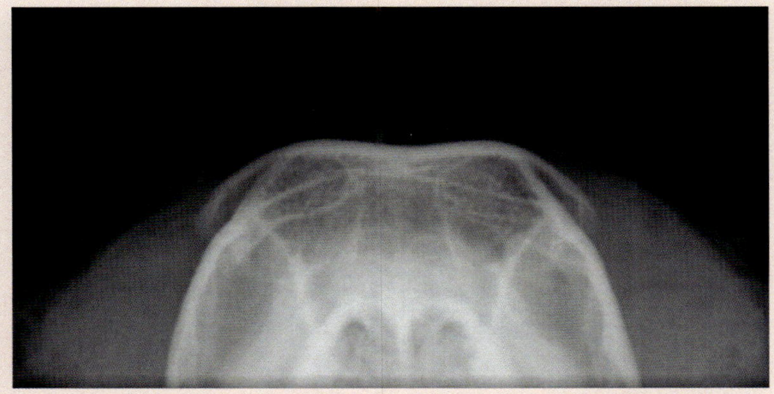

FIGURE 6.27. Rostrocaudal tangential radiograph of the frontal sinuses of a healthy dog. The incorrect positioning of the patient results in the X-ray beam penetrating through the cranial vault and frontal sinuses. The images of both structures add up, which results in a false image of increased radiopacity of the sinuses.

◀ FIGURE 6.26. Ventrodorsal open-mouth radiograph of a healthy dog. The superimposition of the tongue (arrow) creates a false image of mass in the caudal area of the left nasal cavity.

Digital imaging

One of the great advantages of digital radiography is that it has a high contrast resolution in comparison with conventional radiography. The veterinary surgeon who acquires digital radiography equipment for the first time therefore has to get used to "a new way of observing radiographs". Some diagnostic errors can be made during this transition period.

Greater definition of the elements of the lung

In digital radiography, the blood vessels of the lung are very well-defined, which may lead to an incorrect diagnosis of vascular congestion. In some healthy animals, the bronchial walls may also be identified in the medial area of the lung, a finding that would be considered as indicative of a thickening of the bronchial walls, the presence of peribronchial infiltrates or calcification on a conventional radiograph.

Higher pulmonary radiopacity

The lung generally appears less transparent on a digital radiograph, which could be confused with a pathological interstitial pattern. In addition, on a digital radiograph, minimal degrees of lung displacement caused by mediastinal fat or by being in a lateral recumbent position may become more evident and may be similar to a pleural or mediastinal effusion.

Higher tissue contrast

The higher contrast between soft tissues and fat may lead to this latter being mistaken for free peritoneal gas on a digital radiograph of the abdomen. An incorrect diagnosis of pneumoperitoneum may thus be established.

The trabeculae of bones may also appear better defined, which should not be interpreted as a pathological change in the bone marrow.

Overexposure

On highly overexposed digital radiographs, black areas with a loss of image information may appear in the affected area, and are not possible to recover with post-processing tools (fig. 6.28). When these areas appear in the lung, we may mistake them for pulmonary bullae while if they appear in the bone, they may be similar to areas of osteolysis.

Metallic implants

The appearance of an artefact around metallic implants placed in the bone has already been described. It is observed as radiolucent bands around these implants, and may be confused with a sign of mobility or rejection of the material (fig. 6.29). This artefact has already been corrected in many of the current machines and is caused by an excessive use of the edge-enhancement tool.

Excessive post-processing

In general, post-processing tools allow the improvement of the image quality, but when overused they may worsen it and lead to errors (fig. 6.30), in many cases due to an overdiagnosis (we see more than what is actually there).

Excessive zooming

A significant advantage of digital radiography is that we can use the zoom tool to greatly enlarge small areas of the image. However, we should not overuse this tool as we run the risk of losing the global view of the image, which in many cases is essential to establish a correct diagnosis.

Self-assessment cases

http://goo.gl/QJ9PUd

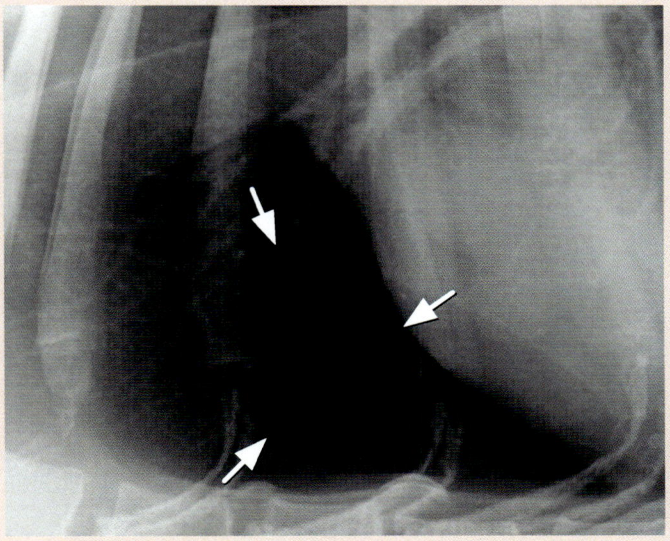

FIGURE 6.28. Enlarged image of the cranioventral area of the thorax of a healthy dog. The arrows indicate an overexposed area of the image (digital), which could be mistaken for an area of hypovascularisation or a pulmonary bulla.

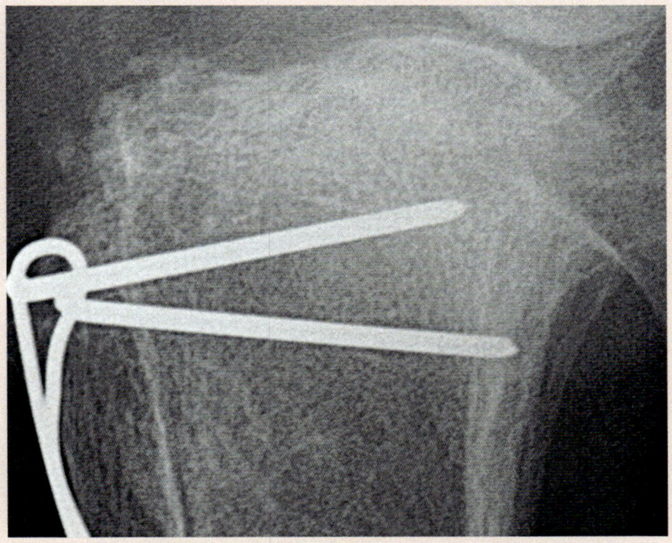

FIGURE 6.29. Enlarged image of the tibia on a mediolateral radiograph of a dog after the placement of pins and a cerclage wire. When the edge-enhancement tool is overused in digital radiography, radiolucent halos may appear around metal implants, which could be mistaken for a sign of rejection or mobility of the material.

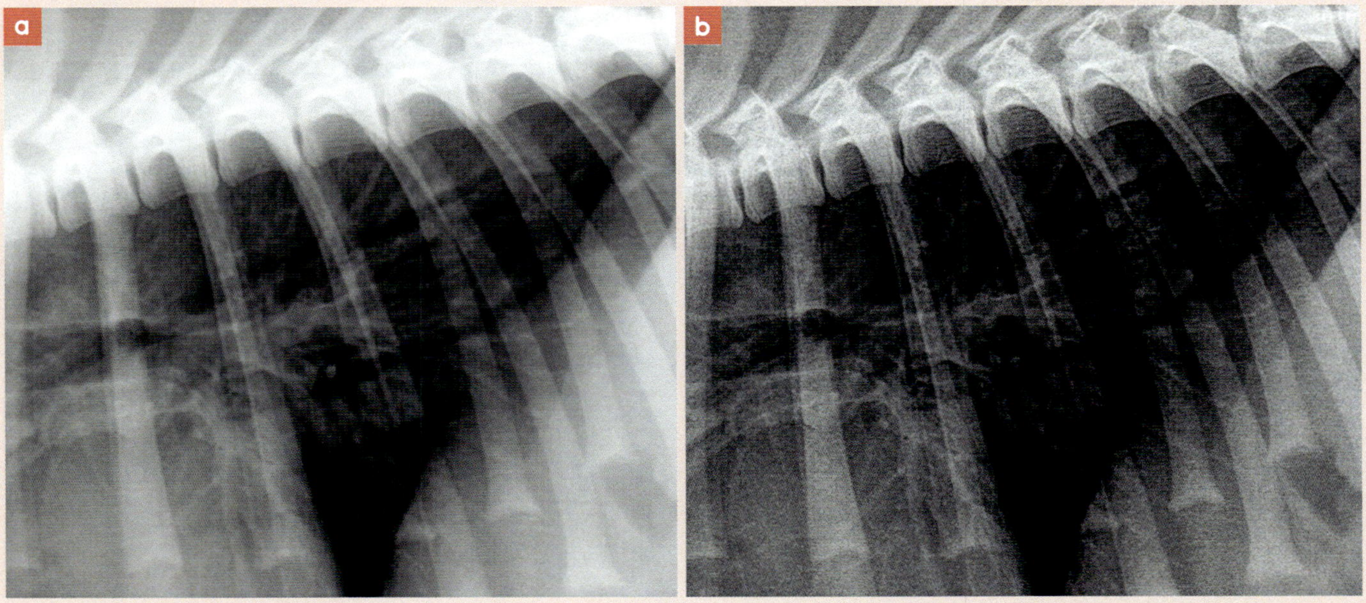

FIGURE 6.30. Enlarged images of the caudodorsal area of a healthy dog. One of them shows the properly processed digital radiograph (a), while the other shows the same image after overuse of the edge enhancement tool (b), which highlights the image of the vessels, bronchial walls and even the lung parenchyma excessively. The overuse of post-processing tools in digital radiography usually leads to diagnostic errors.

Recommended readings

Chapter 1. Abdomen

1. Adams, W.M., Sisterman, L.A., Klauer, J.M., Kirby, B.M., Lin, T.L. Association of intestinal disorders in cats with findings of abdominal radiography. *Journal of the American Veterinary Medical Association*, 2010; 236:880-886.
2. Adin, C.A., Herrgesell, E.J., Nyland, T.G., Hughes, D.M., Gregory, C.R., Kyles, A.E., Cowgill, L.D., Ling, G.V. Antegrade pyelography for suspected ureteral obstruction in cats: 11 cases (1995-2001). *Journal of the Veterinary Medical Association*, 2003; 222:1576-1581.
3. Agut, A., Sánchez-Valverde, M.A., Lasaosa, J.M., Murciano, J., Molina, F. Use of iohexol as a gastrointestinal contrast medium in the dog. *Veterinary Radiology and Ultrasound*, 1993; 34:171-177.
4. Agut, A., Sanchez-Valverde, M.A., Torrecillas, F.E., Murciano, J., Laredo, F.G. Use of iohexol as a gastrointestinal contrast medium in the cat. *Veterinary Radiology and Ultrasound*, 1994; 35:164-168.
5. Allan, F.J., Guilford, W.G., Robertson, I.D., Jones, B.R. Gastric emptying of solid radiopaque markers in healthy dogs. *Veterinary Radiology and Ultrasound*, 1996; 37:336-344.
6. Armbrust, L. The spleen. En: O'Brien, R. and Barr, F. (eds). *BSAVA Manual of Canine and Feline Abdominal Imaging*. British Small Animal Veterinary Association, Gloucester, 2009; pp. 167-176.
7. Atalan, G., Barr, F.J., Holt, P.E. Comparison of ultrasonographic and radiographic measurements of canine prostatic dimensions. *Veterinary Radiology and Ultrasound*, 1999; 40:408-412.
8. Baines, E.A. The peritoneal cavity. En: O'Brien, R. and Barr, F. (eds). *BSAVA Manual of Canine and Feline Abdominal Imaging*. British Small Animal Veterinary Association, Gloucester, 2009; pp. 29-39.
9. Barr, F., O'Brien, R. Approach to abdominal imaging. En: O'Brien, R. and Barr, F. (eds). *BSAVA Manual of Canine and Feline Abdominal Imaging*. British Small Animal Veterinary Association, Gloucester, 2009; pp. 1-4.
10. Bradley, K. The small intestine. En: O'Brien, R. and Barr, F. (eds). *BSAVA Manual of Canine and Feline Abdominal Imaging*. British Small Animal Veterinary Association, Gloucester, 2009; pp. 110-131.
11. Brown, J.C. The urethra. En: Thrall, D.E. (ed). *Textbook of Veterinary Diagnostic Radiology*, 6th edition. Elsevier Saunders, St. Louis, 2013; pp. 744-748.
12. Burk, R.L., Feeney, D.A. *Small Animal Radiology and Ultrasonography. A Diagnostic Atlas and Text*. Elsevier Science, St. Louis, 2003.
13. Costello, M. The male reproductive system. En: O'Brien, R. and Barr, F. (eds). *BSAVA Manual of Canine and Feline Abdominal Imaging*. British Small Animal Veterinary Association, Gloucester, 2009; pp. 237-245.
14. Dennis, R., Kirberger, R.M., Barr, F., Wrigley, R.H. *Handbook of Small Animal Radiology and Ultrasound, 2th Edition*. Churchill Livingstone Elsevier, Edimburg, 2010.
15. Farrow, C.S. Diagnóstico por imagen del perro y el gato. Multimédica ediciones veterinarias, Barcelona, 2005.
16. Feeney, D.A., Johnston, G.R., Klausner, J.S., Perman, V., Leininger, J.R., Tomlinson, M.J. Canine prostatic disease – comparison of radiographic appearance with morphologic and microbiologic findings: 30 cases (1981-1985). *Journal of the American Veterinary Medical Association*, 1987; 190:1018-1026.
17. Frank, P.M. The peritoneal space. En: Thrall, D.E. (ed). *Textbook of Veterinary Diagnostic Radiology*, 6th edition. Elsevier Saunders, St. Louis, 2013; pp. 659-678.
18. Frank, P.M. The stomach. En: Thrall, D.E. (ed). *Textbook of Veterinary Diagnostic Radiology*, 6th edition. Elsevier Saunders, St. Louis, 2013; pp. 769-788.
19. Fraser, J. Abdominal radiography. En: O'Brien, R. and Barr, F. (eds). *BSAVA Manual of Canine and Feline Abdominal Imaging*. British Small Animal Veterinary Association, Gloucester, 2009; pp. 4-17.
20. Frendin, J., Funkquist, B., Hansson, K., Lonnemark M., Carlsten J. Diagnostic imaging of foreign body reactions in dogs with diffuse back pain. *Journal of Small Animal Practice*, 1999; 40:278-285.
21. Gaschen, L. The large intestine and perianal region. En: O'Brien, R. and Barr, F. (eds): *BSAVA Manual of Canine and Feline Abdominal Imaging*. British Small Animal Veterinary Association, Gloucester, 2009; pp. 132-143.
22. Graham, J.P., Lord, P.F., Harrison, J.M. Quantitative estimation of intestinal dilation as a predictor of obstruction in the dog. *Journal of Small Animal Practice*, 1998; 39:521-524.
23. Hammond, G. The female reproductive system. En: O'Brien, R. and Barr, F. (eds). *BSAVA Manual of Canine and Feline Abdominal Imaging*. British Small Animal Veterinary Association, Gloucester, 2009; pp. 222-236.

24. Herrtage, M.E., Dennis, R. Contrast media and techniques. En: Lee, R. (ed). *Manual of Small Animal Diagnostic Imaging.* British Small Animal Veterinary Association, Shurdington, 1995; pp. 147-156.

25. Holloway, A., O'Brien, R. Perirenal effusion in dogs and cats with acute renal failure. *Veterinary Radiology and Ultrasound,* 2007; 48:574-579.

26. Hotston-Moore, A. The bladder and urethra. En: O'Brien, R. and Barr, F. (eds). *BSAVA Manual of Canine and Feline Abdominal Imaging.* British Small Animal Veterinary Association, Gloucester, 2009; pp. 205-221.

27. Kealy, J.K., McAllister, H., Graham, J.P. *Diagnostic Radiology and Ultrasonography of the Dog and Cat,* 5th edition. Saunders Elsevier, St. Louis, 2010.

28. Kinns, J., Nelson, N. The uterus, ovaries and testes. En: Thrall, D.E. (ed). *Textbook of Veterinary Diagnostic Radiology,* 6th edition. Elsevier Saunders, St. Louis, 2013; pp. 757-768.

29. Lamb, C.R. Radiografía de contraste del tracto urinario. *Proceedings del XVII Congreso de AMVAC,* 2000; pp. 105-114.

30. Lamb, C.R. Resolución de problemas: la masa abdominal. *Proceedings del XVII Congreso de AMVAC,* 2000; pp. 115-118.

31. Lattimer, J.C., Essman, S.C. The prostate gland. En: Thrall, D.E. (ed). *Textbook of Veterinary Diagnostic Radiology,* 6th edition. Elsevier Saunders, St. Louis, 2013; pp. 749-756.

32. Llabrés-Díaz, F. The retroperitoneum. En: O'Brien, R. and Barr, F. (eds). *BSAVA Manual of Canine and Feline Abdominal Imaging.* British Small Animal Veterinary Association, Gloucester, 2009; pp. 40-48.

33. Marolf, A.J., Park, R.D. The urinary bladder. En: Thrall, D.E. (ed). *Textbook of Veterinary Diagnostic Radiology,* 6th edition. Elsevier Saunders, St. Louis, 2013; pp. 726-743.

34. Moon, M. The kidneys and ureters. En: O'Brien, R. and Barr, F. (eds). *BSAVA Manual of Canine and Feline Abdominal Imaging.* British Small Animal Veterinary Association, Gloucester, 2009; pp. 185-204.

35. Moon, M. The liver and spleen. En: Thrall, D.E. (ed). *Textbook of Veterinary Diagnostic Radiology,* 6th edition. Elsevier Saunders, St. Louis, 2013; pp. 679-704.

36. Murdoch, D.B. The abdomen. En: Lee, R. (ed). *Manual of Small Animal Diagnostic Imaging.* British Small Animal Veterinary Association, Shurdington, 1995; pp. 68-94.

37. Owens, J.M., Biery, D.N. *Radiographic Interpretation for the Small Animal Clinician,* 2nd edition. Williams & Wilkins, Baltimore, 1999.

38. Penninck, D.G., Feldman, E.C., Nyland, T.G. Radiographic features of canine hyper-adrenocorticism caused by autonomously functioning adrenocortical tumors: 23 cases (1978-1986). *Journal of the American Veterinary Medical Association,* 1988; 192:1604-1608.

39. Petite, A., Busoni, V., Heinen, M.P., Billen, F., Snaps, F. Radiographic and ultrasonographic findings of emphysematous cistitis in four nondiabetic female dogs. *Veterinary Radiology and Ultrasound,* 2006; 47:90-93.

40. Riedesel, E.A. The small bowel. En: Thrall, D.E. (ed). *Textbook of Veterinary Diagnostic Radiology,* 6th edition. Elsevier Saunders, St. Louis, 2013; pp. 789-811.

41. Robertson, I.D., Burbridge, H.M. Pros and cons of barium-impregnated polyethylene spheres in gastrointestinal disease. *Veterinary Clinics of North America: Small Animal Practice,* 2000; 30:449-465.

42. Saunders, W.B., Tobias, K.M. Pneumoperitoneum in dogs and cats: 39 cases (1983-2002). *Journal of the American Veterinary Medical Association,* 2003; 223:462-468.

43. Schwarz, T. The large bowel. En: Thrall, D.E. (ed). *Textbook of Veterinary Diagnostic Radiology,* 6th edition. Elsevier Saunders, St. Louis, 2013; pp. 812-824.

44. Schwarz, T. The liver and gallbladder. En: O'Brien, R. and Barr, F. (eds). *BSAVA Manual of Canine and Feline Abdominal Imaging.* British Small Animal Veterinary Association, Gloucester, 2009; pp. 144-156.

45. Schwarz, T. Urinary system. En: Schwarz, T., Saunders, J. (eds). *Veterinary Computed Tomography.* Wiley-Blackwell, Oxford, 2011; pp. 331-338.

46. Schwarz, T., Störk, C.K., Mellor, D., Sullivan, M. Osteopenia and other radiographic signs in canine hyperadrenocorticism. *Journal of Small Animal Practice,* 2000; 41:491-495.

47. Seiler, G., Mai, W. The stomach. En: O'Brien, R. and Barr, F. (eds). *BSAVA Manual of Canine and Feline Abdominal Imaging.* British Small Animal Veterinary Association, Gloucester, 2009; pp. 87-109.

48. Seiler, G.S. The kidneys and ureters. En: Thrall, D.E. (ed). *Textbook of Veterinary Diagnostic Radiology,* 6th edition. Elsevier Saunders, St. Louis, 2013; pp. 705-725.

49. Sharma, A., Thompson, M.S., Scrivani, P.V., Dykes, N.L., Yeager, A.E., Freer, S.R., Erb, H.N. Comparison of radiography and ultrasonography for diagnosing small-intestinal mechanical obstruction in vomiting dogs. *Veterinary Radiology and Ultrasound,* 2011; 52:248-255.

50. Shiroma, J.T., Gabriel, J.K., Carter, R.L., Scruggs, S.L., Stubbs, P.W. Effect of reproductive status on feline renal size. *Veterinary Radiology and Ultrasound,* 1999; 40: 242-245.

51. Stiffler, K.S., Stevenson, M.A., Mahaffey, M.B., Howerth, E.W., Barsanti, J.A. Intravesical ureterocele with concurrent renal dysfunction in a dog: a case report and proposed classification system. *Journal of the American Animal Hospital Association,* 2002; 38:33-39.

52. Sutherland-Smith, J., Jerram, R.M., Walker A.M., Warman, C. Ectopic ureters and ureteroceles in dogs: presentation, cause, and diagnosis. *Compendium of Continuing Education for Veterinarians,* 2004; 26:303-316.

53. Thrall, D.E. Principles of radiographic interpretation of the abdomen. En: Thrall, D.E. (ed). *Textbook of Veterinary Diagnostic Radiology*, 6th edition. Elsevier Saunders, St. Louis, 2013; pp. 650-658.

54. Wang, K.Y., Samii, V.F., Chew, D.J., McLoughlin, M.A., DiBartola, S.P., Masty, J., Lehman, A.M. Vestibular, vaginal and urethral relationships in spayed and intact normal dogs. *Theriogenology*, 2006; 66:726-35.

55. Wang, K.Y., Samii, V.F., Chew, D.J., McLoughlin, M.A., DiBartola, S.P., Masty, J., Lehman, A.M. Vestibular, vaginal, and urethral relations in spayed dogs with and without lower urinary tract signs. *Journal of Veterinary Internal Medicine*, 2006; 20:1065-73.

56. Zontine, W., Andrews, L. Fatal air embolization as a complication of pneumocystography in two cats. *Journal of the American Veterinary Medical Association*, 1978; 19:8-11.

Chapter 2. Neck and thorax

1. Abbott, J.A. Enfermedad valvular adquirida. En: Tilley, L.P., Smith, F.W.K. Jr., Oyama, M.A., Sleeper, M.M. (eds): *Manual de Cardiología Canina y Felina*, 4ª edición. Multimédica Ediciones Veterinarias, Barcelona, 2009; pp: 95-118.

2. Alexander, K. The pharynx, larynx, and thachea. En: Thrall, D.E. (ed): *Textbook of Veterinary Diagnostic Radiology*, 6th edition. Elsevier Saunders, St. Louis, 2013; pp: 489-499.

3. Bahr, R. The heart and pulmonary vessels. En: Thrall, D.E. (ed): *Textbook of Veterinary Diagnostic Radiology*, 6th edition. Elsevier Saunders, St. Louis, 2013; pp: 585-607.

4. Baines, E. The mediastinum. En: Schwarz, T. and Johnson, V. (eds): *BSAVA Manual of Canine and Feline Thoracic Imaging*. British Small Animal Veterinary Association, Gloucester, 2008; pp: 177-199.

5. Begon, D. La radiografía torácica. *Proceedings del XVII Congreso de AMVAC*, 2000; pp: 53-95.

6. Brinkman, E.L., Biller, D., Armbrust, L. The clinical usefulness of the ventrodorsal versus dorsoventral thoracic radiograph in dogs. *Journal of the American Animal Hospital Association*, 2006; 42:440-449.

7. Buchanan, J.W., Bucheler, J. Vertebral scale system to measure canine heart size in radiographs. *Journal of the American Veterinary Medical Association*, 1995; 206:194-199.

8. Burk, R.L., Feeney D.A. *Small Animal Radiology and Ultrasonography. A Diagnostic Atlas and Text*. Elsevier Science, St. Louis, 2003.

9. Coyne, B.E., Fingland, R.B. Hypoplasia of the trachea in dogs: 103 cases (1974-1990). *Journal of the American Veterinary Medical Association*, 1992; 201:768-772.

10. D'Anjou, M.A., Tidwell, A.S., Hecht, S. Radiographic diagnosis of lung lobe torsion. *Veterinary Radiology and Ultrasound*, 2005; 46:478-484.

11. D'Anjou, M., Schwarz, T. Heart and vessels. En: Schwarz, T., Saunders, J. (eds): *Veterinary Computed Tomography*. Wiley-Blackwell, Oxford, 2011; pp: 229-242.

12. Dennis, R., Kirberger, R.M., Barr, F., Wrigley, R.H. *Handbook of Small Animal Radiology and Ultrasound, 2nd Edition*. Churchill Livingstone Elsevier, Edimburg, 2010.

13. Diana, A., Guglielmini, C., Pivetta, M., Sanacore, A., Di Tommaso, M., Lord, P.F., Cipone, M. Radiographic features of cardiogenic pulmonary edema in dogs with mitral regurgitation: 61 cases (1998-2007). *Journal of the American Veterinary Medical Association*, 2009; 235:1058-1063.

14. Farrow, C.S. *Diagnóstico por imagen del perro y el gato*. Multimédica ediciones veterinarias, Barcelona, 2005.

15. Fasanella, F.J., Shivley, J.M., Wardlaw, J.L., Givaruangsawat, S. Brachycephalic airway obstructive syndrome in dogs: 90 cases (1991-2008). *Journal of the American Veterinary Medical Association*, 2010; 237:1048-1051.

16. Frame, M, King, A. The pleural space. En: Schwarz, T. and Johnson, V. (eds): *BSAVA Manual of Canine and Feline Thoracic Imaging*. British Small Animal Veterinary Association, Gloucester, 2008; pp: 321-339.

17. Fujita, M., Miura, H., Yasuda, D., Hasegawa, D., Orima, H. Tracheal narrowing secondary to airway obstruction in two cats. *Journal of Small Animal Practice*, 2004; 45:29-31.

18. Gadbois, J., d'Anjou, M.A., Dunn, M., Alexander, K., Beauregard, G., D'Astous, J., De Carufel, M., Breton, L., Beauchamp, G. Radiographic abnormalities in cats with feline bronchial disease and intra- and interobserver variability in radiographic interpretation: 40 cases (1999-2006). *Journal of the American Veterinary Medical Association*, 2009; 234:367-375.

19. Gaschen, L. The canine and feline esophagus. En: Thrall, D.E. (ed): *Textbook of Veterinary Diagnostic Radiology*, 6th edition. Elsevier Saunders, St. Louis, 2013; pp: 500-521.

20. Hansson, K., Haggström, J., Kvart, C., Lord, P. Interobserver variability of vertebral heart size measurements in dogs with normal and enlarged hearts. *Veterinary Radiology and Ultrasound*, 2005; 46:122-130.

21. Hayward, N., Schwarz, T., Weisse, C. The trachea. En: Schwarz, T. and Johnson, V. (eds): *BSAVA Manual of Canine and Feline Thoracic Imaging*. British Small Animal Veterinary Association, Gloucester, 2008; pp: 213-227.

22. Herrtage, M.E., Dennis, R. The thorax. En: Lee, R. (ed): *Manual of Small Animal Diagnostic Imaging*. British Small Animal Veterinary Association, Shurdington, 1995; pp: 43-67.

23. Herrtage, M.E., Dennis, R. Contrast media and techniques. En: Lee, R. (ed): *Manual of Small Animal Diagnostic Imaging*. British Small Animal Veterinary Association, Shurdington, 1995; pp: 147-156.

24. Johnson, L. Tracheal collapse. Diagnosis and medical and surgical treatment. *Veterinary Clinics of North America: Small Animal Practice*, 2000; 30:1253-1266.

25. Johnson, L.R. *Cor pulmonale* y tromboembolismo pulmonar. En: Tilley, L.P., Smith, F.W.K. Jr., Oyama, M.A., Sleeper, M.M. (eds): *Manual de Cardiología Canina y Felina*, 4ª edición. Multimédica Ediciones Veterinarias, Barcelona, 2009; pp: 155-160.

26. Johnson, V., Hansson, K., Maï, W., Dukes-McEwan, J., Lester, N., Schwarz, T., Chapman, P., Morandi, F. The heart and major vessels. En: Schwarz, T. and Johnson, V. (eds): *BSAVA Manual of Canine and Feline Thoracic Imaging*. British Small Animal Veterinary Association, Gloucester, 2008; pp: 86-176.

27. Kealy, J.K., McAllister, H., Graham, J.P. *Diagnostic Radiology and Ultrasonography of the Dog and Cat*, 5th edition. Saunders Elsevier, St. Louis, 2010.

28. Kirberger, R.M., Avner, A. The effect of positioning on the appearance of selected cranial thoracic structures in the dog. *Veterinary Radiology and Ultrasound*, 2006; 47:61-68.

29. Lamb, C.R., Tyler, M., Boswood, A., Skelly, B.J., Cain, M. Assessment of the value of the vertebral heart scale in the radiographic diagnosis of cardiac disease in dogs. *Veterinary Record*, 2000; 146:687-690.

30. Lamb, C.R., Wikeley, H., Boswood, A., Pfeiffer, D.U. Use of breed-specific ranges for the vertebral heart scale as an aid to the radiographic diagnosis of cardiac disease in dogs. *Veterinary Record*, 2001; 148:707-711.

31. Leonard, C.D., Johnson, L.R., Bonadio, C.M., Pollard, R.E. Changes in tracheal dimensions during inspiration and expiration in healthy dogs as detected via computed tomography. *American Journal of Veterinary Research*, 2009; 70:986-991.

32. Llabrés-Díaz, F., Petite, A., Saunders, J., Schwarz, T. The thoracic boundaries. En: Schwarz, T. and Johnson, V. (eds): *BSAVA Manual of Canine and Feline Thoracic Imaging*. British Small Animal Veterinary Association, Gloucester, 2008; pp: 340-376.

33. Macready, D.M., Johnson, L.R., Pollard, R.E. Fluoroscopic and radiographic evaluation of tracheal collapse in dogs: 62 cases (2001-2006). *Journal of the American Veterinary Medical Association*, 2007; 230:1870-1876.

34. Maï, W. Pleura. En: Schwarz, T., Saunders, J. (eds): *Veterinary Computed Tomography*. Wiley-Blackwell, Oxford, 2011; pp: 279-284.

35. Maï, W., O'Brien, R., Scrivani, P., Porat-Monseco, Y., Tobin, E., Seiler, G., McConnell, F., Schwarz, T., Zwingenberger, A. The lung parenchyma. En: Schwarz, T. and Johnson, V. (eds): *BSAVA Manual of Canine and Feline Thoracic Imaging*. British Small Animal Veterinary Association, Gloucester, 2008; pp: 242-320.

36. Mantis, P., Johnson, V., Morandi, F. The bronchial tree. En: Schwarz, T. and Johnson, V. (eds): *BSAVA Manual of Canine and Feline Thoracic Imaging*. British Small Animal Veterinary Association, Gloucester, 2008; pp: 228-241.

37. McConnell, F. Basics of thoracic magnetic resonance imaging. En: Schwarz, T. and Johnson, V. (eds): *BSAVA Manual of Canine and Feline Thoracic Imaging*. British Small Animal Veterinary Association, Gloucester, 2008; pp: 71-74.

38. Mims, H.L., Hancock, R.B., Leib, M.S., Waldron, D.R. Primary tracheal collapse in a cat. *Journal of the American Animal Hospital Association*, 2008; 44:149-153.

39. Munro, E.A.C. Thoracic radiology. En: Fuentes, V.L., Swift, S. (eds): *Manual of Small Animal Cardiorespiratory Medicine and Surgery*. British Small Animal Veterinary Association, Shurdington, 1998; pp: 35-51.

40. Murphy, K.A., Brisson, B.A. Evaluation of lung lobe torsion in Pugs: 7 cases (1991-2004). *Journal of the American Veterinary Medical Association*, 2006; 228:86-90.

41. Neath, P.J., Brockman, D.J., King, L.G. Lung lobe torsion in dogs: 22 cases (1981-1999). *Journal of the American Veterinary Medical Association*, 2000; 217:1041-1044.

42. Nemanic, S., London, C.A., Wisner, E.R. Comparison of thoracic radiographs and single breath-hold helical CT for detection of pulmonary nodules in dogs with metastatic neoplasia. *Journal of Veterinary Internal Medicine*, 2006; 20:508-515.

43. Owens, J.M., Biery D.N. *Radiographic Interpretation for the Small Animal Clinician*, 2nd edition. Williams & Wilkins, Baltimore, 1999.

44. Petite, A., Kirberger, R. Mediastinum. En: Schwarz, T., Saunders, J. (eds): *Veterinary Computed Tomography*. Wiley-Blackwell, Oxford, 2011; pp: 249-260.

45. Poteet, B.A. Radiología del corazón. En: Tilley, L.P., Smith, F.W.K. Jr., Oyama, M.A., Sleeper, M.M. (eds): *Manual de Cardiología Canina y Felina*, 4ª edición. Multimédica Ediciones Veterinarias, Barcelona, 2009; pp: 23-43.

46. Rudorf, H., Taeymans, O., Johnson, V. Basics of thoracic radiography and radiology. En: Schwarz, T. and Johnson, V. (eds): *BSAVA Manual of Canine and Feline Thoracic Imaging*. British Small Animal Veterinary Association, Gloucester, 2008; pp: 1-19.

47. Samii, V.F. The thoracic wall. En: Thrall, D.E. (ed): *Textbook of Veterinary Diagnostic Radiology*, 6th edition. Elsevier Saunders, St. Louis, 2013; pp: 522-534.

48. Saunders, J., Vignoli, M., Gielen, I. Thoracic boundaries. En: Schwarz, T., Saunders, J. (eds): *Veterinary Computed Tomography*. Wiley-Blackwell, Oxford, 2011; pp: 285-296.

49. Schwarz, T. Basics of thoracic computed tomography. En: Schwarz, T. and Johnson, V. (eds): *BSAVA Manual of Canine and Feline Thoracic Imaging*. British Small Animal Veterinary Association, Gloucester, 2008; pp: 66-70.

50. Schwarz, T., Johnson, V. Lungs and bronchi. En: Schwarz, T., Saunders, J. (eds): *Veterinary Computed Tomography*. Wiley-Blackwell, Oxford, 2011; pp: 261-277.

51. Schwarz, T., Saunders, J. Trachea. En: Schwarz, T., Saunders, J. (eds): *Veterinary Computed Tomography.* Wiley-Blackwell, Oxford, 2011; pp: 243-248.

52. Seiler, G. Thorax. En: Barr, F., Gaschen, L. (eds): *BSAVA Manual of Canine and Feline Ultrasonography.* British Small Animal Veterinary Association, Gloucester, 2011; pp: 29-36.

53. Seiler, G., Dukes-McEwan, J., Gaschen, L. Basics of thoracic ultrasonography. En: Schwarz, T. and Johnson, V. (eds): *BSAVA Manual of Canine and Feline Thoracic Imaging.* British Small Animal Veterinary Association, Gloucester, 2008; pp: 20-65.

54. Seiler, G., Schwarz, T., Vignoli, M., Rodriguez, D. Computed tomographic features of lung lobe torsion. *Veterinary Radiology and Ultrasound*, 2008; 49:504-8.

55. Strikland, K.N. Cardiopatía congénita. En: Tilley, L.P., Smith, F.W.K. Jr., Oyama, M.A., Sleeper, M.M. (eds): *Manual de Cardiología Canina y Felina*, 4ª edición. Multimédica Ediciones Veterinarias, Barcelona, 2009; pp: 189-209.

56. Taeymans, O., Schwarz, T. Pharynx, larynx and thyroid gland. En: Schwarz, T., Saunders, J. (eds): *Veterinary Computed Tomography.* Wiley-Blackwell, Oxford, 2011; pp: 175-184.

57. Thrall, D.E. Principles of radiographic interpretation of the thorax. En: Thrall, D.E. (ed): *Textbook of Veterinary Diagnostic Radiology*, 6th edition. Elsevier Saunders, St. Louis, 2013; pp: 474-488.

58. Thrall, D.E. The canine and feline lung. En: Thrall, D.E. (ed): *Textbook of Veterinary Diagnostic Radiology*, 6th edition. Elsevier Saunders, St. Louis, 2013; pp: 608-631.

59. Thrall, D.E. The mediastinum. En: Thrall, D.E. (ed): *Textbook of Veterinary Diagnostic Radiology*, 6th edition. Elsevier Saunders, St. Louis, 2013; pp: 550-570.

60. Thrall, D.E. The pleural space. En: Thrall, D.E. (ed): *Textbook of Veterinary Diagnostic Radiology*, 6th edition. Elsevier Saunders, St. Louis, 2013; pp: 571-584.

61. Tobias, A.H., McNiel, E.A. Afecciones pericárdicas y tumores cardiacos. En: Tilley, L.P., Smith, F.W.K. Jr., Oyama, M.A., Sleeper, M.M. (eds): *Manual de Cardiología Canina y Felina*, 4ª edición. Multimédica Ediciones Veterinarias, Barcelona, 2009; pp: 177-188.

62. Wagner, W.M. The oesophagus. En: Schwarz, T. and Johnson, V. (eds): *BSAVA Manual of Canine and Feline Thoracic Imaging.* British Small Animal Veterinary Association, Gloucester, 2008; pp: 200-212.

63. Zekas, L.J., Adams, W.M. Cranial mediastinal cysts in nine cats. *Veterinary Radiology and Ultrasound*, 2002; 43:413-418.

Chapter 3. Appendicular skeleton

1. Adams, G. Radiographic signs of joint disease in dogs and cats. En: Thrall, D.E. (ed): *Textbook of Veterinary Diagnostic Radiology*, 6th edition. Elsevier Saunders, St. Louis, 2013; pp. 319-348.

2. Allan, G., Nicoll, R. Joints - general. En: Barr, F.J., Kirberger, R.M. (eds): *BSAVA Manual of Canine and Feline Musculoskeletal Imaging.* British Small Animal Veterinary Association, Gloucester, 2006; pp. 71-85.

3. Allan, G.S. Radiographic features of feline joint diseases. *Veterinary Clinics of North America: Small Animal Practice*, 2000; 30:281-302.

4. Barr, F. Long bones - juvenile. En: Barr, F.J., Kirberger, R.M. (eds): *BSAVA Manual of Canine and Feline Musculoskeletal Imaging.* British Small Animal Veterinary Association, Gloucester, 2006; pp. 19-31.

5. Barr, F. Soft tissues. En: Barr, F.J., Kirberger, R.M. (eds): *BSAVA Manual of Canine and Feline Musculoskeletal Imaging.* British Small Animal Veterinary Association, Gloucester, 2006; pp. 1-8.

6. Brinker, W.O. *Small Animal Fractures.* Michigan State University Press, East Lansing, 1978.

7. Burk, R.L., Feeney D.A. *Small Animal Radiology and Ultrasonography. A Diagnostic Atlas and Text.* Elsevier Science, St. Louis, 2003.

8. Butterworth, S.J. Long bones - fractures. En: Barr, F.J., Kirberger, R.M. (eds): *BSAVA Manual of Canine and Feline Musculoskeletal Imaging.* British Small Animal Veterinary Association, Gloucester, 2006; pp. 49-70.

9. Davies, J.V., Lee, R. The appendicular skeleton. En: Lee, R. (ed): *Manual of Small Animal Diagnostic Imaging.* British Small Animal Veterinary Association, Shurdington, 1995; pp. 95-135.

10. Dennis, R., Kirberger, R.M., Barr, F., Wrigley, R.H. *Handbook of Small Animal Radiology and Ultrasound, 2nd Edition.* Churchill Livingstone Elsevier, Edimburg, 2010.

11. Dennis, R., Kirberger, R.M., Wrigley, R.H., Barr, F.J. *Handbook of Small Animal Radiological Differential Diagnosis.* W.B. Saunders, London, 2001.

12. Ekman, S., Carlson, C.S. The pathophysiology of osteochondrosis. *Veterinary Clinics of North America: Small Animal Practice*, 1998; 28:17-32.

13. Farrow, C.S. *Diagnóstico por imagen del perro y el gato.* Multimédica ediciones veterinarias, Barcelona, 2005.

14. Frazho, J.K., Graham, J., Peck, J.N., De Haan, J.J. Radiographic evaluation of the anconeal process in skeletally inmature dogs. *Veterinary Surgery*, 2010; 39:829-832.

15. Gavin, P.R., Holmes, S.P. Orthopedic. En: Gavin, P.R., Bagley, R.S. (eds): Practical Small Animal MRI. Wiley-Blackwell, Iowa, 2009; pp. 233-272.

16. Henry, G.A. Fracture healing and complications. En: Thrall, D.E. (ed): *Textbook of Veterinary Diagnostic Radiology*, 6th edition. Elsevier Saunders, St. Louis, 2013; pp. 283-306.

17. Hornof, W.J., Wind, A.P., Wallack, S.T., Schultz, K.S. Canine elbow dysplasia. The early radiographic detection of fragmentation of the coronoid process. *Veterinary Clinics of North America: Small Animal Practice*, 2000; 30:257-266.

18. Innes, J.F., Costello, M., Barr, F.J., Rudorf, H., Barr, A.R.S. Radiographic progression of osteoarthritis of the canine stifle joint: a prospective study. *Veterinary Radiology and Ultrasound*, 2004; 45:143-148.

19. Jackson, L.C., Pacchiana, P.D. Common complications of fracture repair. *Clinical Techniques in Small Animal Practice*, 2004; 19:168-179.

20. Jacobson, L.S., Kirberger, R.M. Canine multiple cartilaginous exostoses: unusual manifestations and a review of the literature. *Journal of the American Animal Hospital Association*, 1996; 32:45-51.

21. Johnson, K. Osteomyelitis in dogs and cats. *Journal of the American Veterinary Medical Association*, 1994; 205:1882-1887.

22. Kealy, J.K., McAllister, H., Graham, J.P. *Diagnostic Radiology and Ultrasonography of the Dog and Cat*, 5th edition. Saunders Elsevier, St. Louis, 2010.

23. Kirberger, R.M. Bones - general. En: Barr, F.J., Kirberger, R.M. (eds): *BSAVA Manual of Canine and Feline Musculoskeletal Imaging*. British Small Animal Veterinary Association, Gloucester, 2006; pp. 9-18.

24. LaFond, E., Breur, G.J., Austin, C.C. Breed susceptibility for developmental orthopedic diseases in dogs. *Journal of the American Animal Hospital Association*, 2002; 38:467-77.

25. Mason, D.R., Schultz, K.S., Samii, V.F., Fujita, Y., Hornof, W.J., Herrgesell, E.J., Long, C.D., Morgan, J.P., Kass, P.H. Sensitivity of radiographic evaluation of radio-ulnar incongruence in the dog in vivo. *Veterinary Surgery*, 2002; 31:125-132.

26. McAllister, H., Tobin, E. Long bones - mature. En: Barr, F.J., Kirberger, R.M. (eds): *BSAVA Manual of Canine and Feline Musculoskeletal Imaging*. British Small Animal Veterinary Association, Gloucester, 2006; pp. 32-48.

27. Morgan, J.P. *Radiology of skeletal disease – principles of diagnosis in the dog*. Iowa State University Press, Iowa, 1981.

28. Nolte, D.M., Fusco, J.V., Peterson, M.E. Incidence of and predisposing factors for nonunion of fractures involving the appendicular skeleton in cats: 18 cases (1998-2002). *Journal of the American Veterinary Medical Association*, 2005; 226:77-82.

29. Owens, J.M., Biery D.N. *Radiographic Interpretation for the Small Animal Clinician*, 2nd edition. Williams & Wilkins, Baltimore, 1999.

30. Pollard, R.E., Wisner, E.R. Orthopedic diseases of young and growing dogs and cats. En: Thrall, D.E. (ed): *Textbook of Veterinary Diagnostic Radiology*, 6th edition. Elsevier Saunders, St. Louis, 2013; pp. 267-282.

31. Salter, R., Harris, W. Injuries involving the epiphyseal plate. *Journal of Bone and Joint Surgery*, 1963; 45:587-622.

32. Samii, V., Gielen, I., Ludewig, E., Adams, W.H., Kiefer, I., van Bree, H., Saunders, J. Joints. En: Schwarz, T., Saunders, J. (eds): *Veterinary Computed Tomography*. Wiley-Blackwell, Oxford, 2011; pp. 387-419.

33. Sande, R. Radiography of orthopedic trauma and fracture repair. *Veterinary Clinics of North America: Small Animal Practice*, 1999; 29:1247-1260.

34. Schultz, R.M., Wisner, E.R. Long bones. En: Schwarz, T., Saunders, J. (eds): *Veterinary Computed Tomography*. Wiley-Blackwell, Oxford, 2011; pp. 381-386.

35. Smith, R.N. Appearance of ossification centres in the kitten. *Journal of Small Animal Practice*, 1968; 9:497-511.

36. Smith, R.N. Fusion of ossification centres in the cat. *Journal of Small Animal Practice*, 1969; 10:523-530.

37. Sumner-Smith, G. Observations on epiphyseal fusion of the canine appendicular skeleton. *Journal of Small Animal Practice*, 1966; 7:303-312.

38. Thrall, D.E. Principles of radiographic interpretation of the appendicular skeleton. En: Thrall, D.E. (ed): *Textbook of Veterinary Diagnostic Radiology*, 6th edition. Elsevier Saunders, St. Louis, 2013; pp. 252-266.

39. Thrall, D.E. Radiographic features of bone tumors and bone infection. En: Thrall, D.E. (ed): *Textbook of Veterinary Diagnostic Radiology*, 6th edition. Elsevier Saunders, St. Louis, 2013; pp. 307-318.

40. Wrigley, R.H. Malignant versus non-malignant bone disease. *Veterinary Clinics of North America: Small Animal Practice*, 2000; 30:315-347.

Chapter 4. Spine

1. Bahr, A. The vertebrae. En: Thrall, D.E. (ed). *Textbook of Veterinary Diagnostic Radiology*, 5th edition. Saunders Elsevier, St. Louis, 2007; pp: 179-193.

2. Begon, D. Radiología en neurología. Proceedings del XVII Congreso de AMVAC, 2000; pp. 43-52.

3. Burk, R.L., Feeney, D.A. The spine. En: *Small Animal Radiology and Ultrasonography. A Diagnostic Atlas and Text*. Elsevier Science, St. Louis, 2003; pp: 661-713.

4. Damur-Djuric, N., Steffen, F., Hassig, J.P., Morgan, J.P., Fluckiger, M.A. Lumbosacral transitional vertebrae in dogs: classification, prevalence and association with sacroiliac morphology. *Veterinary Radiology & Ultrasound*, 2006; 47:32-38.

5. Davies, J.V. Spine-intervertebral disc disease and Wobbler syndrome. En: Barr, F.J. and Kirberger, R.M. (eds). *BSAVA*

Manual of Canine and Feline Musculoskeletal Imaging. British Small Animal Veterinary Association, 2006; pp: 247-256.

6. De Risio, L., Thomas, W.B., Sharp, N.J. Degenerative lumbosacral stenosis. *Veterinary Clinics of North America: Small Animal Practice*, 2000; 30:111-132.
7. Dennis, R., Kirberger, R.M., Barr, F., Wrigley, R.H. Spine. En: *Handbook of Small Animal Radiology and Ultrasound*, 2th Edition. Churchill Livingstone Elsevier, Edimburg, 2010; pp: 115-144.
8. Farrow, C.S. La columna vertebral. En: *Diagnóstico por imagen del perro y el gato*. Gráficas IN – Multimédica, Barcelona, 2005.
9. Fluckiger, M.A., Damur-Djuric, N., Hassig, J.P., Morgan, J.P., Steffen, F. A lumbosacral transitional vertebra in the dog predisposes to cauda equina syndrome. *Veterinary Radiology & Ultrasound*, 2006; 47:39-44.
10. Gibbons, S.E., Macias, C., de Stefani, G.L., Pinchbeck, G.L., McKee, W.M. The value of oblique versus ventrodorsal myelographic views for lesion lateralization in canine thoracolumbar disc disease. *Journal of Small Animal Practice*, 2006; 47:658-662.
11. Kealy, J.K., McAllister, H., Graham, J.P. The skull and the vertebral column. En: *Diagnostic Radiology and Ultrasonography of the Dog and Cat*, 5th edition. Saunders Elsevier, St. Louis, 2010; pp. 447-541.
12. Kirberger, R.M. Spine – general. En: Barr, F.J. and Kirberger, R.M. (eds). *BSAVA Manual of Canine and Feline Musculoskeletal Imaging*. British Small Animal Veterinary Association., 2006; pp. 220-232.
13. Lamb, C.R., Nicholls, A., Targett, M., Mannion, P. Accuracy of survey radiographic diagnosis of intervertebral disc protrusion in dog. *Veterinary Radiology & Ultrasound*, 2002; 43:222-228.
14. Lang, J. Spine - lumbosacral region and cauda equina syndrome. En: Barr, F.J. and Kirberger, R.M. (eds). *BSAVA Manual of Canine and Feline Musculoskeletal Imaging*. British Small Animal Veterinary Association, 2006; pp. 257-271.
15. Lee, R. La columna vertebral. En: Lee, R. (ed). *Manual de diagnóstico por imagen en pequeños animales*. Ediciones S, 1999; pp. 169-182.
16. Lewis, N.D., Coulson, A. *An Atlas of Interpretative Radiographic Anatomy of the Dog and Cat*. Blackwell Science, Oxford, 2002.
17. Llabrés Díaz, F. Practical contrast radiography 4. Myelography. *In Practice*, 2005; 27:502-510.
18. Marioni-Henry, K., Vite, C.H., Newton, L., van Winkle, T.J. Prevalence of diseases of the spinal cord of cats. *Journal of Veterinary Internal Medicine*, 2004; 18: 851-858.
19. McEvoy, F.J. Spine – conditions not related to intervertebral disc disease. En: Barr, F.J. and Kirberger, R.M. (eds): *BSAVA Manual of Canine and Feline Musculoskeletal Imaging*. British Small Animal Veterinary Association, 2006; pp. 233-246.
20. Newitt, A., German, A.J., Barr, F.J. Congenital abnormalities of the feline vertebral column. *Veterinary Radiology & Ultrasound*, 2008; 49:35-41.
21. Owens, J.M., Biery, D.N. Spine. En: *Radiographic Interpretation for the Small Animal Clinician*, 2nd edition. Williams & Wilkins, Baltimore, 1999; pp:. 127-146.
22. Ramerez III, O., Thrall, D.E. A review of imaging techniques for cauda equina syndrome. *Veterinary Radiology & Ultrasound*, 1998; 39:283-296.
23. Scrivani, P.V. Myelographic artefacts. *Veterinary Clinics of North America: Small Animal Practice*, 2000; 30:303-314.
24. Sharp, N.J.H., Wheeler, S.J., Cofone, M. Radiological evaluation of Wobbler syndrome - caudal cervical spondylomyelopathy. *Journal of Small Animal Practice*, 1992; 33:491-499.
25. Squires Bos, A., Brisson, B.A., Holmberg, D.L., Nykamp, S. Use of the ventrodorsal myelographic view to predict lateralization of extruded disk material in small-breed dogs with thoracolumbar intervertebral disk extrusion: 104 cases (2004–2005). *Journal of the American Veterinary Medical Association*, 2007; 230:1860-1865.
26. Waibl, H., Mayrhofer, E., Matis, U., Brunnberg, L., Köstlin, R. *Atlas of Radiographic Anatomy of the Dog*. Parey Verlag, Stuttgart, 2005.
27. Widmer, W.R., Thrall, D.E. Canine and feline intervertebral disc disease, myelography and spinal cord disease. En: Thrall, D.E. (ed): *Textbook of Veterinary Diagnostic Radiology*, 5th edition. Saunders Elsevier, St. Louis, 2007; pp. 194-219.

Chapter 5. Head

1. Benigni, L., Lamb, C. Diagnostic imaging of ear disease in the dog and cat. *In Practice*, 2006; 28:122-130.
2. Bischoff, M.G., Kneller, S.K. Diagnostic imaging of the canine and feline ear. *Veterinary Clinics of North America: Small Animal Practice*, 2004; 34:437-458.
3. Burk, R.L., Feeney, D.A. The skull. En: *Small Animal Radiology and Ultrasonography. A Diagnostic Atlas and Text*. Elsevier Science, St. Louis. 2003; pp. 607-660.
4. Dennis, R., Kirberger, R.M., Barr, F., Wrigley, R.H. Head and neck. En: *Handbook of Small Animal Radiology and Ultrasound*, 2th Edition. Churchill Livingstone Elsevier, Edimburg, 2010; pp. 85-114.
5. Dennis, R. Radiología del cráneo en pequeños animales. Proceedings del XVII Congreso de AMVAC, 2000; pp. 33-42.
6. Dennis, R. Skull – general. En: Barr, F.J. and Kirberger, R.M. (eds). *BSAVA Manual of Canine and Feline Musculoskeletal Imaging*. British Small Animal Veterinary Association, 2006; pp. 173-191.
7. Dickie, A.M., Sullivan, M. The effect of obliquity on the radiographic appearance of the temporomandibular joint in dogs. *Veterinary Radiology & Ultrasound*, 2001; 42:205-217.

8. Farrow, C.S. Cráneo, encéfalo, ojos y oídos. En: *Diagnóstico por imagen del perro y el gato.* Multimédica ediciones veterinarias, Barcelona, 2005; pp. 201-262.
9. Forrest, L.J. Cranial and nasal cavities: canine and feline. En: Thrall, D.E. (ed). *Textbook of Veterinary Diagnostic Radiology*, 5th edition. Saunders Elsevier, St. Louis, 2007; pp: 119-141.
10. Hofer, P., Meisen, N., Bartholdi, S., Kaser-Hotz, B. Radiology corner – A new radiographic view of the feline tympanic bulla. *Veterinary Radiology & Ultrasound,* 1995; 36:14-15.
11. Kealy, J.K., McAllister, H., Graham, J.P. The skull and the vertebral column. En: *Diagnostic Radiology and Ultrasonography of the Dog and Cat,* 5th edition. Saunders Elsevier, St. Louis, 2010; pp. 447-541.
12. Lamb, C.R., Richbell, S., Mantis, P. Radiographic signs in cats with nasal disease. *Journal of Feline Medicine and Surgery,* 2003; 5:227-235.
13. Lamb, C.R. Skull – nasal chambers and frontal sinuses. En: Barr, F.J. and Kirberger, R.M. (eds). *BSAVA Manual of Canine and Feline Musculoskeletal Imaging.* British Small Animal Veterinary Association, 2006; pp. 192-205.
14. Lewis, N.D., Coulson, A. *An Atlas of Interpretative Radiographic Anatomy of the Dog and Cat.* Blackwell Science, Oxford, 2002.
15. Owens, J.M., Biery, D.N. Skull. En: *Radiographic Interpretation for the Small Animal Clinician,* 2nd edition. Williams & Wilkins, Baltimore, 1999; pp. 105-126.
16. Pownder, S., Rose, M., Crawford, J. Radiographic techniques of the nasal cavity and sinuses. *Clinical Techniques in Small Animal Practice,* 2006; 21:46-54.
17. Russo, M., Lamb, C.R., Jakovljevic, S. Distinguishing canine nasal neoplasia and rhinitis by radiography. *Veterinary Radiology & Ultrasound,* 2000; 41:108-124.
18. Saunders, J.H., van Bree, H. Comparison of radiography and computed tomography for the diagnosis of canine nasal aspergillosis. *Veterinary Radiology & Ultrasound,* 2003; 44:414-419.
19. Steenkamp, G. Skull – teeth. En: Barr, F.J. and Kirberger, R.M. (eds). *BSAVA Manual of Canine and Feline Musculoskeletal Imaging.* British Small Animal Veterinary Association, 2006; pp. 206-219.
20. Waibl, H., Mayrhofer, E., Matis, U., Brunnberg, L., Köstlin, R. *Atlas of Radiographic Anatomy of the Dog.* Parey Verlag, Stuttgart, 2005.

Chapter 6. Most common diagnostic errors

1. Baines, E.A., Grandage, J., Herrtage, M.E., Baines, S.J. Radiographic definition of the anticlinal vertebra in the dog. *Veterinary Radiology and Ultrasound,* 2009; 50:69-73.
2. Barr, F., O'Brien, R. Approach to abdominal imaging. En: O'Brien R. and Barr F. (eds): *BSAVA Manual of Canine and Feline Abdominal Imaging.* British Small Animal Veterinary Association, Gloucester, 2009; pp. 1-4.
3. Dennis, R., Kirberger, R.M., Barr, F., Wrigley, R.H. *Handbook of Small Animal Radiology and Ultrasound, 2nd Edition.* Churchill Livingstone Elsevier, Edimburg, 2010.
4. Drost, W.T., Reese, D.J., Hornof, W.J. Digital radiography artifacts. *Veterinary Radiology and Ultrasound,* 2008; 49:S48-56.
5. Kirberger, R.M., Avner, A. The effect of positioning on the appearance of selected cranial thoracic structures in the dog. *Veterinary Radiology and Ultrasound,* 2006; 47:61-68.
6. Rudorf, H., Taeymans, O., Johnson, V. Basics of thoracic radiography and radiology. En: Schwarz, T. and Johnson, V. (eds): *BSAVA Manual of Canine and Feline Thoracic Imaging.* British Small Animal Veterinary Association, Gloucester, 2008; pp. 1-19.
7. Thrall, D.E. Introduction to radiographic interpretation. En: Thrall, D.E. (ed): *Textbook of Veterinary Diagnostic Radiology,* 6th edition. Elsevier Saunders, St. Louis, 2013; pp. 74-86.
8. Thrall, D.E. Principles of radiographic interpretation of the abdomen. En: Thrall, D.E. (ed): *Textbook of Veterinary Diagnostic Radiology,* 6th edition. Elsevier Saunders, St. Louis, 2013; pp. 650-658.
9. Thrall, D.E. Principles of radiographic interpretation of the appendicular skeleton. En: Thrall, D.E. (ed): *Textbook of Veterinary Diagnostic Radiology,* 6th edition. Elsevier Saunders, St. Louis, 2013; pp. 252-266.
10. Thrall, D.E. Principles of radiographic interpretation of the axial skeleton. En: Thrall, D.E. (ed): *Textbook of Veterinary Diagnostic Radiology,* 6th edition. Elsevier Saunders, St. Louis, 2013; pp. 101-113.
11. Thrall, D.E. Principles of radiographic interpretation of the thorax. En: Thrall, D.E. (ed): *Textbook of Veterinary Diagnostic Radiology,* 6th edition. Elsevier Saunders, St. Louis, 2013; pp. 474-488.
12. Thrall, D.E., Robertson, I.D. *Atlas of normal radiographic anatomy and anatomic variants in the dog and cat.* Elsevier-Saunders, St. Louis, 2011.

Index of figures

Chapter 1. Abdomen

Chapter 2. Neck and thorax

Chapter 3. Appendicular skeleton

Chapter 4. Spine

Chapter 5. Head

Chapter 6. Most common diagnostic errors

Published by Servet editorial - Grupo Asís Biomedia S.L.